Chinese Acupuncture and Moxibustion

Chinese Acupuncture and Moxibustion

Chief editor
CHENG XINNONG

FOREIGN LANGUAGES PRESS   BEIJING

First Edition   1987
Sixth Printing   1998

Written by
Deng Liangyue, Gan Yijun, He Shuhui,
Ji Xiaoping, Li Yang, Wang Rufen,
Wang Wenjing, Wang Xuetai, Xu Hengze,
Xue Xiuling and Yuan Jiuling

Edited by
Cheng Youbang, Huang Xinming, Jia Weicheng,
Li Sheng, Qiu Maoliang and Yang Jiasan

ISBN 7-119-00378-X

© Foreign Languages Press, Beijing, 1987

Published by Foreign Languages Press
24 Baiwanzhuang Road, Beijing 100037, China

Distributed by China International Book Trading Corporation
35 Chegongzhuang Xilu, Beijing 100044, China
P.O. Box 399, Beijing, China

Printed in the People's Republic of China

FOREWORD

The science of acupuncture and moxibustion is an important part of traditional Chinese medicine. For thousands of years the Chinese people have appreciated it for its nonpharmaceutical treatment, simple application, wide range of use, good curative effect, and low cost.

As part of Chinese science and culture acupuncture and moxibustion have long been known in the world as a result of cultural exchange between China and other countries. However, a global interest in acupuncture and moxibustion and special enthusiasm for the subject have been growing in the past dozen years. To offer further service to the other people and help acupuncture and moxibustion enrich the world's science and culture, the Ministry of Public Health of China established three international acupuncture training centres in research institutes and colleges of traditional Chinese medicine in Beijing, Shanghai and Nanjing with the support of the Office of the Western Pacific Region of the United Nations' World Health Organization. More than 1,000 foreign students from 120 countries and regions have been trained there in less than ten years. With their strong thirst for knowledge these students were not satisfied with their basic understanding and sought more detailed information. To meet their needs, the three training centres have organized advanced training and research courses.

Chinese Acupuncture and Moxibustion, the textbook for these advanced courses, was compiled by the three training centres, under the supervision of the Ministry of Public Health, in accordance with their teaching programme, acupuncture theory and clinical experience. Professor Cheng Xinnong, well-known specialist of Chinese acupuncture and moxibustion, headed the editorial board for the compilation of this book. Both the Chinese and English editions of *Chinese Acupuncture and Moxibustion* were examined and revised by a number of specialists before publication.

Based on *Essentials of Chinese Acupuncture* and supplemented by the results of many years of teaching and clinical experience, *Chinese Acupuncture and Moxibustion* was continually revised, substantiated and perfected. As a valued scientific gift from the home of acupuncture and moxibustion, this book, we hope, will be a good teacher and helpful friend to students and practitioners of acupuncture and moxibustion in the world.

HU XIMING

Vice-Minister of the Ministry of Public Health,
Director of the State Administration of Traditional Chinese
Medicine, the People's Republic of China
Chairman of the Chinese Acupuncture and Moxibustion Society

September 1987

CONTENTS

Contents   **xiii**

PREFACE

The science of acupuncture and moxibustion is an important component of traditional Chinese medicine used in the prevention and treatment of disease. This therapy has been accepted by the general population for thousands of years. Since the founding of the People's Republic of China, great importance has been attached by the Chinese Government to the investigation of acupuncture and moxibustion. It has thus been greatly popularized and developed and is becoming an increasingly important component of world medicine.

With a view to offering further service to the people of the world, three International Acupuncture Training Centres were established in Beijing, Shanghai and Nanjing. Since 1975, a number of acupuncture training courses have been sponsored for more than one thousand foreign students from one hundred countries and regions, using *Essentials of Chinese Acupuncture** as the textbook. Upon returning to their home countries these students applied what they had learnt to their own practice to good effect. Many practitioners are not satisfied with their understanding of the basic theories and seek more detailed knowledge. Therefore, the Ministry of Public Health has entrusted these three training centres with the task of organizing advanced training and research courses. *Chinese Acupuncture and Moxibustion* has been compiled to serve as the textbook for these courses and as a reference for foreign practitioners in their own study.

Based upon *Essentials of Chinese Acupuncture* and supplemented with many years of teaching and clinical experience, as well as recent research, the book lays emphasis on the integration of theory with practice, in keeping with the great heritage of traditional Chinese medicine. *Chinese Acupuncture and Moxibustion* consists of eighteen chapters. Chapter 1 is a brief history of Chinese acupuncture and moxibustion, giving an outline of its origin and development. Chapters 2 to 4 deal with the basic theories, primarily in relation to yin-yang, five elements, zang-fu, qi, blood, essence and body fluid. Chapters 5 to 10 give an overall description of the 12 regular meridians, 8 extra meridians, 12 divergent meridians, 15 collaterals, 12 muscle meridians, 12 cutaneous regions, acupoints of the 14 meridians and the extra points. Chapters 11 and 12 are concerned with etiology, pathogenesis and diagnostic methods, with emphasis placed on pulse and tongue

---

*Published by the Foreign Languages Press, Beijing, in 1975 and 1980.

diagnosis. Chapter 13 is about differentiation of syndromes according to the eight principles, the theories of qi and blood, meridians and collaterals, and zang-fu organs, with brief differentiation according to the theories of six meridians, wei, qi, ying, xue, and sanjiao. Chapters 14 and 15 cover the techniques of acupuncture and moxibustion in relation to commonly used needling methods and some acupuncture techniques mentioned in *Internal Classic*. Chapter 16 is a general introduction to acupuncture treatment, including general principles and methods of treatment, basic principles for prescription and selection of points, and application of specific points. Chapters 17 and 18 relate to the clinical management of 63 kinds of diseases in internal medicine, gynecology, pediatrics, surgery and ENT. A supplementary section is devoted to ear acupuncture and acupuncture anesthesia.

We are indebted to Wang Dai, Chen Xiuzhen, Zhou Yunxian, Zheng Qiwei and Liang Jingping for their great help in completing this work.

Our thanks also go to the people who helped with the translation: Cha Xiaohu, Du Wei, Guo Gangjun, Huang Guoqi, Huang Wenquan, Jin Huide, Qian Shangsan, Su Zhihong, Tao Jinwen, Wang Huizhu, Xu Bojun, Xu Yao, Yao Yun, Zhang Kai and You Benlin.

We express special appreciation to Fang Tingyu, Su Zhihong, Xie Zhufan and Zhang Kai who edited the English text.

We are grateful to Chen Jirei, Xu Yizhi and Wang Shengai for their valuable editorial assistance.

Thanks are due also to Kuang Peihua and other staff editors of the Foreign Languages Press for the great pains they have taken to check and improve the typescript and proofs.

In conclusion, we sincerely appreciate comments and suggestions from our readers so that we can make revisions in future editions.

August 1, 1987

Chapter 1

A BRIEF HISTORY OF CHINESE ACUPUNCTURE AND MOXIBUSTION

I. THE ORIGIN OF ACUPUNCTURE AND MOXIBUSTION

Acupuncture and moxibustion are an important invention of the Chinese nation which originated as early as in the clan commune period of the primitive society. The activities of human beings appeared in China about 1,700,000 years ago. It was about 100,000 years ago that China entered the clan commune period which lasted till 4,000 years ago. In the ancient literature there were many legends about the origin of acupuncture and moxibustion such as Fu Xi's creation of the therapeutic techniques with stone needles, and Huang Di's invention of acupuncture and moxibustion. The above mentioned Fu Xi and Huang Di in legend actually are the representatives of the clan commune of primitive society.

In the classics of two thousand years ago, it was frequently cited that the acupuncture instruments were made of stone and were named *bian* stone. For example, in *Commentary on the Spring and Autumn Annals*, there is a paragraph in historical records for 550 B.C. saying: "Praise pleasant to hear that does an ill turn is worse than advice unpleasant to hear that acts like a stone." Fu Qian in the second century explained that "stone" here meant *bian* stone. Quan Yuanqi who lived around the 5th-6th centuries pointed out: "*bian* stone is an ancient appliance for external treatment and was known by three names: 1. needle stone; 2. *bian* stone; 3. arrow-headed stone. In fact, they are the same thing. Because there was no iron casting in ancient times, the needles were made of stone." This is correlated with the fact that the stone instruments were extensively used in the primitive society. Primitive period in China was divided into two stages, the Old Stone Age (from remote antiquity to 10,000 years ago) and the New Stone Age (from 10,000-4,000 years ago). In the Old Stone Age the ancestors knew how to use stone knives and scrapers to incise an abscess, drain pus and let blood out for therapeutic purposes. With the accumulation of experiences the indications of the treatment by *bian* stone were gradually increased. In the New Stone Age because of the improvement in their technique of stone manufacturing, the ancient people were able to make *bian* stone as a special tool with more medical usage. In China, a *bian* stone needle 4.5 *cun* long was discovered in the New Stone Age ruins in Duolun County of Inner Mongolia. At one end, it is oval shaped with a semicircular

1

edge used for incising boils and abscesses, and at the other end, it is pyramid shaped with a square base used for bloodletting (see Fig. 1-1). Two more *bian* stones were discovered as funerary objects in a late New Stone Age grave in Rizhao County of Shandong Province. They are 8.3 cm and 9.1 cm in length respectively, with three-edged and cone-shaped ends used for bloodletting and regulating qi circulation. The discovered relics of *bian* stone have provided powerful evidence that acupuncture originated early in the primitive society.

According to the records of Chapter 12 of *Plain Questions*: "The treatment with *bian* stone needle was originated in the east coast of China where the inhabitants lived on fishery, and moxibustion was originated in the north where the people subsisted on animal husbandry. Because it was cold and windy in the northern areas, people had to warm themselves by fire. Living in camps and subsisting on milk, they easily suffered from abdominal pain and distension by cold, suitable to be treated by heat. Through long-term accumulation of experiences, moxibustion therapy and hot compression were created."

II. THE ACADEMIC ACCOMPLISHMENTS OF ANCIENT ACUPUNCTURE AND MOXIBUSTION

From the twenty-first century B.C. when China entered the slave society to 476 B.C., Chinese history went through the Xia, Shang and Western Zhou dynasties and the Spring and Autumn Period. Three thousand years ago in the Shang Dynasty the hieroglyphs of acupuncture and moxibus-

tion appeared in the inscriptions on bones and tortoise shells. Because of the development of bronze casting techniques there appeared bronze medical needles. But *bian* stone was still used as the main tool for treating diseases. During this period the philosophical thinking of yin-yang and five elements was formed, and in the field of medicine the ancient physicians had a preliminary understanding of pulse, blood, body fluid, qi, shen (manifestations of vitality), essence, five sounds, five colours, five flavours, six qi, eight winds, etc., as well as the ideology of relevant adaptation of the human body to natural environment. Thus germinated the sprout of the basic theory of traditional Chinese medicine.

From the Warring States Period (475 B.C.-221 B.C.) to the Qin Dynasty (221 B.C.-207 B.C.) and to the Western Han Dynasty (206 B.C.-A.D. 24), it was the establishing and strengthening stage of the feudal system in China. With the introduction and application of iron instruments, *bian* stone needles were replaced by metal medical needles. This broadened the field of acupuncture practice, bringing about a development of acupuncture by leaps and bounds. As recorded in the book *Miraculous Pivot*, there were nine kinds of metallic needles at that time with different shapes and usage. They are named as nine needles including the needles for puncturing, surgical incision and massage as well. In 1968, in Mancheng County, Hebei Province, an ancient tomb of the Western Han Dynasty buried in 113 B.C. was excavated. Among the relics, there were four golden needles and five decaying silver ones (see Fig. 1-2). These discoveries demonstrate the original shapes of the ancient needles. The doctors of this period treated diseases with multiple techniques. For example, the famous doctor Qin Yueren (or named Bian Que) who lived in about the fifth to fourth century B.C., had a good command of medical knowledge in various clinical branches; he treated patients by needling, moxibustion, herbal decoction, massage and hot compression. He rescued a critically ill prince by acupuncture, and this story went down in history. Another famous doctor Chunyu Yi of the second century B.C. was good at acupuncture-moxibustion and herbal treatment. There is an account of his case reports of twenty-five patients in the book *Historical Records*, in which four cases were treated by acupuncture and moxibustion. In the period of Warring States, ancient doctors began to generalize and summarize medicine and pharmacology, and writings on acupuncture and moxibustion appeared. Two silk scrolls recording meridians and collaterals written in the third century B.C., were discovered in the excavation of the No. 3 Han Tomb at Mawangdui, Hunan Province, which reflected the earliest outlook of the theory of meridians and collaterals. The book *Huangdi's Internal Classic* passed on to now is a medical classic concerning the theory of traditional Chinese medicine, with its authorship ascribed to the ancient Emperor Huangdi. It includes two parts: *Miraculous Pivot*, in another name *Huangdi's Canon of Acupuncture,* and *Plain Questions*. On the basis of previous literature, it takes the theories of yin-yang, five elements, zang-fu, meridians and collaterals, mentality and spirit, qi and blood, body fluid, five emotions and six exogeneous pathogenic factors as the basic knowledge of traditional Chinese medicine, and acupuncture and moxibustion as the main therapeutic technique; it explained the physiology and pathology of the human body, the principles of diagnosis, the prevention and treatment of diseases from the perspective of atheism, holistic conception, the viewpoint of development and change, and the relationship between the human body and the natural environment. This laid a theoretical foundation of Chinese medicine and pharmacology, including acupuncture and moxibustion. During this period also appeared the books *Huangdi's Canon of Eighty-One Difficult Problems* and *Essentials of Points, Acupuncture and Moxibustion,* both related to the fundamental theories of acupuncture and moxibustion, but the latter book has been lost.

From the Eastern Han Dynasty (A.D. 25-220) to the Three Kingdoms Period (220-265), another generalization and summarization of traditional Chinese medicine and pharmacology was made. Many famous doctors paid great attention to the study of acupuncture and moxibustion. For example, Hua Tuo who was the pioneer to apply herbal anesthesia for surgical operations only selected one to two points in acupuncture treatment and took much notice to the propagation of needling sensation. He was ascribed the authorship of *Canon of Moxibustion and Acupuncture Preserved in Pillow* (lost). The outstanding medical doctor Zhang Zhongjing also mentioned the methods of acupuncture, moxibustion, fire needling, warm needling, etc. in his book *Treatise on Febrile and Miscellaneous Diseases*. He stressed very much on combining acupuncture with medicinal herbs as well as applying the treatment according to the differentiation of symptom complex. During this period the basic theories of acupuncture and moxibustion had already been formed, but the locations and names of acupuncture points were neither unified nor systemized.

A bamboo scroll of medicine of the Eastern Han Dynasty which was excavated from Wuwei County in Gansu Province, mistook Zusanli to be located "five cun below the knee."Hua Tuo located Back-Shu points as "one cun bilaterally along the spine," with a great difference in locations and names of the points when compared with other books. Because the earliest acupuncture books contained mistakes and differences, and had missing information, the famous medical doctor Huangfu Mi compiled the book *Systematic Classic of Acupuncture and Moxibustion* in 256-260 by collecting the materials of acupuncture and moxibustion from the ancient books *Plain Questions, Canon of Acupuncture* and *Essentials of Points, Acupuncture and Moxibustion*. The book consists of 12 volumes with 128 chapters, including 349 acupuncture points. He edited and arranged the contents according to the following order: the theories of Zang-Fu, Qi and Blood, channels and collaterals, acupuncture points, the pulse diagnosis, manipulating techniques of acupuncture and moxibustion, and their clinical application in various branches of medicine. It is the earliest exclusive and systemized book on acupuncture and moxibustion which has been one of the most influential works in the history of acupuncture and moxibustion.

During the Jin Dynasty and the Northern and Southern Dynasties (265-581), the chaos was upheaved by wars. The physicians advocated acupuncture and moxibustion therapy very much because of its convenient use in times of turmoil, and the masses of Chinese people also knew something about moxibustion therapy. The famous doctor Ge Hong wrote the book *Prescriptions for Emergencies* to popularize medical knowledge, especially the therapeutic methods of acupuncture and moxibustion. From the Jin Dynasty to the Northern and Southern Dynasties, Xu Xi's family were expert in the art of healing for several generations, including Xu Qiufu, Xu Wenbo and Xu Shuxiang, all well known in the history of acupuncture and moxibustion. In this period there appeared more and more monographs on acupuncture and moxibustion, and charts of acupuncture points, such as *Acupuncture Chart from Lateral and Posterior Views* and *Diagrams of Meridians and Points*.

During the Sui (581-618) and Tang dynasties (618-907), China was undergoing the process of economical and cultural prosperity of the feudal society. The science of acupuncture and moxibustion also had great development. The famous physician Zhen Quan and his contemporary Sun Simiao both had good command of the knowledge of traditional Chinese medicine and made deep study on acupuncture and moxibustion. The Tang government, in the years around 627-649, ordered Zhen Quan and the others to revise the books and charts of acupuncture and moxibustion. Sun Simiao compiled *Prescriptions Worth a Thousand Gold for Emergencies* (650-652), and *A Supplement to the Prescriptions Worth a Thousand Gold* (680-682), in which a great deal of clinical experiences in acupuncture treatment of various schools were included. He also designed and made *Charts of Three Views,* in which "the twelve regular meridians and the eight extra meridians were illustrated in various colours, and there were altogether 650 points." They are the earliest multicoloured charts of meridians and points, but have been lost. In addition, Yang Shangshan of the Tang Dynasty compiled *Acupuncture Points in Internal Classic,* which revised the relevant contents of

Internal Classic; Wang Tao wrote the book *The Medical Secrets of An Official*, in which a host of moxibustion methods of various schools were recorded. During this period there appeared monographs on the treatment of special diseases, for example, the book *Moxibustion Method for Consumptive Diseases* written by Cui Zhidi, in which moxibustion treatment of tuberculosis was described. It has been found that the earliest block-printed edition of acupuncture and moxibustion is *A New Collection of Moxibustion Therapy for Emergency*, which appeared in the year 862, specially describing the moxibustion therapy for emergencies. In the seventh century, acupuncture and moxibustion had already become a special branch of medicine, and those specialized in this field were entitled acupuncturists and moxibustionists. During the Tang Dynasty, the Imperial Medical Bureau responsible for medical education, was divided into four departments of medical specialities and one department of pharmacology. And the department of acupuncture was also one of them, in which there were 1 professor of acupuncture, 1 assistant professor, 10 instructors, 20 technicians and 20 students. The acupuncture professor was in charge of teaching the students the meridian-collaterals and acupuncture points, pulse diagnosis, and manipulating methods of needling.

In the Five Dynasties (907-960), Liao Dynasty (916-1125), Song Dynasty (960-1279), Jin Dynasty (1115-1234) and Yuan Dynasty (1206-1368), the extensive application of printing technique greatly promoted the accumulation of medical literature and speeded up the dissemination and development of Chinese medicine and pharmacology. Supported by the Northern Song government, the famous acupuncturist Wang Weiyi revised the locations of the acupuncture points and their related meridians, and made a supplement to the indications of acupuncture points. In 1026, he wrote the book *Illustrated Manual on the Points for Acupuncture and Moxibustion on a New Bronze Figure*, which was block printed and published by the government. In 1027, two bronze figures designed by Wang Weiyi were manufactured, with the internal organs set inside and the meridians and points engraved on the surface for visual teaching and examination. These achievements and measures promoted the unification of the theoretical knowledge of acupuncture points and meridians. The famous acupuncturist Wang Zhizhong of the Southern Song Dynasty wrote the book *Canon on the Origin of Acupuncture and Moxibustion*, in which he laid stress on practical experiences including folk experiences, exerting a great influence on later generations. The famous doctor Hua Shou of the Yuan Dynasty did textual research on the pathways of meridians and collaterals as well as their relationship with acupuncture points. In 1341 he wrote the book *Exposition of the Fourteen Meridians*, which further developed the theory of meridians and acupuncture points. In this period there were plenty of famous doctors who were good at acupuncture and moxibustion. Some of them laid emphasis on the theory and technique of a particular aspect. So different branches of acupuncture and moxibustion were formed. For example, the publication of *Canon of Acupuncture and Moxibustion for Children's Diseases* (lost), *Moxibustion Methods for Emergencies, The Secret of Moxibustion for Abscess and Ulcer* and so on, showed the deep development of acupuncture and moxibustion into various branches of the clinic. Xi Hong of the early

Southern Song Dynasty who was from a famous acupuncturist family, particularly stressed the manipulating technique of acupuncture. And his contemporary Dou Cai wrote a book entitled *Bian Que's Medical Experiences*, in which he highly praised the scorching moxibustion, and even gave a general anesthesia to avoid pain while applying scorching moxibustion. At the same time, Yang Jie and Zhang Ji observed autopsies, and advocated selecting acupuncture points in the light of anatomical knowledge. He Ruoyu and Dou Hanqin of the Jin and Yuan dynasties suggested that the acupuncture points should be selected according to *ziwuliuzhu* (Chinese two-hour time on the basis of Heavenly Stems and Earthly Branches).

In the Ming Dynasty (1368-1644) acupuncture and moxibustion were worked up to a climax that many problems were studied deeper and broader. There were more famous doctors specialized in this field. Chen Hui of the early stage of Ming Dynasty, Ling Yun of the middle stage, and Yang Jizhou of the later stage, all were known far and wide in China, and exerted a tremendous influence upon the development of acupuncture and moxibustion. The main accomplishments in the Ming Dynasty were: 1. Extensive collection and revision of the literature of acupuncture and moxibustion, e.g. the chapter of acupuncture and moxibustion in the book *Prescriptions for Universal Relief* (1406), *A Complete Collection of Acupuncture and Moxibustion* by Xu Feng in the fifteenth century, *An Exemplary Collection of Acupuncture and Moxibustion* by Gao Wu in 1529, *Compendium of Acupuncture and Moxibustion* in 1601 based on Yang Jizhou's work, *Six Volumes on Acupuncture Prescriptions* by Wu Kun in 1618, and *An Illustrated*

Supplement to Systematic Compilation of the Internal Classic by Zhang Jiebin in 1624, etc. All these works were the summarization of the literature of acupuncture and moxibustion through the ages. 2. Studies on the manipulating methods of acupuncture. On the basis of single manipulation of acupuncture, more than twenty kinds of compound manipulation were developed, and an academical contention was carried out about different manipulation methods. *Questions and Answers Concerning Acupuncture and Moxibustion* by Wang Ji in 1530 was the representative work of that academical dispute. 3. Development of warm moxibustion with moxa stick from burning moxibustion with moxa cone. 4. Sorting out the previous records of acupuncture sites located away from the Fourteen Meridians and formation of a new category of extra points.

From the establishment of the Qing Dynasty to the Opium War (1644-1840), the medical doctors regarded herbal medication as superior to acupuncture, therefore acupuncture and moxibustion gradually turned to a failure. In the eighteenth century Wu Qian and his collaborators compiled the book *Golden Mirror of Medicine* by the imperial order. In this book the chapter "Essentials of Acupuncture and Moxibustion in Verse" took the practical form of rhymed verse with illustrations. Li Xuechuan compiled *The Source of Acupuncture and Moxibustion* (1817), in which selection of acupuncture points according to the differentiation of syndromes was emphasized, acupuncture and herbal medication were equally stressed, and the 361 points on the Fourteen Meridians were systematically listed. Besides these books, there were many publications, but none of them were influential. In 1822, the authorities of the Qing Dynasty declared an order to abolish permanently the acupuncture-moxibustion department from the Imperial Medical College because "acupuncture and moxibustion are not suitable to be applied to the Emperor."

III. MODERN DECLINE AND NEW LIFE OF ACUPUNCTURE AND MOXIBUSTION

Following the Opium War in 1840, China fell into a semifeudal and semicolonial society. The Revolution of 1911 ended the rule of the Qing Dynasty, but the broad masses of Chinese people were in deep distress until the founding of New China, and acupuncture and moxibustion were also trampled upon. Introduction of Western medicine to China should have been a good turn, but the colonists used it as a medium for aggression. They claimed: "Western medicine is vanguard of Christianity and Christianity is the forerunner promoting the sale of goods." With such a purpose, they denounced and depreciated Chinese traditional medicine, and even defamed acupuncture and moxibustion as medical torture and called the acupuncture needle a deadly needle. From 1914, the reactionary government of China continuously yelled to ban traditional medicine and adopted a series of measures to restrict its development, resulting in a decline of Chinese traditional medicine including acupuncture and moxibustion.

Because of the great need of the Chinese people for medical care, acupuncture and moxibustion got its chance to spread among the folk people. Many acupuncturists made unrelenting efforts to protect and develop this great medical legacy by founding acupuncture associations, publishing books and journals on acupuncture, and launching correspondence courses to teach acupuncture. Among those acupuncturists, Cheng Dan'an made a particular contribution. At this period, in addition to inheriting the traditional acupuncture and moxibustion, they made efforts on explaining the theory of acupuncture and moxibustion with modern science and technology. In 1899, Liu Zhongheng wrote a book entitled *Illustration of the Bronze Figure with Chinese and Western Medicine*, paving the way for studying acupuncture through combination of traditional Chinese and Western medicine in the history of acupuncture. In 1934 *The Technique and Principles of Electro-acupuncture* and the *Study of Electro-acupuncture* written by Tang Shicheng et al. started the use of electro-acupuncture in China.

At this period, acupuncture and moxibustion gained its new life in the revolutionary base area led by the Communist Party of China. In October of 1944, after Chairman Mao Zedong made a speech on the United Front of Cultural Work at the meeting of the cultural and educational workers in Shanxi-Gansu-Ningxia border region, many medical doctors trained in Western medicine began to learn and to do research work on acupuncture and moxibustion, and to spread its use in the army of the base area. In April 1945, an acupuncture clinic was opened in the International Peace Hospital in the name of Dr. Norman Bethune in Yan'an. This was the first time that acupuncture and moxibustion entered into a comprehensive hospital. In 1947, the

Health Department of Jinan Military Area Command compiled and published *Practical Acupuncture and Moxibustion*. An acupuncture training course was sponsored by the health school affiliated to the Health Bureau of the People's Government in Northern China in 1948. All these efforts like the seeds spread over the liberated area, and promoted the understanding of acupuncture and moxibustion for Western medical doctors.

IV. REJUVENATION OF ACUPUNCTURE AND MOXIBUSTION IN NEW CHINA

Since the founding of the People's Republic of China, the Chinese Communist Party has paid great attention to inheriting and developing the legacy of traditional Chinese medicine and pharmacology. In 1950 Chairman Mao Zedong adopted an important policy to unite the doctors of both Western and traditional schools; in the same year, Comrade Zhu De wrote an inscription for the book *New Acupuncture*, pointing out, "Chinese acupuncture treatment has a history of thousands of years. It is not only simple and economical, but also very effective for many kinds of diseases. So this is the science. I hope that the doctors of both Western and traditional schools should unite for the further improvement of its technique and science." Comrade Deng Xiaoping also inscribed in the book *Newly Compiled Acupuncture* with the following statement: "It is an important job for us to critically assimilate and systematize our multifarious scientific legacies." With the support and concern of the Party and government leaders, authorities of different levels took a series of measures to develop the great cause of Chinese medicine. In this way acupuncture and moxibustion were unprecedentedly popularized and promoted.

In July 1951, the Experimental Institute of Acupuncture-Moxibustion Therapy affiliated directly to the Ministry of Public Health was set up. It became the Institute of Acupuncture and Moxibustion attached to the Academy of Traditional Chinese Medicine in 1955. Since then the research organizations of traditional Chinese medicine and pharmacology on provincial, municipal and autonomous regional levels have been set up one after the other, in which the research divisions of acupuncture and moxibustion are included. In a few provinces and cities institutes of acupuncture and moxibustion have also been established. There are teaching and research groups of acupuncture and moxibustion in every college of traditional Chinese medicine, and in some of the colleges departments of acupuncture and moxibustion have been founded. In many city hospitals special clinical departments of acupuncture and moxibustion have been set up. Acupuncture and moxibustion have been carried out even in commune hospitals. Many institutes and colleges of Western medicine have put it into the teaching curriculum and taken it as a scientific research item.

To apply modern scientific knowledge to the research work on the basis of exploring and inheriting the traditional acupuncture and moxibustion is the prominent characteristic of the present research on acupuncture and moxibustion. In the early 1950s, the main work was to systematize the basic theory of acupuncture and moxibustion, to observe its clinical indications, and to make a systematic exposition of acupuncture and moxibustion with modern methods. From the later stage of the 1950s to the 1960s, the following were carried out: deep study of the ancient literature, extensive summarization of the clinical effect on various disease entities, propagation of acupuncture anesthesia in clinical use, and experimental research to observe the effect of acupuncture and moxibustion upon the functions of each system and organ. From the 1970s up to now, investigations have been done on the mechanism of acupuncture anesthesia and acupuncture analgesia from the viewpoints of operative surgery, anesthesiology, neuroanatomy, histochemistry, analgesia physiology, biochemistry, psychology and medical electronics, on the phenomena and nature of the meridians from the viewpoint of propagated acupuncture sensation and other angles, and on the relationship between acupuncture points and needling sensation, between acupuncture points and zang-fu organs. Now the accomplishments of acupuncture and moxibustion research gained in China including sorting out of the ancient legacy, the clinical effect and the theoretical research by modern scientific methods are in the forefront of the world.

V.   THE DISSEMINATION OF ACUPUNCTURE AND MOXIBUSTION TO THE WORLD

In the sixth century, acupuncture and moxibustion were introduced to Korea. The Emperor Liangwu sent medical doctors and craftsmen to Baiji in A.D. 541. The Xinluo royal court of Korea in A.D. 693. gave the title of Acupuncture Professor to those who taught acupuncture students. It was also in the sixth century that acupuncture and moxibustion were passed on to Japan. The Chinese Government presented the book *Canon of Acupuncture* to the Mikado of Japan in A.D. 552. Zhi Cong of Wu County brought *Charts of Acupuncture and Moxibustion* and other medical books to Japan. In the seventh century, the Japanese government sent many doctors to China to study Chinese medicine. In A.D. 702 the Japanese government issued an Imperial Order to copy the medical educational system of the Chinese Tang Dynasty and set up a speciality of acupuncture and moxibustion. Since the introduction of Chinese acupuncture and moxibustion to Japan and Korea, acupuncture and moxibustion have been regarded as an important part of their traditional medicine and handed down up to now. With the cultural exchanges between China and foreign countries, acupuncture and moxibustion were also disseminated to Southeast Asia and the continent of India. In the sixth century, Mi Yun from Dun Huang of Gansu Province introduced Hua Tuo's therapeutic methods and prescriptions to Daochang State of north India. In the fourteenth century, Chinese acupuncturist Zou Yin went to Viet Nam to treat diseases for the Vietnamese nobles, and he was given the honour of Magi Doctor. Acupuncture and moxibustion began to be introduced to Europe in the sixteenth century. Later more and more people engaged in the cause of acupuncture and moxibustion. France made an early contribution to spreading this therapy through Europe.

Since the founding of the People's Republic of China, the propagation of acupuncture and moxibustion to the world has been speeded up. In the 1950s, China gave assistance to the Soviet Union and other Eastern European countries in training acupuncturists. Since 1975, at the request of the World Health Organization, the International Acupuncture Training Courses have been run in Beijing, Shanghai and Nanjing, and acupuncturists have been trained for many countries. Up to now, more than one hundred countries have had acupuncturists, and in some countries teaching and scientific research on acupuncture and moxibustion have been carried out with good results. Since its founding in 1979, All-China Association of Acupuncture and Moxibustion has strengthened the connections and exchanges with the corresponding academic organizations of various countries; and China will make greater contributions to international development of acupuncture and moxibustion.

Chapter 2

YIN-YANG AND THE FIVE ELEMENTS

The theories of yin-yang and the five elements were two interpretations of natural phenomena that originated in ancient China. They reflected a primitive concept of materialism and dialectics and played an active role in promoting the development of natural science in China. Ancient physicians applied these two theories to the field of medicine, greatly influencing the formation and development of the theoretical system of traditional Chinese medicine, and guiding clinical work up to the present time.

I. YIN-YANG

The theory of yin-yang is a conceptual framework which was used for observing and analysing the material world in ancient China. The early theory of yin-yang was formed in the Yin and Zhou dynasties (sixteenth century-221 B.C.). The term yin-yang first appeared in *The Book of Changes,* "Yin and yang reflect all the forms and characteristics existing in the universe."

Up to the Spring and Autumn Period (770-476 B.C.) and the Warring States Period (475-221 B.C.), the application of the theory of yin-yang had been deeply rooted in all schools of thought. It was pointed out in Chapter 5 of the book *Plain Questions:* "Yin and yang are the laws of heaven and earth, the great framework of everything, the parents of change, the root and beginning of life and death. . . ."

This quote expresses the idea that all natural events and states of being are rooted in yin and yang, and can be analysed by the theory of yin-yang. The theory of yin-yang, however, does not itself refer to any concrete objective phenomena. It is, rather, a theoretical method for observing and analysing phenomena. Briefly speaking, yin and yang are a philosophical conceptualization, a means to generalize the two opposite principles which may be observed in all related phenomena within the natural world. They may represent two separate phenomena with opposing natures, as well as different and opposite aspects within the same phenomenon. Thus the ancient Chinese people, in the course of their everyday life and work, came to understand that all aspects of the natural world could be seen as having a dual aspect, for example, day and night, brightness and dimness, movement and, stillness, upward and downward direction, heat and cold, etc. The terms yin and yang are applied to express these dual and opposit qualities. Chapter 5 of the book *Plain Questions* states: "Water and fire are symbols of yin and yang." This means that water and fire represent the two

11

primary opposite aspects of a contradiction. Based on the properties of water and fire, everything in the natural environment may be classified as either yin or yang. Those with the basic properties of fire, such as heat, movement, brightness, upward and outward direction, excitement and potency, pertain to yang; those with the basic properties of water, such as coldness, stillness, dimness, downward and inward direction, inhibition and weakness, pertain to yin. Accordingly, within the field of medicine different functions and properties of the body are classified as either yin or yang. For example, the qi of the body which has moving and warming functions is yang, while the qi of the body which has nourishing and moistening functions is yin.

The yin-yang nature of a phenomenon is not absolute but relative. This relativity is reflected in two ways. On the one hand, under certain conditions yin may change into yang and vice versa (the inter-transforming nature of yin and yang), and on the other hand, any phenomenon may be infinitely divided into its yin and yang aspects, reflecting its own inner yin-yang relationship. Day, for example, is yang, while night is yin. Each, however, can be further classified as follows: morning is yang within yang, afternoon yin within yang, the first half of the night yin within yin, and the second half of the night yang within yin. This differentiation of the natural world into its opposite parts can be carried out infinitely.

It can be seen, therefore, that yin and yang are at the same time opposite in nature and yet interdependent. They both oppose and complement each other, and exist within all natural phenomena. Traditional Chinese medicine applies the yin-yang principles of interconnection and continuous transformation to the human body to explain its physiology and pathology and to guide clinical diagnosis and treatment.

1. The Basic Knowledge of the Theory of Yin and Yang

1) The opposition of yin and yang The theory of yin-yang holds that everything in nature has two opposite aspects, namely yin and yang. The opposition of yin and yang is mainly reflected in their ability to struggle with, and thus control each other. For instance, warmth and heat (yang) may dispel cold, while coolness and cold (yin) may lower a high temperature. The yin or yang aspect within any phenomenon will restrict the other through opposition. Under normal conditions in the human body, therefore, a relative physiological balance is maintained through the mutual opposition of yin and yang. If for any reason this mutual opposition results in an excess or deficiency of yin or yang, the relative physiological balance of the body will be destroyed, and disease will arise. Examples are excess of yin leading to deficiency of yang, or hyperactivity of yang leading to deficiency of yin. This is referred to in Chapter 5 of the book *Plain Questions*: "When yin predominates, yang will be diseased; when yang predominates, yin will be diseased."

2) The interdependence of yin and yang Yin and yang oppose each other and yet, at the same time, also have a mutually dependent relationship. Neither can exist in isolation: without yin there can be no yang, without yang no yin. Without upward movement (yang) there can be no downward movement (yin). Without cold (yin) there would be no heat (yang). Both yin and yang are the condition for the other's existence, and this relationship is known as the interdependence of yin and yang. The fifth chapter of *Plain Questions* says, "Yin remains inside to act as a guard for yang, and yang stays outside to act as a servant for yin."

When this is applied to the physiology of the human body, yin corresponds to nutrient substances, and yang to functional activities. The nutrient substances remain in the interior, therefore "yin remains inside," while the functional activities manifest on the exterior, so "yang remains outside." The yang on the exterior is the manifestation of the substantial movement in the interior, so it is known as "the servant of yin." The yin in the interior is the material base for functional activities and is therefore called the "guard of yang." It is stated in the Chapter "Manifestations of Yin and Yang" of *Illustrated Supplement to the Classified Classics*: "Without yang there would be no production of yin; without yin there would be no production of yang."

3) The inter-consuming-supporting relationship of yin and yang The two aspects of yin and yang within any phenomenon are not fixed, but in a state of continuous mutual consumption and support. For instance, the various functional activities (yang) of the body will necessarily consume a certain amount of nutrient substance (yin). This is the process of "consumption of yin leading to gaining of yang." On the other hand, the production of various nutrient substances (yin) will necessarily consume a certain amount of energy (yang). This is the process of "consumption of yang leading to the gaining of yin." Under normal conditions, the inter-consuming-supporting relation of yin and yang is in a state of relative balance. If this relationship goes beyond normal physiological limits, however, the relative

balance of yin and yang will not be maintained, resulting in excess or deficiency of either yin or yang and the occurrence of disease.

4) The inter-transforming relationship of yin and yang The two aspects of yin and yang within any phenomenon are not absolutely static. In certain circumstances, either of the two may transform into its opposite, i.e. yang may transform into yin, and yin into yang. If the inter-consuming-supporting relationship is a process of quantitative change, then the inter-transformation of yin and yang is a process of qualitative change.

The fifth chapter of *Plain Questions* says, "Extreme yin will necessarily produce yang, and extreme yang will necessarily produce yin.... Severe cold will give birth to heat, and severe heat will give birth to cold."

On the one hand, this illustrates the inter-transformation of yin and yang, and on the other hand, the circumstances needed for their transformation. Without the combination of both internal and external factors, the transformation will not occur. Acute febrile disease is an example. Extreme heat severely consumes and damages the anti-pathogenic qi of the organism. After persistent high fever, severe cold manifestations may appear, such as a sudden drop in body temperature, pallor, cold limbs and a fading pulse. If proper emergency treatment is given in time, the yang qi will be resuscitated and there will be an improvement in the pathological condition. with the limbs becoming warm and the complexion and pulse returning to normal. The former is yang transforming into yin, and the latter yin transforming into yang.

5) The infinite divisibility of yin and yang As already mentioned, yin and yang are in a state of constant change. This means that there are relative degrees of both yin and yang. It is stated in the sixth chapter of *Plain Questions*: "Yin and yang could amount to ten in number; they could be extended to one hundred, one thousand, ten thousand or infinity; but although infinitely divisible, yin and yang are based upon only one important principle."

According to circumstances, yin and yang can be amplified into three subdivisions respectively. Chapter 66 of the book *Plain Questions* says, "The qi of yin and yang may be lesser or greater. That is why there are three yin and three yang."

This quotation explains that the qi of yin and yang may be greater or lesser in degree and that there are three sub-divisions of yin and three of yang. Greater Yin is called Taiyin (the third yin), Lesser Yin is called Shaoyin (the second yin), Greater Yang is called Taiyang (the third yang), Scanty Yang is called Shaoyang (the first yang), Extreme Yang is called Yangming (the second yang) and Declining Yin is called Jueyin (the first yin). The three yin and the three yang are a further amplification of yin and yang, and also reflect the consuming-supporting relationship of yin and yang. The differentiation of syndromes applied to the development of febrile diseases is analysed with the application of the Taiyang, Yangming, Shaoyang, Taiyin, Shaoyin and Jueyin categories.

The above mentioned is the basic content of the theory of yin-yang, the cardinal principles of which are explained by the "Yin-Yang Figure" (Taijitu). In this illustration, the white colour indicates yang, and the black colour yin. The opposition and interdependence of yin and yang are illustrated by the curved line showing the inter-consuming-supporting relationship. The white yang area contains a black spot (yin) and the black yin area a white spot (yang) indicating the potential for inter-transformation, yin within yang and yang within yin. This illustration shows that all phenomena are not isolated, but inter-connected, developing and changing.

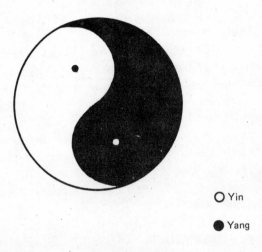

○ Yin

● Yang

Fig. 1 Yin-Yang Figure

2. Application of the Theory of Yin and Yang in Traditional Chinese Medicine

The theory of yin-yang permeates all aspects of the theoretical system of traditional Chinese medicine. It serves to explain the organic structure, physiological functions and pathological changes of the human body, and in addition guides clinical diagnosis and treatment.

1) Yin-yang and the organic structure of the human body   When the theory of yin-yang is applied to explain the organic structure of the human body, the underlying premise is that the human body is an integrated whole. All its organs and tissues are organically connected and can be divided into two opposite aspects, namely yin and yang. In terms of anatomical location, the upper part of the body is yang and the lower part yin; the exterior yang and the interior yin; the lateral aspects of the four limbs yang and the medial aspects yin. According to the nature of their functional activities, the zang organs are yin and the fu organs yang. Furthermore, within each of the zang-fu organs, there are yin and yang aspects; for example, heart-yin and heart-yang, kidney-yin and kidney-yang. Within the meridian system there are two categories: yin meridians and yang meridians. Thus the opposition of yin and yang manifests within all the upper, lower, internal and external organic structures. Each contains yin and yang qualities and all of them can be classified according to yin and yang. Thus, Chapter 25 of the book *Plain Questions* says, "Man has a physical shape which is inseparable from yin and yang."

2) Yin-yang and the physiological functions of the human body   The theory of yin-yang holds that the normal vital activities of the human body are based on the coordination of yin and yang in a unity of opposites. Functional activities pertain to yang and nutrient substances to yin. The various functional activities of the body depend on the support of the nutrient substances. Without nutrient substances, there would be no sustenance for functional activity. At the same time, functional activities are the motive power for the production of nutrient substances in the body. In other words, without the functional activities of the zang-fu organs, water and food cannot be transformed into nutrient substance. In this way, yin and yang within the human body are mutually supportive. They act together to protect the organism from invasion by pathogenic factors and to maintain a relative balance within the body. If yin and yang fail to support each other and become separated, the vital activities of the body will cease. The third chapter of *Plain Questions* says, "When yin is stablized and yang well-conserved, the spirit will be in harmony; separation of yin and yang will cause exhaustion of essential qi."

3) Yin-yang and pathological changes in the human body   The theory of yin-yang is also applied to explain pathological changes. Traditional Chinese medicine considers that the occurrence of disease results from the loss of relative balance between yin and yang, and hence an excess or deficiency of either. The occurrence and development of disease is related both to the antipathogenic qi and to pathogenic factors. There are two types of pathogenic factors: yin and yang. Antipathogenic qi involves yin fluid and yang qi. When yang pathogenic factors cause disease, this may lead to an excess of yang which consumes yin and gives rise to heat syndromes. When yin pathogenic factors cause disease, this may lead to a preponderance of yin which damages yang and gives rise to cold syndromes. When deficiency of yang fails to control yin, deficiency and cold syndromes may appear, in which yang is deficient and yin excessive. When deficiency of yin fluid fails to restrict yang, deficiency and hot syndromes may appear, in which yin is deficient and yang hyperactive.

From the above it can be seen that although the pathological changes that occur in disease are complicated and subject to change, they can be generalized and explained by: "imbalance of yin and yang," "excess of yin leading to cold syndromes," "excess of yang leading to heat syndromes," "deficiency of yang leading to cold syndromes" and "deficiency of yin leading to heat syndromes."

In addition, deficiency of either yang qi or yin fluid may lead to the consumption of the other, known as "mutual consumption of yin and yang." For example, prolonged poor appetite is mainly attributed to weakness of spleen-qi (yang), leading to insufficiency of blood (yin). This is known as "deficiency of both qi and blood due to weakness of yang affecting yin." Another example is haemorrhage, where considerable loss of yin blood usually leads to the syndrome of deficiency of yang, manifesting as chilliness and cold limbs. This is known as "deficiency of both yin and yang resulting from deficiency of yin affecting yang." These pathological changes are all commonly seen in the clinic.

4) Yin-yang as a guide to clinical diagnosis and treatment The root cause for the occurrence and development of disease is imbalance between yin and yang. For this reason, however complicated and changeable the clinical manifestations may be, with a good command of the principle of yin-yang, we may grasp the key linking elements and analyse them effectively. Generally speaking, the nature of any disease does not exceed the scope of analysis by yin-yang. Thus the fifth chapter of *Plain Questions* says, "A good doctor will observe the patient's complexion and feel the pulse, and thus take the first step in determining if it is a yin or a yang disease."

Yin-yang is the basis for the differentiation of syndromes by the eight principles, namely, yin, yang, interior, exterior, cold, heat, deficiency and excess. Exterior, heat and excess are yang, whilst interior, cold and deficiency are yin. In this way, complicated clinical situations can be simplified, and a correct diagnosis given.

Since the root cause for the occurrence and development of disease is imbalance of yin and yang, the basic principle in acupuncture treatment is to adjust yin and yang, making "yin stablized and yang well-conserved" and restoring harmony between them. The fifth chapter of *Miraculous Pivot* says, "The essential technique of needling consists of striking a balance between yin and yang."

From this it can be seen that the basic function of needling is to adjust the qi of yin and yang.

In the clinical application of acupuncture, the theory of yin-yang is applied to determine not only the principles of treatment, but also the selection of points and the technique of needling and moxibustion to be used. For instance, combining points from externally-internally related meridians, as well as combining Yuan-Primary and Luo-Connecting points, is used extensively in clinical practice. Both are methods of selecting points from related yin and yang meridians. In addition, Back-

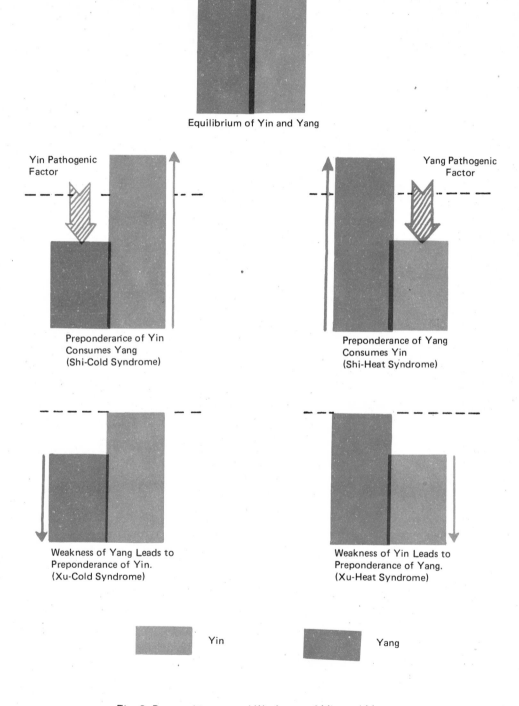

Equilibrium of Yin and Yang

Yin Pathogenic Factor

Yang Pathogenic Factor

Preponderance of Yin
Consumes Yang
(Shi-Cold Syndrome)

Preponderance of Yang
Consumes Yin
(Shi-Heat Syndrome)

Weakness of Yang Leads to
Preponderance of Yin.
(Xu-Cold Syndrome)

Weakness of Yin Leads to
Preponderance of Yang.
(Xu-Heat Syndrome)

Yin   Yang

Fig. 2 Preponderance and Weakness of Yin and Yang

Shu and Front-Mu points are often selected to treat diseases of the zang-fu organs. The related Back-Shu points are mostly selected for diseases of the zang, and the related Front-Mu points for diseases of the fu. Alternatively, a combination of Back-Shu and Front-Mu points is applied to "select Front-Mu points for yang diseases and Back-Shu points for yin diseases," in order to adjust yin and yang in either excess or deficiency. Where acupuncture and moxibustion are used together, apply moxa to the upper part of the body first and the lower part second, and "insert needles deeply with retention for yin diseases, and shallowly without retention for yang diseases."

From this we can see that in acupuncture and moxibustion, the meridians, the points, and techniques for needling and moxibustion are all closely related to the theory of yin and yang, emphasizing the vital role that yin and yang play in both theory and practice.

II. THE FIVE ELEMENTS

The five elements refer to five categories in the natural world, namely wood, fire, earth, metal and water. The theory of the five elements holds that all phenomena in the universe correspond in nature either to wood, fire, earth, metal or water, and that these are in a state of constant motion and change. The theory of the five elements was first formed in China at about the time of the Yin and Zhou dynasties (16th century-221 B.C.). Historically it derives from observations of the natural world made in early times by the Chinese people in the course of their lives and productive labour. Wood, fire, earth, metal and water were considered to be five indispensible materials for the maintenance of life and production, as well as representing five important states that initiated normal changes in the natural world. As said in *A Collection of Ancient Works:* "Food relies on water and fire. Production relies on metal and wood. Earth gives birth to everything. They are used by the people."

Although having different characteristics, the five materials depend on each other and are inseparable. Thus in ancient times, people took these five elements with their mutual relationships to explain all phenomena in the natural world. The primitive concept of the five elements was later developed into a more complex theory, which together with the theory of yin-yang, served as a conceptual method and a theoretical tool for understanding and analysing all phenomena, and ran through various academic classics in ancient times. In traditional Chinese medicine the theory of the five elements is applied to generalise and explain the nature of the zang-fu organs, the inter-relationships between them, and the relation between human beings and the natural world. It thus serves to guide clinical diagnosis and treatment.

1. Classification of Phenomena According to the Five Elements

In early times, the Chinese people recognized that wood, fire, earth, metal and water were indispensible in their daily lives as well as having different natures. For instance, the character of wood is to grow and flourish, the character of fire is to be hot and flare up, the character of earth is to give birth to all things, the character of metal is to descend and be clear, and the character of water is to be cold and to flow downwards. Early doctors applied the theory of the five elements in their extensive study of the physiology and pathology of the zang-fu organs and tissues of the human body, and indeed all phenomena in the natural world that were related to human life. Using analogy, they classified all these, according to their nature, function and form, into the five elements. They applied this theory to explain the complicated physiological and pathological relationships between the zang-fu organs, and between the human body and the external environment. This classification of phenomena was minutely described in the fourth and fifth chapters of *Plain Questions*. The classification of the meridians according to the five elements is based on the nature of the zang-fu organs:

Zang-fu	Meridian	Element
Liver	Foot Jueyin	Wood
Gallbladder	Foot Shaoyang	Wood
Heart	Hand Shaoyin	Fire
Small intestine	Hand Taiyang	Fire
Spleen	Foot Taiyin	Earth
Stomach	Foot Yangming	Earth
Lung	Hand Taiyin	Metal
Large intestine	Hand Yangming	Metal
Kidney	Foot Shaoyin	Water
Bladder	Foot Taiyang	Water
Pericardium	Hand Jueyin	Fire
Sanjiao	Hand Shaoyang	Fire

As for the pericardium and sanjiao, the ancients considered that the pericardium is a protective membrane surrounding the heart, and prevents the heart from being invaded by pathogenic factors. Since the heart pertains to fire, the pericardium also pertains to fire. The table on the next page shows the five categories of things according to the five elements.

2. The Law of Movement of the Five Elements

The law of movement of the five elements mainly manifests in the following ways: interpromoting, interacting, overacting, counteracting, and mutual interaction between mother and son.

Promoting implies promoting growth. Wood promotes fire, fire promotes metal, metal promotes water, and water, in turn, promotes wood. This interpromoting relationship of the five elements is known as the "mother-son" relationship, with each element being the "son" of the element that promotes it, and the "mother" of the one it promotes.

Acting means bringing under control or restraint. In the interacting relationship, wood acts on earth, earth acts on water, water acts on fire, fire acts on metal, and

The Five Categories of Things According to the Five Elements

| Nature | | | | | | | Human Body | | | | | |
Directions	Tastes	Colours	Growth and development factor	Environmental factor	Seasons	Five elements	Zang	Fu	Five sense organs	Five tissues	Emotions	Five notes
East	Sour	Green	Germination	Wind	Spring	Wood	Liver	Gall-bladder	Eye	Tendon	Anger	Jiao
South	Bitter	Red	Growth	Heat	Summer	Fire	Heart	Small intestine	Tongue	Vessel	Joy	Zheng
Middle	Sweet	Yellow	Transformation	Dampness	Late summer	Earth	Spleen	Stomach	Mouth	Muscle	Meditation	Gong
West	Pungent	White	Reaping	Dryness	Autumn	Metal	Lung	Large intestine	Nose	Skin and hair	Grief and melancholy	Shang
North	Salty	Black	Storing	Cold	Winter	Water	Kidney	Bladder	Ear	Bone	Fright and fear	Yu

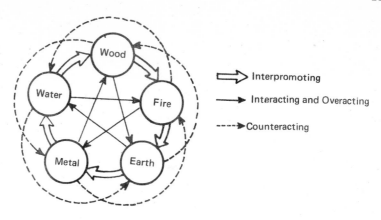

Fig. 3　Interpromoting and Interacting Relationship of the Five Elements

metal in turn acts on wood. Here each of the five elements occupies the role of "being acted upon" (known as "under control") and of "acting upon" (known as "controller"). The interacting relationship is therefore also known as the "intercontrolling" relationship.

Interpromoting and interacting are two inseparable and indispensible aspects of the five elements which both oppose and cooperate with each other. Without promotion there can be no growth and development; without interaction there can be no balance and coordination during development and change. In the promotion of growth there must be control, and in control there must be promotion of growth. The relative balance maintained between promoting and acting thus ensures normal growth and development. When there is excess or insufficiency of any of the five elements, there will be abnormal interpromoting and interacting (known as "overacting" or "counter-acting") and disorders of "the mother affecting the son" and "the son affecting the mother." Overacting can

be likened to launching an attack when a counterpart is weak — it is an excessive acting on the element normally acted upon. It is commonly called "interacting" in the clinic. For example "wood overacting on earth" can also be called "wood acting on earth." The order of overacting is the same as that of acting, except that overacting is not a normal interaction but a harmful condition occurring under particular circumstances. Counteracting means preying upon other elements. The order of counteracting is just the opposite to that of interacting. For instance, under normal conditions, metal acts on wood. In the case of deficiency of metal qi, or hyperactivity of wood-qi, the wood may counteract on metal. Therefore it is stated in Chapter 67 of *Plain Questions:* "When the qi of a given element is in excess, it will overact on the acted element and counteract on the acting element. When the qi of a given element is in deficiency, it will be attacked by the acting element and counteracted by the acted element."

The mutual condition of "affecting

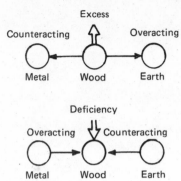

Fig. 4 Overacting and Counteracting among the Five Elements

between mother and son" refers to the phenomenon of abnormal interpromoting between the five elements. The promoted element is considered as the son, and the promoting element as the mother. "Affecting" means influencing in a harmful way, including both "the mother affecting the son" and "the son affecting the mother." The order of "mother affecting the son" is the same as the interpromoting relationship, and the order of "son affecting the mother" is the reverse. Under normal conditions, water promotes wood. Abnormally, "water affecting wood" is known as "the mother affecting the son," and "wood affecting water" is known as the "son affecting the mother."

3. The Application of the Theory of the Five Elements in Traditional Chinese Medicine

When the theory of the five elements is applied in traditional Chinese medicine, the classification of phenomena according to the properties of the five elements and their interpromoting, interacting, overacting and counteracting relationships are used to explain both physiological and pathological phenomena, and to guide clinical diagnosis and treatment.

1) The five elements and the inter-relationship between the zang-fu organs In this theory, each of the internal organs pertains to one of the five elements. The properties of the five elements serve as an analogy to explain some of the physiological functions of the five zang. In addition, the interpromoting and interacting relationships are used to explain some of the interconnections between the zang-fu organs. The liver may serve as an example, it is promoted by the kidney, promotes the heart, is acted on by the lung, and acts on the spleen. The roles of the other organs can also be explained in the same way, and thus an integral relationship between the internal organs is generalised.

The meridians have a close relationship with the zang-fu organs. They are the passages by which the zang-fu organs connect with one another according to the interpromoting and interacting relationships of the five elements. In general, the zang-fu organs connect with each other directly through the meridians, according to the cycles of the five elements. The relationships between the liver, heart, spleen, lung and kidney can serve as an example. In the meridian system, the Liver Meridian of Foot-Jueyin and the Gallbladder Meridian of Foot-Shaoyang run through the heart; the Liver Meridian of Foot Jueyin runs on both sides of the stomach which is externally-internally related with the spleen; the Kidney Meridian of Foot-Shaoyin ascends and runs through the liver; the Liver Meridian of Foot-Jueyin ascends to the lung; the Kidney Meridian of Foot-Shaoyin ascends through the liver and lung, etc. By means of the interconnecting system of the meridians, the five elements maintain a relative balance and coordination.

The theory of the five elements is a naive theory with definite limitations. The laws of interpromoting and interacting can not reflect all the interrelationships between the zang-fu organs and their related tissues. Clinical practice, however, has shown that these laws do reflect certain objective relationships among the five zang organs and can be used to determine diagnosis and treatment.

2) The five elements and pathological relationships among the zang-fu organs   The occurrence of disease is the pathological manifestation of the dysfunction of the zang-fu organs and their related tissues, which may be due to a number of factors. The human body is an organic whole, and both interpromoting and interacting relationships exist among the viscera. Thus when one internal organ is afflicted, other organs and tissues may become involved. This is called "transmission." According to the theory of the five elements, intertransmission may follow either the interpromoting or the interacting cycles.

Transmission following the interpromoting cycle involves disorders of "the mother affecting the son" and "the son affecting the mother." For example, when liver disease is transmitted to the heart, it is called a disorder of "the mother affecting the son," and when liver disease is transmitted to the kidney, it is called a disorder of "the son affecting the mother."

Transmission following the interacting cycle involves "overacting" and "counteracting." When a liver disease is transmitted to the spleen, it is called "wood overacting on earth," and when a liver disease is transmitted to the lung, it is called "wood counteracting on metal."

It must be pointed out that mutual pathological influences among the viscera exist objectively. Some of them can be explained by disorders of "the mother affecting the son," "the son affecting the mother," "overacting" and "counteracting." Therefore the theory may serve to explain those pathological transmissions which are observed in clinical practice.

3) The five elements and clinical diagnosis and treatment   The theory of the five elements is applied to synthesize clinical data obtained through the four diagnostic methods, and determine pathological conditions according to the natures and laws of the five elements. For instance, a patient with redness and pain of the eye and irritability suggests a liver problem; a red complexion accompanied by a bitter taste in the mouth suggests hyperactivity of heart-fire.

In treatment, the five Shu-Points correspond to the five elements. The Jin-Well, Ying-Spring, Shu-Stream, Jing-River and He-Sea points of the yin meridians correspond to wood, fire, earth, metal and water respectively, whilst those of the yang meridians correspond to metal, water, wood, fire and earth respectively. Clinically they are selected for treatment according to the principle of "reinforcing the mother" and "reducing the son." In addition, it is common clinical practice to determine the principle of treatment and selection of points according to pathological influences among the zang-fu organs which follow the cycle of the five elements. For instance, in case of a disharmony between the liver and stomach, "wood overacting on earth," the principle of treatment should be to promote earth and restrain wood. Points such as Zhongwan (Ren 12), Zusanli (S 36) and Taichong (Liv 3) will be selected.

In general, the theories of yin and yang and the five elements both encompass rudimentary concepts of materialism and dialectics, and to some extent reflect the objective laws of nature. They are of prime importance in explaining physiological activities and pathological changes, serving to guide clinical practice. In their clinical application, the two principles are usually related. They supplement each other and cannot be entirely separated. In other words, when applying yin-yang theory, the five elements will be involved; when using the theory of the five elements, yin-yang will be involved. When considering the theories of yin-yang and the five elements, it must be understood that they originated in clinical practice, have played a progressive role in the development of traditional Chinese medicine, and are still guiding clinical practice to a large extent up to the present day. At the same time, owing to the limitations inherent in the historical development of ancient Chinese society, the theories are incomplete and need to be perfected through continuous research and summation in clinical practice.

Chapter 3

THE ZANG-FU ORGANS

Zang-fu is the general term for the organs of the human body, and includes the six zang organs, the six fu organs and the extraordinary fu organs. The heart, lung, spleen, liver, kidney and pericardium are known as the six zang organs. The gallbladder, stomach, small intestine, large intestine, bladder and sanjiao are known as the six fu organs. The brain, marrow, bones, vessels, gallbladder and uterus are known as the "extraordinary fu" organs. Since the pericardium is a protective membrane of the heart, the "extraordinary fu" organs pertain respectively to the other fu organs, it is generally called five zang and six fu organs. The main physiological functions of the zang organs are to manufacture and store essential substances, including vital essence, qi, blood and body fluid. The main physiological functions of the fu organs are to receive and digest food, and transmit and excrete the wastes. The eleventh chapter of *Plain Questions* says: "The so-called five zang organs store pure essential qi without draining it off, and for this reason they can be filled up but cannot be over filled. The six fu organs transmit water and food without storing them, and for this reason they may be over supplied but cannot be filled up."

This description not only describes the functions of the zang-fu organs, but also points out the basic physiological dif-ferences between the zang and the fu organs in their physiological functions.

Although the zang organs are different from the fu organs in terms of physiological activities, there is a structural and functional connection by the way of meridians and collaterals between individual zang and fu organ, between the zang and fu organs collectively; and between the zang-fu organs on the one hand, and the five sense organs and tissues on the other.

The theory of the zang-fu organs considers the physiological functions and pathological changes of the zang and fu organs, as well as their interrelationships. This theory was called "Zang Xiang" by ancient doctors. "Zang" refers to the interior location of the zang-fu organs, and "xiang" denotes their manifestations or "image." In other words, the zang-fu organs are located on the inside of the body, but their physiological activities and pathological changes are reflected on the exterior. The book *Classified Classics* by Zhang Jiebin (1562-1639) states: "The zang-fu organs are situated interiorly and manifested exteriorly; therefore the theory of the zang-fu organs is called Zang Xiang."

There are two main aspects to the theory of the zang-fu organs. Firstly the study of the physiological functions and pathological changes of the zang-fu organs, tissues and their interrelationships. Secondly the physiology and pathology of vital essence, qi, blood and body fluid, as well as the relationship between these on the one hand and the zang-fu organs on the other.

Historically, the development of the theory of the zang-fu organs in the course of extensive medical practice involved three aspects:

1. Ancient anatomical knowledge.

The twelfth chapter of *Miraculous Pivot* says: "A man is about eight *Chi* tall in average; the external size of the body is measurable because its skin and flesh are visible, and also his pulse may be taken in different regions. In addition, when a man dies, his body may be dissected for observation. For this reason, there are established standards by which we determine the hardness and crispness of the zang organs, the size of the fu organs, the quantity of food consumed, the length of the vessels, the clarity and turbidity of the blood, the quantity of qi in the body.... All these aspects of the human body as outlined above are governed by a set of established standards."

In addition, there are some descriptions in the fourteenth, thirty-first and thirty-second chapters of *Miraculous Pivot,* as well as some descriptions in *Classics on Medical Problems.* It can be seen, therefore, that the practice of anatomy in China predates the Christian era. All these are the indispensable foundation of the formation of zang-fu theory.

2. Observation of physiological and pathological phenomena.

An example is the development of the theory that the skin and hair are connected with the nose and lung, through observation of cases of common cold due to invasion of the exterior of the body by pathogenic cold.

Typical symptoms of nasal obstruction, runny nose, chills, fever and cough demonstrate this connection.

3. The summary of rich experience obtained through lengthy clinical practice.

An example is the development of the theory of the kidney dominating bone. In the treatment of fracture, application of the method of tonifying the kidney may hasten the healing of bone.

To summarize, the comparatively integrated theory of the zang-fu organs, which takes the five zang as its core, was formed through a long period of clinical practice and observation.

I.   THE FIVE ZANG ORGANS

1.   The Heart

The heart is situated in the thorax and its meridian connects with the small intestine with which it is internally-externally related. The main physiological functions of the heart are: dominating the blood and vessels, manifesting on the face, housing the mind, and opening into the tongue.

1) Dominating the blood and vessels and manifesting on the face Dominating the blood and vessels means that the heart is the motive force for blood circulation, whilst the vessels are the physical structures which contain and circulate the blood. The blood circulation relies on cooperation between the heart and the vessels, with the heart being of primary importance. In the forty-fourth chapter of *Plain Questions*, it is stated: "The heart dominates the blood and vessels."

The physiological function of the heart in propelling the blood relies on the heart qi. When the heart qi is vigorous, the blood will circulate normally in the vessels to supply the whole body. Since the heart, blood and vessels are interconnected, and there are many vessels on the face, the prosperity or decline of the heart-qi and the amount of blood circulating will be reflected in changes in both the pulse and complexion. If the heart-qi is vigorous and the blood ample, the pulse will be regular and strong and the complexion rosy. When the heart-qi and blood are deficient, the pulse will be thready and weak, and the complexion pale. As the ninth chapter of *Plain Questions* says: "The glory of the heart is manifested on the face, since the blood fills up the vessels."

2) Housing the mind   The word "mind" has the broad meaning of the outward appearance of the vital activities of the whole body, and the narrow meaning of consciousness, e.g. spirit and thinking. The theory of the zang-fu organs holds that thinking is related to the five zang organs, and principally to the physiological functions of the heart. The seventy-first chapter of *Miraculous Pivot* says: "The heart is the residence of the spirit." The eighth chapter in the same book also says: "The mind is responsible for the performance of activities."

This shows that mental activities and thinking have their foundation in the functions of the heart. Spirit, consciousness, thinking, memory and sleep are therefore all related to the function of the heart in housing the mind. Blood is the main material basis for mental activities. It is controlled as well as dominated and regulated by the heart. So the function of the heart in housing the mind is closely related to that of the heart in controlling the blood and vessels. Therefore it is stated in the same chapter, "The heart dominates vessels and the vessels house mind."

3) Opening into the tongue   "Opening"

refers to the close structural, physiological and pathological relationship between a particular zang and one of the sense organs. The tongue is connected to the Heart Meridian interiorly, and via this connection the heart dominates the sense of taste and the speech. When the function of the heart is normal, the tongue will be rosy, moist and lustrous, the sense of taste will be normal, and the tongue will move freely. On the other hand, disorders of the heart will reflect on the tongue. For example, deficiency of heart blood may give rise to a pale tongue; flaring up of heart fire may give rise to redness of the tongue tip and ulceration of the tongue body; stagnation of heart-blood may give rise to a dark, purplish tongue body or purplish spots on the tongue. The saying: "the heart opens into the tongue," and "the tongue is the mirror of the heart" reflect this close physiological and pathological relationship.

Appendix:

The pericardium, known as "xin bao luo," is a membrane surrounding the heart. Its meridian connects with the sanjiao with which it is externally-internally related. Its main function is to protect the heart. When pathogenic qi invades the heart, the pericardium is always the first to be attacked, and invasion of the pericardium by pathogenic qi will often affect the normal function of the heart. For example, invasion of the interior by pathogenic mild heat, which gives rise to symptoms of mental derangement such as coma and delirium, is described as "invasion of the pericardium by pathogenic heat," although the clinical manifestations are the same as those of the heart. For this reason, the pericardium is not generally regarded as an independent organ, but as an attachment to the heart.

2. The Liver

The liver is situated in the right hypochondriac region. Its meridian connects with the gallbladder with which it is internally-externally related. Its main physiological functions are storing blood, maintaining the free flow of qi, controlling the tendons, manifesting in the nails and opening into the eye.

1) Storing blood The liver stores blood and regulates the volume in circulation. The volume of blood circulating in various parts of the body changes according to different physiological needs. During vigorous movement and other daytime activities, the blood is released from the liver, increasing the volume of blood in circulation. During rest and sleep, the volume of blood required decreases, and part of the blood remains in the liver. As Wang Bing said in the explanation on the tenth chapter of *Plain Questions*: "The liver stores blood ... the blood circulates in the vessels during exertion and remains in the liver during rest."

Because of its function of regulating the volume of circulating blood, the liver is closely related to all the activities of the zang-fu organs and tissues. When the liver is diseased, dysfunction of the liver in storing blood will affect the normal activities of the body, and lead to pathological changes of the blood itself. For example, deficiency of liver blood may give rise to blurred vision, spasm and convulsion of the tendons and muscles, numbness of the four limbs, and oligomenorrhoea or even amenorrhoea in females.

2) Maintaining the free flow of qi The liver is responsible for the unrestrained, free going, and harmonious functional activity of all the zang-fu organs, including itself. The normal character of the liver is to "flourish" and to dislike depression. Stagnation of liver qi due to emotional changes may affect the function of the liver in maintaining the free flow of qi, manifesting in the following three ways:

i) The liver and emotional activity

In addition to the heart, emotional activity is closely related to the liver qi. Only when the function of the liver in maintaining the free flow of qi is normal can the qi and blood be harmonious and the mind at ease. Dysfunction of the liver, therefore, is often accompanied by emotional changes such as mental depression or excitement. When liver-qi stagnates, for example, there may be mental depression, paranoia, or even weeping; when liver qi is hyperactive, there may be irascibility, insomnia, dream-disturbed sleep, dizziness and vertigo. Whilst dysfunction of the liver often leads to emotional changes, at the same time prolonged excessive mental irritation often leads to dysfunction of the liver in maintaining the free flow of qi.

ii) The liver function and digestion

The liver function of maintaining the free flow of qi is related not only to the ascending and descending function of the stomach and spleen, but also to the secretion of bile. The liver therefore has an important influence on digestion. Dysfunction of the liver may affect the secretion and excretion of bile, and the digestive function of the spleen and stomach, resulting in dyspepsia. When the liver fails to maintain the free flow of qi, there may be symptoms of stagnation of liver qi such as distending pain of the chest and hypochondrium, mental depression or irascibility. If the descending function of the stomach is affected, there may also be belching, nausea and vomiting, and if the spleen's function of transportation and transformation is affected, there may be abdominal distention and diarrhoea. The former is called "attack of the stomach by liver-qi" and the latter "disharmony of the liver and spleen."

iii) The liver function and qi and blood

The blood circulation relies upon the propelling function of qi. Although the heart and lung play the main role in the circulation of qi and blood, the function of the liver in maintaining the free flow of qi is also needed to prevent stagnation of qi and blood. Stagnation of qi and blood due to the failure of the liver in maintaining the free flow of qi may lead to stuffiness and pressure in the chest, distending or pricking pain in the hypochondriac region, dysmenorrhoea, and even the formation of palpable mass.

3) Controlling the tendons and manifesting in the nails The tendons are the main tissues linking the joints and muscles and dominating the movement of the limbs. Since the liver nourishes the tendons of the whole body to maintain their normal physiological activities, when liver blood is consumed, it may deprive the tendons of nourishment and give rise to weakness of the tendons, numbness of the limbs, and dysfunction of the joints in contraction and relaxation. When the tendons are invaded by pathogenic heat of the liver, there may be convulsion of the four extremities, opisthotonos and clenching of the teeth.

Manifesting in the nails means that the state of the yin and blood of the liver affects not only the movement of the tendons but also the condition of the nails. When liver blood is ample, the tendons and nails are strong, and when liver blood is deficient, the tendons will be weak and the nails soft and thin, withered, or even deformed and chipped. The tenth chapter of *Plain Questions* therefore says: "The liver controls the tendons and manifests in the nails."

4) Opening into the eye In the eightieth chapter of *Miraculous Pivot*, it says: "The essential qi of the five zang and six fu organs flows upward to enter into the eyes to generate vision."

Of the five zang and six fu organs, the liver is the main organ affecting the eyes and vision. The liver stores blood and its meridian ascends to connect with the eyes. Therefore, the seventeenth chapter of *Miracular Pivot* says: "The liver qi is in communication with the eyes."

Whether the liver function is normal or not often reflects on the eye. For example, deficiency of the yin and blood of the liver may lead to dryness of the eyes, blurred vision or even night blindness. Wind heat in the Liver Meridian may give rise to redness, swelling and pain of the eyes.

3.   The Spleen

The spleen is situated in the middle jiao. Its meridian connects with the stomach, with which it is internally-externally related. Its main physiological functions are: governing transportation and transformation, controlling blood, dominating the muscles and limbs, opening into the mouth and manifesting on the lips.

1) Governing transportation and transformation Transportation implies transmission; and transformation implies digestion and absorption. This function of the spleen involves transportation and transformation of water and food on the one hand, and of dampness on the other.

The function of the spleen in transporting and transforming essential substances refers to the digestion, absorption and transmission of nutrient substance. Since water and food are the main source of the nutrient substance required by the body after birth, as well as being the main material base for the manufacture of qi and blood, the spleen is considered to be the main zang organ for the manufacture of qi and blood. When spleen qi is vigorous, digestion, absorption and transmission are normal. Deficiency of spleen qi and dysfunction of the spleen in transportation and transformation may lead to poor appetite, abdominal distention, loose stools, lassitude, emaciation and malnutrition.

The function of the spleen in transporting and transforming dampness refers to the spleen's role in water metabolism. The spleen transports the excess fluid of the meridians, tissues and organs and helps discharge it from the body. It ensures that the various tissues of the body are both properly moistened and at the same time free from retention of dampness. Dysfunction of the spleen in transportation and transformation may lead to retention of dampness, with such clinical manifestations as oedema, diarrhoea, phlegm and retained fluid.

The spleen's functions of transporting and transforming water and food on the one hand, and water damp on the other are interconnected, and failure of the transportation and transformation function may give rise to clinical manifestations of either.

The transportation and transformation function of the spleen relies on spleen qi, which is characterized by ascending. If the spleen qi does not ascend, or indeed sinks, there may be vertigo, blurred vision, prolapse of the rectum after prolonged diarrhoea, or prolapse of various other internal organs. Treatment is aimed at strengthening the ascending function of spleen qi.

2) Controlling blood Controlling blood means that the spleen qi has the function of keeping the blood circulating in the vessels and preventing extravasation. When the spleen qi is strong, the source for the manufacture of blood will also be strong, there will be ample qi and blood in the body, and the blood will be prevented from extravasation. If the spleen qi is weak and fails to control blood, there may be various kinds of haemorrhage, such as bloody stool, uterine bleeding and purpura.

3) Dominating the muscles and four limbs The spleen transports and transforms the essence of food and water to nourish the muscles and the four limbs. Adequate nourishment ensures well-developed muscles and proper function of the limbs. If nourishment is inadequate, the muscles of the four limbs will be weak and soft. The forty-fourth chapter of *Plain Questions* therefore says: "The spleen is in charge of muscles."

4) Opening into the mouth and manifesting on the lips The spleen's function of transportation and transformation is closely related to food intake and the sense of taste. When the spleen functions normally, there will be good appetite and a normal sense of taste; when there is dysfunction of the spleen, there will be poor appetite, impaired sense of taste and a sticky, sweetish sensation in the mouth due to retention of pathogenic damp in the spleen.

The spleen dominates muscles, and the mouth is the aperture of the spleen. For this reason, the lips reflect the condition of the spleen's function of transporting and transforming water and food. When the spleen is healthy, there will be ample qi and blood and the lips will be red and lustrous. Deficiency of spleen qi will lead to deficiency of qi and blood, and the lips will be pale or sallow.

4.   The Lung

The lung, situated in the thorax, communicates with the throat and opens into the nose. It occupies the uppermost position among the zang-fu organs, and is known as the "canopy" of the zang-fu organs. Its meridian connects with the large intestine with which it is internally-externally related. Its main physiological functions are: dominating qi, controlling respiration, dominating dispersing and descending, dominating skin and hair, and regulating the water passages.

1) Dominating qi and controlling respiration Dominating qi has two aspects: dominating the qi of respiration and dominating the qi of the whole body.

Dominating the qi of respiration means that the lung is a respiratory organ through which the qi from the exterior and the qi from the interior are able to mingle. Via the lung, the human body inhales clear qi from the natural environment and exhales waste qi from the interior of the body. This is known as "getting rid of the stale and taking in the fresh." The fifth chapter of *Plain Questions* says: "The qi of heaven is in communication with the lung."

Dominating the qi of the whole body means that the function of the lung in respiration greatly influences the functional activities of the whole body, and is closely related to the formation of pectoral qi, which is formed from the combination of the essential qi of water and food, and the clear qi inhaled by the lung. It accumulates in the chest, ascends to the throat to dominate respiration, and is distributed to the whole body in order to maintain the normal functions of the tissues and organs. The tenth chapter of *Plain Questions* says: "All kinds of qi belong to the lung."

When the function of the lung in dominating qi is normal, the passage of qi will be unobstructed and respiration will be normal and smooth. Deficiency of lung qi may lead to general lassitude, feeble speech, weak respiration and shortness of breath.

2) Dominating dispersing, skin and hair Dispersing here means distributing. It is by the dispersing function of the lung that defensive qi and body fluid are distributed to the whole body to warm and moisten the muscles, skin and hair. The thirtieth chapter of *Miraculous Pivot* says: "Qi refers to the substance that originates in the upper jiao, spreads the essential part of water and food, warms the skin, fills up the body and moistens the hair, like irrigation by fog and dew."

The skin and hair, located on the surface of the body and including the sweat glands, serve as a protective screen to defend the body from exogenous pathogenic factors. The skin and hair are warmed and nourished by defensive qi and body fluid distributed by the lung, which controls respiration. The pores of the skin also have the function of dispersing qi and regulating respiration. For this reason, traditional Chinese medicine says: "the lung dominates skin and hair" and "the pores are the gate of qi."

The close physiological relationship between the lung, skin and hair means that they often affect each other pathologically. For example, exogenous pathogenic factors often invade the lung through the skin and hair, giving rise to symptoms such as aversion to cold, fever, nasal obstruction and cough, reflecting failure of the lung in dispersing. If lung qi is deficient, failure of the lung in dispersing the qi of water and food can result in the skin becoming wan and sallow and lead to deficiency of the anti-pathogenic qi and hence susceptibility to catching cold. When lung qi fails to protect the surface of the body, there may be frequent spontaneous perspiration.

3) The lung dominates descending and regulates the water passages   As a general rule, the upper zang-fu organs have the function of descending, and the lower zang-fu organs the function of ascending. Since the lung is the uppermost zang organ, its qi descends to promote the circulation of qi and body fluid through the body and to conduct them downwards. Dysfunction of the lung in descending may lead to upward perversion of lung qi with symptoms such as cough and shortness of breath.

Regulating the water passages means to regulate the pathways for the circulation and excretion of water. The role of the lung in promoting and maintaining water metabolism depends on the descending function of lung qi. Dysfunction may result in dysuria, oliguria and oedema.

4) Opening into the nose   The nose is the pathway for respiration. The respiratory and olfactory functions of the nose depend on lung qi. When lung qi is normal, the respiration will be free and the sense of smell acute. Dysfunction of the lung in dispersing, for example, due to invasion by wind-cold, will lead to nasal obstruction, runny nose, and anosmia. Excessive pathogenic heat in the lung will lead to shortness of breath and vibration of the ala nasi.

Since the throat is also a gateway of respiration and an organ of speech, through which the Lung Meridian passes, the flow of qi and the speech are directly affected by the state of the lung qi. When the lung is diseased, it usually causes pathological changes in the throat, such as hoarse voice and aphonia.

5.   The Kidney

The kidneys are located at either side of the lumbus, which is therefore described as "the home of the kidney." The Kidney Meridian connects with the bladder with which it is internally-externally related. Its main functions are: to store essence and dominate human reproduction and development, dominate water metabolism and the reception of qi, produce marrow to fill up the brain, dominate bone, manufacture blood, manifest in the hair, open into the ear, and dominate anterior and posterior orifices.

1) Storing essence and dominating development and reproduction   "Essence" is the material base of the human body and of many of its functional activities. Kidney essence consists of two parts: congenital and acquired. Congenital essence is inherited from the parents, and acquired essence is transformed from the essential substances of food by the spleen and stomach. The congenital and acquired essence rely on, and promote, each other. Before birth, congenital essence has prepared the material base for acquired essence. After birth, acquired essence constantly replenishes congenital essence. Of the two, acquired essence is the most important.

The function of the kidney in reproduction and development relies entirely on kidney qi. In other words, the ability to reproduce, grow and develop is related to the prosperity or decline of the essential qi of the kidney.

In childhood the essential qi of the kidney develops gradually and manifests in changes in the skin and hair. It flourishes in adolescence and at this time males will have seminal emission, and females the onset of menstruation, reflecting the ripening of the sexual function. In old age the essential qi of the kidney declines, reproductive ability and sexual function finally disappear, and the body begins to wither. The first chapter of *Plain Questions* says: "At the age of fourteen, a woman will begin to menstruate, her Ren (Conception Vessel) Meridian begins to flow, and the qi in the Chong Meridian begins to flourish. That is why she is capable of becoming pregnant.... At the age of forty-nine, the qi of the Ren Meridian declines, the qi of the Chong Meridian becomes weak and scanty, the sexual energy becomes exhausted and menstruation stops, with the result that her body becomes old and she can no longer become pregnant."

It also says: "At the age of sixteen, the kidney qi of a man becomes even more abundant, his sexual function begins to develop, and he is filled with semen that he can ejaculate. When he has sexual intercourse with a woman, she can have children.... At the age of fifty-six, sexual energy begins to decline, the semen becomes scanty, and the kidney weak, with the result that all parts of the body begin to age. At the age of sixty-four teeth and hair are gone."

These quotations clearly reflect the role played by the kidney in dominating human growth, development and reproduction. This is why the kidney is considered to be "the congenital foundation" and why traditional Chinese medicine attaches such great importance to it.

The essential qi of the kidney includes kidney essence and the kidney qi transformed from kidney essence. The transformation of kidney qi from kidney essence relies on the evaporating function of kidney yang upon kidney yin. Both kidney yin and kidney yang take the essential qi stored in the kidney as their material base. The essential qi of the kidney therefore involves both kidney yin and kidney yang.

Kidney yin is the foundation of the yin fluid of the whole body, which moistens and nourishes the zang-fu organs and tissues. Kidney yang is the foundation of the yang qi of the whole body, which warms and promotes the functions of the zang-fu organs and tissues. Yin and yang are both lodged in the kidney, which was therefore said to be "the house of water and fire" by the ancients. According to their nature, essence is yin, and qi is yang, so kidney essence is sometimes called "kidney yin" and kidney qi is sometimes called "kidney yang." Kidney yin and kidney yang both restrict and promote each other in the human body so as to maintain a dynamic physiological equilibrium. Once this equilibrium is disrupted, pathological changes due to imbalance of yin and yang in the kidney will manifest. If kidney yin is deficient through exhaustion, it will fail to control yang which becomes hyperactive. Typical symptoms are heat sensations of the chest, palms and soles, afternoon fever, night sweats, and seminal emission in males or sexual dreams in females. If kidney yang is deficient, leading to failure in warming and promoting, there may be symptoms such as lack of spirit, coldness and pain in the lumbar region and knees, aversion to cold, cold limbs, and impotence in men and frigidity and infertility in women. If kidney deficiency is not accompanied by obvious cold symptoms, it is usually called "deficiency of kidney qi" or "deficiency of kidney essence."

2) Dominating water metabolism Dominating water metabolism means that the kidney plays an extremely important role in regulating the distribution of body fluid. Such a function relies on the qi activity of the kidney. When the qi activity of the kidney is normal, then the "opening and closing" of the kidney will also be normal. Water is first received by the stomach, and then transmitted by the spleen to the lung which disperses and descends it. Part of the fluid reaches the kidney where it is further divided into two parts — the clear and the turbid by the qi activity of kidney yang. The clear fluid is transmitted up to the lung from which it is circulated to the zang-fu organs and the tissues of the body. The turbid flows into the bladder to form urine which is then excreted. The function of the kidney dominates this whole metabolic process. If the kidney fails to open and close, then disturbance of water metabolism such as oedema or abnormal micturition will occur.

3) Receiving qi Receiving qi means that the kidney assists the lung in its function of receiving and descending the qi. The book *Direct Guidebook of Medicine* states: "The lung is the governor of qi and the kidney is the root of qi."

In other words, respiration depends not only on the descending function of the lung, but also on the kidney's function of reception and control. Only when the kidney qi is strong can the passage of qi in the lung be free, and the respiration smooth and even. If kidney qi is weak, the root of the qi is not firm, and the kidney will fail to receive qi, giving rise to shortness of breath and difficult inhalation which is worse after movement.

4) Dominating bone, manufacturing marrow to fill up the brain and manifesting in the hair The kidney stores essence which produces marrow. The marrow develops in the bone cavities and nourishes their growth and development. When kidney essence is sufficient, the bone marrow has a rich source of production and the bones are well nourished, firm and hard. If the kidney essence is deficient, it will fail to nourish the bones, leading to weakness and soreness of the lumbar region and knees, weakness or even atrophy of the feet, and maldevelopment. Since the kidney dominates bone, and the teeth are the surplus of bone, ample kidney essence will result in strong healthy teeth, whilst deficiency of kidney essence will lead to loose or even falling teeth.

The marrow consists of two parts: spinal marrow and bone marrow. The spinal marrow ascends to connect with the brain, which is formed by the collection of marrow. The thirty-third chapter of *Miraculous Pivot* therefore states: "The brain is the sea of marrow."

Essence and blood promote each other. When the essence is sufficient, then blood will flourish. The nourishment of the hair is dependent on a sufficient supply of blood, but its vitality is rooted in the kidney qi. The hair, therefore, is both the surplus of blood on the one hand, and the outward manifestation of the kidney on the other. Growth or loss of hair, its lustre or withering, are all related to the condition of the kidney qi. During the prime of life, the kidney qi is in a flourishing state and the hair is lustrous; in old age the kidney qi declines and the hair turns white and falls. The tenth chapter of *Plain Questions* states: "The kidney dominates bone and manifests on the hair."

5) Opening into the ear and dominating anterior and posterior orifices The function of the ear in dominating hearing relies on nourishment by the essential qi of the kidney. The ear therefore pertains to the kidney. When the essential qi of the kidney is sufficient, the ear is well nourished and hearing is acute. When the essential qi of the kidney is deficient, it will fail to ascend to the ear leading to tinnitus and deafness.

"Anterior orifice" refers to the urethra and genitalia which have the function of urination and reproduction. "Posterior orifice" refers to the anus which has the function of excreting the faeces. Although the discharge of urine is a function of the bladder, it also relies on the qi activity of the kidney, as do the reproductive function and the excretion of faeces. Decline or deficiency of kidney qi, therefore, may give rise to frequency of micturition, enuresis, oliguria and anuria; seminal emission, impotence, premature ejaculation and infertility in reproduction; and prolonged diarrhoea with prolapse of rectum or constipation.

II.   THE SIX FU ORGANS

1.   The Gallbladder

The gallbladder is attached to the liver with which it is externally-internally related. Its main function is to store bile and continuously excrete it to the intestines to aid digestion. When the function of the gallbladder is normal, its qi descends. Since the bile is bitter in taste and yellow in colour, upward perversion of gallbladder qi may give rise to a bitter taste in the mouth, vomiting of bitter fluid, and failure to aid the stomach and spleen in digestion, resulting in abdominal distention and loose stools. Since this function of the gallbladder is closely related to the liver's function of maintaining

the free flow of qi, it is said that the liver and gallbladder together have the function of maintaining the free flow of qi. Similarly, the relation of the liver to emotional changes is shared by the gallbladder, and this is often taken into account in the clinic when treating symptoms such as fear and palpitations, insomnia and dream-disturbed sleep.

Although the gallbladder is one of the six fu organs, unlike the other five it stores bile and does not receive water or food. For this reason it is also classified as one of the "extraordinary fu."

2.   The Stomach

The stomach is located in the epigastrium. It connects with the oesophagus above, and with the small intestine below. Its upper outlet is the cardia, called *Shangwan*, and its lower outlet is the pylorus—known as *Xiawan*. Between *Shangwan* and *Xiawan* is *Zhongwan*. These three areas together make up the epigastrium. The Stomach Meridian is connected with the spleen with which it is externally-internally related. Its main function is to receive and decompose food. Food enters the mouth, passes through the oesophagus, and is received by the stomach where it is decomposed and transmitted down to the small intestine. Its essential substances are transported and transformed by the spleen to supply the whole body. The stomach and spleen, therefore, act in conjunction and are the main organs carrying out the functions of digestion and absorption. Together they are known as the "acquired foundation."

When the function of the stomach is normal, its qi descends. If the descending function is disturbed, there will be lack of appetite, distending pain in the epigastrium, nausea and vomiting.

3.   The Small Intestine

The small intestine is located in the abdomen. Its upper end connects with the stomach, and its lower end with the large intestine. The Small Intestine Meridian communicates with the heart with which it is externally-internally related. Its main functions are reception and digestion. It receives and further digests the food from the stomach, separates the clear from the turbid, and absorbs essential substance and part of the water from the food, transmitting the residue of the food to the large intestine, and of the water to the bladder. Since the small intestine has the function of separating the clear from the turbid, dysfunction may not only influence digestion, but also give rise to an abnormal bowel movement and disturbance of urination.

4.   The Large Intestine

The large intestine is located in the abdomen. Its upper end connects with the small intestine via the ileocecum, and its lower end is the anus. The Large Intestine Meridian communicates with the lung with which it is externally-internally related. The main function of the large intestine is to receive the waste material sent down from the small intestine, absorb its fluid content, and form the remainder into faeces to be excreted. Pathological changes of the large intestine will lead to dysfunction in this transportation function, resulting in loose stools or constipation.

5.   The Bladder

The bladder is located in the lower abdomen. Its meridian connects with the kidney with which it is externally-internally related. The main function of the bladder is the temporary storage of urine, which is discharged from the body through qi activity when a sufficient quantity has been accumulated. This function of the bladder is performed with the assistance of the kidney qi. Disease of the bladder will lead to symptoms such as anuria, urgency of micturition and dysuria; failure of the bladder to control urine may lead to frequency of micturition, incontinence of urine and enuresis.

6.   The Sanjiao

The sanjiao is located "separately from the zang-fu organs and inside the body." It is divided into three parts: the upper, middle and lower jiao. Its meridian connects with the pericardium with which it is externally-internally related. Its main functions are to govern various forms of qi, and serve as the passage for the flow of yuanqi and body fluid. Yuanqi originates in the kidney, but requires the sanjiao as its pathway for distribution in order to stimulate and promote the functional activities of the zang-fu organs and tissues of the whole body. The chapter "Sixty-sixth Question" of *Classics on Medical Problems*, therefore, says: "The sanjiao is the ambassador of yuanqi. It circulates the three qi and distributes them to the five zang and six fu organs."

The digestion, absorption, distribution and excretion of food and water are performed by the joint efforts of various zang-fu organs, including the sanjiao. The chapter "The Thirty-first Question" in the book of *Classics on Medical Problems* says: "The sanjiao is the passage of water and food."

It is also mentioned in the eighth chapter of *Plain Questions*: "The sanjiao is the irrigation official who builds waterways."

The upper, middle and lower jiao combine with their related zang-fu organs, and each functions differently in order to carry out the digestion, absorption, distribution and excretion of water and food. The upper jiao dominates dispersion and distribution. In other words, in combination with the distributing function of the heart and lung, the upper jiao distributes the essential qi of water and food to the whole body in order to warm and nourish the skin and muscles, tendons and bones, and regulate the skin and pores. This function is described in the eighteenth chapter of *Miraculous Pivot:* "The upper jiao is like a fog."

Here "fog" is used to describe the all-pervading vapour-like state of the clear and light essential qi of water and food.

The middle jiao dominates digestion of water and food. It refers to the functions of the spleen and stomach in digesting food, absorbing essential substance, evaporating body fluid, and transforming nutrient substance into nutrient blood. This function is described in the same chapter: "The middle jiao looks like a froth of bubbles."

"A froth of bubbles" here refers to the appearance of the decomposed state of digested food.

The lower jiao dominates the separation of the clear from the turbid and the discharge of fluid and wastes from the body. This process mainly involves the urinary function of the kidney and bladder, and the defaecation function of the large intestine. The same chapter states: "The lower jiao looks like a drainage ditch."

In other words, the turbid water continuously flows downward to be discharged. If the water passage in the lower jiao is obstructed, there may be urinary retention, dysuria and oedema.

Clinically, the terms upper, middle and lower jiao are often applied to generalise the functions of the internal organs of the chest and abdominal cavity. Above the diaphragm is the upper jiao which includes the heart and lung; between the diaphragm and umbilicus is the middle jiao which includes the spleen and stomach; and below the umbilicus is the lower jiao which includes the kidney, intestines and bladder.

III.   THE EXTRAORDINARY FU ORGANS

The extraordinary fu organs comprise the brain, marrow, bones, vessels, gallbladder and uterus. Since they are different from the five zang and six fu organs, they are called the "extraordinary fu." The bones, marrow, vessles and gallbladder have been discussed in the section on the zang-fu organs, so only the brain and uterus will be considered here.

1.   The Brain

The brain is located in the skull and connects with the spinal marrow. The thirty-third chapter of *Miraculous Pivot* says: "The brain is a sea of marrow. Its upper part lies beneath the scalp at the vertex at point

Baihui (Du 20) and its lower part at point Fengfu (Du 16)."

Baihui and Fengfu are Points of the Du (Governor Vessel) Meridian which ascends the spinal column and enters the brain at point Fengfu. Many points of the Du Meridian, therefore, are indicated in pathological conditions of the brain.

The brain is the organ of spirit, consciousness and thinking. The seventeenth chapter of *Plain Questions* says: "The head is the residence of intelligence."

This means that the brain is related to the activity of thinking. The thirty-third chapter of *Miraculous Pivot* says: "Deficiency of the brain leads to vertigo and dizziness."

It pointed out that hypofunction of the brain may lead to vertigo and blurred vision. Li Shizhen of the Ming Dynasty (1368-1644) clearly indicated that "the brain is the palace of the mind." In the Qing Dynasty (1644-1911), Wang Qingren in his book *Revision of Medical Classics* advanced the theory that "intelligence and memory rely on the brain." He considered that thinking, memory, vision, hearing, smelling and speaking are all dominated by the brain.

Although the ancients had some knowledge of the physiology and pathology of the brain, they ascribed the functions of the brain to various zang-fu organs — the heart, liver and kidney in particular. Many syndromes and treatment of brain disturbances, therefore, are included in the differentiation of syndromes of the zang-fu organs.

2. The Uterus

The uterus, located in the lower abdomen, presides over menstruation and nourishes the foetus. It is closely related to the Kidney,

Chong and Ren (Conception Vessel) meridians. Since the uterus is related to the kidney, its reproductive function is dominated by the kidney qi. Both the Chong and Ren meridians originate from the uterus, the Ren Meridian having the function of regulating the qi of all the yin meridians, and the Chong Meridian the function of regulating the qi and blood of all the twelve regular meridians. When the kidney qi is vigorous and the qi and blood of the Chong and Ren meridians sufficient, menstruation is normal, and the uterus will perform its functions of reproduction and nourishment of the foetus. If the kidney qi is weak, the qi and blood of the Chong and Ren meridians will be deficient, and there will be irregular menstruation, amenorrhoea or infertility. The uterus is also closely connected to the heart, liver and spleen. Since normal menstruation and the nourishment of the foetus rely on the blood, which is dominated by the heart, stored by the liver and controlled by the spleen, dysfunction of these organs may affect the normal function of the uterus.

IV. THE RELATIONSHIPS AMONG THE ZANG-FU ORGANS

Although the zang and fu organs have different physiological functions, there is a very close relationship between them in maintaining the normal functions of the body. An understanding of the theory of the relationships between the zang and fu organs is of great significance in clinical differentation of syndromes and treatment. Interconnected by the meridian system, the zang and fu organs have an internally-externally linked relationship. For example, the meridian of Hand-Taiyin enters the large intestine inferiorly, and goes upward through the diaphragm to connect with the lung. The meridian of Hand-Yangming enters the lung and descends to connect with the large intestine. In this way a close internal relationship between the lung and large intestine is maintained. The heart and small intestine, spleen and stomach, liver and gallbladder and kidney and bladder are similarly closely related, physiologically and pathologically, by means of the yin and yang meridians. The sixty-second chapter of *Plain Questions* therefore says: "The zang organs are all connected with the meridians for the transmission of qi and blood."

From this it can be seen that the functional activities, and internal-external relationships of the zang-fu organs, are based on the meridians system. Without the interconnecting pathways of the meridians, each of the zang-fu organs would become an isolated and static organ, unable to perform its functional activities. This interconnecting function of the meridians is reflected not only by the internal-external connection between the zang and the fu organs, but also by relationships within the zang and the fu organs themselves, thus forming an internal criss-crossing network. For example, the Liver Meridian of Foot-Jueyin has a branch which, "arising from the liver, passes through the diaphragm and flows into the lung," further connecting with the Lung Meridian of Hand-Taiyin and thus forming a connection between the lung and the liver. A branch of the Spleen Meridian of Foot-Taiyin "arises from the stomach, passes through the diaphragm and flows into the heart," where it connects with the Heart Meridian of Hand-Shaoyin, thus forming a connection between the spleen and heart.

There are similar connections between the kidney, heart and lung; stomach, large intestine and small intestine; and between liver and stomach, etc. by means of the meridians and collaterals.

The mutual interconnections between the meridians, zang and fu organs mean that when a particular meridian is diseased due to invasion of pathogenic factors, there may be a transmission of pathological changes to other meridians, and related zang-fu organs, particularly externally-internally related ones. For instance, when the Lung Meridian is invaded by pathogenic factors, it may affect the large intestine, leading to constipation and diarrhoea. When dysfunction of the spleen in transportation and transformation occurs, it may affect the stomach and kidney, giving rise to poor appetite, fullness and distention in the epigastrium, and oedema. In general, only by having a clear understanding of the connections between the meridians by which pathological changes are transmitted, can the practitioner grasp the relationships among the zang-fu organs and determine treatment.

The following is a brief introduction to the relationships between the zang organs, between the zang and fu organs, and between the fu organs.

1. The Relationships Between The Zang Organs

1) **The heart and lung** The heart dominates blood and the lung dominates qi. The circulation of blood relies on the propelling function of qi, and at the same time the qi is attached to the blood to

distribute it through the body. Both the heart and the lung, qi and blood, rely upon each other. Without qi, the blood will stagnate, leading to stagnation of blood; without blood, the qi will have no base to rely upon and will scatter.

Pathologically, deficiency of pectoral qi due to weakness of the lung qi will lead to weakness and stagnation of blood circulation, resulting in stuffiness in the chest, shortness of breath, palpitation, and purplish lips and tongue. Conversely, retardation of blood circulation due to deficiency of heart qi or weakness of heart yang, may impair the function of the lung in dispersing and descending, giving rise to cough, shortness of breath, stuffiness in the chest and a sensation of suffocation.

Both the heart and lung are situated in the upper jiao. During the development of febrile diseases, the pathogenic factors in the lung may not be transmitted to the middle jiao by the normal pathway, but invade the heart directly. This is known as "invasion of the pericardium by pathogenic factors through contrary pathway," showing the mutual connection between heart and lung in pathology.

2) The heart and spleen The heart dominates blood and the spleen controls blood. The function of the spleen in transportation and transformation depends on the propelling force of the yangqi of the heart and kidney. The formation and flourishing of heart blood rely upon the function of the spleen in transporting and transforming the essential substances of food and water. The blood circulating in the vessels therefore, is dominated by the heart and controlled by the spleen.

Pathologically the heart and spleen often affect each other. For example, deficiency of the source of blood due to deficiency of spleen qi, or haemorrhage due to dysfunction of the spleen in controlling blood, may result in consumption of heart blood. Conversely overthinking, which consumes heart blood, may affect the normal function of the spleen in transportation and transformation. Both conditions may give rise to palpitations, insomnia, poor appetite, lassitude and pale complexion, known as "deficiency of both heart and spleen."

3) The heart and liver The heart and liver have a close relationship, not only with regard to emotional activities, but also to blood circulation. The heart dominates blood and the liver stores it. Only when the heart blood is sufficient, can the liver store and regulate its volume in order to meet the physiological needs of the body. The liver maintains the free flow of qi and "dredges" the circulation of qi and blood, ensuring that the blood does not stagnate. This benefits the function of the heart in propelling blood.

Pathologically, the heart and liver influence each other. For instance, deficiency of heart blood often leads to deficiency of liver blood, resulting in palpitations insomnia, dream-disturbed sleep and pale complexion, accompanied by dizziness, blurred and impaired vision, oligomenorrhoea or delayed menstruation. Hyperactivity of liver yang may disturb the heart giving rise to headache, redness of the eyes, and irritability, accompanied by mental restlessness, insomnia and dream-disturbed sleep.

4) The heart and kidney The heart dominates fire, is located in the upper part of the body and belongs to yang. The kidney dominates water, is situated in the lower part of the body and belongs to yin. The relationship between the heart and kidney, therefore, concerns the balance between yin and yang, ascending and descending. Under normal physiological conditions, heart yang descends, together with the kidney yang, to warm kidney yin and kidney water. In contrast, kidney yin ascends, together with heart yin, to moisten heart yang and prevent it from becoming hyperactive. This relationship of mutual communication and restriction is called "harmony of heart and kidney." When water and fire are in harmony, a relative balance between above and below, yin and yang, is maintained, ensuring the normal physiological function of the heart and kidney.

Once the yin-yang balance between the heart and kidney is disrupted, pathological changes will occur. For instance, when deficiency of kidney yin fails to ascend to nourish the heart, it usually leads to hyperactivity of heart yang, giving rise to such manifestations as aching back and seminal emission, with mental restlessness, palpitations, insomnia and dream-disturbed sleep, indicating "disharmony between heart and kidney." When deficiency of kidney yang fails to evaporate fluid which then floods and ascends to depress the function of heart yang, there may be clinical manifestations such as edema, chills, and cold limbs, accompanied by palpitations, shortness of breath and stuffiness in the chest, indicating "retained water afflicting the heart."

The heart dominates blood and the kidney stores essence. Since essence and blood promote each other, there is a mutual causality between consumption of kidney essence and deficiency of heart blood. The heart houses the mind and the kidney essence produces marrow which communicates with the brain — the seat of intelligence. Either deficiency of kidney essence or of heart blood, therefore, may lead to symptoms of disturbance of

consciousness such as insomnia, poor memory and dream-disturbed sleep.

5) The spleen and lung The relationship between the spleen and lung is closely connected with qi and body fluid. The spleen dominates transportation and transformation and is considered to be the source of acquired qi and blood. The strength of the lung qi relies on a continuous supply of the acquired essence of water and food. The condition of the lung qi, therefore, depends greatly on the tonifying action of spleen qi. On the other hand, the function of the spleen in transporting and transforming water fluid also relies on the coordination of the dispersing and descending function of the lung. The twenty-first chapter of *Plain Questions* says: "The spleen spreads the qi for flowing upward to the lung, which regulates the water passages in order to transmit the water fluid down to the bladder."

It pointed out the internal physiological connection between the spleen and the lung. Pathologically, weakness of spleen qi usually leads to deficiency of lung qi, resulting in poor appetite, abdominal distention and emaciation, accompanied by feeble cough, lassitude and dislike of speaking. Dysfunction of the lung in dispersing and descending may lead to accumulation of body fluid and stasis of dampness in the spleen, resulting in cough with much expectoration and stuffiness in the chest, or abdominal distention, borborygmus and oedema.

6) The liver and lung This relationship is mainly manifested in the ascending and descending movement of qi. The lung qi normally descends and the liver qi normally ascends, in order to maintain the harmonious function of the vital activities of the body. If the liver qi is depressed, it may transform into fire which goes upward along the meridian to consume the fluid of the lung, giving rise to such manifestations as hypochondriac pain, irritability, cough and haemoptysis, known as "invasion of the lung by liver fire." Conversely, dysfunction of the lung in descending may lead to pathogenic dryness and heat which descend to consume the yin of the kidney and liver, stirring up hyperactivity of liver yang. In this case, in addition to cough, there may be referred pain in the chest and hypochondriac region, dizziness, headache and redness of the face and eyes.

7) The lung and kidney This association is mainly reflected in the movement of water and qi. Water metabolism is closely related to the functions of the lung and kidney. Dysfunction of the lung in dispersing and descending, or dysfunction of the kidney in evaporating water, may not only affect normal water metabolism, but also influence each other, leading to further and more serious disturbance of water metabolism, and giving rise to such manifestations as cough, shortness of breath, difficulty in lying flat and oedema. In the sixty-first chapter of *Plain Questions* it said, "Therefore when water disease attacks, it will cause oedema in the foot and enlarged abdomen in the lower part of the body, and asthma, with inability to lie flat, in the upper part of the body, due to simultaneous occurrence of both the primary and secondary conditions."

The lung dominates respiration and the kidney dominates reception of qi. Only when the kidney is vigorous can the inhaled qi be sent downward through the lung and be received by the kidney. When kidney qi is deficient, and fails to receive qi, the qi will remain floating above. When prolonged deficiency of lung qi affects the kidney qi, there will be dysfunction of the kidney in reception of qi. Both of these conditions may give rise to shortness of breath which is worse after movement.

The yin fluid of the lung and the kidney nourish each other, and kidney yin is the root of the yin fluid of the whole body. Deficiency of lung yin may injure kidney yin, and deficiency of kidney yin may fail to nourish lung yin. Either may lead to deficiency of yin of both the lung and kidney, resulting in such manifestations as malar flush, afternoon fever, night sweat, dry cough, hoarse voice and weakness and soreness of the lumbar region and knees.

8) The liver and spleen This relationship is mainly reflected in the digestion of water and food, and the circulation of blood.

The spleen dominates transportation and transformation, and the liver maintains the free flow of qi. When the liver performs this function normally, the ascending function of the spleen and the descending function of the stomach will be coordinated to ensure normal digestion, absorption and distribution of food. In addition, if the essential substance of water and food transported and transformed by the spleen is sufficient, liver blood will flourish, as it has a rich source for its production. The liver stores blood and the spleen controls blood. They coordinate their activities to maintain the normal circulation of blood to satisfy the needs of the body.

Pathologically, stagnation of liver qi may affect the spleen's function of transportation and transformation, resulting in hypochondriac pain, mental depression and irritability, accompanied by poor appetite, abdominal fullness and distention, irregular bowel movement and lassitude, known as "stagnation of liver qi leading to deficiency of the spleen," or "disharmony of liver and spleen."

If the spleen qi is weak, it may fail to control blood or lead to dysfunction in transportation and transformation, which causes deficiency of the source of blood. Great loss or insufficiency of blood may lead to deficiency of liver blood, giving rise to poor appetite, emaciation, blurred vision, and oligomenorrhoea or amenorrhoea.

9) The spleen and kidney This connection is mainly reflected in the relationship between congenital and acquired qi. The spleen is considered to be the acquired foundation, and the kidney the congenital foundation. Kidney essence relies on the supply of essential substances of water and food, transported and transformed by the spleen. The spleen's transportation and transformation function in turn relies on the warming and propelling activities of kidney yang. Thus the congenital promotes the acquired, and the acquired nourishes the congenital.

Pathologically, the spleen and kidney influence each other. When kidney yang is deficient, it will fail to warm spleen yang, leading to deficiency of spleen yang. When spleen yang is deficient, it will lead to preponderance of yin and cold in the interior, which may impair kidney yang and cause deficiency if prolonged. Clinically the symptoms may include abdominal fullness, borborygmus, loose stools, soreness and pain of the lumbar region and knees, aversion to cold and cold limbs, known as "deficiency of yang of both spleen and kidney."

10) The liver and kidney The liver stores blood and the kidney stores essence. Liver blood relies on nourishment by kidney essence, and the kidney essence relies on the supply of liver blood. Essence and blood produce and supply each other, hence the saying "essence and blood have the same source," and "the liver and kidney have the same origin."

Pathologically, when deficiency of kidney essence deprives the liver of nourishment, it will lead to deficiency of liver yin, resulting in "deficiency of yin of both liver and kidney." Clinical manifestations may include soreness and weakness of the lumbar region and back, seminal emission, tinnitus, dizziness, vertigo and dryness of the eyes.

If there is hyperactivity of liver yang, there may be headache, redness of the eyes, and irritability. In prolonged cases, if kidney yin is also consumed, there may be soreness and pain of the lumbar region, seminal emission and tinnitus.

2.   The Relationship Between the Zang and the Fu Organs

This refers to the external-internal relationship between the zang and the fu. The zang are yin and the fu yang. Yang dominates the exterior and yin the interior. Via the channels, each zang is externally-internally related to one fu, as follows:

1) The heart and small intestine Pathologically, fire of excess type of the heart channel may transmit pathogenic heat to the small intestine, resulting in oliguria, deep yellow urine and burning sensation during urination, known as "excessive heat in the small-intestine." Conversely, heat in the small intestine may ascend along the channel to affect the heart, leading to symptoms of mental restlessness, redness and ulceration of the tongue, etc.

2) The liver and gallbladder The gallbladder is attached to the liver, and they are externally-internally related through the channels. Bile derives from the liver. Clinically the differentiation of syndromes of the liver and gallbladder cannot completely be separated, and manifestations of both often appear simultaneously. For instance, both excessive liver fire and excessive gallbladder fire may present symptoms of pain in the chest and hypochondrium, bitter taste in the mouth, dryness in the throat, and irritability. In case of damp-heat in the liver and gallbladder, there may be jaundice and bitter taste in the mouth which indicates the extravasation of bile, and hypochondriac pain and mental depression which indicate stagnation of liver qi.

3) The spleen and stomach Both the spleen and stomach are situated in the middle jiao, and are externally-internally related via their channels. The spleen dominates transportation and transformation, and the stomach dominates reception. Reception and digestion of food mainly rely on the stomach, and the absorption and distribution of nutrient substance rely on the spleen. The stomach prepares the food for the spleen to transport and transform, whilst the spleen distributes nutrient substance to assist the stomach in moving body fluid. Dysfunction of the stomach in reception may give rise to poor appetite and an unpleasant and hungry sensation in the stomach. Dysfunction of the spleen in transportation and transformation may often lead to abdominal distension after eating and loose stools.

The spleen dominates ascending and the stomach dominates descending. The spleen distributes the essential substance of water and food up to the heart and lung. The stomach moves the digested water and food downwards. If the spleen qi descends rather than ascends, there may be diarrhoea and prolapse of the rectum. If the stomach qi ascends rather than descends, there may

be nausea, vomiting and hiccups. The physician Ye Tianshi of the Qing Dynasty (1644-1911) said: "The stomach dominates reception, and the spleen dominates transportation and transformation. The spleen is 'favourable' when its ascending function is normal, and the stomach is 'favourable' when its descending function is normal."

The spleen is yin, prefers dryness and dislikes dampness. The stomach is yang, prefers moistness and dislikes dryness. Being yin and yang in nature respectively, each needs the other. When pathogenic dampness invades the spleen, it may injure the transportation and transformation function, and in turn, lead to the production of dampness. When pathogenic heat invades the stomach, it may consume the body fluid in the stomach, and deficiency of stomach yin may stir up heat of deficiency type in the interior. Since the spleen and stomach are mutually connected physiologically, they also affect each other pathologically. For instance, dysfunction of the spleen in transportation and transformation due to retention of dampness may lead to inability to ascend the clear, and affect the stomach function of receiving and descending. Clinical manifestations include poor appetite, nausea, vomiting, and fullness and distension of the epigastrium. Conversely, dysfunction of the stomach in descending the turbid, due to irregular food intake which causes retention of food, may also affect the function of the spleen in transporting, transforming and ascending the clear, giving rise to abdominal distension and diarrhoea.

4) The lung and large intestine When the lung qi descends, the function of the large intestine in transmission is normal and bowel movement free. If the large intestine is obstructed by stasis, it may prevent the lung qi from descending. Clinically, when dysfunction of the lung in descending fails to send down body fluid, there may be difficult bowel movement. If the large intestine is obstructed due to excessive heat, it may lead to dysfunction of the lung qi, resulting in cough and fullness in the chest.

5) The kidney and bladder   The function of the bladder relies on the condition of the kidney qi. Kidney qi assists the bladder in metabolizing body fluid. When the kidney qi is sufficient and its checking function normal, the bladder opens and closes regularly so as to maintain normal water metabolism. When the kidney qi is deficient, disturbance of checking function will lead to irregular opening and closing of the bladder, resulting in dysuria, incontinence of urine, enuresis, and frequency of micturition. Pathological changes in the storage and discharge of urine, therefore, are often related to both the bladder and kidney.

3.   The Relationship Among the Fu Organs

The main function of the six fu organs is transportation and transformation. They play a major role in a series of functional activities of digestion, absorption and excretion. When food enters the stomach, it is digested and sent down to the small intestine for further digestion — separating the clear from the turbid. The clear is the nutrient substance nourishing the whole body, of which the water-fluid part seeps into the bladder. The turbid is the waste matter entering the large intestine. The fluid seeped into the bladder is excreted as urine by the action of qi, and the waste matter in the large intestine is discharged as faeces through the transportation and transformation function.

This process of digestion, absorption and excretion mainly relies on: a) the function of the liver and gallbladder in maintaining the free movement of the digestion, b) the function of the sanjiao in distributing yuanqi and circulating water fluid, and c) the unified functions of the six fu, which transport and transform water and food and continuously receive, digest, transmit and excrete, alternating between emptiness and fullness. They are "favourable" when they are clear and open, and "unfavourable" when they are obstructed. This is stressed in the ancient sayings: "the fu organs are favourable when they are unblocked," and "treatment to remove obstruction in diseases of them plays the same role as the reinforcing method."

The close physiological connections between the six fu organs are also reflected pathologically. For instance, excessive heat in the stomach may consume body fluid, lead to dysfunction of the large intestine in transportation, and result in constipation. Constipation due to dryness in the intestines may affect the stomach's descending function, leading to upward rebellion of stomach qi and hence nausea and vomiting. Hyperactivity of fire in the gallbladder may invade the stomach, giving rise to upward rebellion of stomach qi and hence nausea, vomiting and regurgitation of yellow fluid.

Chapter 4

QI, BLOOD AND BODY FLUID

Qi, blood and body fluid are fundamental substances which maintain the normal vital activities of the human body. They are the material foundation for the physiological functions of the zang-fu organs, tissues and meridians. Qi, blood and body fluid have an independent relationship with the zang-fu organs, the tissues, and the meridians, whilst both theories together combine to explain the physiological functions of human body.

I. QI

According to ancient Chinese thought, qi was the fundamental substance constituting the universe, and all phenomena were produced by the changes and movement of qi. This viewpoint greatly influenced the theory of traditional Chinese medicine. Generally speaking, the word "qi" in traditional Chinese medicine denotes both the essential substances of the human body which maintain its vital activities, and the functional activities of the zang-fu organs and tissues.

Essential substances are the foundation of functional activities. In this sense, qi is too rarefied to be seen and its existence is manifested in the functions of the zang-fu organs. All vital activities of the human body are explained by changes and movement of qi.

1. Classification and Production of Qi

Certain qualitative terms differentiate qi in the human body according to its source, function and distribution. These terms are: yuanqi (primary qi), zongqi (pectoral qi), yingqi (nutrient qi) and weiqi (defensive qi). In terms of their source they may be further classified into congenital qi and acquired qi. Yuanqi, which is derived from congenital essence and inherited from the parents, is referred to as congenital qi. After birth, zongqi, yingqi and weiqi are all derived from food essence, and are therefore known as acquired qi.

Congenital qi and acquired qi are dependent on each other for their production and nourishment. Yuanqi stimulates and promotes the functional activities of the zang-fu organs and the associated tissues of the body, which in turn produce acquired qi. Thus yuanqi is the material foundation for the production of acquired qi. On the other hand, acquired qi continuously nourishes and supplements congenital qi. The relationship is therefore an interdependent one: congenital qi promotes acquired qi, which in turn

46

nourishes congenital qi.

Qi may also describe the functional activities of the zang-fu organs and meridians. It is then referred to, for example, as qi of the heart, liver, lung, spleen, stomach, kidney and meridians. These are discussed further in the relevant chapters.

1)Yuanqi (primary qi) Derived from congenital essence, yuanqi needs to be supplemented and nourished by the qi obtained after birth from food essence. Yuanqi takes root in the kidney and spreads to the entire body via the sanjiao. It stimulates and promotes the functional activities of the zang-fu organs and the associated tissues. The more abundant yuanqi is, the more vigorously the zang-fu organs and the associated tissues will function. The human body will then be healthy and rarely suffer from disease. On the other hand, congenital insufficiency of yuanqi, or deficiency due to a prolonged illness, may lead to various pathological changes.

2) Zongqi (pectoral qi) Zongqi is formed by the combination of qingqi (clean qi) which is inhaled by the lung, and the qi of food essence which is produced by the spleen and stomach. Zongqi is stored in the chest. Its main functions are:

i) To promote the lung's function of controlling respiration. The strength or weakness of speech and respiration are related to the quality of zongqi.

ii) To promote the heart's function of dominating the blood and blood vessels. The circulation of qi and blood, coldness and warmth, and the motor ability of the four limbs and trunk are all associated with zongqi.

3) Yingqi (nutrient qi) Derived from the qi of food essence produced by the spleen and stomach, yingqi circulates in the vessels.

Its primary function is both to produce blood and to circulate with it, providing further nourishment. As yingqi and blood are so closely related, "ying blood" is the term commonly used to refer to their joint functions.

4) Weiqi (defensive qi) Weiqi is also derived from the qi of food essence, but unlike yingqi it circulates outside the vessels. It functions to protect the muscular surface, defend the body against exogenous pathogenic factors, control the opening and closing of the pores, moisten the skin and hair, readjust body temperature, and warm up the zang-fu organs. Defending the body against exogenous pathogenic factors is its principal function, hence the name weiqi.

As mentioned above, the zang-fu and meridians possess their own qi. Originating from yuanqi, zongqi, yingqi and weiqi, the qi of the meridians (which circulates throughout the meridian system) is a combination of the qi of food essence, qingqi inhaled by the lung, and essential qi stored in the kidney. The qi of the meridians, therefore, is referred to as zhengqi or zhenqi (vital qi) flowing in the meridians. According to twenty-seventh chapter of *Plain Questions,* "Zhengqi (vital qi) means the qi of the meridians." As the basis of the functions of the meridians, the qi of the meridians greatly influences the functions of the qi, blood and zang-fu organs of the entire body.

2.   Functions of Qi

Qi acts extensively in the human body by permeating all parts. There is no place that does not have qi nor to which qi does not penetrate. If the movement of qi ceases, the vital activities of the human body will also cease. Abundant qi is the basis of good health and weakness of qi may lead to disease. Hence the statement from the Eighth Problem of *Classic on Medical Problems,* "Qi is the root of the human body; the stem and leaves would dry up without a root." Qi, distributed to various parts of the body, characteristically functions in the following different ways:

1) Promoting function The growth and development of the human body, the physiological activities of the zang-fu and meridians, the circulation of blood and distribution of body fluid, are all dependent on the promoting and stimulating effect of qi. Deficiency of qi impairs this promoting function, and thus produces pathological changes such as retarded growth and development, hypofunction of the zang-fu organs and meridians, impaired blood circulation, dysfunction in transforming and distributing body fluid, and production of phlegm dampness in the interior.

2) Warming function The normal temperature of the body is maintained and readjusted by qi. According to the Twenty-second Problem of *Classic on Medical Problems,* "Qi dominates warming." The forty-seventh chapter of *Miraculous Pivot* says: "Weiqi warms up the muscles..." Insufficiency of yang qi may impair its warming effect, giving rise to aversion to cold, and cold sensations of the four limbs.

3) Defensive function Qi defends the body surface against exogenous pathogenic factors. The seventy-second chapter of *Plain Questions* therefore states: "The existence of the antipathogenic qi in the interior prevents the pathogenic factor from invading." Qi also combats pathogenic factors once disease occurs, and brings about recovery by eliminating the invading pathogenic factors.

4) Checking function Qi checks, controls and regulates certain bodily substances and metabolic products. For instance, qi controls blood by keeping it circulating in the vessels, and checks sweating, urination and seminal emission. If this checking function of qi is impaired, spontaneous sweating, incontinence of urine, premature ejaculation and spermatorrhoea may occur.

5) Qihua (activities of qi) Qihua has two meanings. Firstly it refers to the process of mutual transformation among essence, qi, body fluid and blood. According to the fifth chapter of *Plain Questions,* "Essence is transformed into qi." In his annotation of the same chapter, Wang Bing, a physician in the Tang Dynasty says: "The activities of qi produce essence; a harmonious supply of food essence enables the body to grow." These statements explain the mutual transformation of essence and qi.

Secondly, qihua implies certain functional activities of the zang-fu organs. According to the eighth chapter of *Plain Questions,* "The bladder stores body fluid, which is then excreted by the activities of qi." The activities of qi here refer to the function of the bladder in discharging urine.

6) Nourishing function This refers to yingqi—the nutrient substance formed from food. Yingqi, which circulates in the blood vessels, is a part of blood and provides nourishment to the whole body.

Although these six functions of qi are different, they cooperate with and supplement each other.

II. BLOOD

Blood is a red liquid circulating in the vessels, and is a vital nutrient substance in the body.

1.   Formation and Circulation of Blood

As the fundamental substances required in blood formation originate from food essence produced by the spleen and stomach, these two organs are regarded as the source of qi and blood. The thirtieth chapter of *Miraculous Pivot* holds: "When the middle jiao receives food essence it will transform it into red fluid which is called blood."

The seventy-first chapter of the same book also says: "Yingqi flows into the vessels to be transformed into blood." Essence and blood may also transform into each other. The book *Zhang's General Medicine* states: "If blood is not consumed, it turns into essence in the kidney; if essence does not leak out, it is transformed into blood in the liver." Taking food essence and kidney essence as the material basis, blood is formed by the functional activities of zang-fu organs such as the spleen, stomach, heart, lung, liver and kidney.

After being formed, blood normally circulates in the vessels throughout the body, and is acted upon jointly by the heart, liver and spleen. The heart dominates the blood and vessels, and the propelling force of heart qi is the basis of blood circulation. The spleen qi controls blood and prevents extravasation. The liver promotes the free flow of qi, stores blood and regulates its volume. The coordination of these three organs ensures continuous blood circulation in the vessels throughout the body. Dysfunction of any of them may cause abnormal blood circulation. Deficiency of heart qi, for instance, may lead to stagnation of heart blood. Dysfunction of the spleen in controlling blood may lead to bloody stools, uterine or subcutaneous bleeding, and ecchymoses.

2.   Functions of Blood

Blood circulates throughout the body, passing through the five zang and six fu in the interior, and the skin, muscles, tendons and bones on the exterior. In this way blood nourishes and moistens the various tissues and organs of the body. The Twenty-second Problem of *Classic on Medical Problems* generalises this function of blood, saying: "Blood dominates nourishment and moisture." The nourishing and moistening function of blood manifests clearly in the movement of the eye and four limbs. According to the tenth chapter of *Plain Questions*, "When the liver receives blood, it gives rise to vision; when the feet receive blood they are capable of walking; when the palms receive blood they are capable of holding; and when the fingers receive blood they are capable of grasping."

The forty-seventh chapter of *Miraculous Pivot* says: "When the blood is in harmony... the tendons and bones will be strong and the joints will function smoothly." Insufficiency of blood may impair its nourishing and moistening function, and give rise to symptoms such as impaired vision, dryness of the eyes, motor impairment of the joints, numbness of the four limbs and dryness and itchiness of the skin.

Blood is the material foundation for mental activities. A sufficient blood supply ensures clear consciousness and a vigorous spirit. The twenty-sixth chapter of *Plain Questions* states: "Qi and blood are the foundation for human mental activities." The thirty-second chapter of *Miraculous Pivot* says: "Harmonious circulation of blood ensures a vigorous spirit." These quotations explain the close relationship between blood and mental activities. Deficiency of blood, therefore, may produce mental disorders. An example is deficiency of heart or liver blood which may result in mental restlessness, with symptoms such as palpitation, insomnia and dream-disturbed sleep.

III. BODY FLUID

Body fluid is a collective term for all the normal fluids of the body. These are saliva, gastric juice, intestinal juice and the liquids in the joint cavities, as well as tears, nasal discharge, sweat and urine.

1. Formation and Distribution of Body Fluid

Body fluid is formed from food and drink after its digestion and absorption by the spleen and stomach. The distribution and excretion of body fluid principally rely on the spleen's function of transportation, the lung's function of dispersing and descending and regulating water passages, and the kidney's function of controlling urination and separating the clear and the turbid. Of these three organs, the kidney is the most important. The twenty-first chapter of *Plain Questions* explains the formation and distribution of body fluid by saying: "After food enters the stomach, the qi of food essence and water is transmitted to the spleen, which spreads it to the lung. The lung regulates the water passages and transmits the qi of water to the bladder below. The qi of water then spreads in four directions and travels along the meridians of the five zang

organs." When talking about the sanjiao as the pathway of body fluid, the eighth chapter of *Plain Questions* states: "The sanjiao is the irrigation official who builds waterways."

In addition, fluids sent downwards from the stomach continue to be absorbed by the small and large intestines. A part of the fluid, after passing through the spleen, lung and sanjiao, is excreted from the skin and hair as sweat. Another part of the fluid is sent downwards to the bladder via the waterways of the sanjiao, and excreted from the body as urine, with the assistance of the qi of the kidney and bladder. Acted upon by all these zang-fu, body fluid reaches the skin and hair on the exterior, and penetrates the zang-fu in the interior, thus nourishing all the tissues and organs throughout the body.

To conclude, the formation, distribution and excretion of body fluid is a complicated process resulting from the coordinated activities of many of the zang-fu, especially the lung, spleen and kidney. Pathological changes of these organs may consequently affect the formation, distribution and excretion of body fluid. For example, if there is insufficient formation or excessive loss, body fluid may be damaged or consumed. A disturbance in distribution of body fluid may lead to its accumulation, resulting in retained fluid and oedema, or the formation of phlegm. Pathological changes of body fluid may, in turn, impair the functions of many zang-fu organs, for example invasion of the heart by retained water produces palpitations; retention of fluid in the lung results in cough with asthmatic breathing; dryness of the lung due to consumption of body fluid leads to unproductive cough; dryness of the stomach causes thirst; and dryness of the intestines leads to constipation.

2.   Functions of Body Fluid (Jingye)

Body fluid moistens and nourishes various parts of the body. There are noticeable differences, however, in the nature, form and location of different types of body fluid. Clear and thin fluids are referred to as "jing," whilst thick and heavy fluids are known as "ye." "Jing" is distributed on the muscular surface, and has the function of warming and nourishing the muscles and moistening the skin. "Ye" is stored in the joints and orifices and has the function of moistening the joints, strengthening the brain and marrow and nourishing the orifices. As both "jing" and "ye" are normal fluids in the body and are derived from the same source—the qi of food essence—they may be transformed into each other. Generally they are referred to together by the term "jingye" (body fluid).

IV.   THE RELATIONSHIP BETWEEN QI, BLOOD AND BODY FLUID

Although qi, blood and body fluid have their respective natures, they coordinate with, promote and restrain one another in their functional activities. Their close and complicated relationships often manifest in physiology and pathology, and are important in determining treatment on the basis of differentiation of syndromes.

1.   The Relationship Between Qi and Blood

Both qi and blood are the material foundation for the functional activities of the body. They originate from food essence and from essential qi in the kidney, and their production depends on the functional activities of the lung, spleen and kidney. Qi mainly provides warmth and motive force, whilst blood provides nourishment and moisture. This is described in the Twenty-second Problem of *Classic on Medical Problems*, "Qi dominates warmth while blood dominates nourishment." Qi is considered to be yang, while blood is yin. Their relationship may be summarized by the statement: "Qi is the commander of blood and blood is the mother of qi." "Qi is the commander of blood" means that blood cannot be separated from qi in its formation and circulation. The material basis of blood is yin essence, the transformation of which into blood depends on qi. Qi functions well in transforming yin essence into blood if it is abundant. Conversely, this function of qi is weakened if qi is dificient, so deficiency of qi may lead to deficiency of blood. For this reason, when treating disorders resulting from blood deficiency, qi tonics are sometimes added to the prescription. Since the heart qi dominates blood circulation, the lung qi ensures normal distribution and the liver qi takes charge of the free flow of qi of the entire body, the blood circulation depends on the functional activities of these three organs. This is described as "qi circulation leading to blood circulation." Either weakness in propelling blood due to qi deficiency, or retardation of qi circulation, may cause disorders of blood circulation, or even stagnation of blood. That is why in order to obtain good therapeutic effects in the treatment of blood stagnation, herbs which circulate qi, and qi tonics, are often prescribed in combination with herbs to activate blood circulation and remove stasis. The controlling function of qi ensures the normal circulation of blood in the vessels and prevents extravasation. Deficiency of qi may impair this function of controlling blood, leading to various types of haemorrhage. This is known as "qi fails to control blood." To stop haemorrhage due to qi deficiency, the method of tonifying qi must be used.

"Blood is the mother of qi" refers to the fact that qi is "attached" to blood, and that qi does not function well in promoting the physiological activities of various parts of the body unless it receives sufficient nourishment from blood. In cases of massive bleeding, there will also be loss of qi, which is known as "qi follows blood in becoming exhausted."

2. The Relationship Between Qi and Body Fluid

Qi differs from body fluid in nature, form and functional activities. There are similarities between them, however, in their formation, circulation and distribution. Both originate from food essence and circulate throughout the body.

The formation, distribution and excretion of body fluid depend upon qi circulation, and cannot be separated from the activities of the qi of zang-fu organs such as the lung, liver, kidney, sanjiao and bladder. Impairment of the activities of the qi of these organs may result in pathological changes, for example, insufficient production or accumulation of body fluid. If the qi of these zang-fu organs is deficient, and unable to exert its controlling function, there may be loss of body fluid. On the other hand, accumulation of body fluid may hinder qi circulation and affect the functions of certain zang-fu organs. Profuse loss of body fluid may also lead to massive dissipation of qi.

3. The Relationship Between Blood and Body Fluid

Since both blood and body fluid are liquids and their main function is to nourish and moisten, they are considered yin. Body fluid is an important part of blood, and when it passes out of the vessels, it forms body fluid. As body fluid and blood can be transformed into each other, there is a saying: "Body fluid and blood are of the same origin." Recurrent or severe bleeding may injure body fluid and result in thirst, scanty urination and dry skin. Severe consumption or loss of body fluid may also affect the source of blood, manifesting as exhaustion of both body fluid and blood. For this reason, it is not advisable to use diaphoretics for haemorrhagic patients. The method of breaking the blood (in which powerful drugs are administered to dissolve blood sludge) or the bleeding method, should be avoided in treating patients with consumption of body fluid due to excessive sweating. The sixty-first chapter of *Miraculous Pivot* states: "The first contraindication refers to a patient who is emaciated; the second to a patient after severe loss of blood; the third to a patient after severe perspiration; the fourth to a patient after severe diarrhoea; the fifth to a patient after loss of blood following childbirth. The reducing method is contraindicated in all these circumstances." The same essay also points out that care should be taken in the acupuncture clinic when treating patients who are emaciated due to deficiency of qi, or severe consumption of qi, blood and body fluid.

Chapter 5

THE MERIDIANS AND COLLATERALS

The meridians and collaterals are pathways in which the qi and blood of the human body are circulated. They pertain to the zang-fu organs interiorly and extend over the body exteriorly, forming a network and linking the tissues and organs into an organic whole. The meridians, which constitute the main trunks, run longitudinally and interiorly within the body; while the collaterals, which represent branches of the meridians, run transversely and superficially from the meridians. They are collectively termed Jingluo (meridians and collaterals) in traditional Chinese medicine. This system of meridians and collaterals includes the twelve regular meridians, eight extra meridians, fifteen collaterals, twelve divergent meridians, twelve muscle regions and twelve cutaneous regions.

It is said in Chapter 33 of *Miraculous Pivot* that "internally, the twelve regular meridians connect with the zang-fu organs, and externally with the joints, limbs and other superficial tissues of the body." The meridians and collaterals are distributed both interiorly and exteriorly over the body, transporting qi and blood to nourish the zang-fu organs, skin, muscles, tendons and bones. Normal functioning of various organs is thus ensured, and a relative equilibrium maintained. It is stated in Chapter 10 of *Miraculous Pivot* that "so

important are the meridians and collaterals which determine life and death in the treatment of all diseases and the regulation of deficiency and excess conditions that one must gain a thorough understanding of them. The importance of studying the theory of meridians and collaterals can indeed never be overemphasized.

The theory of meridians and collaterals was systematized by the ancient Chinese people in their prolonged clinical practice. Its formation is generally considered to be in relation to the observation of the symptoms and signs of diseases and the transmission of needling sensation, the application of Tuina (Chinese remedial massage), Daoying (ancient deep breathing exercises), and ancient anatomical knowledge. Just like the other basic traditional Chinese medical theories, such as that of the zang-fu organs, of qi and blood, etc., the theory of meridians and collaterals is of great significance in guiding diagnosis and treatment in traditional Chinese medicine, and acupuncture in particular.

I. THE BASIC CONCEPT OF THE MERIDIANS AND COLLATERALS

Responsible for the circulation of qi and

blood and distributed both interiorly and exteriorly across the body, the meridians and collaterals have an extensive coverage in contents. The following is a general description of their nomenclature, functions, distribution and the order of the cyclic flow of qi and blood.

1. The Nomenclature of the Meridians and Collaterals and Their Composition

The twelve regular meridians include the three yin meridians of the hand (the Lung Meridian of Hand-Taiyin, the Pericardium Meridian of Hand-Jueyin and the Heart Meridian of Hand-Shaoyin), the three yang meridians of the hand (the Large Intestine Meridian of Hand-Yangming, the Sanjiao (Triple Energizer) Meridian of Hand-Shaoyang and the Small Intestine Meridian of Hand-Taiyang), the three yang meridians of the foot (the Stomach Meridian of Foot-Yangming, the Gallbladder Meridian of Foot-Shaoyang and the Bladder Meridian of Foot-Taiyang), and the three yin meridians of the foot (the Spleen Meridian of Foot-Taiyin, the Liver Meridian of Foot-Jueyin and the Kidney Meridian of Foot-Shaoyin). They are called the twelve regular meridians because they are the major trunks in the system. The nomenclature of the twelve regular meridians is based on the three factors: a) hand or foot, b) yin or yang, and c) a zang or fu organ. Both the upper limbs (hands) and lower limbs (feet) are divided into six regions, which are supplied respectively by the three yin (Taiyin, Shaoyin and Jueyin) and three yang (Yangming, Taiyang and Shaoyang) meridians. There exists an exterior-interior relationship between the three yin and three yang meridians:

$$\text{yin}\begin{cases}\text{Taiyin-----Yangming}\\\text{Jueyin-----Shaoyang}\\\text{Shaoyin-----Taiyang}\end{cases}\text{yang}$$

In accordance with the fact that the zang organs pertain to yin, the fu organs to yang, and the medial aspect is attributed to yin, the lateral aspect, to yang, the meridians that pertain to the zang organs are yin meridians, which are mainly distributed on the medial aspect of the four limbs. Those distributed on the medial aspect of the upper limbs are three yin meridians of the hand; while those distributed on the medial aspect of the lower limbs are three yin meridians of the foot. The meridians that pertain to the fu organs are yang meridians, which mainly travel along the lateral aspect of the four limbs. Those travelling along the lateral aspect of the upper limbs are three yang meridians of the hand; while those travelling along the lateral aspect of the lower limbs are the three yang meridians of the foot.

The eight extra meridians, different from the twelve regular meridians, are called the extra meridians in short. Their nomenclature is explained as follows. Du means governing. Running along the midline of the back, the Du (Governor Vessel) Meridian governs all the yang meridians. Ren means fostering and responsibility. Going along the midline of the abdomen, the Ren (Conception Vessel) Meridian is responsible for all the yin meridians. Chong means a vital pass. As it regulates the flow of qi and blood in the twelve regular meridians, the Chong Meridian is called "the sea of the twelve primary meridians." Dai means a girdle. The Dai Meridian goes around the waist, binding up all the meridians. Qiao means the heel. The one starting from below the external malleolus is the Yangqiao Meridian, while the one starting from below the internal malleolus is the Yinqiao

Meridian. Wei denotes connection and network. The Yangwei Meridian connects and networks the exterior yang of the whole body, while the Yinwei Meridian connects and networks the interior yin of the whole body. Besides, the twelve divergent meridians are those going out from the regular meridians and the fifteen collaterals are branches arising from the regular meridians. Connected with their own relating regular meridians, the twelve muscle regions and cutaneous regions of the twelve regular meridians are named after hand or foot, three yin or three yang respectively as well.

The whole system of the meridians and collaterals is shown in the following table.

2.　Functions of the Meridians and Collaterals

The network of the meridians and collaterals is closely connected with the tissues and organs of the body, and plays an important role in human physiology, pathology, prevention and treatment of ailments.

1) Transporting qi and blood and regulating yin and yang Under normal conditions, the system of the meridians and collaterals functions to transport qi and blood and regulate the balance between yin and yang of the whole body. Chapter 47 in *Miraculous Pivot* says: "The meridians and collaterals transport blood and qi to adjust yin and yang, nourish tendons and bones, and improve joint function." The meridians and collaterals are passages for the circulation of qi and blood. Transversely and longitudinally, they cross with each other in both the interior and exterior of the body. "Nutrient qi flows inside the meridians and defensive qi runs outside the meridians," thus the interior and the exterior, the upper and lower portions and the left and right sides of the body are kept in a close association, and a relative equilibrium of normal life activities is maintained.

2) Resisting pathogens and reflecting symptoms and signs Under pathological conditions, the system of the meridians and collaterals exerts its functions of combatting pathogens and reflecting systemic or local symptoms and signs. Chapter 71 in *Miraculous Pivot* points out, "When the lung and heart are involved in a pathogenic invasion, the pathogenic qi lingers in both elbows; when the liver is involved, it lingers in both axillae; when the spleen is involved, it stays in both groins; when the kidney is involved, it stays in both popliteal fossae." This classical exposition shows that various symptoms and signs of diseases of the internal organs may find their way to the particular location where the corresponding meridians traverse. Occasionally, disorders of internal organs may give rise to reactionary signs on the face or in the five sense organs. For instance, flare-up of the heart fire may cause ulceration on the tongue; pervere ascension of the liver fire may lead to congestion and swelling of the eye; deficiency of kidney qi may result in decrease of hearing, etc. Besides, when the antipathogenic qi is deficient and pathogenic qi predominant, the meridians and collaterals may serve as passages for pathogen transmission. Disorders of meridians and collaterals developing from the exterior may traverse inward to impair the internal organs in the interior. Conversely, diseases of internal organs may affect the meridians and collaterals, as is described in Chapter 22 of *Plain Questions*, "In a case of

Table 2. Classification of Meridians and Collaterals

```
                                    ┌ Lung — Hand-Taiyin ------ Lieque (L 7)
                        Three Yin  ┤ Pericardium — Hand-Jueyin --- Neiguan (P 6)
                                    └ Heart — Hand-Shaoyin ------ Tongli (H 5)
              Hand
                                    ┌ Large Intestine — Hand-Yangming ------ Pianli (L I 6)
                        Three Yang ┤ Sanjiao — Hand-Shaoyang ------ Waiguan (S J 5)
                                    └ Small Intestine — Hand-Taiyang ------ Zhizen (S I 7)

                        ------ (The Major Collateral of the Spleen) ------ Dabao (Sp 21)

                                    ┌ Spleen — Foot-Taiyin ------ Gongsun (Sp 4)
  Twelve                 Three Yin ┤ Liver — Foot-Jueyin -------- Ligou (Liv 5)
  Regular                           └ Kidney — Foot-Shaoyin ------ Dazhong (K 4)          Fifteen
  Meridians  Foot                                                                         Collaterals
                                    ┌ Stomach — Foot-Yangming ----- Fenglong (S 40)
                        Three Yang ┤ Gallbladder — Foot-Shaoyang --- Guangming (G 37)
                                    └ Bladder — Foot-Taiyang --- Feiyang (B 58)
```

```
              ┌ Du Meridian --- Collateral of Du Meridian ------ Changqiang (Du 1)
              │ Ren Meridian --- Collateral of Ren Meridian ---- Jiuwei (Ren 5)
  Eight       │ Chong Meridian      ┐
  Extra      ┤ Dai Meridian         │
  Meridians   │ Yangqiao Meridian    ├ meet with the above 14 meridians
              │ Yinqiao Meridian     │
              │ Yangwei Meridian     │
              └ Yinwei Meridian     ┘
```

Meridians

```
  Twelve
  Divergent
  Meridians  ┐
              │ Same as the twelve Regular Meridians, fit to                    Collaterals
              │ the hand and foot, three yin and three yang
  Twelve      │
  Muscle      ┘
  Regions
```

```
  Twelve
  Cutaneous — Regionalized on the body surface according to the
  Regions      distribution of meridians and collaterals
               Minute Collaterals --- split from collaterals and
                                     distributed all over the body
```

liver disease, the pain in both hypochondria may extend to the lower abdomen," and "a patient with a heart disease may have pain in the chest, fullness of the costal region, pain in the hypochondrium, back, shoulder, and even in the medial aspect of both arms."

3) Transmitting needling sensation and regulating deficiency and excess conditions In the treatment and prevention of disease, the system of the meridians and collaterals assumes the responsibility of transmitting needling sensation and regulating deficiency or excess conditions. When acumoxibustion therapy is applied, stimulation of the acupoints is transmitted to the relevant zang-fu organs. Consequently, normal free flow of qi and blood is restored, the functions of zang-fu organs regulated, and diseases cured. It is said in *Precious Supplementary Prescriptions* that "located on the courses of the meridians and collaterals, acupoints usher qi to the distant sites to achieve curative aims." Chapter 5 in *Miraculous Pivot* states, "The key point in acupuncture treatment is to know how to regulate yin and yang," meaning that the therapeutic action of acupuncture and moxibustion is realized mainly through the function of meridians and collaterals in regulating yin and yang. "The arrival of qi," a phenomenon in acupuncture, is the functional manifestation of the meridians and collaterals in transmitting needling sensation. Therapeutic results are closely related to "the arrival of qi." Therefore, the first chapter in *Miraculous Pivot* points out, "In acupuncture, the arrival of qi is essential to obtaining therapeutic effects." And Chapter 9 in *Miracular Pivot* says, "Acupuncture treatment must aim at regulating the flow of qi." To induce "the arrival of qi" and to employ the reinforcing and reducing methods in acupuncture are simply for the purpose of regulating the flow of qi, and neither of them can be successful without the transmissive function of the meridians and collaterals.

3. Distribution of the Fourteen Meridians

The twelve regular meridians together with the Du and Ren Meridians are called "the fourteen meridians." The twelve regular meridians are distributed symmetrically at the left and right sides of the body. Both the Du and Ren Meridians emerge from the perineum, and ascend respectively along the midlines of the front and back of the body.

Distribution in the Limbs:

The medial aspect of the limbs attributes to yin, the lateral to yang. Each limb is supplied by the three yin and three yang meridians. On the upper limbs, the anterior border of the medial aspect and the radial end of the thumb are supplied by the meridian of Hand-Taiyin; the middle of the medial aspect and the radial end of the middle finger by the meridian of Hand-Jueyin; the posterior border of the medial aspect and the radial end of the small finger by the meridian of Hand-Shaoyin, while the meridian of Hand-Yangming goes from the radial end of the index finger to the anterior border of the lateral aspect; the meridian of Hand-Shaoyang from the ulnar end of the index finger to the middle of the lateral aspect, the meridian of Hand-Taiyang from the ulnar end of the small finger to the posterior border of the lateral aspect. On the lower limbs, the anterior border of the lateral aspect and the lateral end of the second toe are supplied by the meridian of Foot-Yangming; the middle of the lateral side and the lateral end of the fourth toe by the meridian of Foot-Shaoyang; the posterior border of the lateral aspect and the lateral end of the little toe by the meridian of Foot-Taiyang, while the meridian of Foot-Taiyin runs from the medial end of the great toe to the middle of the medial aspect of the lower limb and further goes round to its anterior border; the meridian of Foot-Jueyin goes from the lateral end of the great toe to the anterior border of the medial aspect of the lower limb and further shifts to the middle; and the meridian of Foot-Shaoyin starts under the little toe, crosses the sole and further goes along the posterior border of the medial aspect of the lower limb.

Distribution in the Body Trunk:

In the thoracic and abdominal regions, the Ren Meridian is situated on the midline. The first line lateral to it is the Kidney Meridian of Foot-Shaoyin, the second lateral line is the Stomach Meridian of Foot-Yangming, and the Lung Meridian of Hand-Taiyin and the Spleen Meridian of Foot-Taiyin correspond to the third line. The Gallbladder Meridian of Foot-Shaoyang is located at the lateral side of the hypochondrium and the lumbar region, while the Liver Meridian of Foot-Jueyin is in the region of the anterior external genitalia and hypochondrium. On the back, the Du Meridian stays in the middle, while both the first and second lines lateral to the Du Meridian are the Bladder Meridian of Foot-Taiyang.

Distribution in the Head, Face and Neck:

The Yangming Meridians of Hand and Foot run in the facial region; and the Shaoyang Meridian of Hand and Foot travel in the lateral aspect of the head. The Du Meridian goes along the midline of the neck and head, while the Bladder Meridian of Foot-Taiyang runs on both sides of the Du Meridian.

Among the twelve regular meridians, the yin meridians pertaining to the zang organs communicate with the fu organs, while the yang meridians pertaining to the fu organs communicate with the zang organs, thus forming an exterior-interior relation between yin and yang, the zang and fu organs. The zang organs (the lung, heart and pericardium) that are situated in the chest are connected with the yin meridians of the hand, while those (the spleen, liver and kidney) in the abdomen are linked with the yin meridians of the foot. The six fu organs, however, are related to yang meridians in accordance with their respective exterior-interior relations. All the three yang meridians of the hand and foot traverse the head and facial regions. In this way, between the twelve regular meridians and the head, face, chest and abdomen a specific relationship is established. Chapter 38 of *Miraculous Pivot* states, "The three yin meridians of the hand go from the chest to the hand; the three yang meridians of the hand run from the hand to the head; the three yang meridians of the foot travel from the head to the foot; and the three yin meridians of the foot go from the foot to the abdomen." The meridians of the hand and foot are connected with each other, forming an interminable circulation of yin and yang.

Not only do the twelve regular meridians have their fixed courses, but also they cross at given places as follows: the yin meridians (the interior meridians) meet the yang meridians (the exterior meridians) in the four limbs; the yin meridians meet the yin meridians bearing the same name on the head and face; and the three yin meridians of the hand and the three yin meridians of the foot meet in the chest.

4. Cyclical Flow of Qi in the Twelve Regular Meridians

The twelve regular meridians link one another in a fixed order. A cyclical flow of qi is maintained by the connection of the meridians of the hand and foot, yin and yang, exterior and interior. See the following table.

The Cyclical Flow of Qi in the Twelve Regular Meridians

(———➤pertaining and communicative ←- - - ——exterior and interior relations)

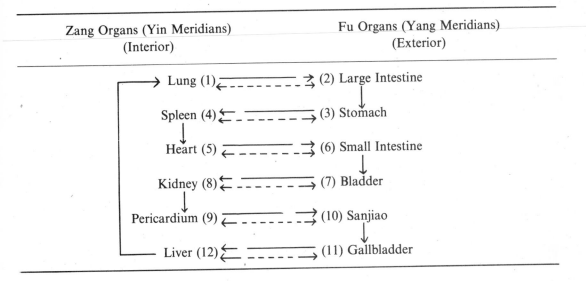

Zang Organs (Yin Meridians) (Interior)	Fu Organs (Yang Meridians) (Exterior)
Lung (1)	(2) Large Intestine
Spleen (4)	(3) Stomach
Heart (5)	(6) Small Intestine
Kidney (8)	(7) Bladder
Pericardium (9)	(10) Sanjiao
Liver (12)	(11) Gallbladder

II.   THE TWELVE REGULAR MERIDIANS

As the major part in the meridian system, the twelve regular meridians share the following features. Each with its own acupoints is distributed on a fixed portion of the body surface; each pertains to either a zang or a fu organ (those that pertain to the zang organ communicating with the fu organ, and vice versa); among the meridians exists an exterior-interior relation of mutual connection; and each meridian presents its pathological manifestation(s), in case its qi fails in a smooth flow. The courses of the twelve regular meridians are described respectively in their circulative order as follows.

1. The Lung Meridian of Hand-Taiyin

The Lung Meridian of Hand-Taiyin originates from the middle *jiao*, running downward to connect with the large intestine (1). Winding back, it goes along the upper orifice of the stomach (2), passes through the diaphragm (3), and enters the lung, its pertaining organ (4). From the lung system, which refers to the portion of the lung communicating with the throat, it comes out transversely (Zhongfu, L 1) (5). Descending along the medial aspect of the upper arm, it passes in front of the Heart Meridian of Hand-Shaoyin and the Pericardium Meridian of Hand-Jueyin (6), and reaches the cubital fossa (7). Then it goes continuously downward along the anterior border of the radial side in the medial aspect of the forearm (8) and enters *cunkou* (the radial artery at the wrist for pulse palpation) (9). Passing the thenar eminence (10), it goes along its radial border (11), ending at the medial side of the tip of the thumb (Shaoshang, L 11) (12).

The branch proximal to the wrist emerges from Lieque (L 7) (13) and runs directly to the radial side of the tip of the index finger (Shangyang, L I 1) where it links with the Large Intestine Meridian of Hand-Yangming. (See Fig. 5)

2. The Large Intestine Meridian of Hand-Yangming

The Large Intestine Meridian of Hand-Yangming starts from the tip of the index finger (Shangyang, L I · 1) (1). Running upward along the radial side of the index finger and passing through the interspace of the 1st and 2nd metacarpal bones (Hegu, L I 4), it dips into the depression between the tendons of m. extensor pollicis longus and brevis (2). Then, following the lateral anterior aspect of the forearm (3), it reaches the lateral side of the elbow (4). From there, it ascends along the lateral anterior aspect of the upper arm (5) to the highest point of the shoulder (Jianyu, L I 15) (6). Then, along the anterior border of the acromion (7), it goes up to the 7th cervical vertebra (the confluence of the three yang meridians of the hand and foot) (Dazhui, Du 14) (8), and descends to the supraclavicular fossa (9) to connect with the lung (10). It then passes through the diaphragm (11) and enters the large intestine, its pertaining organ (12).

The branch from the supraclavicular fossa runs upward to the neck (13), passes through the cheek (14) and enters the gums of the lower teeth (15). Then it curves around the upper lip and crosses the opposite meridian at the philtrum. From there, the left meridian goes to the right and the right meridian to the left, to both sides of the nose (Yingxiang, L I 20), where the Large Intestine Meridian links with the Stomach Meridian of Foot-Yangming (16). (See Fig.6)

3. The Stomach Meridian of Foot-Yangming

The Stomach Meridian of Foot-Yangming starts from the lateral side of ala nasi (Yingxiang, L I 20) (1). It ascends to the bridge of the nose, where it meets the Bladder Meridian of Foot-Taiyang (Jingming, B 1) (2). Turning downward along the lateral side of nose (Chengqi, S 1) (3), it enters the upper gum (4). Reemerging, it curves around the lips (5) and descends to meet the Ren Meridian at the mentolabial

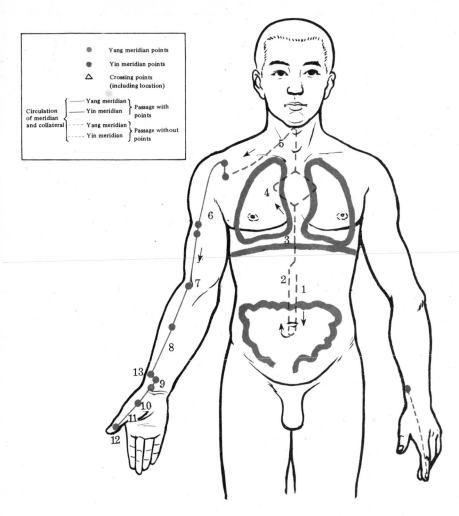

Fig. 5. The Lung Meridian of Hand-Taiyin

groove (Chengjiang, Ren 24) (6). Then it runs posterolaterally across the lower portion of the cheek at Daying (S 5) (7). Winding along the angle of the mandible (Jiache, S 6) (8), it ascends in front of the ear and traverses Shangguan (G 3) (9). Then it follows the anterior hairline (10) and reaches the forehead (11).

The facial branch emerging in front of Daying (S 5) runs downward to Renying (S 9) (12). From there it goes along the throat and enters the supraclavicular fossa (13).

Descending, it passes through the diaphragm (14), enters the stomach, its pertaining organ, and connects with the spleen (15).

The straight portion of the meridian arising from the supraclavicular fossa runs downward (16), passing through the nipple. It descends by the umbilicus and enters Qichong (S 30) on the lateral side of the lower abdomen (17).

The branch from the lower orifice of the stomach (18) descends inside the abdomen and joins the previous portion of the

Fig. 6 The Large Intestine Meridian
of Hand-Yangming

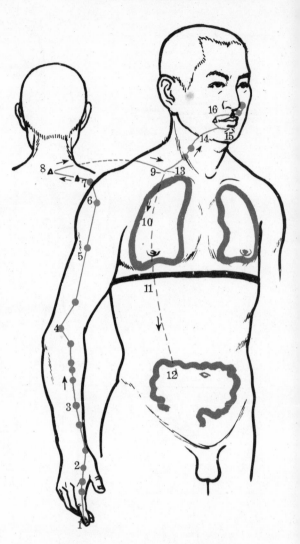

meridian at Qichong (S 30). Running downward, traversing Biguan (S 31) (19), and further through Femur-Futu (S 32) (20), it reaches the knee (21). From there, it continues downward along the anterior border of the lateral aspect of the tibia (22), passes through the dorsum of the foot (23), and reaches the lateral side of the tip of the 2nd toe (Lidui, S 45) (24).

The tibial branch emerges from Zusanli (S 36), 3 cun below the knee (25), and enters the lateral side of the middle toe (26).

The branch from the dorsum of the foot arises from Chongyang (S 42) (27) and terminates at the medial side of the tip of the great toe (Yinbai, Sp 1), where it links with the Spleen Meridian of Foot-Taiyin. (See Fig. 7)

4.   The Spleen Meridian of Foot-Taiyin

The Spleen Meridian of Foot-Taiyin starts from the tip of the big toe (Yinbai, Sp 1) (1). It runs along the medial aspect of the foot at the junction of the red and white skin (2), and ascends in front of the medial malleolus (3) up to the medial aspect of the leg (4). It follows the posterior aspect of the tibia (5), crosses and goes in front of the Liver Meridian of Foot-Jueyin (6). Passing through the anterior medial aspect of the

knee and thigh (7), it enters the abdomen (8), then the spleen, its pertaining organ, and connects with the stomach (9). From there it ascends, passing through the diaphragm (10) and running alongside the esophagus (11). When it reaches the root of the tongue it spreads over its lower surface (12).

The branch from the stomach goes upward through the diaphragm (13), and flows into the heart to link with the Heart Meridian of Hand-Shaoyin (14). (See Fig. 8)

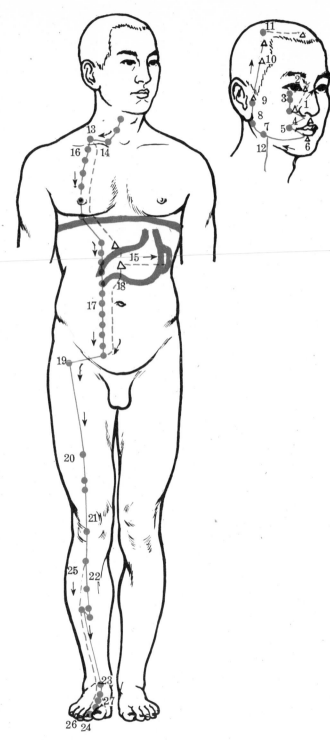

Fig. 7 The Stomach Meridian of Foot-Yangming

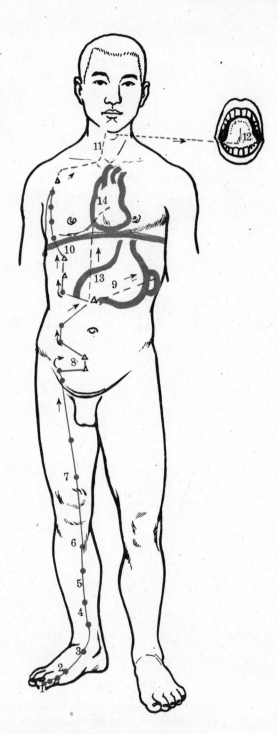

Fig. 8 The Spleen Meridian of Foot-Taiyin

5.   The Heart Meridian of Hand-Shaoyin

The Heart Meridian of Hand-Shaoyin originates from the heart. Emerging, it spreads over the "heart system" (i.e., the tissues connecting the heart with the other zang-fu organs) (1). It passes through the diaphragm to connect with the small intestine (2).

The ascending portion of the meridian from the "heart system" (3) runs alongside the esophagus (4) to connect with the "eye system" (i.e., the tissues connecting the eyes with the brain) (5).

The straight portion of the meridian from the "heart system" goes upward to the lung (6). Then it turns downward and emerges from the axilla (Jiquan, H 1). From there it goes along the posterior border of the medial aspect of the upper arm behind the Lung

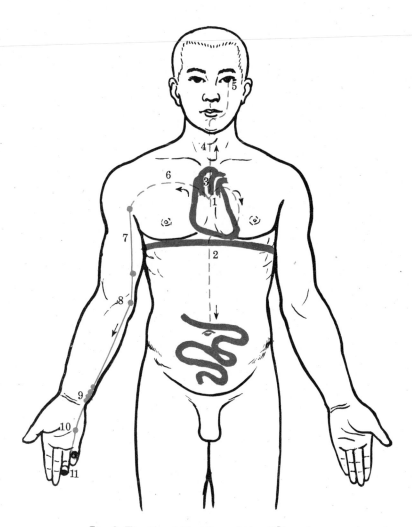

Fig. 9 The Heart Meridian of Hand-Shaoyin

Meridian of Hand-Taiyin and the Pericardium Meridian of Hand-Jueyin (7) down to the cubital fossa (8). From there it descends along the posterior border of the medial aspect of the forearm to the pisiform region proximal to the palm (9) and enters the palm (10). Then it follows the medial aspect of the little finger to its tip (Shaochong, H 9) (11) and links with the Small Intestine Meridian of Hand-Taiyang. (See Fig. 9)

6. The Small Intestine Meridian of Hand-Taiyang

The Small Intestine Meridian of Hand-Taiyang starts from the ulnar side of the tip of the little finger (Shaoze, S I 1) (1). Following the ulnar side of the dorsum of the hand it reaches the wrist where it emerges from the styloid process of the ulna (2). From there it ascends along the posterior aspect of the forearm (3), passes between the olecranon of the ulna and the medial epicondyle of the humerus, and runs along the posterior border of the lateral aspect of the upper arm (4) to the shoulder joint (5). Circling around the scapular region (6), it meets Dazhui (Du 14) on the superior aspect of the shoulder (7). Then, turning downward to the supraclavicular fossa (8), it connects with the heart (9). From there it descends along the esophagus (10), passes through the diaphragm (11), reaches the stomach (12), and finally enters the small intestine, its pertaining organ (13).

The branch from the supraclavicular fossa (14) ascends to the neck (15), and further to the cheek (16). Via the outer canthus (17), it enters the ear (Tinggong, S I 19) (18).

The branch from the neck (19) runs upward to the infraorbital region (Quanliao,

S I 18) and further to the lateral side of the nose. Then it reaches the inner canthus (Jingming, B 1) to link with the Bladder Meridian of Foot-Taiyang (20). (See Fig. 10)

7. The Bladder Meridian of Foot-Taiyang

The Bladder Meridian of Foot-Taiyang starts from the inner canthus (Jingming, B 1) (1). Ascending to the forehead (2), it joins the Du Meridian at the vertex (Baihui, Du 20) (3), where a branch arises, running to the temple (4).

The straight portion of the meridian enters and communicates with the brain from the vertex (5). It then emerges and bifurcates to descend along the posterior aspect of the neck (6). Running downward alongside the medial aspect of the scapula region and parallel to the vertebral column (7), it reaches the lumbar region (8), where it enters the body cavity via the paravertebral muscle (9) to connect with the kidney (10) and join its pertaining organ, the bladder (11).

The branch of the lumber region descends through the gluteal region (12) and ends in the popliteal fossa (13).

The branch from the posterior aspect of the neck runs straight downward along the medial border of the scapula (14). Passing through the gluteal region (Huantiao, G 30) (15) downward along the lateral aspect of the thigh (16), it meets the preceding branch descending from the lumbar region in the popliteal fossa (17). From there it descends to the leg (18) and further to the posterior aspect of the external malleolus (19). Then, running along the tuberosity of the 5th metatarsal bone (20), it reaches the lateral side of the tip of the little toe (Zhiyin, B 67),

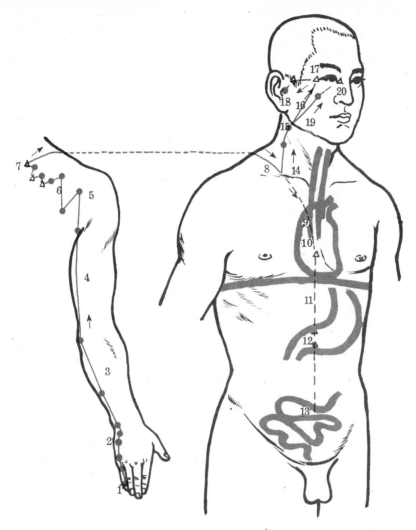

Fig. 10 The Small Intestine Meridian of Hand-Taiyang

where it links with the Kidney Meridian of Foot-Shaoyin (21). (See Fig. 11)

8. The Kidney Meridian of Foot-Shaoyin

The Kidney Meridian of Foot-Shaoyin starts from the inferior aspect of the small toe (1) and runs obliquely towards the sole (Yongquan, K 1). Emerging from the lower

aspect of the tuberosity of the navicular bone (2) and running behind the medial malleolus (3), it enters the heel (4). Then it ascends along the medial side of the leg (5) to the medial side of the popliteal fossa (6) and goes further upward along the postero-medial aspect of the thigh (7) towards the vertebral column (Changqiang, Du 1), where it enters the kidney, its pertaining organ (8), and connects with the bladder (9).

The straight portion of the meridian

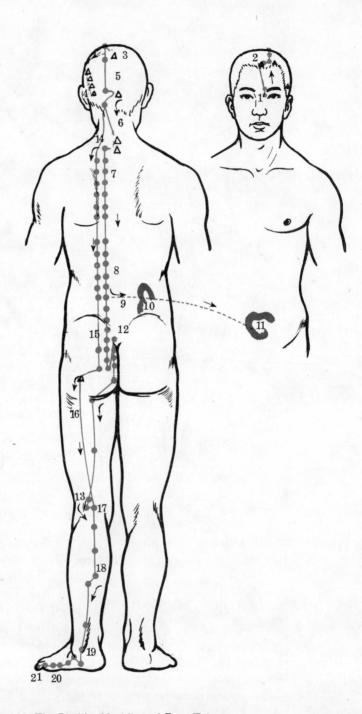

Fig. 11 The Bladder Meridian of Foot-Taiyang

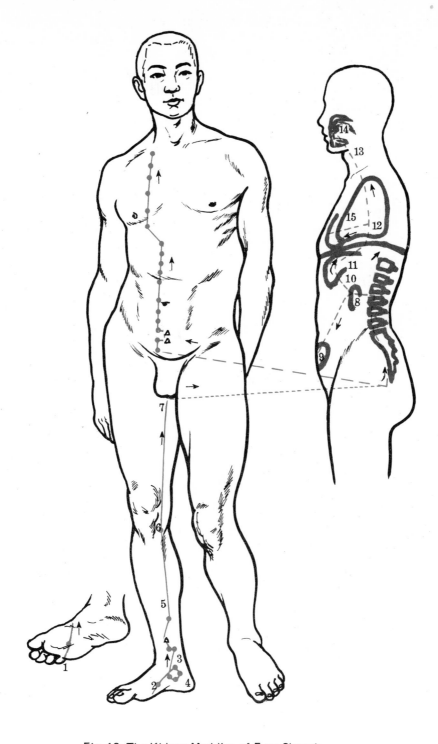

Fig. 12 The Kidney Meridian of Foot-Shaoyin

reemerges from the kidney (10). Ascending and passing through the liver and diaphragm (11), it enters the lung (12), runs along the throat (13) and terminates at the root of the tongue (14).

A branch springs from the lung, joins the heart and runs into the chest to link with the Pericardium Meridian of Hand-Jueyin (15). (See Fig. 12)

9. The Pericardium Meridian of Hand-Jueyin

The Pericardium Meridian of Hand-Jueyin originates from the chest. Emerging,

it enters its pertaining organ, the pericardium (1). Then, it descends through the diaphragm (2) to the abdomen, connecting successively with the upper, middle and lower *jiao* (i.e., *sanjiao*) (3).

A branch arising from the chest runs inside the chest (4), emerges from the costal region at a point 3 cun below the anterior axillary fold (Tianchi P 1) (5) and ascends to the axilla (6). Following the medial aspect of the upper arm, it runs downward between

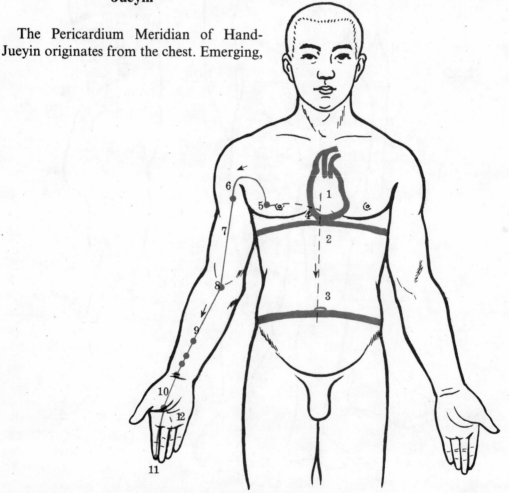

Fig. 13 The Pericardium Meridian of Hand-Jueyin

the Lung Meridian of Hand-Taiyin and the Heart Meridian of Hand-Shaoyin (7) to the cubital fossa (8), further downward to the forearm between the two tendons (the tendons of m. palmaris longus and m. flexor carpi radialis) (9), ending in the palm (10). From there it passes along the middle finger right down to its tip (Zhongchong P 9) (11).

Another branch arises from the palm at Laogong (P 8) (12), runs along the ring finger to its tip (Guanchong, S J 1) and links with the Sanjiao Meridian of Hand-Shaoyang. (See Fig. 13)

10. The Sanjiao Meridian of Hand-Shaoyang

The Sanjiao Meridian of Hand-Shaoyang originates from the tip of the ring finger (Guanchong S J 1) (1), running upward between the 4th and 5th metacarpal bones (2) along the dorsal aspect of the wrist (3) to the lateral aspect of the forearm between the radius and ulna (4). Passing through the olecranon (5) and along the lateral aspect of the upper arm (6), it reaches the shoulder region (7), where it goes across and passes behind the Gallbladder Meridian of Foot-Shaoyang (8). Winding over to the supraclavicular fossa (9), it spreads in the chest to connect with the pericardium (10). It then descends through the diaphragm down to the abdomen, and joins its pertaining organ, the upper, middle and lower *jiao* (i.e., *sanjiao*) (11).

A branch originates from the chest (12). Running upward, it emerges from the supraclavicular fossa (13). From there it ascends to the neck (14), running along the posterior border of the ear (15), and further to the corner of the anterior hairline (16). Then it turns downward to the cheek and

terminates in the infraorbital region (17).

The auricular branch arises from the retroauricular region and enters the ear (18). Then it emerges in front of the ear, crosses the previous branch at the cheek and reaches the outer canthus (Sizhukong, S J 23) to link with the Gallbladder Meridian of Foot-Shaoyang (19). (See Fig. 14)

11. The Gallbladder Meridian of Foot-Shaoyang

The Gallbladder Meridian of Foot-Shaoyang originates from the outer canthus (Tongziliao, G 1) (1), ascends to the corner of the forehead (Hanyan, G 4) (2), then curves downward to the retroauricular region (Fengchi, G 20) (3) and runs along the side of the neck in front of the Sanjiao Meridian of Hand-Shaoyang to the shoulder (4). Turning back, it traverses and passes behind the Sanjiao Meridian of Hand-Shaoyang down to the supraclavicular fossa (5).

The retroauricular branch arises from the retroauricular region (6) and enters the ear. It then comes out and passes the preauricular region (7) to the posterior aspect of the outer canthus (8).

The branch arising from the outer canthus (9) runs downward to Daying (S 5) (10) and meets the Sanjiao Meridian of Hand-Shaoyang in the infraorbital region (11). Then, passing through Jiache (S 6) (12), it descends to the neck and enters the supraclavicular fossa where it meets the main meridian (13). From there it further descends into the chest (14), passes through the diaphragm to connect with the liver (15) and enters its pertaining organ, the gallbladder (16). Then it runs inside the hypochondriac region (17), comes out from

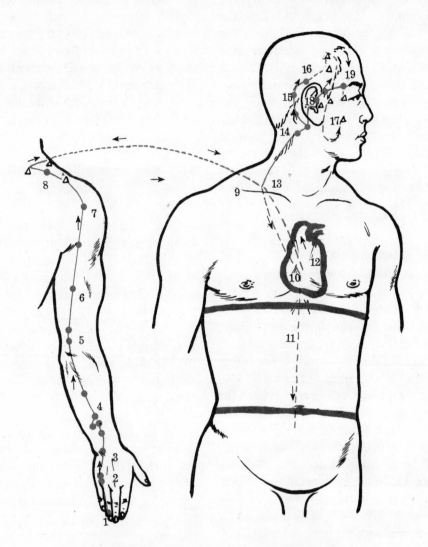

Fig. 14 The Sanjiao Meridian of Hand-Shaoyang

the lateral side of the lower abdomen near the femoral artery at the inguinal region (18). From there it runs superficially along the margin of the pubic hair (19) and goes transversely into the hip region (Huantiao, G 30) (20).

The straight portion of the channel runs downward from the supraclavicular fossa (21), passes in front of the axilla (22) along the lateral aspect of the chest (23) and through the free ends of the floating ribs (24) to the hip region where it meets the previous branch (25). Then it descends along the lateral aspect of the thigh (26) to the lateral side of the knee (27). Going further downward along the anterior aspect of the fibula (28) all the way to its lower end (Xuanzhong, G 39) (29), it reaches the

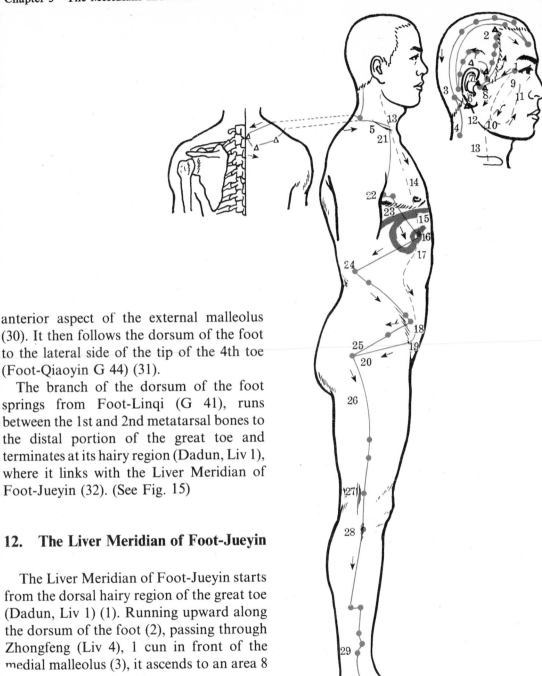

anterior aspect of the external malleolus
(30). It then follows the dorsum of the foot
to the lateral side of the tip of the 4th toe
(Foot-Qiaoyin G 44) (31).

The branch of the dorsum of the foot
springs from Foot-Linqi (G 41), runs
between the 1st and 2nd metatarsal bones to
the distal portion of the great toe and
terminates at its hairy region (Dadun, Liv 1),
where it links with the Liver Meridian of
Foot-Jueyin (32). (See Fig. 15)

12.   The Liver Meridian of Foot-Jueyin

The Liver Meridian of Foot-Jueyin starts
from the dorsal hairy region of the great toe
(Dadun, Liv 1) (1). Running upward along
the dorsum of the foot (2), passing through
Zhongfeng (Liv 4), 1 cun in front of the
medial malleolus (3), it ascends to an area 8

Fig. 15 The Gallbladder Meridian of Foot-Shaoyang

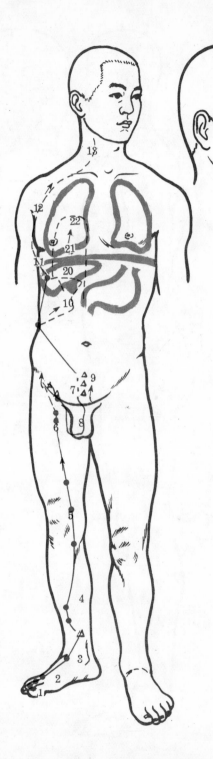

Fig. 16 The Liver Meridian of Foot-Jueyin

cun above the medial malleolus, where it runs across and behind the Spleen Meridian of Foot-Taiyin (4). Then it runs further upward to the medial side of the knee (5) and along the medial aspect of the thigh (6) to the pubic hair region (7), where it curves around the external genitalia (8) and goes up to the lower abdomen (9). It then runs upward and curves around the stomach to enter the liver, its pertaining organ, and connects with the gallbladder (10). From there it continues to ascend, passing through the diaphragm (11), and branching out in the costal and hypochondriac region (12). Then it ascends along the posterior aspect of the throat (13) to the nasopharynx (14) and connects with the "eye system" (15). Running further upward, it emerges from the forehead (16) and meets the Du Meridian at the vertex.

The branch which arises from the "eye system" runs downward into the cheek (18) and curves around the inner surface of the lips (19).

The branch arising from the liver (20) passes through the diaphragm (21), runs into the lung and links with the Lung Meridian of Hand-Taiyin (22). (See Fig. 16)

III. THE EIGHT EXTRA MERIDIANS

The eight extra meridians are the Du, Ren, Chong, Dai, Yangqiao, Yinqiao, Yangwei and Yinwei meridians. They are different from the twelve regular meridians because none of them pertains to the zang organs and communicates with the fu organs or pertains to the fu organs and communicates with the zang organs. And they are not exteriorly-interiorly related. Apart from the Du and Ren Meridians which have their own acupoints, the extra meridians share their points with other regular meridians. Strengthening the association among the meridians, they assume the responsibility to control, join, store, and regulate the qi and blood of each meridian.

Running along the midline of the back and ascending to the head and face, the Du Meridian meets all the yang meridians. It is therefore described as "the sea of the yang meridians." Its function is to govern the qi of all the yang meridians.

Running along the midline of the abdomen and the chest, going upward to the chin, the Ren Meridian meets all the yin meridians. Thus it is called "the sea of the yin meridians." Its function is to receive and bear the qi of the yin meridians.

The Chong Meridian runs parallel to the Kidney Meridian of Foot-Shaoyin up to the infra-orbital region. Meeting all the twelve regular meridians, it is termed "the sea of the twelve regular meridians" or "the sea of blood." Its function is to reservoir the qi and blood of the twelve regular meridians.

The Dai Meridian, which originates in the hypochondrium and goes around the waist

Table 4. Distribution of the Eight Extra Meridians and Their Connecting Meridians

Eight Extra Meridian	Area Supplied	Their Connecting Meridians
Du Meridian	Posterior Midline	Foot-Yangming and Ren
Ren Meridian	Anterior Midline	Foot-Yangming and Du
Chong Meridian	1st lateral line of the abdomen	Foot-Shaoyin
Dai Meridian	lateral side of the lumbar region	Foot-Shaoyang
Yangqiao Meridian	Lateral side of the lower extremities, shoulder and head	Hand and Foot-Taiyang, Hand and Foot-Yangming and Foot-Shaoyang
Yinqiao Meridian	Medial aspect of the lower extremities and eye	Foot-Shaoyin and Foot-Taiyang
Yangwei Meridian	Lateral aspect of the lower extremities, shoulder and vertex	Hand and Foot-Taiyang, Du, Hand and Foot-Shaoyang and Foot-Yangming
Yinwei Meridian	Medial aspect of the lower extremities, 3rd lateral line of the abdomen and neck	Foot-Shaoyin, Foot-Taiyin, Foot-Jueyin and Ren

as a girdle, performs a function of binding up all the meridians.

The Yangqiao Meridian starts in the lateral aspect of the heel and merges into the meridian of Foot-Taiyang to ascend, while the Yinqiao Meridian starts in the medial aspect of the heel and merges into the meridian of Foot-Shaoyin to go upwards.

Following their own courses, the two meridians meet each other at the inner canthus. Motion regulation of the lower limbs is their joint function.

The Yangwei Meridian is connected with all the yang meridians and dominates the exterior of the whole body; the Yinwei Meridian is connected with all the yin

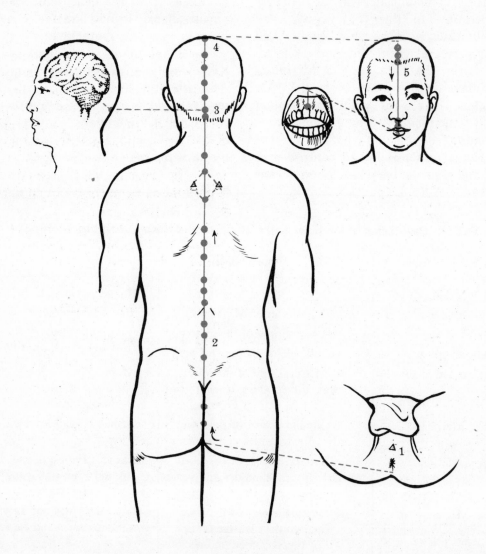

Fig. 17 The Du Meridian

meridians and dominates the interior of the whole body. The two meridians regulate the flow of qi in the yin and yang meridians, and help maintain coordination and equilibrium between the yin and yang meridians.

Du Meridian

The Du Meridian arises from the lower abdomen and emerges from the perineum (1). Then it runs posteriorly along the interior of the spinal column (2) to Fengfu (Du 16) at the nape, where it enters the brain (3). It further ascends to the vertex (4) and winds along the forehead to the columnella of the nose (5).

The coalescent points of the Du Meridian are Fengmen (B 12) and Huiyin (Ren 1). (See Fig. 17)

Ren Meridian

The Ren Meridian starts from the inside of the lower abdomen and emerges from the perineum (1). It goes anteriorly to the pubic region (2) and ascends along the interior of the abdomen, passing through Guanyuan (Ren 4) and the other points along the front midline (3) to the throat (4). Ascending further, it curves around the lips (5), passes through the cheek and enters the infraorbital region (Chengqi, S 1).

The coalescent points of the Ren Meridian are Chengqi (S 1), Yinjiao (Du 28). (See Fig. 18)

Chong Meridian

The Chong Meridian starts from the inside of the lower abdomen and emerges at

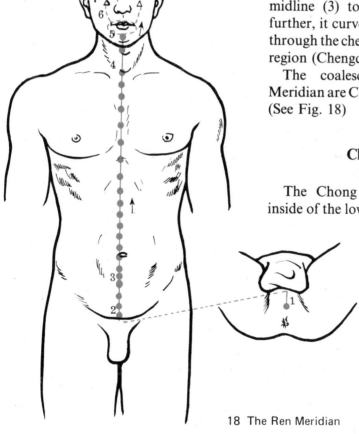

18 The Ren Meridian

the perineum (1). Ascending, it runs inside of the spinal column (2), where its superficial branch passes through the region of Qichong (S 30) and communicates with the Kidney Meridian of Foot-Shaoyin. Running along the both sides of the abdomen, it goes up to the throat and curves around the lips (5).

The coalescent points of the Chong Meridian are Huiyin (Ren 1), Henggu (K 11), Dahe (K 12), Qixue (K 13), Simen (K 14), Zhongzhu (K 15), Huangshu (K 16), Shangqu (K 17), Shiguan (K 18), Yindu (K 19), Futonggu (K 20) and Youmen (K 21). (See Fig. 19)

Dai Meridian

The Dai Meridian originates below the hypochondriac region and runs obliquely downward through Daimai (G 26), Wushu (G 27), and Weidao (G 28) (1). It runs transversely around the waist like a belt (2).

The coalescent points of the Dai Meridian are Daimai (G 26), Wushu (G 27), and Weidao (G 28). (See Fig. 20)

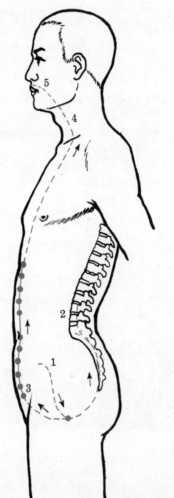

Fig. 19 The Chong Meridian

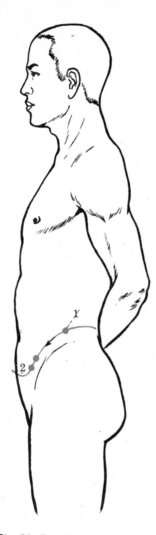

Fig. 20 The Dai Meridian

Yangqiao Meridian

The Yangqiao Meridian starts from the lateral side of the heel (Shenmai, B 62), Pushen (B 61) (1). It runs upward along the external malleolus (2) and passes the posterior border of the fibula. It then goes onwards along the lateral side of the thigh and posterior side of the hypochondrium to the posterior axillary fold. From there, it winds over to the shoulder and ascends along the neck to the corner of the mouth. Then it enters the inner canthus (Jingming, B 1) to communicate with the Yinqiao Meridian. Running further upward along the Bladder Meridian of Foot-Taiyang to the forehead, it meets the Gallbladder Meridian of Foot-Shaoyang at Fengchi (G 20) (3).

The coalescent points of the Yangqiao Meridian are Shenmai (B 62), Pushen (B 61), Fuyang (B 59), Femur-Juliao (G 29), Naoshu (S I 10), Jiaoyu (L I 15), Jugu (L I 16), Dicang (S 4), Nose-Juliao (S 3), Chengqi (S 1), Jingming (B 1) and Fengchi (G 20). (See Fig. 21)

Yinqiao Meridian

The Yinqiao Meridian starts from the posterior aspect of the navicular bone (Zhaohai, K 6) (1). Ascending to the upper portion of the medial malleolus (2), it runs straight upward along the posterior border of the medial aspect of the thigh (3) to the external genitalia (4). Then it goes upward along the chest (5) to the supraclavicular fossa (6) and runs further upward lateral to the Adam's apple in front of Renying (S 9) (7) and then along the zygoma (8). From there, it reaches the inner canthus (Jingming, B 1) and communicates with the Yangqiao Meridian (9).

The coalescent points of the Yinqiao Meridian are Zhaohai (K 6), and Jiaoxin (K 8). (See Fig. 21)

Yangwei Meridian

The Yangwei Meridian originates from the heel (Jinmen, B 63) (1) and emerges from the external malleolus (2). Ascending along the Gallbladder Meridian of Foot-Shaoyang, it passes through the hip region (3). Then it runs further upward along the

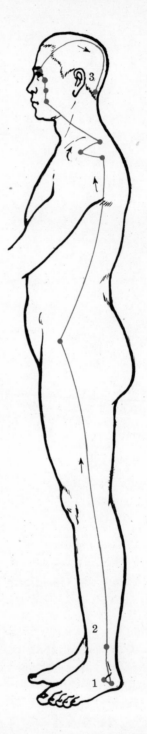

Fig. 21 The Yangqiao and Yinqiao Meridians

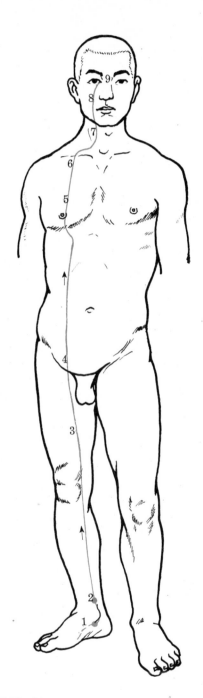

Fig. 21 The Yangqiao and Yinqiao Meridians

posterior aspect of the hypochondriac and costal regions (4) and the posterior aspect of the axilla to the shoulder (5) and to the forehead (6). It then turns backward to the back of the neck, where it communicates with the Du Meridian (Fengfu, Du 16, Yamen, Du 15) (7).

The coalescent points of the Yangwei Meridian are Jinmen (B 63), Yangjiao (G 35), Naoshu (S I 10), Tianliao (S J 15), Jianjing (G 21), Benshen (G 13), Yangbai (G 14), Toulinqi (G 15), Muchuang (G 16), Zhengying (G 17), Chengling (G 18), Naokong (G 19), Fengchi (G 20), Fengfu (Du 16) and Yamen (Du 15). (See Fig. 22)

Yinwei Meridian

The Yinwei Meridian starts from the medial aspect of the leg (Zhubin, K 9) (1), and ascends along the medial aspect of the thigh to the abdomen (2) to communicate with the Spleen Meridian of Foot-Taiyin (3). Then it runs along the chest (4) and communicates with the Ren Meridian at the neck (Tiantu, Ren 22), Lianquan, (Ren 23) (5).

The coalescent points of the Yinwei Meridian are Zhubin (K 9), Fushe (Sp 13), Daheng (Sp 15), Fuai (Sp 16), Qimen (Liv 14), Tiantu (Ren 22) and Lianquan (Ren 23). (See Fig. 22)

IV. THE TWELVE DIVERGENT MERIDIANS AND FIFTEEN COLLATERALS

The Divergent Meridians and Collaterals branch out from the twelve regular

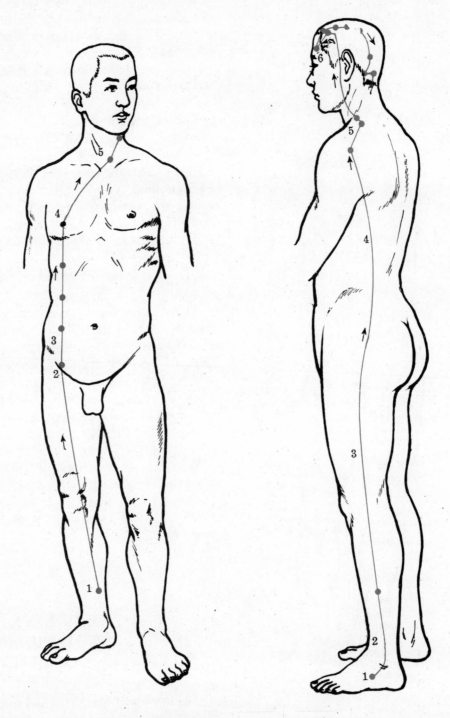

Fig. 22 The Yangwei and Yinwei Meridians

meridians. The divergent meridians mainly run deeper in the body, with the collaterals being mostly distributed on the body surface. They both strengthen and connect the internally-externally related meridians. The divergent meridians govern the inside of the body, so they do not have points of their pertaining organs, while the collaterals control the body surface, each of them has a Luo (Connecting) point, effective to certain diseases. The distribution of the twelve divergent meridians and fifteen collaterals are described as follows:

The Twelve Divergent Meridians:

The twelve divergent meridians, which branch out from the twelve regular meridians, are mainly distributed on the chest, abdomen and head. Their function is to connect internally-externally related meridians, strengthen their relation with the zang-fu organs and serve as the extension of regular meridians. The distribution of the Divergent Meridians is summarized as follows:

Most of them derive from the regular meridians at the regions of four limbs and then enter the thoracic and abdominal cavities. The Yin and Yang Divergent Meridians run parallelly inside the body and emerge from the neck. In the head region, the Yin Divergent Meridians connect the Yang Divergent Meridians and then join the regular meridians. Thus the twelve Divergent Meridians can be paired into six confluences according to their internal and external relationship.

The Divergent Meridians mainly run deeper in the body, supplementing the pathway that the regular meridians do not reach. There are no points located on the Divergent Meridians.

1.   The First Confluence

1) Divergent Meridian of the Bladder Meridian of Foot Taiyang   After deriving from the Bladder Meridian in the popliteal fossa, it proceeds to a point five cun below the sacrum. Winding round to the anal region, it connects with the bladder and disperses in the kidneys. Then it follows the spine and disperses in the cardiac region and finally emerges at the neck and converges with the Bladder Meridian of Foot Taiyang. (See Fig. 23)

2) Divergent Meridian of the Kidney Meridian of Foot Shaoyin   After deriving from the Kidney Meridian in the popliteal fossa, it intersects the Divergent Meridian of the Bladder Meridian on the thigh. It then runs upward, connecting with the kidney and crossing the Dai Meridian at about the level of the 7th thoracic vertebra. Further it ascends to the root of the tongue and finally, emerges at the nape to join the Bladder Meridian of Foot Taiyang. (See Fig. 23)

2.   The Second Confluence

1) Divergent Meridian of the Stomach Meridian of Foot Yangming   After deriving from the Stomach Meridian on the thigh, it enters the abdomen, connects with the stomach and disperses in the spleen. It then ascends through the heart and alongside the esophagus to reach the mouth. It then runs upward beside the nose and connects with the eye before finally joining the Stomach Meridian of Foot Yangming. (See Fig. 24)

2) Divergent Meridian of the Spleen Meridian of Foot Taiyin   After deriving from the Spleen Meridian on the thigh, it converges with the Divergent Meridian of the Stomach Meridian of Foot Yangming

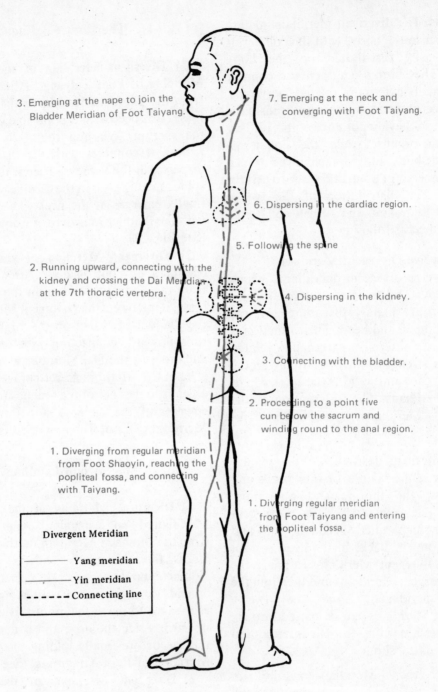

3. Emerging at the nape to join the Bladder Meridian of Foot Taiyang.

7. Emerging at the neck and converging with Foot Taiyang.

6. Dispersing in the cardiac region.

5. Following the spine

2. Running upward, connecting with the kidney and crossing the Dai Meridian at the 7th thoracic vertebra.

4. Dispersing in the kidney.

3. Connecting with the bladder.

2. Proceeding to a point five cun below the sacrum and winding round to the anal region.

1. Diverging from regular meridian from Foot Shaoyin, reaching the popliteal fossa, and connecting with Taiyang.

1. Diverging regular meridian from Foot Taiyang and entering the popliteal fossa.

Divergent Meridian

——————— Yang meridian

————————— Yin meridian

- - - - - - - Connecting line

Fig. 23 Divergent Meridians of Foot-Taiyang and Foot-Shaoyin

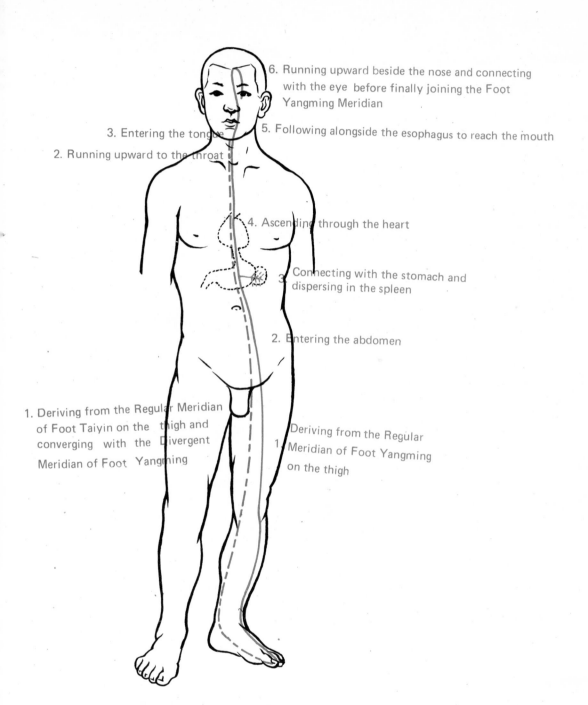

6. Running upward beside the nose and connecting with the eye before finally joining the Foot Yangming Meridian

3. Entering the tongue

5. Following alongside the esophagus to reach the mouth

2. Running upward to the throat

4. Ascending through the heart

3. Connecting with the stomach and dispersing in the spleen

2. Entering the abdomen

1. Deriving from the Regular Meridian of Foot Taiyin on the thigh and converging with the Divergent Meridian of Foot Yangming

1. Deriving from the Regular Meridian of Foot Yangming on the thigh

Fig. 24 Divergent Meridians of Foot-Yangming and Foot-Tiayin

and runs upward to the throat, and finally enters the tongue. (See Fig. 24)

3.   The Third Confluence

1) Divergent Meridian of the Gallbladder Meridian of Foot Shaoyang After deriving from the Gallbladder Meridian on the thigh, it crosses over the hip joint and enters the lower abdomen in the pelvic region and converges with the Divergent Meridian of the Liver Meridian. Then, it crosses between the lower ribs, connects with the gallbladder and spreads through the liver. Proceeding further upward, it crosses the heart and esophagus and disperses in the face. It then connects with the eye and rejoins the Gallbladder Meridian of Foot Shaoyang at the outer canthus. (See Fig. 25)

2) Divergent Meridian of the Liver Meridian of Foot Jueyin After derving from the Liver Channel on the instep, it runs upward to the pubic region, and converges with the Gallbladder Meridian of Foot Shaoyang. (See Fig. 25)

4.   The Fourth Confluence

1) Divergent Meridian of the Small Intestine Meridian of Hand Taiyang After deriving from the Small Intestine Meridian at the shoulder joint, it enters the axilla, crosses the heart and runs downward to the abdomen to link up with the Small Intestine Meridian. (See Fig. 26)

2) Divergent Meridian of the Heart Meridian of Hand Shaoyin After deriving from the Heart Meridian in the axillary fossa, it enters the chest and connects with the heart. Then it runs upward across the throat and emerges on the face, and joins the Small Intestine Meridian at the inner canthus. (See Fig. 26)

5.   The Fifth Confluence

1) Divergent Meridian of the Large Intestine Meridian of Hand Yangming After deriving from the Large Intestine Meridian on the hand, it continues upward, crossing the arm and shoulder to reach the breast. A branch separates at the top of the shoulder and enters the spine at the nape. It runs downward to connect with the large intestine and lung. Another branch runs upward from the shoulder along the throat and emerges at the supraclavicular fossa; there it rejoins the Large Intestine Meridian. (See Fig. 27)

2) Divergent Meridian of the Lung Meridian of Hand Taiyin After deriving from the Lung Meridian at the axilla, it runs anterior to the Pericardium Meridian of Hand Taiyin into the chest, and there it connects with the lung and then disperses in the large intestine. A branch extends upward from the lung and emerges at the clavicle, it ascends across the throat and converges with the Large Intestine Meridian. (See Fig. 27)

6.   The Sixth Confluence

1) Divergent Meridian of the Sanjiao (Triple Energizer) Meridian of Hand Shaoyang After deriving from the Sanjiao Meridian at the vertex, it descends into the supraclavicular fossa crosses the upper *jiao*, middle *jiao* and lower *jiao* and finally disperses in the chest. (See Fig. 28)

2) Divergent Meridian of the Pericardium

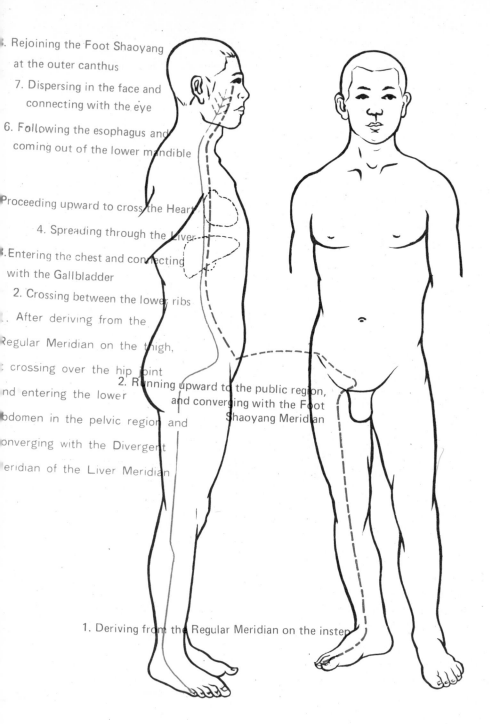

. Rejoining the Foot Shaoyang
  at the outer canthus
    7. Dispersing in the face and
      connecting with the eye
6. Following the esophagus and
  coming out of the lower mandible

Proceeding upward to cross the Heart

    4. Spreading through the Liver

.Entering the chest and connecting
 with the Gallbladder
  2. Crossing between the lower ribs
. After deriving from the
Regular Meridian on the thigh,
 crossing over the hip joint
              2. Running upward to the public region,
nd entering the lower   and converging with the Foot
              Shaoyang Meridian
odomen in the pelvic region and
onverging with the Divergent
eridian of the Liver Meridian

    1. Deriving from the Regular Meridian on the instep

Fig. 25 Divergent Meridians of Foot-Shaoyang and Foot-Jueyin

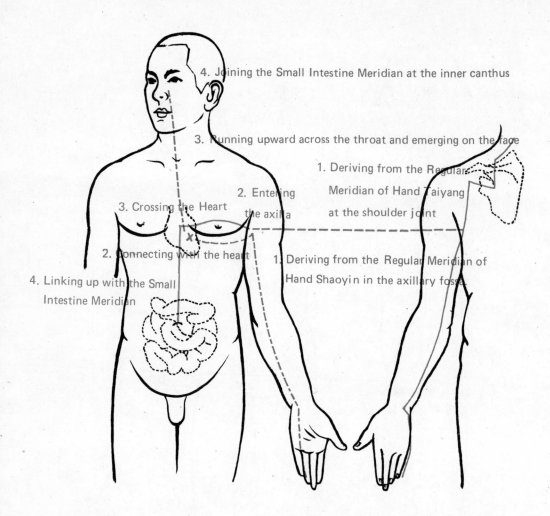

4. Joining the Small Intestine Meridian at the inner canthus

3. Running upward across the throat and emerging on the face

1. Deriving from the Regular Meridian of Hand Taiyang at the shoulder joint

2. Entering the axilla

3. Crossing the Heart

2. Connecting with the heart

1. Deriving from the Regular Meridian of Hand Shaoyin in the axillary fossa

4. Linking up with the Small Intestine Meridian

Fig. 26 Divergent Meridians of Hand-Taiyang and Hand-Shaoyin

Meridian of Hand Jueyin After deriving from the Pericardium Channel at a point three cun below the axilla, it enters the chest and communicates with the Sanjiao. A branch ascends across the throat and emerges behind the ear and then converges with the Sanjiao Meridian. (See Fig. 28)

The fifteen collaterals:

The fifteen collaterals include the twelve collaterals separating from the twelve regular meridians, the collaterals of the Ren and Du and the major collateral of the spleen. They are distributed superficially over the four limbs and in the anterior, posterior and lateral aspects of the body. Their function is to connect the externally-internally related meridians and transport the local qi and blood so as to promote the free circulation of qi and blood of the meridians.

The distribution of the fifteen collaterals may be summarized as follows:

Each of the collaterals has a Luo (Connecting) point, pertaining to the meridian where it derives. The collaterals on the four limbs not only run to the externally-internally related meridians but also possess other tributaries. The collaterals on the trunk and collateral of the Ren Meridian disperse in the abdominal region. The Collateral of Du Meridian disperses in the head and joins with the Bladder Meridian on

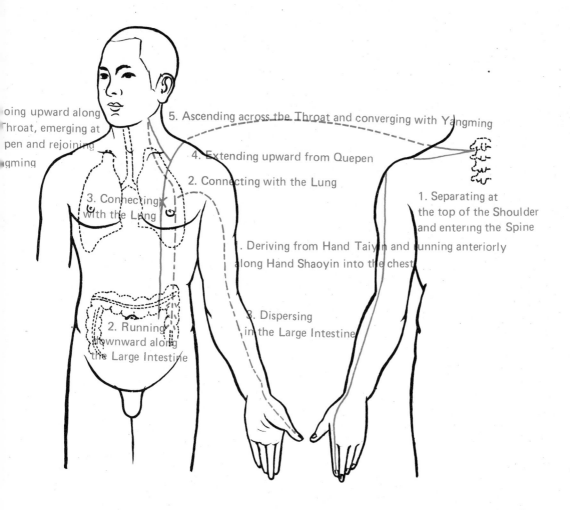

oing upward along Throat, emerging at pen and rejoining gming

5. Ascending across the Throat and converging with Yangming

4. Extending upward from Quepen

2. Connecting with the Lung

3. Connecting with the Lung

1. Separating at the top of the Shoulder and entering the Spine

. Deriving from Hand Taiyin and running anteriorly along Hand Shaoyin into the chest

2. Running downward along the Large Intestine

3. Dispersing in the Large Intestine

Fig. 27 The Schematic Diagram for the Divergent Meridians of Hand-Yangming and Hand-Taiyin

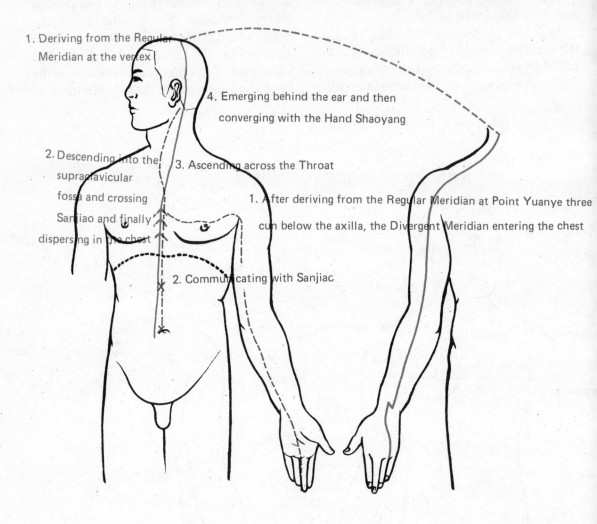

1. Deriving from the Regular Meridian at the vertex

4. Emerging behind the ear and then converging with the Hand Shaoyang

2. Descending into the supraclavicular fossa and crossing Sanjiao and finally dispersing in the chest

3. Ascending across the Throat

1. After deriving from the Regular Meridian at Point Yuanye three cun below the axilla, the Divergent Meridian entering the chest

2. Communicating with Sanjiao

Fig. 28 Divergent Meridians of Hand-Shaoyang and Hand-Jueyin

the back. The major collateral of the spleen disperses in the chest and hypochondrium. All the collaterals possess the function of transporting qi to different parts of the body. Besides, there are many smaller branches and subbranches which are called Minute Collaterals and Superficial Collaterals respectively. These Minute and Superficial Collaterals are distributed all over the body, possessing the function of transporting qi and blood to the body surface.

1.   The Three Yin Collaterals of Hand

1) The Collateral of the Lung Meridian of Hand Taiyin   It arises from Lieque (L 7) and runs to the Large Intestine Meridian of Hand Yangming. Another branch follows the Lung Meridian of Hand Taiyin into the palm of the hand and spreads through the thenar eminence. (See Fig. 29)

2) The Collateral of the Heart Meridian of Hand Shaoyin   It branches out at Tongli (H 5). One cun above the transverse crease of the wrist, it connects with the Small Intestine Meridian of Hand Taiyang. About one and a half cun above the wrist, it again follows the meridian and enters the heart; it then runs to the root of the tongue and connects with the eye. (See Fig. 29)

3) The Collateral of Pericardium Meridian of Hand Jueyin   It begins from Neiguan (P 6). Two cun above the wrist, disperses between the two tendons and runs along the Pericardium Meridian to the Pericardium, and finally connects with the heart. (See Fig. 29)

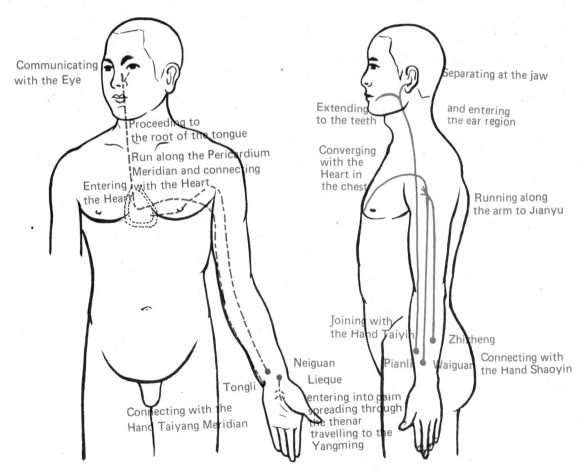

Fig. 29 The Three Yin Collaterals of Hand and Three Yang Collaterals of Hand

2. The Three Yang Collaterals of Hand

1) The Collateral of the Large Intestine Meridian of Hand Yangming It starts from Pianli (L I 6) and joins the Lung Meridian of Hand Taiyin three cun above the wrist. Another branch runs along the arm to Jianyu (L I 15), crosses the jaw and extends to the teeth. Still another branch derives at the jaw and enters the ear to join the Chong Meridian. (See Fig. 29)

2) The Collateral of the Small Intestine Meridian of Hand Taiyang It originates from Zhizheng (S I 7). Five cun above the wrist, it connects with the Heart Meridian. Another branch runs upward, crosses the elbow and connects with Jianyu (L I 15). (See Fig. 29)

3) The Collateral of the Sanjiao Meridian of Hand Shaoyang It arises from Waiguan (S J 5), two cun above the dorsum of the wrist, it travels up the posterior aspect of the arm and over the shoulder, disperses in the chest, converging with the Pericardium Meridian. (See Fig. 29)

3. The Three Yang Collaterals of Foot

1) The Collateral of the Stomach Meridian of Foot Yangming It starts from Fenglong (S 40), eight cun above the external malleolus, it connects with the Spleen Meridian. A branch runs along the lateral aspect of the tibia upward to the top of the head, and converges with the other Yang Meridians on the head and neck. From there it runs downward to connect with the throat. (See Fig. 30)

2) The Collateral of the Bladder Meridian of Foot Taiyang It arises from Feiyang (B 58), seven cun above the external malleolus, it connects with the Kidney Meridian.

3) The Collateral of the Gallbladder Meridian of Foot Shaoyang It begins from Guangming (G 37), five cun above the external malleolus, it joins the Liver Meridian, and then runs downward and disperses over the dorsum of the foot. (See Fig. 30)

4. The Three Yin Collaterals of Foot

1) The Collateral of the Spleen Meridian of Foot Taiyin It branches out at Gongsun (Sp 4), one cun posterior to the base of the first metatarsal bone, and then joins the Stomach Meridian. A branch runs upward to the abdomen and connects with the stomach and intestines. (See Fig. 30)

2) The Collateral of the Kidney Meridian of Foot Shaoyin It originates from Dazhong (K 4) on the posterior aspect of internal malleolus, it crosses the heel, and joins the Bladder Meridian. A branch follows the Kidney Meridian upward to a point below the pericardium and then pierces through the lumbar vertebrae.

3) The Collateral of the Liver Meridian of Foot Jueyin It starts from Ligou (Liv 5), five cun above the internal malleolus and connects with the Gallbladder Meridian. A branch runs up the leg to the genitals. (See Fig. 30)

5. The Collaterals of the Ren and Du Meridians and the Major Collateral of the Spleen

1) The Collateral of the Ren Meridian It separates from the Du Meridian at the lower end of the sternum. From Jiuwei (Ren 15), it spreads over the abdomen. (See Fig. 31)

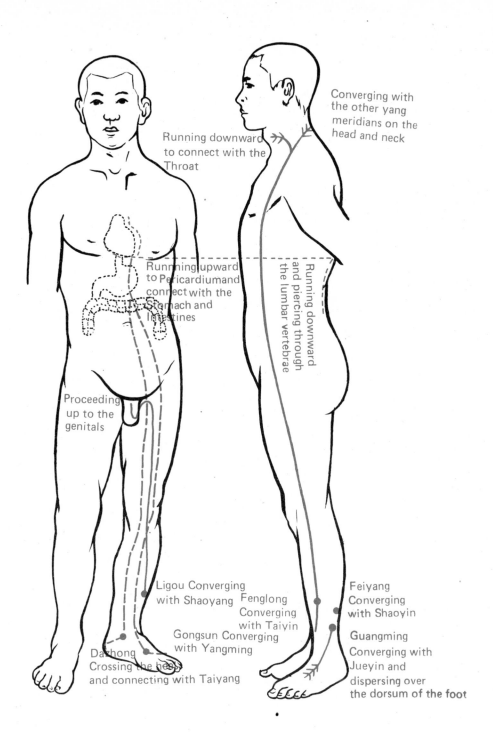

Converging with
the other yang
meridians on the
head and neck

Running downward
to connect with the
Throat

Running downward
and piercing through
the lumbar vertebrae

Running upward
to Pericardiumand
connect with the
Stomach and
Intestines

Proceeding
up to the
genitals

Ligou Converging
with Shaoyang

Fenglong
Converging
with Taiyin

Gongsun Converging
with Yangming

Dazhong
Crossing the heel
and connecting with Taiyang

Feiyang
Converging
with Shaoyin

Guangming
Converging with
Jueyin and
dispersing over
the dorsum of the foot

Fig. 30 The Three Yang Collaterals of Foot and Three Yin Collaterals of Foot

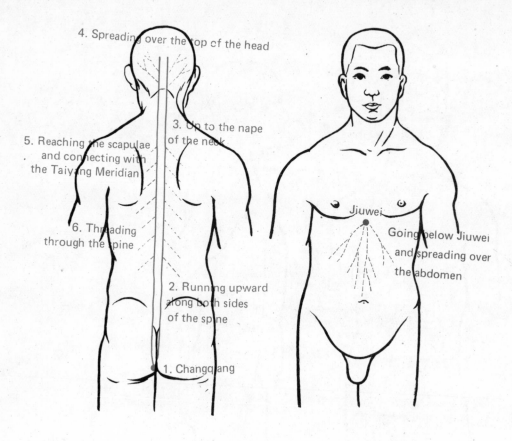

4. Spreading over the top of the head

5. Reaching the scapulae and connecting with the Taiyang Meridian

3. Up to the nape of the neck

6. Threading through the spine

2. Running upward along both sides of the spine

1. Changqiang

Jiuwei

Going below Jiuwei and spreading over the abdomen

Fig. 31 The Collaterals of Ren and Du Meridians

2) The Collateral of Du Meridian It arises from Changqiang (Du 1)in the perineum, runs upward along both sides of the spine to the nape, and spreads over the top of the head. When it gets to the scapular regions, it connects with the Bladder Meridian and pierces through the spine. (See Fig. 31)

3) The Major Collateral of the Spleen It begins from Dabao (Sp 21), emerges at three cun below Yuanye (G 22) and spreads through the chest and hypochondriac region, gathering the blood all over the body. (See Fig. 32)

V. THE TWELVE MUSCLE REGIONS AND TWELVE CUTANEOUS REGIONS

The muscle regions and cutaneous regions are the sites where the qi and blood of the meridians nourish the muscles, tendons and skin. Similar to the twelve regular meridians, they are also divided into three hand yin and three hand yang, three foot yin and three foot yang. The muscle regions are deeply distributed under the skin, while the cutaneous regions are located in the superficial layers of the skin. As cutaneous regions cover an extensive area, they are generally known as cutaneous regions of six meridians.

1.   The Twelve Muscle Regions

The twelve Muscle Regions, the conduits which distribute the qi and blood of the twelve regular meridians to nourish the muscles, possess the function of connecting all the bones and joints of the body and maintaining the normal range of motion. The distribution is described as follows:

The Muscle Regions originate from the extremities of the limbs and ascend to the head and trunk, but do not reach zang and fu organs. Thus, they are not related to the zang-fu organs, and flow of qi and blood. The three yang Muscle Regions of the foot are distributed in the anterior, lateral and posterior aspects of the trunk, all connecting with the eyes; the three yin Muscle Regions of the foot connect with the genital region; the three yang Muscle Regions of the hand connect with the angle of forehead; the three

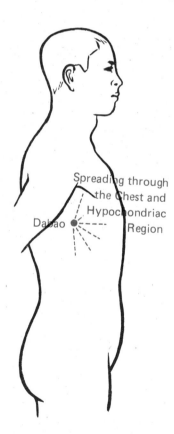

Fig. 32 The Major Collateral of the Spleen

yin Muscle Regions of the hand connect with the thoracic cavity. In the treatment of diseases, the Muscle Regions are mainly indicated in muscular problems, such as the Bi syndrome, contracture, stiffness, spasm and muscular atrophy. In Chapter 13 of *Miraculous Pivot,* it says, "Where there is pain, there is an acupoint." That means muscle problems can be treated by needling the local points.

1) Three Yang Muscle Regions of Foot

a) Muscle Region of Foot Taiyang (Bladder) It starts from the little toe, ascends to knot at external malleolus and then at the knee. A lower branch separates below the external malleolus, extending to the heel, and runs upward to knot at the lateral aspect of the popliteal fossa. Another branch starts at the convergence of the medial and lateral heads of the gastrocnemius muscle and ascends to knot at the medial side of the popliteal fossa. These two branches join in the gluteal region and then ascend along the side of the spine to the nape, where a branch enters the root of the tongue. Above the neck, the straight portion knots with the occipital bone and crosses over the top of the head to knot at the nose bridge. A branch spreads around the eye and knots at the side of below the nose. Another branch extends from the lateral side of the posterior axillary fold to knot with Jianyu (L I 15). Another branch enters the chest below the axilla, emerges from the supraclavicular fossa and then knots at Wangu (G 12) behind the ear. Still, another branch emerges from the supraclavicular fossa and traverses the face to come out beside the nose. (See Fig. 33)

b) Muscle Region of Foot Shaoyang (Gallbladder) It originates from the fourth toe, knots with the external malleolus. Then it ascends along the lateral side of the tibia where it knots with the knee. A branch begins at the upper part of the fibula and continues upward along the thigh. One of its subbranches runs anteriorly, knotting above Futu (S 32). Another subbranch runs posteriorly and knots with the sacrum. The straight branch ascends across the ribs, dispersing around and anterior to the axilla, connecting first at the breast region and then knottinᵍ at Quepen (S 12). Another branch extends from the axilla upward across the clavicle, emerging in front of the Foot Taiyang (Bladder) Muscle Region where it continues upward behind the ear to the temple. Then, it proceeds up to the vertex to join its bilateral counterpart. A branch descends from the temple across the cheek and then knots beside the bridge of the nose. A subbranch knots with the outer canthus. (See Fig. 34)

c) Muscle Region of Foot Yangming (Stomach) It arises from the second, middle and fourth toes, knots at the dorsum of the foot, and ascends obliquely along the lateral aspect of the leg where it disperses at the tibia and then knots at the lateral aspect of the knee. Ascending directly to knot at the hip joint, it extends to the lower ribs to connect with the spine. The straight branch runs along the tibia and knots at the knee. A subbranch connects with the fibula, and joins with the Foot Shaoyang (Gallbladder). From the knee, it ascends across the thigh and knots in the pelvic region. Dispersing upward on the abdomen and knotting at Quepen (S 12), it extends to the neck and mouth, meeting at the side of the nose and knotting below the nose. Above, it joins with the Foot Taiyang (Bladder) to form a muscular net around the eye. A subbranch separates at the jaw and knots in front of the ear. (See Fig. 35)

2) Three Yin Muscle Regions of Foot

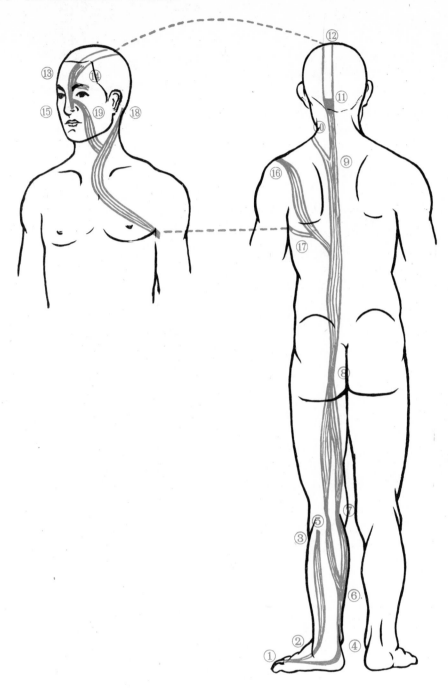

Fig. 33 Muscle Region of Foot-Taiyang

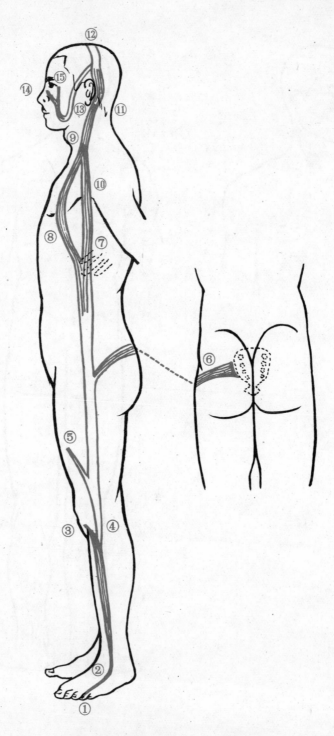

Fig. 34 Muscle Region of Foot-Shaoyang

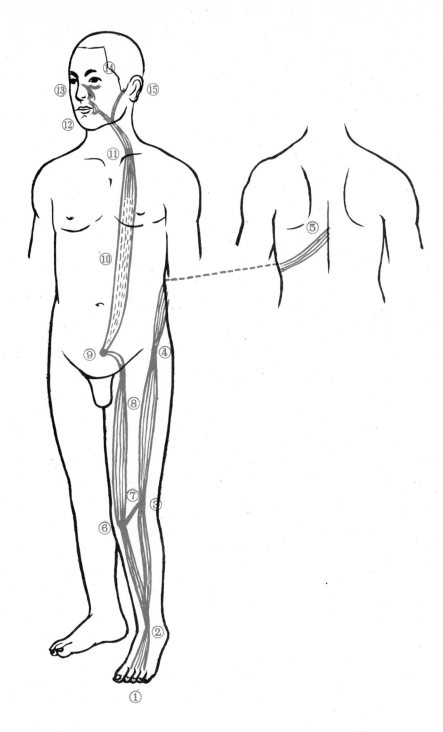

Fig. 35 Muscle Region of Foot-Yangming

a) Muscle Region of Foot Taiyin (Spleen) It starts from the medial side of the big toe and knots at the internal malleolus. Continuing upward and knotting at the medial side of the knee, it traverses the medial aspect of the thigh, and knots at the hip. Then it joins with the external genitalia and extends to the abdomen, knotting with the umbilicus. From there, it enters the abdominal cavity, knots with the ribs, and disperses through the chest. An internal branch adheres to the spine. (See Fig. 36)

b) Muscle Region of Foot Jueyin (Liver) It originates from the dorsum of the big toe and knots anterior to the internal malleolus. Then it runs upward along the medial side of the tibia and knots at the lower, medial aspect of the knee. From there, it runs upward along the medial aspect of the thigh to the genital region, where it converges with other Muscle Regions. (See Fig. 37)

c) Muscle Region of Foot Shaoyin (Kidney) It begins beneath the little toe. Together with the Muscle Region of Foot Taiyin, it runs obliquely below the internal malleolus and knots at the heel, converging with Muscle Region of Foot Taiyang (Bladder), knotting at the lower, medial aspect of the knee, it joins with Muscle Region of Foot Taiyin (Spleen) and ascends along the medial aspect of the thigh to knot at the genital region. A branch proceeds upward along the side of the spine to the nape and knots with the occipital bone, converging with the Muscle Region of Foot Taiyang (Bladder). (See Fig. 38)

3) Three Hand Yang Muscle Regions
a) Muscle Region of Hand Taiyang (Small Intestine) It starts from the tip of the small finger, knots at the dorsum of the wrist, and proceeds up along the forearm to knot at the medial condyle of the humerus in the elbow. Then it continues up along the arm and knots below the axilla. A branch runs behind the axilla, curves around the scapula and emerges in front of the Foot Taiyang (Bladder) on the neck, knotting behind the ear. A branch separates behind the auricle and enters the ear. Emerging above the auricle, the straight branch descends across the face and knots beneath the mandible, then continues upward to link the outer canthus. Another branch starts at the mandible, ascends around the teeth and in front of the ear, connects the outer canthus and knots at the angle of the forehead. (See Fig. 39)

b) Muscle Region of Hand Shaoyang (Sanjiao) It starts from the extremity of the fourth finger and knots at the dorsum of the wrist. Then, it ascends along the forearm and knots at the olecranon of the elbow. Proceeding upward along the lateral aspect of the upper arm, it crosses the shoulder and the neck, then converges with the Muscle Region of Hand Taiyang (Small Intestine). A branch splits out at the angle of the mandible and connects with the root of the tongue. Another branch proceeds upward in front of the ear to the outer canthus, then crosses the temple and connects at the corner of the forehead. (See Fig. 40)

c) Muscle Region of Hand Yangming (Large Intestine) It begins from the extremity of the index finger and knots at the dorsum of the wrist. Then it goes upward along the forearm, and knots at the lateral aspect of the elbow. Continuing up the arm, it knots at Jianyu (L I 15). A branch moves around the scapula and attaches to the spine. The straight branch continues from Jianyu (L I 15) to the neck, where a branch separates and knots at the side of the nose. The straight branch continues upward and emerges in front of Muscle Meridian of Hand Taiyang (Small Intestine). Then it

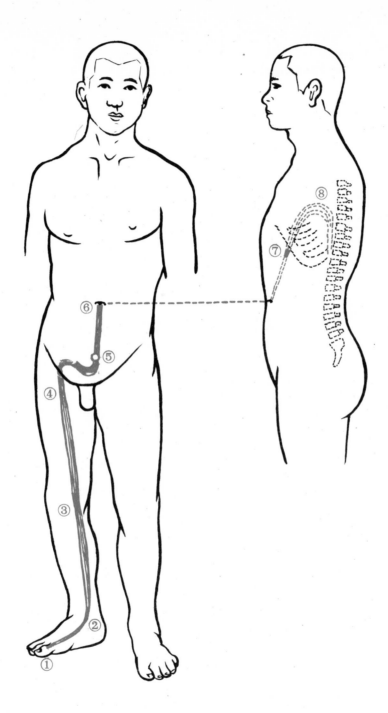

Fig. 36 Muscle Region of Foot-Taiyin

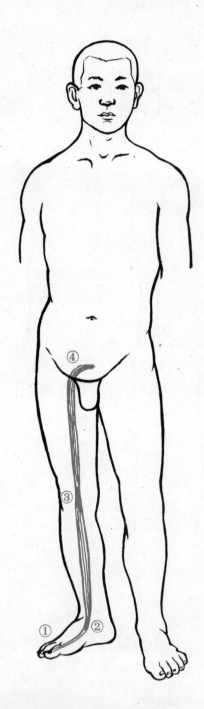

Fig. 37 Muscle Region of Foot-Jueyin

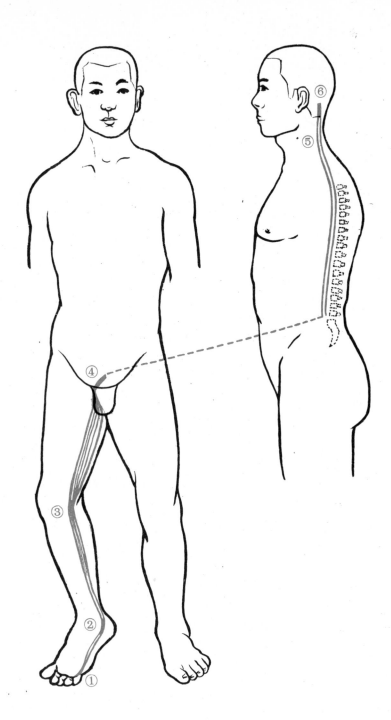

Fig. 38　Muscle Region of Foot-Shaoyin

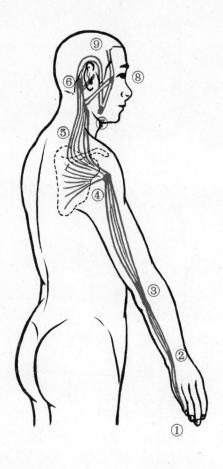

Fig. 39 Muscle Region от Hand-Taiyang

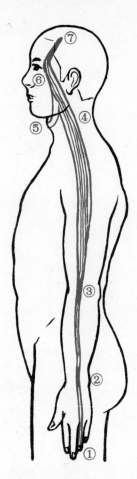

Fig. 40 Muscle Region of Hand-Shaoyang

crosses over the head, connecting at the mandible on the opposite side of the face. (See Fig. 41)

4) Three Hand Yin Muscle Regions

a) Muscle Region of Hand Taiyin (Lung) It arises from the tip of the thumb and knots at the lower thenar eminence. Proceeding up laterally to the pulse and along the forearm, it knots at the elbow, then ascends along the medial aspect of the arm and enters the chest below the axilla. Emerging from Quepen (S 12), it knots anteriorly to Jianyu (L I 15).

Above, it knots with the clavicle, and below it knots in the chest, dispersing over the diaphragm and converging again at the lowest rib. (See Fig. 42)

b) Muscle Region of Hand Jueyin (Pericardium) It arises from the palmar aspect of the middle finger and follows the Muscle Region of Hand Taiyin (Lung) upward. It first knots at the medial aspect of the elbow, and afterwards below the axilla. Then it descends, dispersing at the front and back sides of the ribs. A branch enters the chest below the axilla and spreads over the

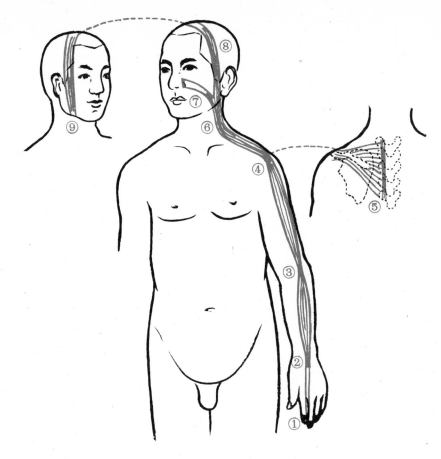

Fig. 41 Muscle Region of Hand-Yangming

chest, knotting in the thoracic diaphragm. (See Fig. 43)

c) Muscle Region of Hand Shaoyin (Heart)   It begins from the medial side of the small finger, knots first at the pisiform bone of the hand, and afterward at the medial aspect of the elbow. Continuing upward and entering the chest below the axilla, it crosses the Muscle Region of Hand Taiyin (Lung) in the breast region and knots in the chest. Then it descends across the thoracic diaphragm to connect with the umbilicus. (See Fig. 44)

2. The Twelve Cutaneous Regions

The twelve cutaneous regions refer to the sites through which the qi and blood of the meridians are transfered to the body surface. In the ancient medical classics in Chapter 56 of *Plain Questions,* it says, "The Cutaneous Regions are the part of meridian system located in the superficial layers of the body. The Cutaneous Regions are marked by the regular meridians." In other words, the cutaneous regions are

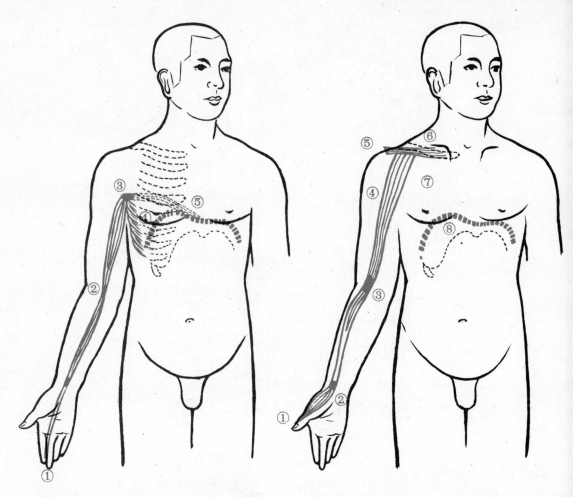

Fig. 43 Muscle Region of Hand-Jueyin   Fig. 42 Muscle Region of Hand-Taiyin

twelve distinct areas on the body surface within the domains of the twelve regular meridians. It is also known as cutaneous regions of six meridians when the Hand and Foot meridians are combined into six pairs. Since the cutaneous regions are the most superficial part of the body tissues, they bear the protective function of the organism. When this function is lost, the exogenous pathogen may penetrate the skin to invade the collaterals and gain access to meridians and zang-fu organs. In Chapter 56 of *Plain Questions*, it says, "Skin is the place where the meridians are distributed. When the pathogen attacks the skin, the sweat pores will open, and then the pathogen may advance toward the collaterals, meridians and zang-fu organs through the sweat pore." The transmitting order of a disease is: Skin — collaterals — meridians — zang organs — fu organs. Conversely, symptoms and signs of internal diseases can also be

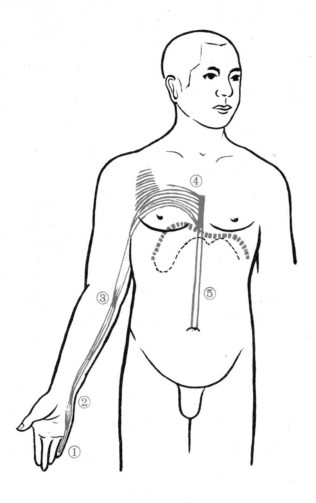

Fig. 44 Muscle Region of Hand-Shaoyin

projected onto the skin through meridians and collaterals. It says again in Chapter 56 of *Plain Questions*, "Blue-coloured skin signifies local pain. Dark-coloured skin indicates blockage of qi and blood. Yellow to red coloured skin refers to heat syndromes, and white coloured skin to cold syndromes." Obviously, colour changes of the skin can tell presence of internal disorders. Therapeutically, the cutaneous regions of paired meridians are interactive. There are meridians of Hand-Yangming and Foot-Yangming. The meridian of Hand-Yangming starts at the hand and goes to the head, while the meridian of Foot-Yangming originates in the head and runs to the foot. They are diagnostically and therapeutically interactive.

Chapter 6

AN INTRODUCTION TO ACUPOINTS

Acupoints are the specific sites through which the qi of the zang-fu organs and meridians is transported to the body surface. The Chinese characters "腧穴" for an acupoint mean respectively "transportation" and "hole." In the medical literature of the past dynasties, acupoints, the sites where acupuncture treatment is applied, have other terms such as "qi point" and "aperture." Acupoints are not only the pathways for the circulation of qi and blood, but also the loci of response to diseases. In acupuncture and moxibustion treatment, proper techniques are applied on the acupoints to regulate the functional activities of the body, strengthen body resistence so as to prevent and treat diseases. Medical practitioners of past ages have left plentiful recordings describing the locations and indications of acupoints, formulating a systematical theory.

I. CLASSIFICATION AND NOMENCLATURE OF ACUPOINTS

1. Classification of Acupoints

There are numerous acupoints distributed over the human body. A great deal of work has been accomplished by medical workers in the past to generalize and systematize acupoints, which have been classified either "by meridians" or "by body parts." Generally speaking, acupoints fall into the following three categories in terms of their evolution.

1) Acupoints of the fourteen meridians Also known as "regular points," acupoints of the fourteen meridians are distributed along the twelve regular meridians, the Du (Governor Vessel) and the Ren (Conception Vessel) Meridians, totally amounting to 361. According to ancient medical records, the acupoints of this category are the crystallization of rich clinical experience of medical workers in the past. All the points in this category can be used to treat disorders of the related meridians and collaterals. They are the most commonly used points and form the main part of all acupoints. Those of the twelve regular meridians are distributed symmetrically in pairs on the left and right sides of the body, while those of the Du and the Ren Meridians are single ones, aligning on the posterior and anterior midlines respectively.

2) Extraordinary Points Extraordinary points are named "extra points" in short. They are experiential points with specific names and definite locations, but are not attributed to the fourteen meridians. They are effective in the treatment of certain diseases. Although scattered over the body, they are still related to the meridians system, for example, Yintang (Extra 1) is related to the Du Meridian, Lanwei (Extra 18) to the Stomach Meridian of Foot-Yangming. A survey of the ancient acupuncture literature has revealed that some regular points were developed from the extraordinary points. Examples are Gaohuang (B 43), which was added to the regular points in *Illustrated Manual of Acupoints on the Bronze Figure* and Meichong (B 3), which was added to the regular points in *Classic of Health-Promoting Acupuncture*. Both were formerly extraordinary points. Therefore, extraordinary points are said to be the preceding counterparts of regular points. Clinically, they are the supplement to regular points.

3) Ashi Points   Ashi Points are also called "reflexing points," "unfixed points" or "tender spots." Chapter 13 of *Miraculous Pivot* says, "Tender spots can be used as acupoints," and this was the primary method for point selection in early acupuncture and moxibustion treatments. Without specific names and definite locations, Ashi Points are considered to represent the earliest stage of acupoint evolution. Clinically, they are mostly used for pain syndromes.

2. Nomenclature of Acupoints

Acupoints of the fourteen meridians have their definite locations and names. It is stated in Chapter 5 of *Plain Questions*, "Acupoints are the sites into which qi and blood are infused. Each has its own location and name." *Precious Supplementary Prescriptions* further points out, "Each point is named with profound significance," which indicates that the name of each point has its own meaning.

Most of the acupoints are nominated by way of analogy. The flow of qi and blood is similized by that of water; the prominence and depression of the tendons and bones are compared to mountains and valleys; the characteristic local shape of the body is signified by certain animals or utensils; and the acupoint functions are analogized by architectural structures, astronomical or meteorological phenomena. Examples are as follows.

1) Names bearing analogy to water flow, mountains and valleys   Quchi (L I 11, Crooked Pond), Chize (L 5, Ulnar Marsh), Shaohai (H 3, Young Sea), Taiyuan (L 9, Great Deep Pool), Zhigou (S J 6, Limb Ditch), Jingqu (L 8, Channel Ditch), Sidu (S J 9, Four Rivers), Fuliu (K 7, Continuing Water Flow), Houxi (S I 3, Back Stream), Zhongzhu (S J 3, Middle Water Margin), Hegu (L I 4, Connected Valleys), Chengshan (B 57, Sustaining Mountain), Liangqiu (S 34, Hill Ridge), Qiuxu (G 40, Large Mound), Yanglingquan (G 34, Yang Mound Spring).

2) Names bearing analogy to animals, plants or utensils   Yuji (L 10, Fish Border), Dubi (S 35, Calf Nose), Jiuwei (Ren 15, Turtledove Tail), Futu (S 32, Prostrate Rabbit), Zanzhu (B 2, Assembled Bamboo), Dazhu (B 11, Large Shuttle), Jiache (S 6, Cheek Vehicle), Quepen (S 12, Depression Basin), Tianding (L I 17, Heavenly Cooking Vessel).

3) Names bearing analogy to architectural structure   Shenmen (H 7, Spiritual Gate), Qihu (S 13, Qi Gate), Yingchuang (S 16, Chest Window), Tianyou (S J 16, Heaven Window), Tiantu (Ren 22, Heaven Chimney), Quyuan (S I 13, Curved Wall), Tinggong (S I 19, Hearing Palace), Neiting

(S 44, Interior Courtyard), Zhongfu (L 1, Central Mansion), Qishe (S 11, Qi Residence), Dicang (S 4, Earth Granary), Kufang (S 14, Storehouse), Zhishi (B 52, Will Chamber), Yutang (Ren 18, Jade Palace), Bulang (K 22, Step Corridor), Lingtai (Du 10, Spirit Platform), Neiguan (P 6, Medial Pass), Juque (Ren 14, Great Palace Gate), Fengshi (G 31, Windy Fair),

Xiongxiang (Sp 19, Chest Village), Jianjing (G 21, Shoulder Well).

4) Names bearing analogy to astronomical and meteorological phenomena Riyue (G 24, Sun and Moon), Shangxing (Du 23, Upper Star), Taiyi (S 23, Grand Yi "the second of the ten Heavenly Stems"), Taibai (Sp 3, Venus), Xuanji (Ren 21, The 2nd and 3rd stars of the Big Dipper), Fengchi (G 20,

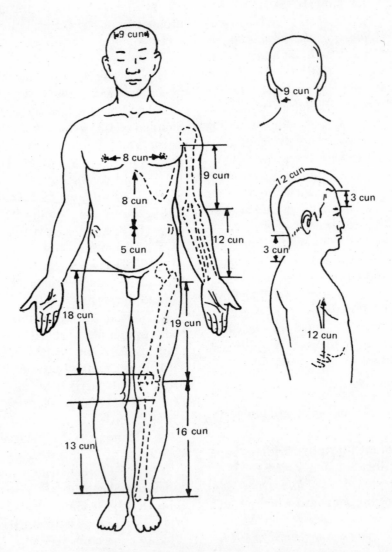

Fig. 45 The Running Course of the Meridian

Wind Pool), Yunmen (L 2, Cloud Door).

5) Points named according to anatomical terms   Zhongwan (Ren 12, Middle Stomach), Henggu (K 11, Pubis), Jianyu (L I 15, Shoulder Corner), Binao (L I 14, Arm Muscle Prominence), Zhouliao (L I 12, Elbow Foramen), Wangu (S I 4, Wrist Bone), Biguan (S 31, Thigh Joint), Juegu (G 39, External Malleolus).

6) Points named according to their therapeutic properties   Feishu (B 13, Lung Point), Guangming (G 37, Brightness), Chengqi (S I, Tear Receiver), Chengjiang (Ren 24, Fluid Receiver), Qihai (Ren 6, Sea of Qi), Xuehai (Sp 10, Sea of Blood), Guangyuan (Ren 4, Storage of Primary Qi), Jingming (B 1, Brightening Eyes), Yingxiang (L I 20, Welcome Fragrance).

II. METHODS OF LOCATING ACUPOINTS

Location of acupoints, whether accurate or not, will affect the therapeutic results. Great importance therefore has been attached to precise location of acupoints by medical practitioners in past ages.

In the chapter Lyrics of Acupuncture and Profundities of *Compendium of Acupuncture and Moxibustion*, it is said, "Methods of locating points are based on standard measurements. An acupuncturist should first of all have a clear idea of these measurements and patient's body build, and then observe the anatomical landmarks on the patient. Some points should be located with the limbs flexed, some with the body in a lying position...."

At present, commonly used in clinics are three methods of acupoint location, i.e.,

proportional measurement, anatomical landmarks, and finger measurement.

1. Proportional Measurements

The earliest record of proportional measurement can be found in Chapter 14 of *Miraculous Pivot*. In the light of this record, the width or length of various portions of the human body are divided respectively into definite numbers of equal units as the standards for the proportional measurement. These standards are applicable on any patient of different sexes, ages and body sizes. See Fig. 45 and Table 5 for details.

2. Anatomical Landmarks

Various anatomical landmarks on the body surface are the basis for locating points. Those landmarks fall into two categories.

1) Fixed landmarks   Fixed landmarks are those that would not change with body movement. They include the five sense organs, hair, nails, nipple, umbilicus, and prominence and depression of the bones. With them, it is easy to locate points. The proportional measurement is established on the basis of these anatomical landmarks. However, points that are adjacent to or on such landmarks can be located directly. Examples are Yintang (Extra 1) between the two eyebrows, Suliao (Du 25) on the tip of the nose, and Shenque (Ren 8) in the centre of the umbilicus.

2) Moving landmarks   Moving landmarks refer to those that will appear only when a body part keeps in a specific position. For instances, when the arm is

Table 5 Standards for Proportional Measurement

Body Part	Distance	Proportional Measurement	Method	Explanation
Head	From the anterior hairline to the posterior hairline	12 cun	Longitudinal measurement	The distance from the glabella to the anterior hairline is taken as 3 cun. The distance from Dazhui (Du 14) to the posterior hairline is taken as 3 cun. If the anterior and posterior hairlines are indistinguishable, the distance from the glabella to Dazhui (Du 14) then is taken as 18 cun.
	Between the two mastoid processes	9 cun	Transverse measurement	The transverse measurement is also used to localize other points on the head.
Chest and Abdomen	From the sternocostal angle to the centre of the umbilicus	8 cun	Longitudinal measurement	The longitudinal measurement of the chest and the hypochondriac region is generally based on the intercostal space.
	Between the centre of the umbilicus and the upper border of symphysis pubis	5 cun		
	Between the two nipples	8 cun	Transverse measurement	The distance between the bilateral Quepen (S 12) can be used as the substitute of the transverse measurement of the two nipples.
Back	Between the medial border of the scapula and the posterior midline	3 cun	Transverse measurement	The longitudinal measurement on the back is based on the spinous processes of the vertebral column. In clinical practice, the lower angle of the scapula is about at the same level of the 7th thoracic vertebra, the iliac spine is about at the same level of the 4th lumbar vertebra.

Continued

Region		cun		Notes
Lateral Side of the Chest	From the end of the axillary fold on the lateral side of the chest to the tip of the 11th rib	12 cun	Longitudinal measurement	
Upper Extremities	Between the end of the axillary fold and the transverse cubital crease	9 cun	Longitudinal measurement	Used for the three Yin and the three Yang Meridians of the Hand.
	Between the transverse cubital crease and the transverse wrist crease	12 cun		
	From the level of the upper border of symphysis pubis to the medial epicondyle of femur	18 cun	Longitudinal measurement	Used for the three Yin Meridians of the Foot.
Lower Extremities	From the lower border of the medial condyle of tibia to the tip of medial malleolus	13 cun		
	From the prominence of the great trochanter to the middle of patella	19 cun	Longitudinal measurement	1. Used for the three Yang Meridians of the Foot. 2. The distance from the gluteal crease to the centre of patella is taken as 14 cun. 3. The anterior level of the centre of the patella is about the same level of Dubi(S 35), and the posterior level, about the same level of Weizhong(B 40).
	Between the centre of patella and the tip of lateral malleolus	16 cun		
	From the tip of the lateral malleolus to the heel	3 cun		

flexed and the cubital crease appears, Quchi (L I 11) can be located; and when a fist is made and the transverse palmar crease appears, Houxi (S I 3) can be located. Also employed in clinic are some simple methods of point location. For example, to locate Baihui (Du 20) directly above the apexes of the ears, or Fengshi (G 31) when at attention.

3. Finger Measurement

The length and width of the patient's finger(s) are taken as a standard for point location. The following three methods are commonly used in clinic.

1) Middle finger measurement When the patient's middle finger is flexed, the distance between the two medial ends of the creases of the interphalangeal joints is taken as one cun. This method is employed for measuring the vertical distance to locate the limb points of the yang meridians, or for measuring the horizontal distance to locate the points on the back. (See Fig. 46)

also employed for measuring the vertical distance to locate the points on the limbs. (See Fig. 47)

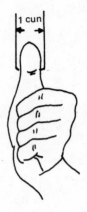

Fig. 47

3) Four-Finger Measurement The width of the four fingers. (index, middle, ring and little) close together at the level of the dorsal skin crease of the proximal interphalangeal joint of the middle finger is taken as three cun. It is used to locate the points on the limb and in the abdominal region. (See Fig. 48)

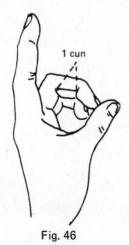

Fig. 46

2) Thumb Measurement The width of the interphalangeal joint of the patient's thumb is taken as one cun. The method is

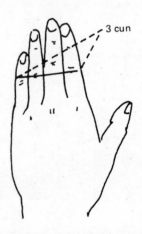

Fig. 48

III. SPECIFIC POINTS

Specific points refer to those of the fourteen meridians that have special properties and are grouped under special names. In view of their locations, they can be classified into two major groups: one on the limbs, and the other one on the head and the trunk.

1. Specific Points on the Limbs

1) Five Shu Points Each of the twelve regular meridians has, below the elbow or knee, five specific points, namely, Jing-Well, Ying-Spring, Shu-Stream, Jing-River and He-Sea, which are termed Five Shu points in general. They are situated in the above order from the distal extremities to the elbow or knee. It is said in the first chapter of *Miraculous Pivot* that "the qi of the twelve regular meridians and fifteen collaterals flow all over the body. The flow of qi running in the meridians from the extremities to the elbow or knee is flourishing gradually." The names of the five shu points image the flow of meridian qi as the flow of water. The Jing-Well point is situated in the place where the meridian qi starts to bubble. The Ying-Spring point is where the meridian qi starts to gush. The Shu-Stream point is where the meridian qi flourishes. The Jing-River point is where the meridian qi is pouring abundantly. Finally, the He-Sea point signifies the confluence of rivers in the sea, where the meridian qi is the most flourishing.

In addition, each of the six fu organs has another He-Sea point in the three yang meridians of the foot, known as the Lower He-Sea point. Chapter 4 of *Miracular Pivot* says, "The Lower He-Sea Points of the stomach, large intestine, small intestine, sanjiao, bladder and gallbladder are Zusanli (S 36), Shangjuxu (S 37), Xiajuxu (S 39), Weiyang (B 39), Weizhong (B 40) and Yanglingquan (G 34) respectively. Among these points, Zusanli (S 36), Weizhong (B 40) and Yanglingquan (G 34) overlap with the relevant He-Sea points in the Five Shu points. The Lower He-Sea points are mostly employed to treat the disorders of the six fu organs in clinic.

2) Yuan-Primary Points Each of the twelve regular meridians has a Yuan-Primary Point, which is located on the limbs. The Chinese character "原" (yuan) means primary qi in this context. The chapter "The 66th Medical Problem" in *Classic of Medical Problems* describes the relation between the Yuan-Primary Points and Yuan-Primary Qi.

The Yuan-Primary Qi, originating below the umbilicus and between the kidneys, is dispersed to the zang-fu organs and further to the limbs via Sanjiao. The sites where the Yuan-Primary Qi is retained are Yuan-Primary Points, which are used to treat disorders of the zang-fu organs. In the yin meridians, the Yuan-Primary Points overlap with the Shu-Stream Points of the Five Shu Points. Each yang meridian, however, has its Yuan-Primary Point other than the Shu-Stream Point.

3) Luo-Connecting Points Each of twelve regular meridians has, on the limbs, a Luo-Connecting Point to link its exteriorly-interiorly related meridian. Each of the Du and Ren meridians, and the Major Collateral of the Spleen has its Luo-Connecting Point on the trunk. They are termed "the Fifteen Luo-Connecting

Points." A Luo-Connecting Point is used to treat disorders involving the two exteriorly-interiorly related meridians and those in the area supplied by the two meridians.

4) Xi-Cleft Points The Xi-Cleft Point is the site where the qi and blood of the meridian are deeply converged. Each of the twelve regular meridians and the four extra meridians (Yinqiao, Yangqiao, Yinwei and Yangwei) has a Xi-Cleft Point on the limbs, amounting to sixteen in all. The Xi-Cleft Point is used to treat acute disorders in the area supplied by its pertaining meridian and those of its pertaining zang or fu organ.

5) Eight Confluent Points Eight Confluent Points refer to the eight points on the limbs where the regular meridians communicate with the eight extra meridians. They are Neiguan (P 6), Gongsun (Sp 4), Houxi (S I 3), Shenmai (B 62), Waiguan (S J 5), Zulinqi (G 41), Lieque (L 7) and Zhaohai (K 6), which are respectively connected with the Yinwei, Chong, Du, Yangqiao, Yangwei, Dai, Ren and Yinqiao Meridians. The Eight Confluent Points are used to treat a variety of disorders of the corresponding eight extra meridians.

2. Specific Points on the Head and Trunk

1) Back-Shu Points Back-Shu Points are specific points on the back where the qi of the respective zang-fu organs is infused. It is stated in Chapter 51 of *Miraculous Pivot* that "in the Back-Shu Points you are looking for the reactionary spots of tenderness and soreness, or the points on which pressure exerted relieves pain and discomforts of the patient." Situated close to their respectively related zang-fu organs, the Back-Shu points

present abnormal reactions to the dysfunction of their corresponding zang-fu organs. They are often used for disorders of the internal organs.

2) Front-Mu Points Front-Mu points are those points on the chest and abdomen where the qi of the respective zang-fu organs is infused and converged. Located close to their corresponding zang-fu organs, the Front-Mu points play a significant role in the diagnosis and treatment of the disorders of the internal organs.

3) Crossing Points Crossing points are those at the intersections of two or more meridians. Distributed mainly on the head, face and trunk, and amounting to over ninety in total. They are key points used to treat meridian disorders of the areas where they are located.

Appendix

Eight Influential Points

The Eight Influential Points are first recorded in the chapter "The 45th Medical Problem" of *Classic on Medical Problems*. They are Zhangmen (Liv 13), Zhongwan (Ren 12), Yanglingquan (G 34), Juegu, or Xuanzhong (G 39), Geshu (B 17), Dazhu (B 11), Taiyuan (L 9), and Tanzhong (Ren 17), which respectively dominate the zang organs, fu organs, qi, blood, tendon, vessel, bone and marrow. They coincide with some other specific points. Clinically, the corresponding Influential Point can be employed to treat disorders of the zang organs, fu organs, qi, blood, tendon, vessel, bone or marrow.

IV. AN OUTLINE OF THE THERAPEUTIC PROPERTIES OF THE POINTS OF THE FOURTEEN MERIDIANS

The therapeutic properties of the points of the fourteen meridians are generalized on the basis of the principle that the course of a meridian is amenable to treatment. Each of the points has its own therapeutic feature owing to its particular location and pertaining meridian. Generally speaking, however, all the points can be used to treat disorders of the areas where they are located, and those adjacent to their location. These are known respectively as the local and adjacent points with therapeutic properties. In addition, some of the points can be used to treat disorders of the areas far away from where they are located. These are known as the remote or distal points with therapeutic properties.

1. The Remote Therapeutic Properties of the Points

The remote therapeutic properties of the points form a major regularity which is established on the basis of the meridian theory. Among the points of the fourteen meridians, those located on the limbs, especially below the elbow and knee joints, are effective not only for local disorders but also for disorders of the remote zang-fu organs and tissues on the course of their pertaining meridians. Some even have systemic therapeutic properties. For example, Lieque (L 7) treats disorders not only on the upper limbs but also in the vertex, chest, lung and throat as well as exogeneous diseases; Yanglingquan (G 34)

is effective not only for diseases of the lower limbs but also for hypochondrium, biliary, hepatic, and mental disorders as well as tendon abnormalities such as spasm and convulsion. For detailed information, see Table 6.

2. The Local and Adjacent Therapeutic Properties of the Points

All the points in the body share a common feature in terms of their therapeutic properties, namely, all have local and adjacent therapeutic properties. Each point located on a particular site is able to treat disorders of this area and of nearby organs. For example, Yingxiang (L I 20) and Kouheliao (L I 19) located beside the nose, and the neighboring points Shangxing (Du 23), Tongtian (B 7) can all be effective to nasal disorders. Zhongwan (Ren 12) and Liangmen (S 21) located in the epigastric region, and the nearby points Zhangmen (Liv 13) and Qihai (Ren 6) are used for gastric disorders. The therapeutic properties of the points on the head, face and trunk are judged according to this principle, so are those of the points on both the Ren and Du meridians and those of the points situated bilaterally along the above two extra meridians. Owing to the special distribution of the Ren and Du meridians, their points have more systemic influence. The local and adjacent therapeutic properties of the points on the head, face and trunk are generalized in Table 7.

The remote, adjacent, and local therapeutic property of these points are determined by how far away their effects reach from the location of points themselves. The therapeutic properties, remote, adjacent, or local points, are nevertheless characterized

Table 6. Indications of Points of the Extremities with Relation to Meridians.

Name of the Meridian \ Indications	Meridian	Indications of Individual Meridian	Indications of Two Meridians in Common	Indications of Three Meridians in Common
The Three Yin Meridians of Hand	The Lung Meridian of Hand-Taiyin	Disorders of the lung and throat		Disorders of Chest
	The Pericardium Meridian of Hand-Jueyin	Disorders of the heart and stomach	Mental illness	
	The Heart Meridian of Hand-Shaoyin	Disorders of the heart		
The Three Yang Meridian of Hand	The Large Intestine Meridian of Hand-Yangming	Disorders of the forehead, face, nose, mouth and teeth		Disorders of the eye, throat and febrile diseases
	The Sanjiao Meridian of Hand-Shaoyang	Disorders of the temporal and hypochondriac regions	Disorders of the ear	
	The Small Intestine Meridian of Hand-Taiyang	Disorders of the occipital region and scapular region and mental illness		
The Three Yang Meridians of Foot	The Stomach Meridian of Foot-Yangming	Disorders of the face, mouth, teeth, throat, stomach and intestine		Mental illness, febrile diseases
	The Gallbladder Meridian of Foot-Shaoyang	Disorders of the ear, temporal and hypochondriac regions	Disorders of the eyes	

		Disorders of the external genitalia, gynaecological diseases
	The Gallbladder Meridian of Foot-Taiyang	Disorders of the neck, dorso-lumbar region. (Back-Shu Points also for zang-fu disorders.)
	The Spleen Meridian of Foot-Taiyin	Disorders of the spleen and stomach
The Three Yin Meridians of Foot	The Liver Meridian of Foot-Jueyin	Disorders of the liver
	The Kidney Meridian of Foot-Shaoyin	Disorders of the kidney, lung and throat

Indications of Ren and Du Meridians

Meridian	Indications of Individual Meridian	Indications of Two Meridians In Common
Ren Meridian	Prolapse of Yang, collapse. (It is also for general tonification.)	Disorders of zang-fu organs, mental illness, gynaecological disorders
Du Meridian	Apoplexy, coma, febrile diseases, disorders of the head and face	

by functional regulation. Clinical practice has proven that puncturing certain points may bring forth biphasic regulation on diversified functional abnormalities of the body. For instance, puncturing Tianshu (S 25) relieves both diarrhea and constipation; puncturing Neiguan (P 6) corrects both tachycardia and bradycardia. In addition to the general therapeutic properties of points, clinical attention should also be paid to the special therapeutic properties of some points. Examples are Dazhui (Du 14), which has an antipyretic effect, and Zhiyin (B 67),

which is indicated in malposition of a fetus.

To summarize all the points of a particular meridian are indicated in the disorders of that particular meridian. Points of the exteriorly-interiorly related meridians can be combined to treat disorders of those meridians. Neighbouring points will have similar therapeutic properties. The therapeutic properties of the points on the limbs should be catagorized meridian by meridian, those points of the head, face and trunk, should be recognized in light of their locations.

Table 7. Indications of Points on the Head, Face and Trunk with Relation to Their Locations

Locations of Points	Indications
Head, face, neck	Disorders of the brain, eye, ear, nose, mouth, teeth and throat
Chest, upper dorsal region (corresponding to the region between the 1st and 7th thoracic vertebrae)	Disorders of the lung and heart
Upper abdomen, lower dorsal region (corresponding to the region between the 8th thoracic and the 1st lumbar vertebrae)	Disorders of the liver, gallbladder, spleen and stomach
Lower abdomen, lumbosacral region (corresponding to the region between the 2nd lumbar and the 4th sacral vertebrae)	Disorders of the kidney, intestine, bladder and genital organs

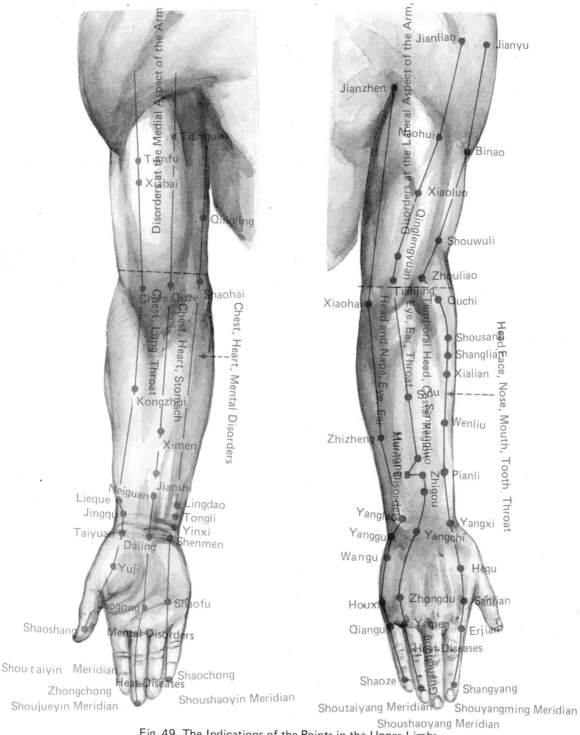

Fig. 49 The Indications of the Points in the Upper Limbs

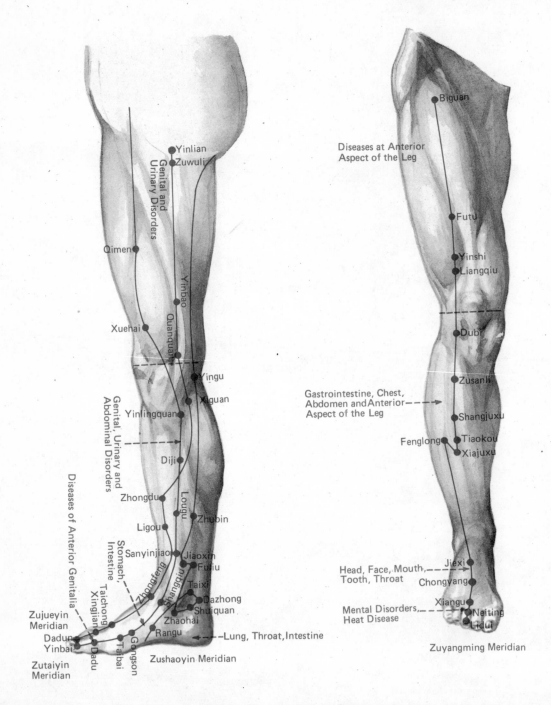

Fig. 50 The Therapeutic Properties of the Points at the Lower Limbs

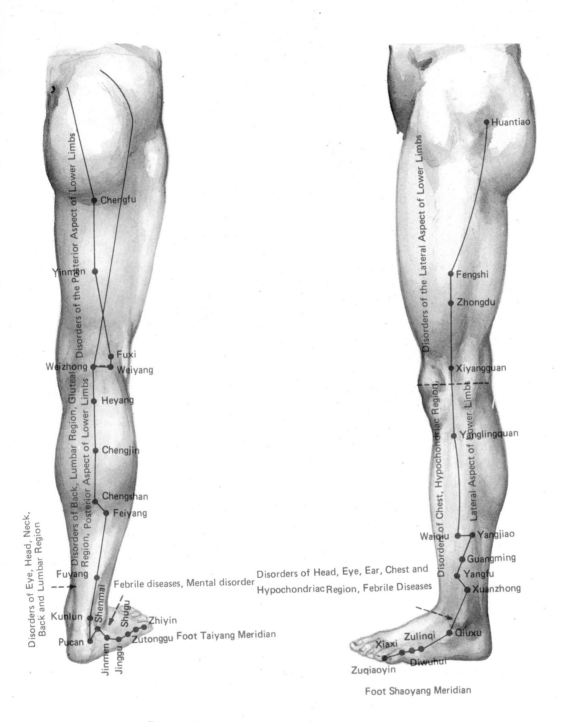

Fig. 51 The Indications of the Points in the Lower Limbs

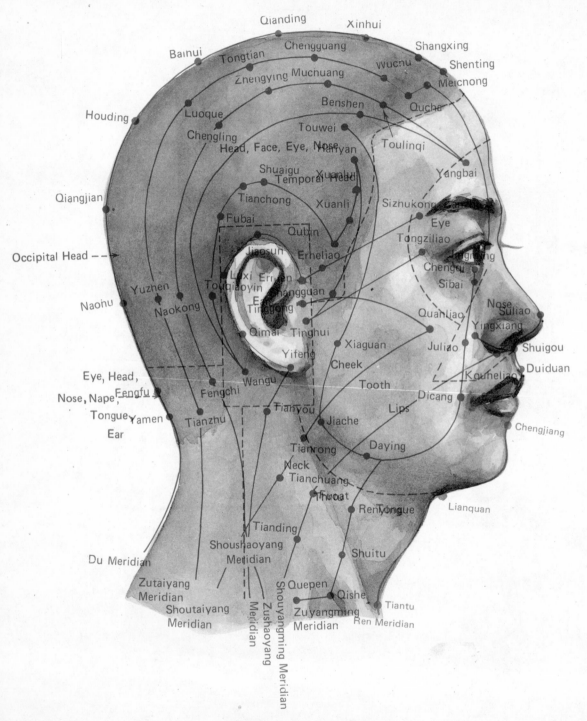

Fig. 52 The Therapeutic Properties of the Points on the Head and Face

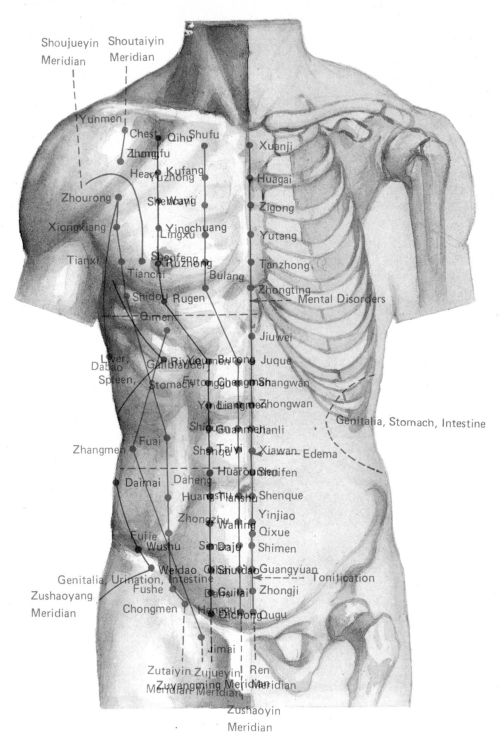

Fig. 53 The Therapeutic Properties of the Points at the Chest and Abdomen

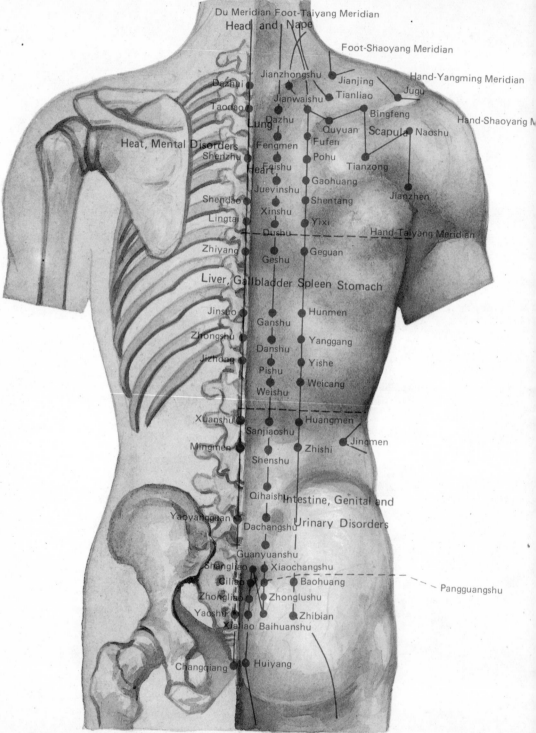

Fig. 54 The Therapeutic Properties of the Points on the Back and at the Lumbar Region

Chapter 7

ACUPOINTS OF THE TAIYIN AND YANGMING MERIDIAN

The Lung Meridian of Hand-Taiyin running from the chest to the hand, and the Large Intestine Meridian of Hand-Yangming going from the hand to the head, are exteriorly-interiorly related, so are the Stomach Meridian of Foot-Yangming travelling from the head to the foot and the Spleen Meridian of Foot-Taiyin travelling from the foot to the abdomen (chest). The four meridians are mainly distributed on the extremities and in the anterior aspect of the trunk. Their acupoints are described as follows.

I. THE LUNG MERIDIAN OF HAND-TAIYIN

1. Zhongfu (Front-Mu Point of the Lung, L1)

Location: Laterosuperior to the sternum at the lateral side of the first intercostal space, 6 cun lateral to the Ren Meridian. (See Fig. 55)

Indications: Cough, asthma, pain in the chest, shoulder and back, fullness of the chest.

Method: Puncture obliquely 0.5-0.8 inch towards the lateral aspect of the chest. To avoid injuring the lung, never puncture deeply towards the medial aspect. Moxibustion is applicable.

Regional anatomy

Vasculature: Superolaterally, the axillary artery and vein, the thoracoacromial artery and vein.

Innervation: The intermediate supra-clavicular nerve, the branches of the anterior thoracic nerve, and the lateral cutaneous branch of the first intercostal nerve.

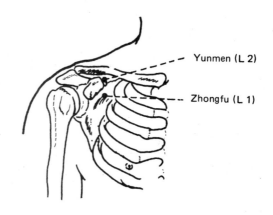

Yunmen (L 2)

Zhongfu (L 1)

Fig. 55

2. Yunmen (L 2)

Location: In the depression below the acromial extremity of the clavicle, 6 cun lateral to the Ren Meridian. (See Fig. 55)

Indications: Cough, asthma, pain in the chest, shoulder and arm, fullness in the chest.

Method: Puncture obliquely 0.5-0.8 inch towards the lateral aspect of the chest. To avoid injuring the lung, never puncture deeply towards the medial aspect. Moxibustion is applicable.

Regional anatomy

Vasculature: The cephalic vein, the thoracoacromial artery and vein; inferiorly, the axillary artery.

Innervation: The intermediate and lateral supraclavicular nerve, the branches of the anterior thoracic nerve, and the lateral cord of the brachial plexus.

3. Tianfu (L 3)

Location: On the medial aspect of the upper arm, 3 cun below the end of axillary fold, on the radial side of m. biceps brachii. (See Col. Fig. 1)

Indications: Asthma, epistaxis, pain in the medial aspect of the upper arm.

Method: Puncture perpendicularly 0.5-1 inch.

Regional anatomy

Vasculature: The cephalic vein and muscular branches of the brachial artery and vein.

Innervation: The lateral brachial cutaneous nerve at the place where the musculo-cutaneous nerve passes through.

4. Xiabai (L 4)

Location: On the medial aspect of the upper arm, 1 cun below Tainfu (L 3), on the radial side of m. biceps brachii. (See Col. Fig. 1)

Indications: Cough, fullness in the chest, pain in the medial aspect of the upper arm.

Method: Puncture perpendicularly 0.5-1 inch. Moxibustion is applicable.

Regional anatomy

Vasculature: The cephalic vein and muscular branches of the brachial artery and vein.

Innervation: The lateral brachial cutaneous nerve at the place where the musculo-cutaneous nerve passes through.

5. Chize (He-Sea Point, L 5)

Location: On the cubital crease, on the radial side of the tendon of m. biceps brachii. This point is located with the elbow slightly flexed. (See Fig. 56)

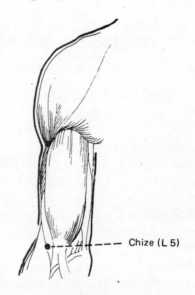

Chize (L 5)

Fig. 56

Indication: Cough, hemoptysis, after-noon fever, asthma, sore throat, fullness in the chest, infantile convulsions, spasmodic pain of the elbow and arm, mastitis.

Method: Puncture perpendicularly 0.5-1 inch.

Regional anatomy

Vasculature: The branches of the radial recurrent artery and vein, the cephalic vein.

Innervation: The lateral antebrachial cutaneous nerve and the radial nerve.

Indications: Cough, pain in the chest, asthma, hemoptysis, sore throat, spasmodic pain of the elbow and arm.

Method: Puncture perpendicularly 0.5-1 inch. Moxibustion is applicable.

Regional anatomy

Vasculature: The cephalic vein, the radial artery and vein.

Innervation: The lateral antebrachial cutaneous nerve and the superficial ramus of the radial nerve.

6.   Kongzui (Xi-Cleft Point, L 6)

Location: On the palmar aspect of the forearm, on the line joining Taiyuan (L 9) and Chize (L 5), 7 cun above the transverse crease of the wrist. (See Fig. 57)

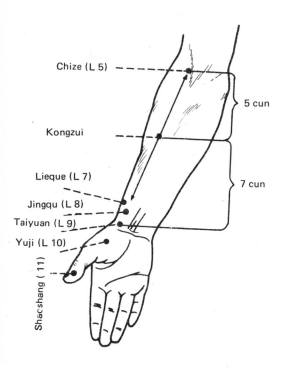

Fig. 57

7.   Lieque   (Luo-Connecting   Point, Confluent Point, L 7)

Location: Superior to the styloid process of the radius, 1.5 cun above the transverse crease of the wrist. (See Fig. 57)   When the index fingers and thumbs of both hands are crossed with the index finger of one hand placed on the styloid process of the radius of the other, the point is in the depression right under the tip of the index finger. (See Fig. 58)

Indications: Headache, migraine, neck rigidity, cough, asthma, sore throat, facial paralysis, toothache, pain and weakness of the wrist.

Method: Puncture 0.3-0.5 inch obliquely upward. Moxibustion is applicable.

Regional anatomy

Vasculature: The cephalic vein, branches of the radial artery and vein.

Innervation: The lateral antebrachial cutaneous nerve and the superficial ramus of the radial nerve.

8.   Jingqu (Jing-River Piont, L 8)

Location: 1 cun above the transverse crease of the wrist in the depression on the

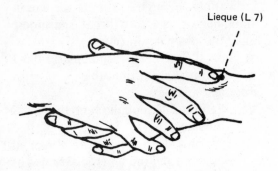

Lieque (L 7)

Fig. 58

lateral side of the radial artery. (See Fig. 57)

Indications: Cough, asthma, fever, pain in the chest, sore throat, pain in the wrist.

Method: Puncture perpendicularly 0.1-0.3 inch. Avoid puncturing the radial artery.

Regional anatomy

Vasculature: Laterally, the radial artery and vein.

Innervation: The lateral antebrachial cutaneous nerve and the superficial ramus of the radial nerve.

9. Taiyuan (Shu-Stream and Yuan-Primary Point, Influential Point of Vessels, L 9)

Location: At the radial end of the transverse crease of the wrist, in the depression on the lateral side of the radial artery. (See Fig. 57)

Indications: Cough, asthma, hemoptysis, sore throat, palpitation, pain in the chest, wrist and arm.

Method: Puncture perpendicularly 0.2-0.3 inch. Avoid puncturing the radial artery. Moxibustion is applicable.

Regional anatomy

Vasculature: The radial artery and vein.

Innervation: The lateral antebrachial cutaneous nerve and the superficial ramus of the radial nerve.

10.   Yuji (Ying-Spring Point, L 10)

Location: On the radial aspect of the midpoint of the first metacarpal bone, on the junction of the red and white skin (i.e., the junction of the dorsum and palm of the hand). (See Fig. 57)

Indications: Cough, hemoptysis, sore throat, loss of voice, fever, feverish sensation in the palm.

Method: Puncture perpendicularly 0.5-0.8 inch. Moxibustion is applicable.

Regional anatomy

Vasculature: Venules of the thumb draining to the cephalic vein.

Innervation: The superficial ramus of the radial nerve.

11.   Shaoshang (Jing-Well Point, L 11)

Location: On the radial side of the thumb, about 0.1 cun posterior to the corner of the nail. (See Fig. 57)

Indication: Sore throat, cough, asthma, epistaxis, fever, loss of consciousness, mania, spasmodic pain of the thumb.

Method: Puncture 0.1 inch, or prick the point to cause bleeding.

Regional anatomy

Vasculature: The arterial and venous network formed by the palmar digital proprial artery and veins.

Innervation: The terminal nerve network formed by the mixed branches of the lateral antebrachial cutaneous nerve and the superficial ramus of the radial nerve as well as the palmar digital proprial nerve of the median nerve.

II. THE LARGE INTESTINE MERIDIAN OF HAND-YANGMING

1. Shangyang (Jing-Well Point, L I 1)

Location: On the radial side of the index finger, about 0.1 cun posterior to the corner of the nail. (See Fig. 59)

Indications: Toothache, sore throat, swelling of the submandibular region, numbness of fingers, febrile diseases with anhidrosis, loss of consciousness.

Method: Puncture 0.1 inch, or prick the point to cause bleeding.

Regional anatomy

Vasculature: The arterial and venous network formed by the dorsal digital arteries and veins.

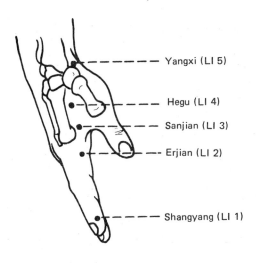

Fig. 59

2. Erjian (Ying-Spring Point, L I 2)

Location: On the radial side of the index finger, distal to the metacarpal-phalangeal joint, at the junction of the red and white skin. The point is located with the finger slightly flexed. (See Fig. 59)

Indications: Blurring of vision, Epistaxis, toothache, sore throat, febrile diseases.

Method: Puncture perpendicularly 0.2-0.3 inch. Moxibustion is applicable.

Regional anatomy

Vasculature: The dorsal digital and plamar digital proprial arteries and veins derived from the radial artery and vein.

Innervation: The dorsal digital nerve of the radial nerve, and the palmar digital proprial nerve of the median nerve.

3. Sanjian (Shu-Stream Point, L I 3)

Location: When a loose fist is made, the point is on the radial side of the index finger, in the depression proximal to the head of the second metacarpal bone. (See Fig. 59)

Indications: Toothache, ophthalmalgia, sore throat, redness and swelling of fingers and the dorsum of the hand.

Method: Puncture perpendicularly 0.5-0.8 inch. Moxibustion is applicable.

Regional anatomy

Vasculature: The dorsal venous network of the hand and the branch of the first dorsal metacarpal artery.

Innervation: The superficial ramus of radial nerve.

Innervation: The palmar digital proprial nerve derived from the median nerve.

4. Hegu (Yuan-Primary Point, L I 4)

Location: On the dorsum of the hand, between the 1st and 2nd metacarpal bones, approximately in the middle of the 2nd metacarpal bone on the radial side. (See Fig. 59) Or, place in coincident position the transverse crease of the interphalangeal joint of the thumb with the margin of the web between the thumb and the index finger of the other hand. The point is where the tip of the thumb touches. (See Fig. 60)

Indications: Headache, pain in the neck, redness, swelling and pain of the eye, epistaxis, nasal obstruction, rhinorrhea, toothache, deafness, swelling of the face, sore throat, parotitis, trismus, facial paralysis, febrile diseases with anhidrosis, hidrosis, abdominal pain, dysentery, constipation, amenorrhea, delayed labour, infantile convulsion, pain, weakness and motor impairment of the upper limbs.

Method: Puncture perpendicularly 0.5-1 inch. Moxibustion is applicable. Acupuncture and moxibustion are contraindicated in pregnant women.

Regional anatomy

Vasculature: The venous network of the dorsum of the hand.

Innervation: The superficial ramus of the radial nerve.

5. Yangxi (Jing-River Point, L I 5)

Location: On the radial side of the wrist. When the thumb is tilted upward, it is in the depression between the tendons of m. extensor pollicis longus and brevis. (See Fig. 59)

Indications: Headache, redness, pain and swelling of the eye, toothache, sore throat, pain of the wrist.

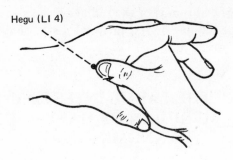

Hegu (LI 4)

Fig. 60

Method: Puncture perpendicularly 0.3-0.5 inch. Moxibustion is applicable.

Regional anatomy

Vasculature: The cephalic vein, the radial artery and its dorsal carpal branch.

Innervation: The superficial ramus of the radial nerve.

6. Pianli (Luo-Connecting Point, L I 6)

Location: With the elbow flexed and the radial side of arm upward, the point is on the line joining Yangxi (L I 5) and Quchi (L I 11), 3 cun above Yangxi (L I 5). (See Fig. 61)

Indications: Redness of the eye, tinnitus, deafness, epistaxis, aching of the hand and arm, sore throat, edema.

Method: Puncture perpendicularly or obliquely 0.5-0.8 inch. Moxibustion is applicable.

Regional anatomy

Vasculature: The cephalic vein.

Innervation: On the radial side, the lateral antebrachial cutaneous nerve and the superficial ramus of the radial nerve; on the ulnar side, the posterior antebrachial cutaneous nerve and the posterior antebrachial interosseous nerve.

7.   Wenliu (Xi-Cleft Point, L I 7)

Location: With the elbow flexed and the radial side of arm upward, the point is on the line joining Yangxi (L I 5) and Quchi (L I 11), 5 cun above Yangxi (L I 5). (See Fig. 61)

Indications: Headache, swelling of the face, sore throat, borborygmus, abdominal pain, aching of the shoulder and arm.

Method: Puncture perpendicularly 0.5-1.0 inch. Moxibustion is applicable.

Regional anatomy

Vasculature: The muscular branch of the radial artery, the cephalic vein.

Innervation: The posterior antebrachial cutaneous nerve and the deep ramus of the radial nerve.

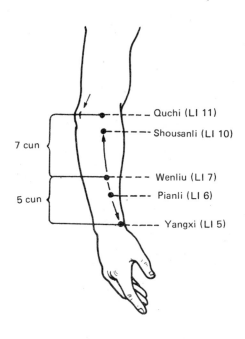

7 cun

5 cun

---- Quchi (LI 11)

--- Shousanli (LI 10)

--- Wenliu (LI 7)

--- Pianli (LI 6)

---- Yangxi (LI 5)

Fig. 61

8.   Xialian (L I 8)

Location: On the line joining Yangxi (L I 5) and Quchi (L I 11), 4 cun below Quchi (L I 5). (See Col Fig. 2)

Indications: Abdominal pain, borborygmus, pain in the elbow and arm, motor impairment of the upper limbs.

Method: Puncture perpendicularly 0.5-1.0 inch. Moxibustion is applicable.

Regional anatomy: See Wenliu (L I 7)

9.   Shanglian (L I 9)

Location: On the line joining Yangxi (L I 5) and Quchi (L I 11), 3 cun below Quchi (L I 5). (See Col Fig. 2)

Indications: Aching of the shoulder and arm, motor impairment of the upper limbs, numbness of the hand and arm, borborygmus, abdominal pain.

Method: Puncture perpendicularly 0.5-1.0 inch. Moxibustion is applicable.

Regional anatomy: See Wenliu (L I 7).

10.   Shousanli (L I 10)

Location: On the line joining Yangxi (L I 5) and Quchi (L I 11), 2 cun below Quchi (L I 5). (See Fig. 61)

Indications: Abdominal pain, diarrhea, toothache, swelling of the cheek, motor impairment of the upper limbs, pain in the shoulder and back.

Method: Puncture perpendicularly 0.8-1.2 inches. Moxibustion is applicable.

Regional anatomy

Vasculature: The branches of the radial recurrent artery and vein.

Innervation: See Wenliu (L I 7).

11.　Quchi (He-Sea Point, L I 11)

Location: When the elbow is flexed, the point is in the depression at the lateral end of the transverse cubital crease, midway between Chize (L 5) and the lateral epicondyle of the humerus. (See Fig. 61)

Indications: Sore throat, toothache, redness and pain of the eye, scrofula, urticaria, motor impairment of the upper extremities, abdominal pain, vomiting, diarrhea, febrile diseases.

Method: Puncture perpendicularly 1.0-1.5 inches. Moxibustion is applicable.

Regional anatomy

Vasculature: The branches of the radial recurrent artery and vein.

Innervation: The posterior antebrachial cutaneous nerve; deeper, on the medial side, the radial nerve.

12.　Zhouliao (L I 12)

Location: When the elbow is flexed, the point is superior to the lateral epicondyle of the humerus, about 1 cun superolateral to Quchi (L I 11), on the medial border of the humerus. (See Col. Fig. 2)

Indications: Pain, numbness and contracture of the elbow and arm.

Method: Puncture perpendicularly 0.5-1.0 inch. Moxibustion is applicable.

Regional anatomy

Vasculature: The radial collateral artery and vein.

Innervation: The posterior antebrachial cutaneous nerve; deeper, on the medial side, the radial nerve.

13.　Shouwuli (L I 13)

Location: Superior to the lateral epicondyle of the humerus, on the line joining Quchi (L I 11) and Jianyu (L I 15), 3 cun above Quchi (L I 11). (See Col Fig. 2)

Indications: Contracture and pain of the elbow and arm, scrofula.

Method: Puncture perpendicularly 0.5-1.0 inch. Avoid injuring the artery. Moxibustion is applicable.

Regional anatomy

Vasculature: The radial collateral artery and vein.

Innervation: The posterior antebrachial cutaneous nerve; deeper, the radial nerve.

14.　Binao (L I 14)

Location: On the line joining Quchi (L I 11) and Jianyu (L I 15), 7 cun above Quchi, on the radial side of the humerus, superior to the lower end of m. deltoideus. (See Col. Fig. 2)

Indications: Pain in the shoulder and arm, rigidity of the neck, scrofula.

Method: Puncture perpendicularly or obliquely upward 0.8-1.5 inches. Moxibustion is applicable.

Regional anatomy

Vasculature: The branches of posterior circumflex humeral artery and vein, the deep brachial artery and vein.

Innervation: The posterior brachial cutaneous nerve; deeper, the radial nerve.

15.　Jianyu (L I 15)

Location: Antero-inferior to the acromion, on the upper portion of m. deltoideus.

When the arm is in full abduction, the point is in the depression appearing at the anterior border of the acromioclavicular joint. (See Fig. 62)

Indications: Pain in the shoulder and arm, motor impairment of the upper extremities, rubella, scrofula.

Method: Puncture perpendicularly or obliquely 0.8-1.5 inches. Moxibustion is applicable.

Regional anatomy

Vasculature: The posterior circumflex artery and vein.

Innervation: The lateral supraclavicular nerve and axillary nerve.

16.   Jugu (L I 16)

Location: In the upper aspect of the shoulder, in the depression between the acromial extremity of the clavicle and the scapular spine. (See Col. Fig. 2)

Indications: Pain and motor impairment

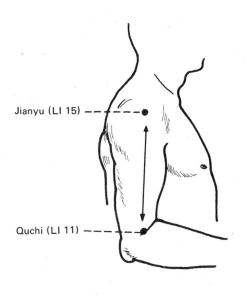

Fig.62

of the upper extremities, pain in the shoulder and back.

Method: Puncture perpendicularly 0.5-0.7 inch. Moxibustion is applicable.

Regional Anatomy

Vasculature: Deeper, the suprascapular artery and vein.

Innervation: Superficially, the lateral supraclavicular nerve, the branch of the accessory nerve; deeper, the suprascapular nerve.

17.   Tianding (L I 17)

Location: On the lateral side of the neck, 1 cun below Neck-Futu (L I 18), on the posterior border of m. sternocleidomastoideus. (See Col. Fig. 2)

Indications: Sudden loss of voice, sore throat, scrofula, goiter.

Method: Puncture perpendicularly 0.3-0.5 inch. Moxibustion is applicable.

Regional anatomy

Vasculature: The external jugular vein.

Innervation: Superficially, the supraclavicular nerve. It is on the posterior border of m. sternocleidomastoideus just where the cutaneous cervical nerve emerges. Deeper, the phrenic nerve.

18.   Futu (L I 18)

Location: On the lateral side of the neck, level with the tip of Adam's apple, between the sternal head and clavicular head of m. sternocleidomastoideus. (See Col. Fig. 2)

Indications: Cough, asthma, sore throat, sudden loss of voice, scrofula, goiter.

Method: Puncture perpendicularly 0.3-0.5 inch. Moxibustion is applicable.

Regional anatomy

Vasculature: Deeper, on the medial side, the ascending cervical artery and vein.

Innervation: The great auricular nerve, cutaneous cervical nerve, lesser occipital nerve and accessory nerve.

19.   Kouheliao (L I 19)

Location: Right below the lateral margin of the nostril, 0.5 cun lateral to Renzhong (Shuigou, Du 26). (See Col. Fig. 2)

Indications: Nasal obstruction, epistaxis, deviation of the mouth.

Method:Puncture obliquely 0.2-0.3 inch.

Regional anatomy

Vasculature: The superior labial branches of the facial artery and vein.

Innervation: The anastomotic branch of the facial nerve and the infraorbital nerve.

20.   Yingxiang (L I 20)

Location: In the nasolabial groove, at the

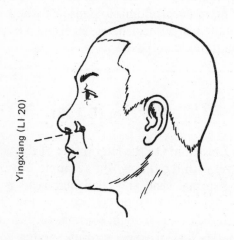

Fig. 63

level of the midpoint of the lateral border of ala nasi. (See Fig. 63)

Indications: Nasal obstruction, hyposmia, epistaxis, rhinorrhea, deviation of the mouth, itching and swelling of the face.

Method: Puncture obliquely or subcutaneously 0.3-0.5 inch.

Regional anatomy

Vasculature: The facial artery and vein, the branches of the infraorbital artery and vein.

Innervation: The anastomotic branch of the facial and infraorbital nerves.

III.   THE STOMACH MERIDIAN OF FOOT-YANGMING

1.   Chengqi (S 1)

Location: With the eyes looking straight forward, the point is directly below the pupil, between the eyeball and the infraorbital ridge. (See Fig. 64)

Indications: Redness, swelling and pain of the eye, lacrimation, night blindness, twitching of eyelids, facial paralysis.

Method: Push the eyeball upward with the left thumb and puncture perpendicularly and slowly 0.5-1.0 inch along the infraorbital ridge. It is not advisable to manipulate the needle with large amplitude.

Regional anatomy

Vasculature: The branches of the infraorbital and ophthalmic arteries and veins.

Innervation: The branch of the infraorbital nerve, the inferior branch of the oculomotor nerve and the muscular branch of the facial nerve.

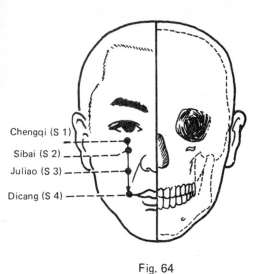

Chengqi (S 1)
Sibai (S 2)
Juliao (S 3)
Dicang (S 4)

Fig. 64

2.　Sibai (S 2)

Location: Below Chengqi (S 1), in the depression at the infraorbital foramen. (See Fig. 64)

Indications: Redness, pain and itching of the eye, facial paralysis, twitching of eye lids, pain in the face.

Method: Puncture perpendicularly 0.2-0.3 inch. It is not advisable to puncture deeply.

Regional anatomy

Vasculature: The branches of facial artery and vein, the infraorbital artery and vein.

Innervation: The branches of the facial nerve. The point is right on the course of the infraorbital nerve.

3.　Juliao (S 3)

Location: Directly below Sibai (S 2), at the level of the lower border of ala nasi, on the lateral side of the nasolabial groove. (See Fig. 64)

Indications: Facial paralysis, twitching of eyelids, epistaxis, toothache, swelling of lips and cheek.

Method: Puncture perpendicularly 0.3-0.5 inch. Moxibustion is applicable.

Regional anatomy

Vasculature: The branches of the facial and infraorbital arteries and veins.

Innervation: The branches of the facial and infraorbital nerves.

4.　Dicang (S 4)

Location: Lateral to the corner of the mouth, directly below Juliao (S 3). (See Fig. 64)

Indications: Deviation of the mouth, salivation, twitching of eyelids.

Method: Puncture subcutaneously 1.0-1.5 inches with the tip of the needle directed towards Jiache (S 6). Moxibustion is applicable.

Regional anatomy

Vasculature: The facial artery and vein.

Innervation: Superficially, the branches of the facial and infraorbital nerves; deeper, the terminal branch of the buccal nerve.

5.　Daying (S 5)

Location: Anterior to the angle of mandible, on the anterior border of the attached portion of m. masseter, in the groove-like depression appearing when the cheek is bulged. (See Col. Fig. 3)

Indications: Facial paralysis, trismus, swelling of the cheek, pain in the face, toothache.

Method: Avoid puncturing the artery. Puncture obliquely 0.3-0.5 inch. Moxibustion is applicable.

Regional anatomy

Vasculature: Anteriorly, the facial artery and vein.

Innervation: The facial and buccal nerves.

6.   Jiache (S 6)

Location: One finger-breadth anterior and superior to the lower angle of the mandible where m. masseter attaches at the prominence of the muscle when the teeth are clenched. (See Fig. 65)

Indications: Facial paralysis, toothache, swelling of the cheek and face, mumps, trismus.

Method: Puncture perpendicularly 0.3-0.5 inch, or subcutaneously with the tip of the needle directed towards Dicang (S 4). Moxibustion is applicable.

Regional anatomy

Vasculature: The masseteric artery.

Innervation: The great auricular nerve, facial nerve and masseteric nerve.

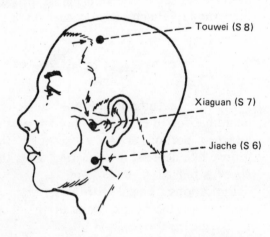

Fig. 65

7.   Xiaguan (S 7)

Location: At the lower border of the zygomatic arch, in the depression anterior to the condyloid process of the mandible. This point is located with the mouth closed. (See Fig. 65)

Indications: Deafness, tinnitus, otorrhea, toothache, facial paralysis, pain of the face, motor impairment of the jaw.

Method: Puncture perpendicularly 0.3-0.5 inch. Moxibustion is applicable.

Regional anatomy

Vasculature: Superficially, the transverse facial artery and vein; in the deepest layer, the maxillary artery and vein.

Innervation: The zygomatic branch of the facial nerve and the branches of the auriculotemporal nerve.

8.   Touwei (S 8)

Location: 0.5 cun within the anterior hairline at the corner of the forehead, 4.5 cun lateral to Shenting (Du 24). (See Fig. 65)

Indications: Headache, blurrmg of vision, ophthalmalgia, lacrimation.

Method: Puncture   0.5-1.0   inch subcutaneously.

Regional anatomy

Vasculature: The frontal branches of the superficial temporal artery and vein.

Innervation: The branch of the auriculo-temporal nerve and the temporal branch of the facial nerve.

9.   Renying (S 9)

Location: Level with the tip of Adam's apple, just on the course of the common

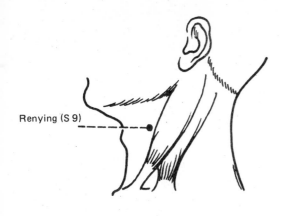

Renying (S 9)

Fig. 66

carotid artery, on the anterior border of m. sternocleidomastoideus. (See Fig. 66)

Indications: Sore throat, asthma, goiter, dizziness, flushing of the face.

Method: Avoid puncturing the common carotid artery, puncture perpendicularly 0.3-0.5 inch.

Regional anatomy

Vasculature: The superior thyroid artery on the bifurcation of the internal and the external carotid artery.

Innervation: Superficially, the cutaneous cervical nerve, the cervical branch of the facial nerve; deeper, the sympathetic trunk; laterally, the descending branch of the hypoglossal nerve and the vagus nerve.

10.   Shuitu (S 10)

Location: At the midpoint of the line joining Renying (S 9) and Qishe (S 11), on the anterior border of m. sternocleidomastoideus. (See Col. Fig. 3)

Indications: Sore throat, asthma, cough.

Method: Puncture perpendicularly 0.3-0.5 inch. Moxibustion is applicable.

Regional anatomy

Vasculature: The common carotid artery.

Innervation: Superficially, the cutaneous cervical nerve; deeper, the superior cardiac nerve issued from the sympathetic nerve and the sympathetic trunk.

11.   Qishe (S 11)

Location: At the superior border of the sternal extremity of the clavicle, between the sternal head and clavicular head of m. sternocleidomastoideus. (See Col. Fig. 3)

Indications: Sore throat, pain and rigidity of the neck, asthma, hiccup, goiter.

Method: Puncture perpendicularly 0.3-0.5 inch. Moxibustion is applicable.

Regional anatomy

Vasculature: Superficially, the anterior jugular vein; deeper, the common carotid artery.

Innervation: The medial supraclavicular nerve and the muscular branch of ansa hypoglossi.

12.   Quepen (S 12)

Location: In the midpoint of the supraclavicular fossa, 4 cun lateral to Ren Meridian. (See Col. Fig. 3)

Indications: Cough, asthma, sore throat, pain in the supraclavicular fossa.

Method: Avoid puncturing the artery. Puncture perpendicularly 0.3-0.5 inch. Deep puncture is not advisable. Moxibustion is applicable.

Regional anatomy

Vasculature: Superiorly, the transverse cervical artery.

Innervation: Superficially, the intermediate supraclavicular nerve; deeper, the supraclavicular portion of brachial plexus.

13. Qihu (S 13)

Location: At the lower border of the middle of the clavicle, 4 cun lateral to the Ren Meridian. (See Col. Fig. 3)

Indications: Fullness in the chest, asthma, cough, hiccup, pain in the chest and hypochondrium.

Method: Puncture obliquely 0.3-0.5 inch. Moxibustion is applicable.

Regional anatomy

Vasculature: The branches of the thoracoacromial artery and vein; superiorly, the subclavicular vein.

Innervation: The branches of the supraclavicular nerve and the anterior thoracic nerve.

14. Kufang (S 14)

Location: In the first intercostal space, 4 cun lateral to the Ren Meridian. (See Col. Fig. 3)

Indications: Sensation of fullness and pain in the chest, cough.

Method: Puncture obliquely 0.3-0.5 inch. Moxibustion is applicable.

Regional anatomy

Vasculature: The thoracoacromial artery and vein and the branches of the lateral thoracic artery and vein.

Innervation: The branch of the anterior thoracic nerve.

15. Wuyi (S 15)

Location: In the second intercostal space,

4 cun lateral to the Ren Meridian (See Col. Fig. 3)

Indications: Fullness and pain in the chest and the costal region, cough, asthma, mastitis.

Method: Puncture obliquely 0.3-0.5 inch. Moxibustion is applicable.

Regional anatomy

Vasculature: See Kufang (S 14).

Innervation: On the course of the branch of m. pectoralis major derived from the anterior thoracic nerve.

16. Yingchuang (S 16)

Location: In the third intercostal space, 4 cun lateral to the Ren Meridian. (See Col. Fig. 3)

Indications: Fullness and pain in the chest and hypochondrium, cough, asthma, mastitis.

Method: Puncture obliquely 0.3-0.5 inch. Moxibustion is applicable.

Regional anatomy

Vasculature: The lateral thoracic artery and vein.

Innervation: The branch of the anterior thoracic nerve.

17. Ruzhong (S 17)

Location: In the fourth intercostal space, in the centre of the nipple. (See Col. Fig. 3)

Acupuncture and moxibustion on this point are contraindicated. This point serves only as a landmark for locating points on the chest and abdomen.

Regional anatomy

Innervation: The anterior and lateral cutaneous branches of the fourth intercostal nerve.

18.   Rugen (S 18)

Location: In the fifth intercostal space, directly below the nipple. (See Fig. 67)

Indications: Pain in the chest, cough, asthma, mastitis, insufficient lactation.

Method: Puncture obliquely 0.3-0.5 inch. Moxibustion is applicable.

Regional anatomy

Vasculature: The branches of the intercostal artery and vein.

Innervation: The branch of the fifth intercostal nerve.

19.   Burong (S 19)

Location: 6 cun above the umbilicus, 2 cun lateral to Juque (Ren 14). (Col. Fig. 3)

Indications: Abdominal distension, vomiting, gastric pain, anorexia.

Method: Puncture perpendicularly 0.5-0.8 inch. Moxibustion is applicable.

Regional anatomy

Vasculature: The branches of the seventh intercostal artery and vein, the branches of the superior epigastric artery and vein.

Innervation: The branch of the seventh intercostal nerve.

20.   Chengman (S 20)

Location: 5 cun above the umbilicus, 2 cun lateral to Shangwan (Ren 13). (See Col. Fig. 3)

Indications: Gastric pain, abdominal distension, vomiting, anorexia.

Method: Puncture perpendicularly 0.5-

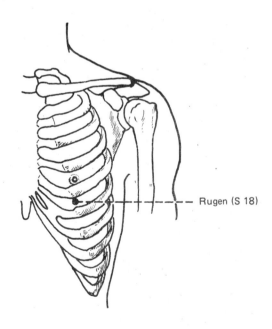

Rugen (S 18)

Fig. 67

1.0 inch. Moxibustion is applicable.
Regional anatomy: See Burong (S 19)

21.   Liangmen (S 21)

Location: 4 cun above the umbilicus, 2
cun lateral to Zhongwan (Ren 12). (See Fig.
68)
Indications: Gastric pain, vomiting,
anorexia, abdominal distension, diarrhea.
Method: Puncture perpendicularly 0.8-
1.0 inch. Moxibustion is applicable.
Regional anatomy
Vasculature: The branches of the eighth
intercostal and superior epigastric arteries
and veins.
Innervation: The branch of the eighth
intercostal nerve.

22.   Guanmen (S 22)

Location: 3 cun above the umbilicus, 2
cun lateral to Jianli (Ren 11). (Col. Fig. 3)
Indications: Abdominal distension and
pain, anorexia, borborygmus, diarrhea,
edema.
Method: Puncture perpendicularly 0.8-
1.0 inch. Moxibustion is applicable.
Regional anatomy: See Liangmen (S 21)

23.   Taiyi (S 23)

Location: 2 cun above the umbilicus, 2
cun lateral to Xiawan (Ren 10). (See Col.
Fig. 3)
Indications: Gastric pain, irritability,
mania, indigestion.
Method: Puncture perpendicularly 0.7-
1.0 inch. Moxibustion is applicable.

Regional anatomy
Vasculature: The branches of the eighth
and ninth intercostal and inferior epigastric
arteries and veins.
Innervation: The branches of the eighth
and ninth intercostal nerves.

24.   Huaroumen (S 24)

Location: 1 cun above the umbilicus, 2
cun lateral to Shuifen (Ren 9). (See Col.
Fig. 3)
Indications: Gastric pain, vomiting,
mania.
Method: Puncture perpendicularly 0.7-
1.0 inch. Moxibustion is applicable.
Regional anatomy
Vasculature: The branches of the ninth
intercostal and inferior epigastric arteries
and veins.
Innervation: The branch of the ninth
intercostal nerve.

25.   Tianshu (Front-Mu Point of the
Large Intestine, S 25)

Location: 2 cun lateral to the centre of the
umbilicus. (See Fig. 68)
Indications: Abdominal pain and distension, borborygmus, pain around the
umbilicus, constipation, diarrhea, dysentery, irregular menstruation, edema.
Method: Puncture perpendicularly 0.7-
1.2 inches. Moxibustion is applicable.
Regional anatomy
Vasculature: The branches of the tenth
intercostal and inferior epigastric arteries
and veins.
Innervation: The branch of the tenth
intercostal nerve.

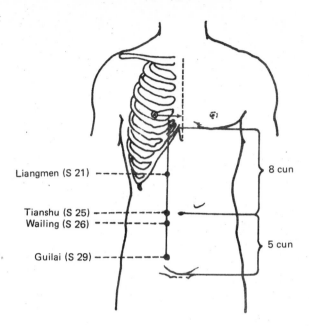

Liangmen (S 21)

8 cun

Tianshu (S 25)
Wailing (S 26)

5 cun

Guilai (S 29)

Fig. 68

26.   Wailing (S 26)

Location: 1 cun below the umbilicus, 2 cun lateral to Yinjiao (Ren 7). (See Fig. 68)

Indications: Abdominal pain, hernia, dysmenorrhea.

Method: Puncture perpendicularly 0.7-1.2 inches. Moxibustion is applicable.

Regional anatomy: See Tianshu (S 25)

27.   Daju (S 27)

Location: 2 cun below the umbilicus, 2 cun lateral to Shimen (Ren 5). (Col. Fig. 3)

Indications: Lower abdominal distension, dysuria, hernia, seminal emission, premature ejaculation.

Method: Puncture perpendicularly 0.7-1.2 inches. Moxibustion is applicable.

Regional anatomy

Vasculature: The branches of the eleventh intercostal artery and vein; laterally, the inferior epigastric artery and vein.

Innervation: The eleventh intercostal nerve.

28.   Shuidao (S 28)

Location: 3 cun below the umbilicus, 2 cun lateral to Guanyuan (Ren 4). (See Col. Fig. 3)

Indications: Lower abdominal distension, retention of urine, edema, hernia, dysmenorrhea, sterility.

Method: Puncture perpendicularly 0.7-1.2 inches. Moxibustion is applicable.

Regional anatomy

Vasculature: The branches of the subcostal artery and vein; laterally, the inferior epigastric artery and vein.

Innervation: A branch of the subcostal nerve.

29.   Guilai (S 29)

Location: 4 cun below the umbilicus, 2 cun lateral to Zhongji (Ren 3). (See Fig. 68)

Indications: Abdominal pain, hernia, dysmenorrhea, irregular menstruation, amenorrhea, leucorrhea, prolapse of the uterus.

Method: Puncture perpendicularly 0.7-1.2 inches. Moxibustion is applicable.

Regional anatomy

Vasculature: Laterally, the inferior epigastric artery and vein.

Innervation: The iliohypogastric nerve.

30.   Qichong (S 30)

Location: 5 cun below the umbilicus, 2 cun lateral to Qugu (Ren 2). (See Col. Fig. 3)

Indications: Abdominal pain, borborygmus, hernia, swelling and pain of the external genitalia, impotence, dysmenorrhea, irregular menstruation.

Method: Puncture perpendicularly 0.5-1.0 inch. Moxibustion is applicable.

Regional anatomy

Vasculature: The branches of the superficial epigastric artery and vein. Laterally, the inferior epigastric artery and vein.

Innervation: The pathway of the ilioinguinal nerve.

31.   Biguan (S 31)

Location: At the crossing point of the line drawn directly down from the anterior superior iliac spine and the line level with the lower border of the symphysis pubis, in the depression on the lateral side of m. sartorius when the thigh is flexed. (See Fig. 69)

Indications: Pain in the thigh, muscular atrophy, motor impairment, numbness and pain of the lower extremities.

Method: Puncture perpendicularly 1.0-1.5 inches. Moxibustion is applicable.

Regional anatomy

Vasculature: Deeper, the branches of the lateral circumflex femoral artery and vein.

Innervation: The lateral femoral cutaneous nerve.

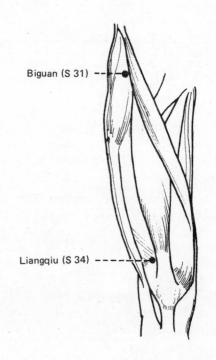

Biguan (S 31)

Liangqiu (S 34)

Fig. 69

32. Futu (S 32)

Location: On the line connecting the anterior superior iliac spine and lateral border of the patella, 6 cun above the laterosuperior border of the patella, in m. rectus femoris. (See Col. Fig. 4)

Indications: Pain in the lumbar and iliac region, coldness of the knee, paralysis or motor impairment and pain of the lower extremities, beriberi.

Method: Puncture perpendicularly 1.0-1.5 inches. Moxibustion is applicable.

Regional anatomy

Vasculature: The branches of the lateral circumflex femoral artery and vein.

Innervation: The anterior and lateral femoral cutaneous nerves.

33. Yinshi (S 33)

Location: When the knee is flexed, the point is 3 cun above the laterosuperior border of the patella, on the line joining the laterosuperior border of the patella and the anterior superior iliac spine. (See Col. Fig. 4)

Indications: Numbness, soreness, motor impairment of the leg and knee, motor impairment of the lower extremities.

Method: Puncture perpendicularly 0.7-1.0 inch. Moxibustion is applicable.

Regional anatomy

Vasculature: The descending branch of the lateral circumflex femoral artery.

Innervation: The anterior and lateral femoral cutaneous nerves.

34. Liangqiu (Xi-Cleft Point, S 34)

Location: When the knee is flexed, the point is 2 cun above the laterosuperior border of the patella. (See Fig. 69)

Indications: Pain and numbness of the knee, gastric pain, mastitis, motor impairment of the lower extremities.

Method: Puncture perpendicularly 0.5-1.0 inch. Moxibustion is applicable.

Regional anatomy: See Yinshi (S 33)

35. Dubi (S 35)

Location: When the knee is flexed, the point is at the lower border of the patella, in the depression lateral to the patellar ligament. (See Fig. 70)

Indications: Pain, numbness and motor impairment of the knee, beriberi.

Method: Puncture perpendicularly 0.7-1.0 inch. Moxibustion is applicable.

Regional anatomy

Vasculature: The arterial and venous network around the knee joint.

Innervation: The lateral sural cutaneous nerve and the articular branch of the common peroneal nerve.

36. Zusanli (He-Sea Point, S 36)

Location: 3 cun below Dubi (S 35), one finger-breadth from the anterior crest of the tibia, in m. tibialis anterior. (See Fig. 70)

Indications: Gastric pain, vomiting hiccup, abdominal distension, borborygmus, diarrhea, dysentery, constipation, mastitis, enteritis, aching of the knee joint and leg, beriberi, edema, cough, asthma, emaciation due to general deficiency, indigestion, apoplexy, hemiplegia, dizziness, insomnia, mania.

Method: Puncture perpendicularly 0.5-1.2 inches. Moxibustion is applicable.

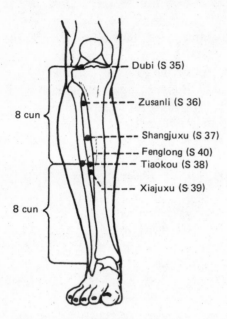

Fig. 70

Regional anatomy

Vasculature: The anterior tibial artery and vein.

Innervation: Superficially, the lateral sural cutaneous nerve and the cutaneous branch of the saphenous nerve; deeper, the deep peroneal nerve.

37. Shangjuxu (The Lower He-Sea Point of the Large Intestine, S 37)

Location: 3 cun below Zusanli (S 36), one finger-breadth from the anterior crest of the tibia, in m. tibialis anterior. (See Fig. 70)

Indications: Abdominal pain and distension, borborygmus, diarrhea, dysentery, constipation, enteritis, paralysis due to stroke, beriberi.

Method: Puncture perpendicularly 0.5-1.2 inches. Moxibustion is applicable.

Regional anatomy: See Zusanli (S 36)

38. Tiaokou (S 38)

Location: 2 cun below Shangjuxu (S 37), midway between Dubi (S 35) and Jiexi (S 41). (See Fig. 70)

Indications: Numbness, soreness and pain of the knee and leg, weakness and motor impairment of the foot, pain and motor impairment of the shoulder, abdominal pain.

Method: Puncture perpendicularly 0.5-1.0 inch. Moxibustion is applicable.

Regional anatomy: See Zusanli (S 36)

39. Xiajuxu (The Lower He-Sea Point of the Small Intestine, S 39)

Location: 3 cun below Shangjuxu (S 37), one finger-breadth from the anterior crest of the tibia, in m. tibialis anterior. (See Fig. 70)

Indications: Lower abdominal pain, backache referring to the testis, mastitis, numbness and paralysis of the lower extremities.

Method: Puncture perpendicularly 0.5-1.0 inch. Moxibustion is applicable.

Regional anatomy

Vasculature: The anterior tibial artery and vein.

Innervation: The branches of the superficial peroneal nerve and the deep peroneal nerve.

40. Fenglong (Luo-Connecting Point, S 40)

Location: 8 cun superior to the external malleolus, about one finger-breadth lateral to Tiaokou (S 38). (See Fig. 70)

Indications: Headache, dizziness and vertigo, cough, asthma, excessive sputum, pain in the chest, constipation, mania, epilepsy, muscular atrophy, motor impairment, pain, swelling or paralysis of the lower extremities.

Method: Puncture perpendicularly 0.5-1.0 inch. Moxibustion is applicable.

Regional anatomy

Vasculature: The branches of the anterior tibial artery and vein.

Innervation: The superficial peroneal nerve.

41.   Jiexi (Jing-River Point, S 41)

Location: On the dorsum of the foot, at the midpoint of the transverse crease of the ankle joint, in the depression between the tendons of m. extensor digitorum longus and hallucis longus, approximately at the level of the tip of the external malleolus. (See Fig. 71)

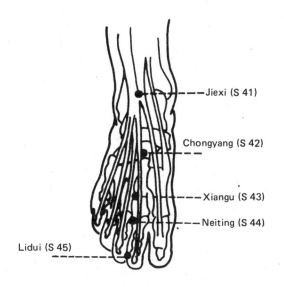

Jiexi (S 41)

Chongyang (S 42)

Xiangu (S 43)

Neiting (S 44)

Lidui (S 45)

Fig. 71

Indications: Pain of the ankle joint, muscular atrophy, motor impairment, pain and paralysis of the lower extremities, epilepsy, headache, dizziness and vertigo, abdominal distension, constipation.

Method: Puncture perpendicularly 0.5-0.7 inch. Moxibustion is applicable.

Regional anatomy

Vasculature: The anterior tibial artery vein.

Innervation: The superficial and deep peroneal nerves.

42.   Chongyang (Yuan-Primary Point, S 42)

Location: Distal to Jiexi (S 41), at the highest point of the dorsum of the foot, in the depression between the second and third metatarsal bones and the cuneiform bone. (See Fig. 71)

Indications: Pain of the upper teeth, redness and swelling of the dorsum of the foot, facial paralysis, muscular atrophy and motor impairment of the foot.

Method: Avoid puncturing the artery. Puncture perpendicularly 0.3-0.5 inch. Moxibustion is applicable.

Regional anatomy

Vasculature: The dorsal artery and vein of foot, the dorsal venous network of foot.

Innervation: Superficially, the medial dorsal cutaneous nerve of foot derived from the superficial peroneal nerve; deeper, the deep peroneal nerve.

43.   Xiangu (Shu-Stream Point, S 43)

Location: In the depression distal to the junction of the second and third metatarsal bones. (See Fig. 71)

Indications: Facial or general edema, abdominal pain, borborygmus, swelling and pain of the dorsum of the foot.

Method: Puncture perpendicularly 0.3-0.5 inch. Moxibustion is applicable.

Regional anatomy

Vasculature: The dorsal venous network of foot.

Innervation: The medial dorsal cutaneous nerve of foot.

44. Neiting (Ying-Spring Point, S 44)

Location: Proximal to the web margin between the second and third toes, in the depression distal and lateral to the second metatarsodigital joint. (See Fig. 71)

Indications: Toothache, pain in the face, deviation of the mouth, sore throat, epistaxis, gastric pain, acid regurgitation, abdominal distension, diarrhea, dysentery, constipation, swelling and pain of the dorsum of the foot, febrile diseases.

Method: Puncture perpendicularly 0.3-0.5 inch. Moxibustion is applicable.

Regional anatomy

Vasculature: The dorsal venous network of foot.

Innervation: Just where the lateral branch of the medial dorsal cutaneous nerve divides into dorsal digital nerves.

45. Lidui (Jing-Well Point, S 45)

Location: On the lateral side of the 2nd toe, 0.1 cun posterior to the corner of the nail. (See Fig. 71)

Indications: Facial swelling, deviation of the mouth, epistaxis, toothache, sore throat and hoarse voice, abdominal distension,

coldness in the leg and foot, febrile diseases, dream-disturbed sleep, mania.

Method: Puncture subcutaneously 0.1 inch. Moxibustion is applicable.

Regional anatomy

Vasculature: The arterial and venous network formed by the dorsal digital artery and vein of foot.

Innervation: The dorsal digital nerve derived from the superficial peroneal nerve.

IV. THE SPLEEN MERIDIAN OF FOOT-TAIYIN

1. Yinbai (Jing-Well Point, Sp 1)

Location: On the medial side of the great toe, 0.1 cun posterior to the corner of the nail. (See Fig. 72)

Indications: Abdominal distension, bloody stools, menorrhagia, uterine bleeding, mental disorders, dream-disturbed sleep, convulsion.

Method: Puncture subcutaneously 0.1 inch. Moxibustion is applicable.

Regional anatomy

Vasculature: The dorsal digital artery.

Innervation: On the anastomosis of the dorsal digital nerve derived from the superficial peroneal nerve and the plantar digital proprial nerve.

2. Dadu (Ying-Spring Point, Sp 2)

Location: On the medial side of the great toe, distal and inferior to the first metatarsodigital joint, at the junction of the red and white skin. (See Fig. 72)

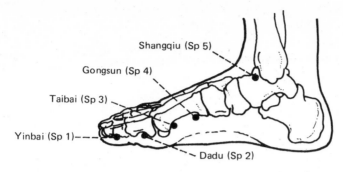

Fig. 72

Indications: Abdominal distension, gastric pain, constipation, febrile diseases with anhidrosis.

Method: Puncture perpendicularly 0.1-0.3 inch. Moxibustion is applicable.

Regional anatomy

Vasculature: The branches of the medial plantar artery and vein.

Innervation: The plantar digital proprial nerve derived from the medial plantar nerve.

3.   Taibai (Shu-Stream and Yuan-Primary Point, Sp 3)

Location: Proximal and inferior to the head of the first metatarsal bone, at the junction of the red and white skin. (See Fig. 72)

Indications: Gastric pain, abdominal distension, constipation, dysentery, vomiting, diarrhea, borborygmus, sluggishness, beriberi.

Method: Puncture perpendicularly 0.3-0.5 inch. Moxibustion is applicable.

Regional anatomy

Vasculature: The dorsal venous network of the foot, the medial plantar artery and the branches of the medial tarsal artery.

Innervation: The branches of the saphenous nerve and superficial peroneal nerve.

4.   Gongsun (Luo-Connecting Point, Confluent Point, Sp 4)

Location: In the depression distal and inferior to the base of the first metatarsal bone, at the junction of the red and white skin. (See Fig. 72)

Indications: Gastric pain, vomiting, abdominal pain and distension, diarrhea, dysentery, borborygmus.

Method: Puncture perpendicularly 0.5-0.8 inch. Moxibustion is applicable.

Regional anatomy

Vasculature: The medial tarsal artery and the dorsal venous network of the foot.

Innervation: The saphenous nerve and the branch of the superficial peroneal nerve.

5.   Shangqiu (Jing-River Point, Sp 5)

Location: In the depression distal and inferior to the medial malleolus, midway between the tuberosity of the navicular bone and the tip of the medial malleolus. (See Fig. 72)

Indications: Abdominal distension, constipation, diarrhea, borborygmus, pain and rigidity of the tongue, pain in the foot and ankle, hemorrhoid.

Method: Puncture perpendicularly 0.2-0.3 inch. Moxibustion is applicable.

Regional anatomy

Vasculature: The medial tarsal artery and the great saphenous vein.

Innervation: The medial crural cutaneous nerve and the branch of the superficial peroneal nerve.

6. Sanyinjiao (Sp 6)

Location: 3 cun directly above the tip of the medial malleolus, on the posterior border of the medial aspect of the tibia. (See Fig. 73)

Indications: Abdominal pain, borborygmus, abdominal distension, diarrhea, dysmenorrhea, irregular menstruation, uterine bleeding, morbid leukorrhea, prolapse of the uterus, sterility, delayed labour, nocturnal emission, impotence, enuresis, dysuria, edema, hernia, pain in the external genitalia, muscular atrophy, motor impairment, paralysis and pain of the lower extremities, headache, dizziness and vertigo, insomnia.

Method: Puncture perpendicularly 0.5-1.0 inch. Moxibustion is applicable. Acupuncture on this point is contraindicated in pregnant women.

Regional anatomy

Vasculature: The great saphenous vein, the posterior tibial artery and vein.

Innervation: Superficially, the medial crural cutaneous nerve; deeper, in the posterior aspect, the tibial nerve.

7. Lougu (Sp 7)

Location: 3 cun above Sanyinjiao (Sp 6) on the line joining the tip of the medial

malleolus and Yinlingquan (Sp 9). (See Fig. 73)

Indications: Abdominal distension, borborygmus, coldness, numbness and paralysis of the knee and leg.

Method: Puncture perpendicularly 0.5-1.0 inch. Moxibustion is applicable.

Regional anatomy: See Sanyinjiao (Sp 6).

8. Diji (Xi-Cleft Point, Sp 8)

Location: 3 cun below Yinlingquan (Sp 9), on the line connecting Yinlingquan (Sp 9) and the medial malleolus. (See Fig. 73)

Indications: Abdominal pain and distension, diarrhea, edema, dysuria, nocturnal emission, irregular menstruation, dysmenorrhea.

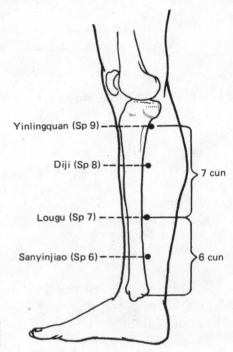

Yinlingquan (Sp 9)

Diji (Sp 8)

7 cun

Lougu (Sp 7)

Sanyinjiao (Sp 6)

6 cun

Fig. 73

Method: Puncture perpendicularly 0.5-
1.0 inch. Moxibustion is applicable.
Regional anatomy
Vasculature: Anteriorly, the great saphenous vein and the branch of the genu
suprema artery; deeper, the posterior tibial
artery and vein.
Innervation: See Sanyinjiao (Sp 6).

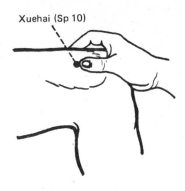

Xuehai (Sp 10)

Fig. 74

9.   Yinlingquan (He-Sea Point, Sp 9)

Location: On the lower border of the
medial condyle of the tibia, in the depression
on the medial border of the tibia. (See
Fig. 73)
Indications: Abdominal pain and distension, diarrhea, dysentery, edema, jaundice,
dysuria, enuresis, incontinence of urine, pain
in the external genitalia, dysmenorrhea, pain
in the knee.
Method: Puncture perpendicularly 0.5-
1.0 inch. Moxibustion is applicable.
Regional anatomy
Vasculature: Anteriorly, the great saphenous vein, the genu suprema artery; deeper,
the posterior tibial artery and vein.
Innervation: Superficially, the medial
crural cutaneous nerve; deeper, the tibial
nerve.

forming an angle of 45° with the index
finger. The point is where the tip of your
thumb rests. (See Fig. 74)
Indications: Irregular menstruation, dysmenorrhea, uterine bleeding, amenorrhea,
urticaria, eczema, erysipelas, pain in the
medial aspect of the thigh.
Method: Puncture perpendicularly 0.5-
1.2 inches. Moxibustion is applicable.
Regional anatomy
Vasculature: The muscular branches of
the femoral artery and vein.
Innervation: The anterior femoral cutaneous nerve and the muscular branch of the
femoral nerve.

10.   Xuehai (Sp 10)

Location: When the knee is flexed, the
point is 2 cun above the mediosuperior
border of the patella, on the bulge of the
medial portion of m. quadriceps femoris. Or
when the patient's knee is flexed, cup your
right palm to his left knee, with the thumb on
the medial side and with the other four
fingers directed proximally, and the thumb

11.   Jimen (Sp 11)

Location: 6 cun above Xuehai (Sp 10), on
the line drawn from Xuehai (Sp 10) to
Chongmen (Sp 12). (See Col. Fig. 5)
Indications: Dysuria, enuresis, pain and
swelling in the inguinal region, muscular
atrophy, motor impairment, pain and
paralysis of the lower extremities.
Method: Puncture perpendicularly 0.5-
1.0 inch. Moxibustion is applicable.

Regional anatomy

Vasculature: Superficially, the great saphenous vein; deeper on the lateral side, the femoral artery and vein.

Innervation: The anterior femoral cutaneous nerve; deeper, the saphenous nerve.

12. Chongmen (Sp 12)

Location: Superior to the lateral end of the inguinal groove, on the lateral side of the femoral artery, at the level of the upper border of symphysis pubis, 3.5 cun lateral to Qugu (Ren 2). (See Col. Fig. 6)

Indications: Abdominal pain, hernia, dysuria.

Method: Avoid puncturing the artery. Puncture perpendicularly 0.5-1.0 inch. Moxibustion is applicable.

Regional anatomy

Vasculature: On the medial side, the femoral artery.

Innervation: Just where the femoral nerve traverses.

13. Fushe (Sp 13)

Location: 0.7 cun laterosuperior to Chongmen (Sp 12), 4 cun lateral to the Ren Meridian. (See Col. Fig. 6)

Indications: Lower abdominal pain, hernia.

Method: Puncture perpendicularly 0.5-1.0 inch. Moxibustion is applicable.

Regional anatomy

Innervation: The ilioinguinal nerve.

14. Fujie (Sp 14)

Location: 1.3 cun below Daheng (Sp 15), 4 cun lateral to the Ren Meridian, on the lateral side of m. rectus abdominis. (See Col. Fig. 6)

Indications: Pain around the umbilical region, abdominal distension, hernia, diarrhea, constipation.

Method: Puncture perpendicularly 0.5-1.0 inch. Moxibustion is applicable.

Regional anatomy

Vasculature: The eleventh intercostal artery and vein.

Innervation: The eleventh intercostal nerve.

15. Daheng (Sp 15)

Location: 4 cun lateral to the center of the umbilicus, lateral to m. rectus abdominis. (See Fig. 75)

Indications: Abdominal pain and distension, diarrhea, dysentery, constipation.

Method: Puncture perpendicularly 0.7-1.2 inches. Moxibustion is applicable.

Regional anatomy

Vasculature: The tenth intercostal artery and vein.

Innervation: The tenth intercostal nerve.

16. Fuai (Sp 16)

Location: 3 cun above Daheng (Sp 15), 4 cun lateral to Jianli (Ren 11). (Col. Fig. 6)

Indications: Abdominal pain, indigestion, constipation, dysentery.

Method: Puncture perpendicularly 0.5-1.0 inch. Moxibustion is applicable.

Regional anatomy

Vasculature: The eighth intercostal artery and vein.

Innervation: The eighth intercostal nerve.

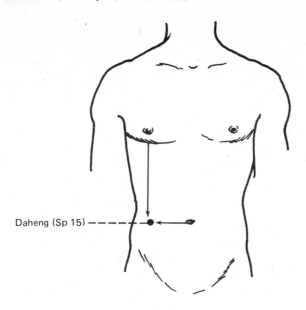

Daheng (Sp 15)

Fig. 75

17.   Shidou (Sp 17)

Location: In the fifth intercostal space, 6 cun lateral to the Ren Meridian. (See Col. Fig. 6)

Indications: Fullness and pain in the chest and hypochondriac region.

Method: Puncture obliquely 0.3-0.5 inch. Moxibustion is applicable.

Regional anatomy

Vasculature: The thoracoepigastric vein.

Innervation: The lateral cutaneous branch of the fifth intercostal nerve.

18.   Tianxi (Sp 18)

Location: In the fourth intercostal space, 6 cun lateral to the Ren Meridian. (See Col. Fig. 6)

Indications: Fullness and pain in the chest and hypochondrium, cough, hiccup, mastitis, insufficient lactation.

Method: Puncture obliquely 0.3-0.5 inch. Moxibustion is applicable.

Regional anatomy

Vasculature: The branches of the lateral thoracic artery and vein, the thoracoepigastric artery and vein, the fourth intercostal artery and vein.

Innervation: The lateral cutaneous branch of the fourth intercostal nerve.

19.   Xiongxiang (Sp 19)

Location: In the third intercostal space, 6 cun lateral to the Ren Meridian. (See Col. Fig. 6)

Indications: Fullness and pain in the chest and hypochondriac region.

Method: Puncture obliquely 0.3-0.5 inch. Moxibustion is applicable.

Regional anatomy

Vasculature: The lateral thoracic artery and vein, the third intercostal artery and vein.

Innervation: The lateral cutaneous branch of the third intercostal nerve.

20. Zhourong (Sp 20)

Location: In the second intercostal space, 6 cun lateral to the Ren Meridian. (See Col. Fig. 6)

Indications: Fullness in the chest and hypochondriac region, cough, hiccup.

Method: Puncture obliquely 0.3-0.5 inch. Moxibustion is applicable.

Regional anatomy

Vasculature: The lateral thoracic artery and vein, the second intercostal artery and vein.

Innervation: The muscular branch of the anterior thoracic nerve, the lateral cutaneous branch of the second intercostal nerve.

21. Dabao (Major Luo-Connecting Point of the Spleen, Sp 21)

Location: On the mid-axillary line, 6 cun below the axilla, midway between the axilla and the free end of the eleventh rib. (See Col. Fig. 6)

Indications: Pain in the chest and hypochondriac region, asthma, general aching and weakness.

Method: Puncture obliquely 0.3-0.5 inch. Moxibustion is applicable.

Regional anatomy

Vasculature: The thoracodorsal artery and vein, the seventh intercostal artery and vein.

Innervation: The seventh intercostal nerve and the terminal branch of the long thoracic nerve.

Chapter 8

ACUPOINTS OF THE SHAOYIN AND TAIYANG MERIDIAN

The Heart Meridian of Hand-Shaoyin going from the chest to the hand and the Small Intestine Meridian of Hand-Taiyang going from the hand to the head are exteriorly and interiorly related, so are the Bladder Meridian of Foot-Taiyang running from the head to the foot and the Kidney Meridian of Foot-Shaoyin running from the foot to the abdomen (chest). The four meridians are mainly distributed on the extremities and in the posterior aspect of the trunk. Their acupoints are described as follows:

I. THE HEART MERIDIAN OF HAND-SHAOYIN

1. Jiquan (H 1)

Location: When the upper arm is abducted, the point is in the centre of the axilla, on the medial side of the axillary artery. (See Col. Fig. 7)

Indications: Pain in the costal and cardiac regions, scrofula, cold pain of the elbow and arm, dryness of the throat.

Method: Avoid puncturing the axillary artery. Puncture perpendicularly 0.5-1.0 inch. Moxibustion is applicable.

Regional anatomy
Vasculature: Laterally, the axillary artery.
Innervation: The ulnar nerve, median nerve and medial brachial cutaneous nerve.

2. Qingling (H 2)

Location: When the elbow is flexed, the point is 3 cun above the medial end of the transverse cubital crease (Shaohai H 3), in the groove medial to m. biceps brachii. (See Col. Fig. 7)

Indications: Pain in the cardiac and hypochondriac regions, shoulder and arm.

Method: Puncture perpendicularly 0.3-0.5 inch. Moxibustion is applicable.

Regional anatomy
Vasculature: The basilic vein, the superior ulnar collateral artery.
Innervation: The medial antebrachial cutaneous nerve, the medial brachial cutaneous nerve and the ulnar nerve.

3. Shaohai (He-Sea Point, H 3)

Location: When the elbow is flexed into a right angle, the point is in the depression between the medial end of the transverse cubital crease and the medial epicondyle of the humerus. (See Fig. 76)

Indications: Cardiac pain, spasmodic pain and numbness of the hand and arm, tremor of the hand, scrofula, pain in the axilla and hypochondriac region.

Method: Puncture perpendicularly 0.5-1.0 inch. Moxibustion is applicable.

Regional anatomy

Vasculature: The basilic vein, the inferior ulnar collateral artery, the ulnar recurrent artery and vein.

Innervation: The medial antebrachial cutaneous nerve.

4. Lingdao (Jing-River Point, H 4)

Location: When the palm faces upward, the point is on the radial side of the tendon of

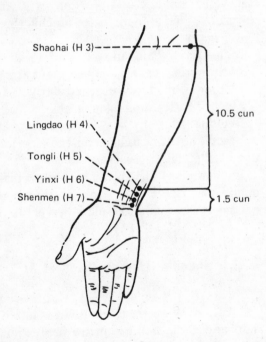

Fig. 76

m. flexor carpi ulnaris, 1.5 cun above the transverse crease of the wrist. (See Fig. 76)

Indications: Cardiac pain, spasmodic pain of the elbow and arm, sudden loss of voice.

Method: Puncture perpendicularly 0.3-0.5 inch. Moxibustion is applicable.

Regional anatomy

Vasculature: The ulnar artery.

Innervation: The medial antebrachial cutaneous nerve; on the ulnar side, the ulnar nerve.

5. Tongli (Luo-Connecting Point, H 5)

Location: When the palm faces upward, the point is on the radial side of the tendon of m. flexor carpi ulnaris, 1 cun above the transverse crease of the wrist. (See Fig. 76)

Indications: Palpitation, dizziness, blurring of vision, sore throat, sudden loss of voice, aphasia with stiffness of the tongue, pain in the wrist and elbow.

Method: Puncture perpendicularly 0.3-0.5 inch. Moxibustion is applicable.

Regional anatomy: See Lingdao (H 4).

6. Yinxi (Xi-Cleft Point, H 6)

Location: When the palm faces upward, the point is on the radial side of the tendon of m. flexor carpi ulnaris, 0.5 cun above the transverse crease of the wrist. (See Fig. 76)

Indications: Cardiac pain, hysteria, night sweating, hemoptysis, epistaxis, sudden loss of voice.

Method: Puncture perpendicularly 0.3-0.5 inch. Moxibustion is applicable.

Regional anatomy: See Lingdao (H 4).

7. Shenmen (Shu-Stream and Yuan-Primary Point, H 7)

Location: At the ulnar end of the transverse crease of the wrist, in the depression on the radial side of the tendon of m. flexor carpi ulnaris. (See Fig. 76)

Indications: Cardiac pain, irritability, palpitation, hysteria, amnesia, insomnia, mania, epilepsy, dementia, pain in the hypochondriac region, feverish sensation in the palm, yellowish sclera.

Method: Puncture perpendicularly 0.3-0.5 inch. Moxibustion is applicable.

Regional anatomy: See Lingdao (H 4).

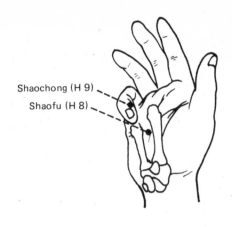

Shaochong (H 9)
Shaofu (H 8)

Fig. 77

8. Shaofu (Ying-Spring Point, H 8)

Location: When the palm faces upward, the point is between the fourth and fifth metacarpal bones. When a fist is made, the point is where the tip of the little finger rests. (See Fig. 77)

Indications: Palpitation, pain in the chest, spasmodic pain of the little finger, feverish sensation in the palm, enuresis, dysuria, pruritus of the external genitalia.

Method: Puncture perpendicularly 0.3-0.5 inch. Moxibustion is applicable.

Regional anatomy

Vasculature: The common palmar digital artery and vein.

Innervation: The fourth common palmar digital nerve derived from the ulnar nerve.

9. Shaochong (Jing-Well Point, H 9)

Location: On the radial side of the little finger, about 0.1 cun posterior to the corner of the nail. (See Fig. 77)

Indications: Palpitation, cardiac pain, pain in the chest and hypochondriac regions, mania, febrile diseases, loss of consciousness.

Method: Puncture subcutaneously 0.1 inch, or prick with a three-edged needle to cause bleeding. Moxibustion is applicable.

Regional anatomy

Vasculature: The arterial and venous network formed by the palmar digital proprial artery and vein.

Innervation: The palmar digital proprial nerve derived from the ulnar nerve.

II.   THE SMALL INTESTINE MERIDIAN OF HAND-TAIYANG

1.   Shaoze (Jing-Well Point, S I 1)

Location: On the ulnar side of the little finger, about 0.1 cun posterior to the corner of the nail. (See Fig. 78)

Indications: Headache, febrile diseases, loss of consciousness, insufficient lactation, sore throat, redness of the eye, cloudiness of the cornea.

Method: Puncture subcutaneously 0.1 inch, or prick the point to cause bleeding. Moxibustion is applicable.

Regional anatomy

Vasculature: The arterial and venous network formed by the palmar digital proprial artery and vein and the dorsal digital artery and vein.

Innervation: The palmar digital proprial nerve and the dorsal digital nerve derived from the ulnar nerve.

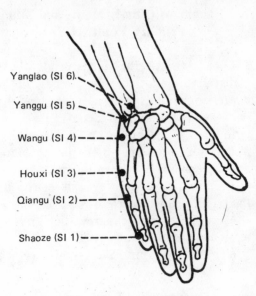

Fig. 78

2.   Qiangu (Ying-Spring Point, S I 2)

Location: When a loose fist is made, the point is on the ulnar side, distal to the fifth metacarpophalangeal joint, at the junction of the red and white skin. (See Fig. 78)

Indications: Numbness of the fingers, febrile diseases, tinnitus, headache, reddish urine.

Method: Puncture perpendicularly 0.3-0.5 inch. Moxibustion is applicable.

Regional anatomy

Vasculature: The dorsal digital artery and vein arising from the ulnar artery and vein.

Innervation: The dorsal digital nerve and palmar digital proprial nerve derived from the ulnar nerve.

Indications: Pain and rigidity of the neck, tinnitus, deafness, sore throat, mania, malaria, acute lumbar sprain, night sweating, febrile diseases, contracture and numbness of the fingers, pain in the shoulder and elbow.

Method: Puncture perpendicularly 0.5-0.7 inch. Moxibustion is applicable.

Regional anatomy

Vasculature: The dorsal digital artery and vein, the dorsal venous network of the hand.

Innervation: The dorsal branch derived from the ulnar nerve.

3. Houxi (Shu-Stream Point, One of the Eight Confluent Points, S I 3)

Location: When a loose fist is made, the point is on the ulnar side, proximal to the fifth metacarpophalangeal joint, at the end of the transverse crease and the junction of the red and white skin. (See Fig. 78)

4.   Wangu (Yuan-Primary Point, S I 4)

Location: On the ulnar side of the palm, in the depression between the base of the fifth metacarpal bone and the triquetral bone. (See Fig. 78)

Indications: Febrile diseases with anhidrosis, headache, rigidity of the neck, contracture of the fingers, pain in the wrist, jaundice.

Method: Puncture perpendiculary 0.3-0.5 inch. Moxibustion is applicable.

Regional anatomy

Vasculature: The posterior carpal artery (the branch of the ulnar artery), the dorsal venous network of the hand.

Innervation: The dorsal branch of the ulnar nerve.

5.   Yanggu (Jing-River Point, S I 5)

Location: At the ulnar end of the transverse crease on the dorsal aspect of the wrist, in the depression between the styloid process of the ulna and the triquetral bone. (See Fig. 78)

Indications: Swelling of the neck and submandibular region, pain of the hand and wrist, febrile diseases.

Method: Puncture perpendicularly 0.3-0.5 inch. Moxibustion is applicable.

Regional anatomy

Vasculature: The posterior carpal artery.

Innervation: The dorsal branch of the ulnar nerve.

6.   Yanglao (Xi-Cleft Point, S I 6)

Location: Dorsal to the head of the ulna. When the palm faces the chest, the point is in the bony cleft on the radial side of the styloid process of the ulna. (See Figs. 78 and 79)

Indications: Blurring of vision, pain in the shoulder, elbow and arm.

Method: Puncture perpendicularly 0.3-0.5 inch. Moxibustion is applicable.

Regional anatomy

Vasculature: The terminal branches of the posterior interosseous artery and vein, the dorsal venous network of the wrist.

Innervation: The anastomotic branches of the posterior antebrachial cutaneous nerve and the dorsal branch of the ulnar nerve.

7.   Zhizheng (Luo-Connecting Point, S I 7)

Location: On the line joining Yanggu (S I 5) and Xiaohai (S I 8), 5 cun above Yanggu (S I 5). (See Fig. 80)

Indications: Neck rigidity, headache, dizziness, spasmodic pain in the elbow and fingers, febrile diseases, mania.

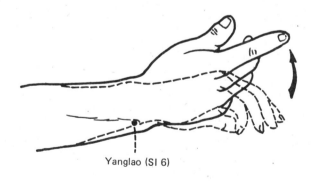

Yanglao (SI 6)

Fig. 79

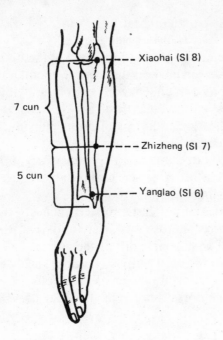

7 cun

5 cun

— — Xiaohai (SI 8)

— — Zhizheng (SI 7)

— — Yanglao (SI 6)

Fig. 80

Method: Puncture perpendicularly 0.5-0.8 inch. Moxibustion is applicable.

Regional anatomy

Vasculature: The terminal branches of the posterior interosseous artery and vein.

Innervation: Superficially, the branch of the medial antebrachial cutaneous nerve; deeper, on the radial side, the posterior interosseous nerve.

8. Xiaohai (He-Sea Point, S I 8)

Location: When the elbow is flexed, the point is located in the depression between the olecranon of the ulna and the medial epicondyle of the humerus.   (See Figs. 80 and 81)

Indications: Headache, swelling of the cheek, pain in the nape, shoulder, arm and elbow, epilepsy.

Method: Puncture perpendicularly 0.3-0.5 inch. Moxibustion is applicable.

Regional anatomy

Vasculature: The superior and inferior ulnar collateral arteries and veins, the ulnar recurrent artery and vein.

Innervation: The branches of the medial antebrachial cutaneous nerve, the ulnar nerve.

9. Jianzhen (S I 9)

Location: Posterior and inferior to the shoulder joint. When the arm is adducted, the point is 1 cun above the posterior end of the axillary fold. (See Fig. 82)

Indications: Pain in the scapular region, motor impairment of the hand and arm.

Method: Puncture perpendicularly 0.5-1.0 inch. Moxibustion is applicable.

Regional anatomy

Vasculature: The circumflex scapular artery and vein.

Innervation: The branch of the axillary

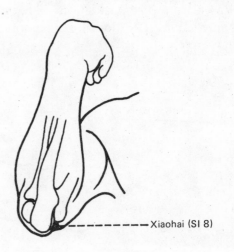

— — — — — — — — — —Xiaohai (SI 8)

Fig. 81

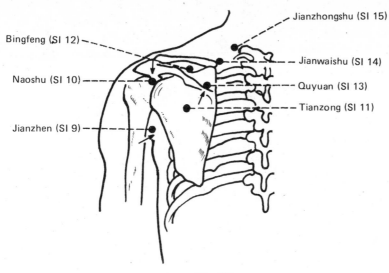

Fig. 82

nerve; deeper in the superior aspect, the radial nerve.

10. Naoshu (S I 10)

Location: When the arm is adducted, the point is directly above Jianzhen (S I 9), in the depression inferior to the scapular spine. (See Fig. 82)

Indications: Swelling of the shoulder, aching and weakness of the shoulder and arm.

Method: Puncture perpendicularly 0.5-1.0 inch. Moxibustion is applicable.

Regional anatomy

Vasculature: The posterior circumflex humeral artery and vein; deeper, the suprascapular artery and vein.

Innervation: The posterior cutaneous nerve of the arm, the axillary nerve; deeper, the suprascapular nerve.

11. Tianzong (S I 11)

Location: In the infrascapular fossa, at the junction of the upper and middle third of the distance between the lower border of the scapular spine and the inferior angle of the scapula. (See Fig. 82)

Indications: Pain in the scapular region, pain in the lateroposterior aspect of the elbow and arm, asthma.

Method: Puncture perpendicularly or obliquely 0.5-1.0 inch. Moxibustion is applicable.

Regional anatomy

Vasculature: The muscular branches of the circumflex scapular artery and vein.

Innervation: The suprascapular nerve.

12. Bingfeng (S I 12)

Location: In   the   centre   of   the suprascapular fossa, directly above Tianzong (S I 11). When the arm is lifted, the point is at the site of the depression. (See Fig. 82)

Indications: Pain in the scapular region, numbness and aching of the upper extremities, motor impairment of the shoulder and arm.

Method: Puncture perpendicularly 0.5-0.7 inch. Moxibustion is applicable.

Regional anatomy

Vasculature: The suprascapular artery and vein.

Innervation: The lateral suprascapular nerve and accessory nerve; deeper, the suprascapular nerve.

13. Quyuan (S I 13)

Location: On the medial extremity of the suprascapular fossa, about midway between Naoshu (S I 10) and the spinous process of the second thoracic vertebra. (See Fig. 82)

Indications: Pain and stiffness of the scapular region.

Method: Puncture perpendicularly 0.3-0.5 inch. Moxibustion is applicable.

Regional anatomy

Vasculature: Superficially, the descending branches of the transverse cervical artery and vein; deeper, the muscular branch of the suprascapular artery and vein.

Innervation: Superficially, the lateral branch of the posterior ramus of the second thoracic nerve, the accessory nerve; deeper, the muscular branch of the suprascapular nerve.

14. Jianwaishu (S I 14)

Location: 3 cun lateral to the lower border of the spinous process of the first thoracic vertebra where Taodao (Du 13) is located. (See Fig. 82)

Indications: Aching of the shoulder and back, pain and rigidity of the neck.

Method: Puncture obliquely 0.3-0.7 inch. Moxibustion is applicable.

Regional anatomy

Vasculature: Deeper, the transverse cervical artery and vein.

Innervation: Superficially, the medial cutaneous branches of the posterior rami of the first and second thoracic nerves, the accessory nerve; deeper, the dorsal scapular nerve.

15. Jianzhongshu (S I 15)

Location: 2 cun lateral to the lower border of the spinous process of the seventh cervical vertebra (Dazhui, Du 14). (See Fig. 82)

Indications: Cough, asthma, pain in the shoulder and back, hemoptysis.

Method: Puncture obliquely 0.3-0.6 inch. Moxibustion is applicable.

Regional anatomy: See Jianwaishu (S I 14).

16. Tianchuang (S I 16)

Location: In the lateral aspect of the neck, in the posterior border of m. sternocleido-mastoideus, posterosuperior to Futu (L I 18). (See Col. Fig. 8)

Indications: Sore throat, sudden loss of voice, deafness, tinnitus, stiffness and pain of the neck.

Method: Puncture perpendicularly 0.3-0.7 inch. Moxibustion is applicable.

Regional anatomy

Vasculature: The ascending cervical artery.

Innervation: The cutaneous cervical nerve, the emerging portion of the great auricular nerve.

17.   Tianrong (S I 17)

Location: Posterior to the angle of mandible, in the depression on the anterior border of m. sternocleidomastoideus. (See Fig. 83)

Indications: Deafness, tinnitus, sore throat, swelling of the cheek, foreign body sensation in the throat, goiter.

Method: Puncture perpendicularly 0.5-0.7 inch. Moxibustion is applicable.

Regional anatomy

Vasculature: Anteriorly, the external jugular vein; deeper, the internal carotid artery and internal jugular vein.

Innervation: Superficially, the anterior branch of the great auricular nerve, the cervical branch of the facial nerve; deeper,

the superior cervical ganglion of the sympathetic trunk.

18.   Quanliao (S I 18)

Location: Directly below the outer canthus, in the depression on the lower border of zygoma. (See Fig. 84)

Indications: Facial paralysis, twitching of eyelids, pain in the face, toothache, swelling of the cheek, yellowish sclera.

Method: Puncture perpendicularly 0.5-0.8 inch.

Regional anatomy

Vasculature: The branches of the transverse facial artery and vein.

Innervation: The facial and infraorbital nerves.

19.   Tinggong (S I 19)

Location: Anterior to the tragus and posterior to the condyloid process of the

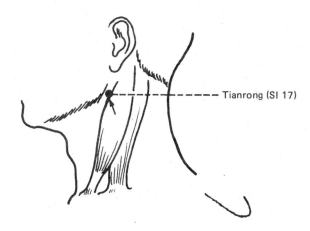

Tianrong (SI 17)

Fig. 83

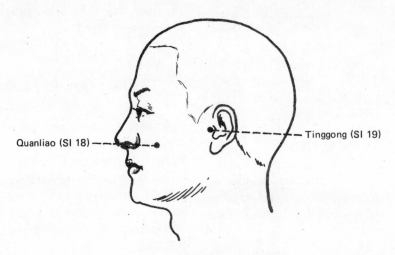

Quanliao (SI 18) —————— Tinggong (SI 19)

Fig. 84

mandible, in the depression formed when the mouth is open. (See Fig. 84)

Indications: Deafness, tinnitus, otorrhea, motor impairment of the mandibular joint, toothache.

Method: Puncture perpendicularly 0.5-1.0 inch when the mouth is open. Moxibustion is applicable.

Regional anatomy

Vasculature: The auricular branches of the superficial temporal artery and vein.

Innervation: The branch of the facial nerve, the auriculotemporal nerve.

III. THE BLADDER MERIDIAN OF FOOT-TAIYANG

1. Jingming (B 1)

Location: 0.1 cun superior to the inner canthus. (See Fig. 85)

Indications: Redness, swelling and pain of the eye, itching of the canthus, lacrimation,

night blindness, colour blindness, blurring of vision, myopia.

Method: Ask the patient to close his eyes when pushing gently the eyeball to the lateral side. Puncture slowly perpendicularly 0.3-0.7 inch along the orbital wall. It is not advisable to twist or lift and thrust the needle vigorously. To avoid bleeding, press the puncturing site for a few seconds after withdrawal of the needle. Moxibustion is forbidden.

Regional anatomy

Vasculature: The angular artery and vein, deeper, superiorly, the ophthalmic artery and vein.

Innervation: Superficially, the supratrochlear and infratrochlear nerves; deeper, the branches of the oculomotor nerve, the ophthalmic nerve.

2. Zanzhu (B 2)

Location: On the medial extremity of the eyebrow, or on the supraorbital notch. (See Fig. 85)

Indications: Headache, blurring and failing of vision, pain in the supraorbital region, lacrimation, redness, swelling and pain of the eye, twitching of eyelids, glaucoma.

Method: Puncture subcutaneously 0.3-0.5 inch, or prick with three-edged needle to cause bleeding.

Regional anatomy

Vasculature: The frontal artery and vein.

Innervation: The medial branch of the frontal nerve.

3.   Meichong (B 3)

Location: Directly above the medial end of the eyebrow, 0.5 cun within the anterior hairline, between Shenting (Du 24) and Quchai (B 4). (See Col. Fig. 9)

Indications: Headache, giddiness, epilepsy, nasal obstruction.

Method: Puncture subcutaneously 0.3-0.5 inch.

Regional anatomy: See Zanzhu (B 2).

4.   Quchai (B 4)

Location: 1.5 cun lateral to Shenting (Du 24) at the junction of the medial third and lateral two-thirds of the distance from Shenting (Du 24) to Touwei (S 8). (See Col. Fig. 9)

Indications: Headache, nasal obstruction, epistaxis, blurring and failing of vision.

Method: Puncture subcutaneously 0.3-0.5 inch. Moxibustion is applicable.

Regional anatomy

Vasculature: The frontal artery and vein.

Innervation: The lateral branch of the frontal nerve.

5.   Wuchu (B 5)

Location: 1.5 cun lateral to Shangxing (Du 23), or 0.5 cun directly above Quchai (B 4). (See Col. Fig. 9)

Indications: Headache, blurring of vision, epilepsy, convulsion.

Method: Puncture subcutaneously 0.3-0.5

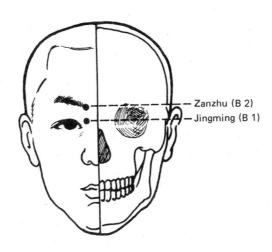

— Zanzhu (B 2)
— Jingming (B 1)

Fig. 85

inch. Moxibustion is applicable.

Regional anatomy: See Quchai (B 4).

6. Chengguang (B 6)

Location: 1.5 cun posterior to Wuchu (B 5), 1.5 cun lateral to the Du Meridian. (See Col. Fig. 9)

Indications: Headache, blurring of vision, nasal obstruction.

Method: Puncture subcutaneously 0.3-0.5 inch.

Regional anatomy

Vasculature: The anastomotic network of the frontal artery and vein, the superficial temporal artery and vein, the occipital artery and vein.

Innervation: The anastomotic branch of the lateral branch of the frontal nerve and the great occipital nerve.

7. Tongtian (B 7)

Location: 1.5 cun posterior to Chengguang (B 6), 1.5 cun lateral to the Du Meridian. (See Col. Fig. 9)

Indications: Headache, giddiness, nasal obstruction, epistaxis, rhinorrhea.

Method: Puncture subcutaneously 0.3-0.5 inch. Moxibustion is applicable.

Regional anatomy

Vasculature: The superficial temporal artery and vein and the occipital artery and vein.

Innervation: The branch of the great occipital nerve.

8. Luoque (B 8)

Location: 1.5 cun posterior to Tongtian (B 7), 1.5 cun lateral to the Du Meridian. (See Col. Fig. 9)

Indications: Dizziness, blurring of vision, tinnitus, mania.

Method: Puncture subcutaneously 0.3-0.5 inch.

Regional anatomy

Vasculature: The branches of the occipital artery and vein.

Innervation: The branch of the great occipital nerve.

9. Yuzhen (B 9)

Location: 1.3 cun lateral to Naohu (Du 17), on the lateral side of the superior border of the external occipital protuberance. (See Col. Fig. 9)

Indications: Headache and neck pain, dizziness, ophthalmalgia, nasal obstruction.

Method: Puncture subcutaneously 0.3-0.5 inch. Moxibustion is applicable.

Regional anatomy

Vasculature: The occipital artery and vein.

Innervation: The branch of the great occipital nerve.

10. Tianzhu (B 10)

Location: 1.3 cun lateral to Yamen (Du 15), in the depression on the lateral aspect of m. trapezius. (See Col. Fig. 9)

Indications: Headache, nasal obstruction, sore throat, neck rigidity, pain in the shoulder and back.

Method: Puncture perpendicularly 0.5-0.8 inch.

Regional anatomy

Vasculature: The occipital artery and vein.

Innervation: The great occipital nerve.

11. Dazhu (Influential Point of Bone, B 11)

Location: 1.5 cun lateral to Taodao (Du 13), at the level of the lower border of the spinous process of the first thoracic vertebra.

Indications: Headache, pain in the neck and back, pain and soreness in the scapular region, cough, fever, neck rigidity.

Method: Puncture obliquely 0.5-0.7 inch. Moxibustion is applicable.

Regional anatomy

Vasculature: The medial cutaneous branches of the posterior branches of the intercostal artery and vein.

Innervation: The medial cutaneous branches of the posterior rami of the first and second thoracic nerves; deeper, their lateral cutaneous branches.

12. Fengmen (B 12)

Location: 1.5 cun lateral to the Du Meridian, at the level of the lower border of the spinous process of the second thoracic vertebra. (See Fig. 86)

Indications: Common cold, cough, fever and headache, neck rigidity, backache.

Method: Puncture obliquely 0.5-0.7 inch. Moxibustion is applicable.

Regional anatomy

Vasculature: The medial cutaneous branches of the posterior branches of the intercostal artery and vein.

Innervation: Superficially, the medial cutaneous branches of the posterior rami of the second and third thoracic nerves; deeper, their lateral cutaneous branches.

13. Feishu (Back-Shu Point of the Lung, B 13)

Location: 1.5 cun lateral to Shenzhu (Du 12), at the level of the lower border of the spinous process of the third thoracic vertebra. (See Fig. 86)

Indications: Cough, asthma, chest pain, spitting of blood, afternoon fever, night sweating.

Method: Puncture obliquely 0.5-0.7 inch. Moxibustion is applicable.

Regional anatomy

Vasculature: The medial cutaneous branches of the posterior branches of the intercostal artery and vein.

Innervation: The medial cutaneous branches of the posterior rami of the third and fourth thoracic nerves; deeper, their lateral branches.

14. Jueyinshu (Back-Shu Point of the Pericardium, B 14)

Location: 1.5 cun lateral to the Du Meridian, at the level of the lower border of the spinous process of the fourth thoracic vertebra. (See Col. Fig. 9)

Indications: Cough, cardiac pain, palpitation, stuffy chest, vomiting.

Method: Puncture obliquely 0.5-0.7 inch. Moxibustion is applicable.

Regional anatomy

Vasculature: The medial cutaneous branches of the posterior branches of the intercostal artery and vein.

Innervation: The medial cutaneous branches of the posterior rami of the fourth or fifth thoracic nerves; deeper, their lateral branches.

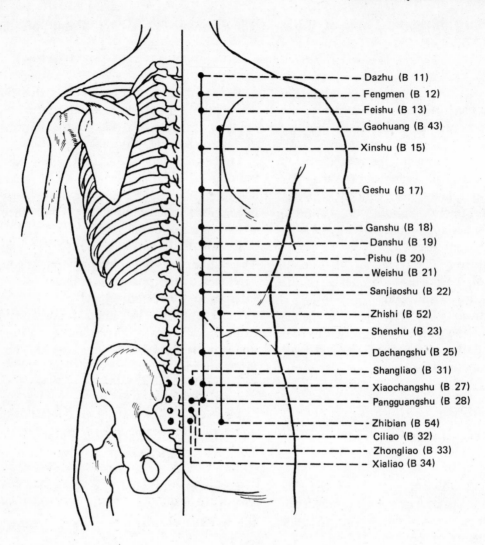

Dazhu (B 11)
Fengmen (B 12)
Feishu (B 13)
Gaohuang (B 43)
Xinshu (B 15)

Geshu (B 17)

Ganshu (B 18)
Danshu (B 19)
Pishu (B 20)
Weishu (B 21)
Sanjiaoshu (B 22)

Zhishi (B 52)
Shenshu (B 23)

Dachangshu (B 25)
Shangliao (B 31)
Xiaochangshu (B 27)
Pangguangshu (B 28)

Zhibian (B 54)
Ciliao (B 32)
Zhongliao (B 33)
Xialiao (B 34)

Fig. 86

15. Xinshu (Back-Shu Point of the Heart, B 15)

Location: 1.5 cun lateral to Shendao (Du 11), at the level of the lower border of the spinous process of the fifth thoracic vertebra. (See Fig. 86)

Indications: Cardiac pain, panic, loss of memory, palpitation, cough, spitting of blood, nocturnal emission, night sweating, mania, epilepsy.

Method: Puncture obliquely 0.5-0.7 inch. Moxibustion is applicable.

Regional anatomy

Vasculature: The medial cutaneous

branches of the posterior branches of the intercostal artery and vein.

Innervation: The medial cutaneous branches of the posterior rami of the fifth and sixth thoracic nerves; deeper, their lateral branches.

16.   Dushu (B 16)

Location: 1.5 cun lateral to Lingtai (Du 10), at the level of the lower border of the spinous process of the sixth thoracic vertebra. (See Col. Fig. 9)

Method: Puncture obliquely 0.5-0.7 inch. Moxibustion is applicable.

Regional anatomy

Vasculature: The medial branches of the posterior branches of the intercostal artery and vein, the descending branch of the transverse cervical artery.

Innervation: The dorsal scapular nerve, the medial cutaneous branches of the dorsal rami of the sixth and seventh thoracic nerves; deeper, their lateral branches.

17.   Geshu (Influential Point of Blood, B 17)

Location: 1.5 cun lateral to Zhiyang (Du 9), at the level of the lower border of the spinous process of the seventh thoracic vertebra. (See Fig. 86)

Indications: Vomiting, hiccup, belching, difficulty in swallowing, asthma, cough, spitting of blood, afternoon fever, night sweating, measles.

Method: Puncture obliquely 0.5-0.7 inch. Moxibustion is applicable.

Regional anatomy

Vasculature: The medial branches of the

posterior branches of the intercostal artery and vein.

Innervation: The medial branches of the posterior rami of the seventh and eighth thoracic nerves; deeper, their lateral branches.

18.   Ganshu (Back-Shu Point of the Liver, B 18)

Location: 1.5 cun lateral to Jinsuo (Du 8), at the level of the lower border of the spinous process of the ninth thoracic vertebra. (See Fig. 86)

Indications: Jaundice, pain in the hypochondriac region, redness of the eye, blurring of vision, night blindness, mental disorders, epilepsy, backache, spitting of blood, epistaxis.

Method: Puncture obliquely 0.5-0.7 inch. Moxibustion is applicable.

Regional anatomy

Vasculature: The medial branches of the posterior branches of the intercostal artery and vein.

Innervation: The medial cutaneous branches of the posterior rami of the ninth and tenth thoracic nerves; deeper, their lateral branches.

19.   Danshu (Back-Shu Point of the Gallbladder, B 19)

Location: 1.5 cun lateral to Zhongshu (Du 7), at the level of the lower border of the spinous process of the tenth thoracic vertebra. (See Fig. 86)

Indications: Jaundice, bitter taste of the mouth, pain in the chest and hypochondriac region, pulmonary tuberculosis, afternoon fever.

Method: Puncture obliquely 0.5-0.8 inch. Moxibustion is applicable.

Regional anatomy

Musculature: M. latissimus dorsi, the site between m. longissimus and m. iliocostalis.

Vasculature: The medial branches of the posterior branches of the intercostal artery and vein.

Innervation: The medial cutaneous branches of the posterior rami of the tenth and eleventh thoracic nerves; deeper, their lateral branches.

20. Pishu (Back-Shu Point of the Spleen, B 20)

Location: 1.5 cun lateral to Jizhong (Du 6), at the level of the lower border of the spinous process of the eleventh thoracic vertebra. (See Fig. 86)

Indications: Epigastric pain, abdominal distension, jaundice, vomiting, diarrhea, dysentery, bloody stools, profuse menstruation, edema, anorexia, backache.

Method: Puncture obliquely 0.5-0.7 inch. Moxibustion is applicable.

Regional anatomy

Vasculature: The medial branches of the posterior branches of the intercostal artery and vein.

Innervation: The medial cutaneous branches of the posterior rami of the eleventh and twelfth thoracic nerves; deeper, their lateral branches.

21. Weishu (Back-Shu Point of the Stomach, B 21)

Location: 1.5 cun lateral to the Du Meridian, at the level of the lower border of the spinous process of the twelfth thoracic vertebra. (See Fig. 86)

Indications: Pain in the chest and hypochondriac and epigastric regions, anorexia, abdominal distension, borborygmus, diarrhea, nausea, vomiting.

Method: Puncture obliquely 0.5-0.8 inch. Moxibustion is applicable.

Regional anatomy

Vasculature: The medial branches of the posterior branches of the subcostal artery and vein.

Innervation: The medial cutaneous branch of the posterior ramus of the twelfth thoracic nerve; deeper, its lateral branch.

22. Sanjiaoshu (Back-Shu Point of Sanjiao, B 22)

Location: 1.5 cun lateral to Xuanshu (Du 5), at the level of the lower border of the spinous process of the first lumbar vertebra. (See Fig. 86)

Indications: Borborygmus, abdominal distension, indigestion, vomiting, diarrhea, dysentery, edema, pain and stiffness of the lower back.

Method: Puncture perpendicularly 0.5-1.0 inch. Moxibustion is applicable.

Regional anatomy

Vasculature: The posterior branches of the first lumber artery and vein.

Innervation: The lateral cutaneous branch of the posterior ramus of the tenth thoracic nerve; deeper, the lateral branch of the posterior ramus of the first lumbar nerve.

23. Shenshu (Back-Shu Point of the Kidney, B 23)

Location: 1.5 cun lateral to Mingmen (Du 4), at the level of the lower border of the spinous process of the second lumbar vertebra. (See Fig. 86)

Indications: Nocturnal emission, impotence, enuresis, irregular menstruation, leukorrhea, low back pain, weakness of the knee, blurring of vision, dizziness, tinnitus, deafness, edema, asthma, diarrhea.

Method: Puncture perpendicularly 1-1.2 inches. Moxibustion is applicable.

Regional anatomy

Vasculature: The posterior branches of the second lumbar artery and vein.

Innervation: The lateral branch of the posterior ramus of the first lumbar nerve; deeper, its lateral branch.

24.   Qihaishu (B 24)

Location: 1.5 cun lateral to the Du Meridian, at the level of the lower border of the spinous process of the third lumbar vertebra. (See Col. Fig. 9)

Indications: Low back pain, irregular menstruation, dysmenorrhea, asthma.

Method: Puncture perpendicularly 0.8-1.2 inches. Moxibustion is applicable.

Regional anatomy

Vasculature: The posterior branch of the third lumbar artery and vein.

Innervation: The lateral cutaneous branch of the posterior ramus of the second lumbar nerve.

25.   Dachangshu (Back-Shu Point of the Large Intestine, B 25)

Location: 1.5 cun lateral to Yaoyangguan (Du 3), at the level of the lower border of the spinous process of the fourth lumbar vertebra. (See Fig. 86)

Indications: Low back pain, borborygmus, abdominal distension, diarrhea, constipation, muscular atrophy, pain, numbness and motor impairment of the lower extremities, sciatica.

Method: Puncture perpendicularly 0.8-1.2 inches. Moxibustion is applicable.

Regional anatomy

Vasculature: The posterior branch of the fourth lumbar artery and vein.

Innervation: The posterior ramus of the third lumbar nerve.

26.   Guanyuanshu (B 26)

Location: 1.5 cun lateral to the Du Meridian, at the level of the lower border of the spinous process of the fifth lumbar vertebra. (See Col. Fig. 9)

Indications: Low back pain, abdominal distension, diarrhea, enuresis, sciatica, frequent urination.

Method: Puncture perpendicularly 0.8-1.2 inches. Moxibustion is applicable.

Regional anatomy

Vasculature: The posterior branches of the lowest lumbar artery and vein.

Innervation: The posterior ramus of the fifth lumbar nerve.

27.   Xiaochangshu (Back-Shu Point of the Small Intestine, B 27)

Location: 1.5 cun lateral to the Du Meridian, at the level of the first posterior sacral foramen. (See Fig. 86)

Indications: Lower abdominal pain and distension, dysentery, nocturnal emission, hematuria, enuresis, morbid leukorrhea, lower back pain, sciatica.

Method: Puncture perpendicularly 0.8-1.2 inches. Moxibustion is applicable.

Regional anatomy

Vasculature: The posterior branches of the lateral sacral artery and vein.

Innervation: The lateral branch of the posterior ramus of the first sacral nerve.

28. Pangguangshu (Back-Shu Point of the Bladder, B 28)

Location: 1.5 cun lateral to the Du Meridian, at the level of the second posterior sacral foramen. (See Fig. 86)

Indications: Retention of urine, enuresis, frequent urination, diarrhea, constipation, stiffness and pain of the lower back. (See Fig. 86)

Method: Puncture perpendicularly 0.8-1.2 inches. Moxibustion is applicable.

Regional anatomy

Vasculature: The posterior branches of the lateral sacral artery and vein.

Innervation: The lateral branches of the posterior rami of the first and second sacral nerves.

29. Zhonglushu (B 29)

Location: 1.5 cun lateral to the Du Meridian, at the level of the third posterior sacral foramen. (See Col. Fig. 9)

Indications: Dysentery, hernia, stiffness and pain of the lower back.

Method: Puncture perpendicularly 0.8-1.2 inches. Moxibustion is applicable.

Regional anatomy

Vasculature: The posterior branches of the lateral sacral artery and vein, the branches of the inferior gluteal artery and vein.

Innervation: The lateral branches of the

posterior rami of the third and fourth sacral nerves.

30. Baihuanshu (B 30)

Location: 1.5 cun lateral to the Du Meridian, at the level of the fourth posterior sacral foramen. (See Col. Fig. 9)

Indications: Enuresis, pain due to hernia, morbid leukorrhea, irregular menstruation, cold sensation and pain of the lower back, dysuria, constipation, tenesmus, prolapse of the rectum.

Method: Puncture perpendicularly 0.8-1.2 inches.

Regional anatomy

Vasculature: The inferior gluteal artery and vein; deeper, the internal pudendal artery and vein.

Innervation: The lateral branches of the posterior rami of the third and fourth sacral nerves, the inferior gluteal nerve.

31. Shangliao (B 31)

Location: In the first posterior sacral foramen. (See Fig. 86)

Indications: Low back pain, dysuria, constipation, irregular menstruation, morbid leukorrhea, prolapse of the uterus.

Method: Puncture perpendicularly 0.8-1.2 inches. Moxibustion is applicable.

Regional anatomy

Vasculature: The posterior branches of the lateral sacral artery and vein.

Innervation: At the site where the posterior ramus of the first sacral nerve passes.

32.   Ciliao (B 32)

Location: In the second posterior sacral foramen. (See Fig. 86)

Indications: Low back pain, hernia, irregular menstruation, leukorrhea, dysmenorrhea, nocturnal emission, impotence, enuresis, dysuria, muscular atrophy, pain, numbness and motor impairment of the lower extremities.

Method: Puncture perpendicularly 0.8-1.2 inches. Moxibustion is applicable.

Regional anatomy

Vasculature: The posterior branches of the lateral sacral artery and vein.

Innervation: The posterior ramus of the second sacral nerve.

33.   Zhongliao (B 33)

Location: In the third posterior sacral foramen. (See Fig. 86)

Indications: Low back pain, constipation, diarrhea, dysuria, irregular menstruation, morbid leukorrhea.

Method: Puncture perpendicularly 0.8-1.2 inches. Moxibustion is applicable.

Regional anatomy

Vasculature:The posterior branches of the lateral sacral artery and vein.

Innervation: On the course of the posterior ramus of the third sacral nerve.

34.   Xialiao (B 34)

Location: In the fourth posterior sacral foramen. (See Fig. 86)

Indications: Low back pain, lower abdominal pain, dysuria, constipation, morbid leukorrhea.

Method: Puncture perpendicularly 0.8-1.2 inches. Moxibustion is applicable.

Regional anatomy

Vasculature: The branches of the inferior gluteal artery and vein.

Innervation: On the course of the posterior ramus of the fourth sacral nerve.

35.   Huiyang (B 35)

Location: On either side of the tip of the coccyx, 0.5 cun lateral to the Du Meridian. (See Col. Fig. 9)

Indications: Dysentery, bloody stools, diarrhea, hemorrhoids, impotence, morbid leukorrhea.

Method: Puncture perpendicularly 0.5-1.0 inch. Moxibustion is applicable.

Regional anatomy

Vasculature: The branches of the inferior gluteal artery and vein.

Innervation: The coccygeal nerve.

36.   Chengfu (B 36)

Location: In the middle of the transverse gluteal fold. Locate the point in prone position. (See Col. Fig. 9)

Indications: Pain in the lower back and gluteal region, constipation, muscular atrophy, pain, numbness and motor impairment of the lower extremities.

Method: Puncture perpendicularly 1.0-1.5 inches. Moxibustion is applicable.

Regional anatomy

Vasculature: The artery and vein running alongside the sciatic nerve.

Innervation: The posterior femoral cutaneous nerve; deeper, the sciatic nerve.

37.   Yinmen (B 37)

Location: 6 cun below Chengfu (B 36) on the line joining Chengfu (B 36) and Weizhong (B 40). (See Col. Fig. 10)

Indications: Pain in the lower back and thigh, muscular atrophy, pain, numbness and motor impairment of the lower extremities, hemiplegia.

Method: Puncture perpendicularly 1.0-2.0 inches. Moxibustion is applicable.

Regional anatomy

Vasculature: Laterally, the third perforating branches of the deep femoral artery and vein.

Innervation: The posterior femoral cutaneous nerve; deeper, the sciatic nerve.

38.   Fuxi (B 38)

Location: 1 cun above Weiyang (B 39) on the medial side of the tendon of m. biceps femoris. The point is located with the knee slightly flexed. (See Col. Fig. 10)

Indications: Numbness of the gluteal and femoral regions, contracture of the tendons in the popliteal fossa.

Method: Puncture perpendicularly 0.5-1.0 inch. Moxibustion is applicable.

Regional anatomy

Vasculature: The superolateral genicular artery and vein.

Innervation: The posterior femoral cutaneous nerve and the common peroneal nerve.

39.   Weiyang (Lower He-Sea Point of Sanjiao, B 39)

Location: Lateral to Weizhong (B 40), on the medial border of the tendon of m. biceps femoris. (See Fig. 87)

Indications: Stiffness and pain of the lower back, distension and fullness of the lower abdomen, edema, dysuria, cramp of the leg and foot.

Method: Puncture perpendicularly 0.5-1.0 inch. Moxibustion is applicable.

Regional anatomy: See Fuxi (B 38).

40.   Weizhong (He-Sea Point, B 40)

Location: Midpoint of the transverse crease of the popliteal fossa, between the tendons of m. biceps femoris and m. semitendinosus. (See Fig. 87)

Indications: Low back pain, motor impairment of the hip joint, contracture of the tendons in the popliteal fossa, muscular atrophy, pain, numbness and motor impairment of the lower extremities, hemiplegia, abdominal pain, vomiting, diarrhea, erysipelas.

Method: Puncture perpendicularly 0.5-1.0 inch, or prick the popliteal vein with three-edged needle to cause bleeding.

Regional anatomy

Vasculature: Superficially, the femoro-popliteal vein; deeper and medially, the popliteal vein; deepest, the popliteal artery.

Innervation: The posterior femoral cutaneous nerve, the tibial nerve.

41.   Fufen (B 41)

Location: 3 cun lateral to the Du Meridian, at the level of the lower border of the spinous process of the second thoracic vertebra, on the spinal border of the scapula. (See Col. Fig. 9)

Indications: Stiffness and pain of the shoulder, back and neck, numbness of the elbow and arm.

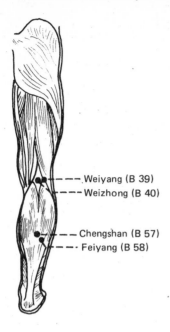

—— Weiyang (B 39)

--- Weizhong (B 40)

— — Chengshan (B 57)

— — · Feiyang (B 58)

Fig. 87

Method: Puncture perpendicularly 0.3-0.5 inch. Moxibustion is applicable.

Regional anatomy

Vasculature: The descending branch of the transverse cervical artery, the posterior branches of the intercostal artery and vein.

Innervation: The lateral branches of the posterior rami of the first and second thoracic nerves; deeper, the dorsal scapular nerve.

42.   Pohu (B 42)

Location: 3 cun lateral to the Du Meridian, at the level of the lower border of the spinous process of the third thoracic vertebra, on the spinal border of the scapula. (See Col. Fig. 9)

Indications: Pulmonary tuberculosis, hemoptysis, cough, asthma, neck rigidity, pain in the shoulder and back.

Method: Puncture obliquely 0.3-0.5 inch. Moxibustion is applicable.

Regional anatomy

Vasculature: The posterior branch of the intercostal artery, the descending branch of the transverse cervical artery.

Innervation: The medial cutaneous branches of the posterior rami of the second and third thoracic nerves; deeper, their lateral branches and the dorsoscapular nerve.

43.   Gaohuangshu (B 43)

Location: 3 cun lateral to the Du Meridian, at the level of the lower border of the spinous process of the fourth thoracic vertebra, on the spinal border of the scapula. (See Fig. 86)

Indications: Pulmonary tuberculosis, cough, asthma, spitting of blood, night sweating, poor memory, nocturnal emission.

Method: Puncture perpendicularly 0.3-0.5 inch. Moxibustion is applicable.

Regional anatomy

Vasculature: The posterior branch of the intercostal artery and the descending branch of the transverse cervical artery.

Innervation: The medial cutaneous branches of the posterior rami of the second and third thoracic nerves; deeper, their lateral branches and the dorsoscapular nerve.

44.   Shentang (B 44)

Location: 3 cun lateral to Shendao (Du 11), at the level of the lower border of the spinous process of the fifth thoracic vertebra, on the spinal border of the scapula. (See Col. Fig. 9)

Indications: Asthma, cardiac pain, palpitation, stuffy chest, cough, stiffness and pain of the back.

Method: Puncture obliquely 0.3-0.5 inch. Moxibustion is applicable.

Regional anatomy

Vasculature: The posterior branches of the intercostal artery and vein, the descending branch of the transverse cervical artery.

Innervation: The medial cutaneous branches of the posterior rami of the fourth and fifth thoracic nerves; deeper, their lateral branches and the dorsoscapular nerve.

45.   Yixi (B 45)

Location: 3 cun lateral to Lingtai (Du 10), at the level of the lower border of the spinous process of the sixth thoracic vertebra, on the spinal border of the scapula. (See Col. Fig. 9)

Indications: Cough, asthma, pain of the shoulder and back.

Method: Puncture obliquely downward 0.3-0.5 inch. Moxibustion is applicable.

Regional anatomy

Vasculature: The posterior branches of the intercostal artery and vein.

Innervation: The medial cutaneous branches of the posterior rami of the fifth and sixth thoracic nerves; deeper, their lateral branches.

46.   Geguan (B 46)

Location: 3 cun lateral to Zhiyang (Du 9), at the level of the lower border of the spinous process of the seventh thoracic vertebra, approximately at the level of the inferior angle of the scapula.(Col. Fig. 9)

Indications: Dysphagia, hiccup, vomiting, belching, pain and stiffness of the back.

Method: Puncture obliquely 0.3-0.5 inch. Moxibustion is applicable.

Regional anatomy

Vasculature: The posterior branches of the intercostal artery and vein.

Innervation: The medial cutaneous branches of the posterior rami of the sixth and seventh thoracic nerves; deeper, their lateral branches.

47.   Hunmen (B 47)

Location: 3 cun lateral to Jinsuo (Du 8), at the level of the lower border of the spinous process of the ninth thoracic vertebra. (See Col. Fig. 9)

Indications: Pain in the chest and hypochondriac region, back pain, vomiting, diarrhea.

Method: Puncture obliquely 0.3-0.5 inch. Moxibustion is applicable.

Regional anatomy

Vasculature: The posterior branches of the intercostal artery and vein.

Innervation: The lateral cutaneous branches of the posterior rami of the seventh and eighth thoracic nerves.

48.   Yanggang (B 48)

Location: 3 cun lateral to Zhongshu (Du 7), at the level of the lower border of the spinous process of the tenth thoracic vertebra. (See Col. Fig. 9)

Indications: Borborygmus, abdominal pain, diarrhea, pain in the hypochondriac region, jaundice.

Method: Puncture obliquely 0.3-0.5 inch. Moxibustion is applicable.

Regional anatomy
Vasculature: The posterior branches of the intercostal artery and vein.
Innervation: The lateral cutaneous branches of the posterior rami of the eighth and ninth thoracic nerves.

49.   Yishe (B 49)

Location: 3 cun lateral to Jizhong (Du 6), at the level of the lower border of the spinous process of the eleventh thoracic vertebra. (See Col. Fig. 9)
Indications: Abdominal distension, borborygmus, vomiting, diarrhea, difficulty in swallowing.
Method: Puncture obliquely 0.3-0.5 inch. Moxibustion is applicable.
Regional anatomy
Vasculature: The posterior branches of the intercostal artery and vein.
Innervation: The lateral branches of the posterior rami of the tenth and eleventh thoracic nerves.

50.   Weicang (B 50)

Location: 3 cun lateral to the Du Meridian, at the level of the lower border of the spinous process of the twelfth thoracic vertebra. (See Col. Fig. 9)
Indications: Abdominal distension, pain in the epigastric region and back, infantile indigestion.
Method: Puncture obliquely 0.3-0.5 inch. Moxibustion is applicable.
Regional anatomy
Vasculature: The posterior branches of the subcostal artery and vein.
Innervation: The lateral cutaneous branches of the posterior ramus of the eleventh thoracic nerve.

51.   Huangmen (B 51)

Location: 3 cun lateral to Xuanshu (Du 5), at the level of the lower border of the spinous process of the first lumbar vertebra. (See Col. Fig. 9)
Indications: Abdominal pain, constipation, abdominal mass.
Method: Puncture obliquely 0.3-0.5 inch. Moxibustion is applicable.
Regional anatomy
Vasculature: The posterior branches of the first lumbar artery and vein.
Innervation: The lateral branch of the posterior ramus of the twelfth thoracic nerve.

52.   Zhishi (B 52)

Location: 3 cun lateral to Mingmen (Du 4), at the level of the lower border of the spinous process of the second lumbar vertebra. (See Fig. 86)
Indications: Nocturnal emission, impotence, enuresis, frequency of urination, dysuria, irregular menstruation, pain in the back and knee, edema.
Method: Puncture perpendicularly 0.5-1.0 inch. Moxibustion is applicable.
Regional anatomy
Vasculature: The posterior branches of the second lumbar artery and vein.
Innervation: The lateral branch of the posterior ramus of the twelfth thoracic nerve and the lateral branch of the first lumbar nerve.

53.   Baohuang (B 53)

Location: 3 cun lateral to the Du Meridian, at the level of the second sacral posterior foramen. (See Col. Fig. 9)

Indications: Borborygmus, abdominal distension, pain in the lower back, anuria.

Method: Puncture perpendicularly 0.8-1.2 inches. Moxibustion is applicable.

Regional anatomy

Vasculature: The superior gluteal artery and vein.

Innervation: The superior cluneal nerves; deeper, the superior gluteal nerve.

54.   Zhibian (B 54)

Location: Lateral to the hiatus of the sacrum, 3 cun lateral to Yaoshu (Du 2). (See Fig. 86)

Indications: Pain in the lumbosacral region, muscular atrophy, motor impairment of the lower extremities, dysuria, swelling around external genitalia, hemorrhoids, constipation.

Method: Puncture perpendicularly 1.5-2.0 inches. Moxibustion is applicable.

Regional anatomy

Vasculature: The inferior gluteal artery and vein.

Innervation: The inferior gluteal nerve, the posterior femoral cutaneous nerve and the sciatic nerve.

55.   Heyang (B 55)

Location: 2 cun directly below Weizhong (B 40), between the medial and lateral heads of m. gastrocnemius, on the line joining Weizhong (B 40) and Chengshan (B 57). (See Col. Fig. 9)

Indications: Low back pain, pain and paralysis of the lower extremities.

Method: Puncture perpendicularly 0.7-1.0 inch. Moxibustion is applicable.

Regional anatomy

Vasculature: The small saphenous vein; deeper, the popliteal artery and vein.

Innervation: The medial sural cutaneous nerve; deeper, the tibial nerve.

56.   Chengjin (B 56)

Location: Midway between Heyang (B 55) and Chengshan (B 57), in the centre of the belly of m. gastrocnemius. (Col. Fig. 9)

Indications: Spasm of the gastrocnemius, hemorrhoids, acute lower back pain.

Method: Puncture perpendicularly 0.8-1.2 inches. Moxibustion is applicable.

Regional anatomy

Vasculature: The small saphenous vein; deeper, the posterior tibial artery and vein.

Innervation: The medial sural cutaneous nerve; deeper, the tibial nerve.

57.   Chengshan (B 57)

Location: Directly below the belly of m. gastrocnemius, on the line joining Weizhong (B 40) and tendo calcaneus, about 8 cun below Weizhong (B 40). (See Fig. 87)

Indications: Low back pain, spasm of the gastrocnemius, hemorrhoids, constipation, beriberi.

Method: Puncture perpendicularly 0.8-1.2 inches. Moxibustion is applicable.

Regional anatomy: See Chengjin (B 56).

58.   Feiyang (Luo-Connecting Point, B 58)

Location: 7 cun directly above Kunlun (B 60), on the posterior border of fibula, about 1 cun inferior and lateral to Chengshan (B 57). (See Fig. 87)

Indications: Headache, blurring of vision, nasal obstruction, epistaxis, back pain, hemorrhoids, weakness of the leg.

Method: Puncture perpendicularly 0.7-1.0 inch. Moxibustion is applicable.

Regional anatomy

Innervation: The lateral sural cutaneous nerve.

59.   Fuyang (Xi-Cleft Point of the Yangqiao Meridian, B 59)

Location: 3 cun directly above Kunlun (B 60). (See Fig. 88)

Indications: Heavy sensation of the head, headache, low back pain, redness and swelling of the external malleolus, paralysis of the lower extremities.

Method: Puncture perpendicularly 0.5-1.0 inch. Moxibustion is applicable.

Regional anatomy

Vasculature: The small saphenous vein; deeper, the terminal branch of the peroneal artery.

Innervation: The sural nerve.

60.   Kunlun (Jing-River Point, B 60)

Location: In the depression between the external malleolus and tendo calcaneus. (See Fig. 88)

Indications: Headache, blurring of vision, neck rigidity, epistaxis, pain in the shoulder, back and arm, swelling and pain of the heel, difficult labour, epilepsy.

Method: Puncture perpendicularly 0.5-1.0 inch. Moxibustion is applicable.

Regional anatomy

Vasculature: The small saphenous vein, the posteroexternal malleolar artery and vein.

Innervation: The sural nerve.

61.   Pucan (B 61)

Location: Posterior and inferior to the external malleolus, directly below Kunlun (B 60), in the depression of calcaneum at the junction of the red and white skin. (See Fig. 88)

Indications: Muscular atrophy and weakness of the lower extremities, pain in the heel.

Method: Puncture perpendicularly 0.3-0.5 inch. Moxibustion is applicable.

Regional anatomy

Vasculature: The external calcaneal branches of the peroneal artery and vein.

Innervation: The external calcaneal branch of the sural nerve.

62.   Shènmai (Confluent Point, B 62)

Location: In the depression directly below the external malleolus. (See Fig. 88)

Indications: Epilepsy, mania, headache, dizziness, insomnia, backache, aching of the leg.

Method: Puncture perpendicularly 0.3-0.5 inch. Moxibustion is applicable.

Regional anatomy

Vasculature: The external malleolar arterial network.

Innervation: The sural nerve.

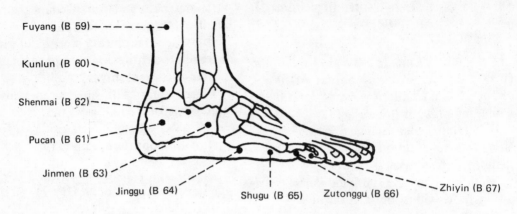

Fuyang (B 59)

Kunlun (B 60)

Shenmai (B 62)

Pucan (B 61)

Jinmen (B 63)

Jinggu (B 64)

Shugu (B 65)

Zutonggu (B 66)

Zhiyin (B 67)

Fig. 88

63. Jinmen (Xi-Cleft Point, B 63)

Location: Anterior and inferior to Shenmai (B 62), in the depression lateral to the cuboid bone. (See Fig. 88)

Indications: Mania, epilepsy, infantile convulsion, backache, pain in the external malleolus, motor impairment and pain of the lower extremities.

Method: Puncture perpendicularly 0.3-0.5 inch. Moxibustion is applicable.

Regional anatomy

Vasculature: The lateral plantar artery and vein.

Innervation: The lateral dorsal cutaneous nerve of foot; deeper, the lateral plantar nerve.

64. Jinggu (Yuan-Primary Point, B 64)

Location: Below the tuberosity of the fifth metatarsal bone, at the junction of the red and white skin. (See Fig. 88)

Indications: Headache, neck rigidity, pain in the lower back and thigh, epilepsy.

Method: Puncture perpendicularly 0.3-

0.5 inch. Moxibustion is applicable.

Regional anatomy: See Jinmen (B 63).

65. Shugu (Shu-Stream Point, B 65)

Location: Posterior to the head of the fifth metatarsal bone, at the junction of the red and white skin. (See Fig. 88)

Indications: Mania, headache, neck rigidity, blurring of vision, backache, pain in the lower extremities.

Method: Puncture perpendicularly 0.3-0.5 inch. Moxibustion is applicable.

Regional anatomy

Vasculature: The fourth common plantar digital artery and vein.

Innervation: The fourth common plantar digital nerve and the lateral dorsal cutaneous nerve of foot.

66. Zutonggu (Ying-Spring Point, B 66)

Location: In the depression anterior to the fifth metatarsophalangeal joint. (See Fig. 88)

Indications: Headache, neck rigidity, blurring of vision, epistaxis, mania.

Method: Puncture perpendicularly 0.2-0.3 inch. Moxibustion is applicable.

Regional anatomy

Vasculature: The plantar digital artery and vein.

Innervation: The plantar digital proprial nerve and the lateral dorsal cutaneous nerve of foot.

67. Zhiyin (Jing-Well Point, B 67)

Location: On the lateral side of the small toe, about 0.1 cun posterior to the corner of the nail. (See Fig. 88)

Indications: Headache, nasal obstruction, epistaxis, ophthalmalgia, malposition of fetus, difficult labour, detention of afterbirth, feverish sensation in the sole.

Method: Puncture superficially 0.1 inch. Moxibustion is applicable.

Regional anatomy

Vasculature: The network formed by the dorsal digital artery and plantar digital proprial artery.

Innervation: The plantar digital proprial nerve and the lateral dorsal cutaneous nerve of foot.

IV. THE KIDNEY MERIDIAN OF FOOT-SHAOYIN

1. Yongquan (Jing-Well Point, K 1)

Location: On the sole, in the depression when the foot is in plantar flexion, approximately at the junction of the anterior

third and posterior two thirds of the sole. (See Fig. 89)

Indications: Headache, blurring of vision, dizziness, sore throat, dryness of the tongue, loss of voice, dysuria, infantile convulsions, feverish sensation in the sole, loss of consciousness.

Method: Puncture perpendicularly 0.3-0.5 inch. Moxibustion is applicable.

Regional anatomy

Vasculature: Deeper, the plantar arterial arch.

Innervation: The second common plantar digital nerve.

2. Rangu (Ying-Spring Point, K 2)

Location: Anterior and inferior to the medial malleolus, in the depression on the lower border of the tuberosity of the navicular bone. (See Fig. 90)

Indications: Pruritus vulvae, prolapse of uterus, irregular menstruation, nocturnal

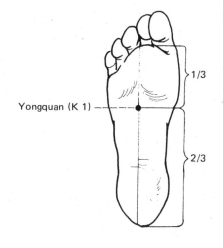

Yongquan (K 1)

1/3

2/3

Fig. 89

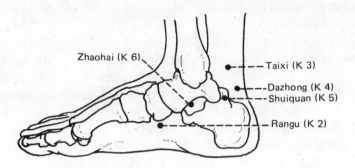

Fig. 90

emission, hemoptysis, thirst, diarrhea, swelling and pain of the dorsum of foot, acute infantile omphalitis.

Method: Puncture perpendicularly 0.3-0.5 inch. Moxibustion is applicable.

Regional anatomy

Vasculature: The branches of the medial plantar and medial tarsal arteries.

Innervation: The terminal branch of the medial crural cutaneous nerve, the medial plantar nerve.

3. Taixi (Shu-Stream and Yuan-Primary Point, K 3)

Location: In the depression between the medial malleolus and tendo calcaneus, at the level with the tip of the medial malleolus. (See Fig. 90)

Indications: Sore throat, toothache, deafness, tinnitus, dizziness, spitting of blood, asthma, thirst, irregular menstruation, insomnia, nocturnal emission, impotence, frequency of micturition, pain in the lower back.

Method: Puncture perpendicularly 0.3-0.5 inch. Moxibustion is applicable.

Regional anatomy

Vasculature: Anteriorly, the posterior tibial artery and vein.

Innervation: The medial crural cutaneous nerve, on the course of the tibial nerve.

4. Dazhong (Luo-Connecting Point, K 4)

Location: Posterior and inferior to the medial malleolus, in the depression medial to the attachment of tendo calcaneus. (See Fig. 90)

Indications: Spitting of blood, asthma, stiffness and pain of the lower back, dysuria, constipation, pain in the heel, dementia.

Method: Puncture perpendicularly 0.3-0.5 inch. Moxibustion is applicable.

Regional anatomy

Vasculature: The medial calcaneal branch of the posterior tibial artery.

Innervation: The medial crural cutaneous nerve, on the course of the medial calcaneal ramus derived from the tibial nerve.

5. Shuiquan (Xi-Cleft Point, K 5)

Location: 1 cun directly below Taixi (K 3) in the depression anterior and superior to the medial side of the tuberosity of the calcaneum. (See Fig. 90)

Indications: Amenorrhea, irregular menstruation, dysmenorrhea, prolapse of uterus, dysuria, blurring of vision.

Method: Puncture perpendicularly 0.3-0.5 inch. Moxibustion is applicable.

Regional anatomy: See Dazhong (K 4).

6.   Zhaohai (the Eight Confluent Point, K 6)

Location: In the depression of the lower border of the medial malleolus, or 1 cun below the medial malleolus. (See Fig. 90)

Indications: Irregular menstruation, morbid leukorrhea, prolapse of uterus, pruritus vulvae, frequency of micturition, retention of urine, constipation, epilepsy, insomnia, sore throat, asthma.

Method: Puncture perpendicularly 0.3-0.5 inch. Moxibustion is applicable.

Regional anatomy

Vasculature: Posteriorly, the posterior tibial artery and vein.

Innervation: The medial crural cutaneous nerve; deeper, the tibial nerve.

7.   Fuliu (Jing-River Point, K 7)

Location: 2 cun directly above Taixi (K 3), on the anterior border of tendo calcaneus. (See Fig. 91)

Indications: Edema, abdominal distension, diarrhea, borborygmus, muscular atrophy of the leg, night sweating, spontaneous sweating, febrile diseases without sweating.

Method: Puncture perpendicularly 0.5-0.7 inch. Moxibustion is applicable.

Regional anatomy

Vasculature: Deeper, anteriorly, the posterior tibial artery and vein.

Innervation: The medial sural and medial crural cutaneous nerves; deeper, the tibial nerve.

8.   Jiaoxin (Xi-Cleft Point of the Yinqiao Meridian, K 8)

Location: 0.5 cun anterior to Fuliu (K 7), 2 cun above Taixi (K 3) posterior to the medial border of tibia. (See Fig. 91)

Indications: Irregular menstruation, dysmenorrhea, uterine bleeding, prolapse of uterus, diarrhea, constipation, pain and swelling of testis.

Method: Puncture perpendicularly 0.5-0.7 inch. Moxibustion is applicable.

Regional anatomy

Vasculature: Deeper, the posterior tibial artery and vein.

Innervation: The medial crural cutaneous nerve; deeper, the tibial nerve.

9.   Zhubin (Xi-Cleft Point of the Yinwei Meridian, K 9)

Location: 5 cun directly above Taixi (K 3) at the lower end of the belly of m. gastrocnemius, on the line drawn from Taixi (K 3) to Yingu (K 10). (See Fig. 91)

Indications: Mental disorders, pain in the foot and lower leg, hernia.

Method: Puncture perpendicularly 0.5-0.7 inch. Moxibustion is applicable.

Regional anatomy

Vasculature: Deeper, the posterior tibial artery and vein.

Innervation: The medial sural and medial crural cutaneous nerves; deeper, the tibial nerve.

10. Yingu (He-Sea Point, K 10)

Location: When the knee is flexed, the point is on the medial side of the popliteal fossa, between the tendons of m. semitendinosus and semimembranosus, at the level with Weizhong (B 40). (See Fig. 91)

Indications: Impotence, hernia, uterine bleeding, dysuria, pain in the knee and popliteal fossa, mental disorders.

Method: Puncture perpendicularly 0.8-1.0 inch. Moxibustion is applicable.

Regional anatomy

Vasculature: The medial superior genicular artery and vein.

Innervation: The medial femoral cutaneous nerve.

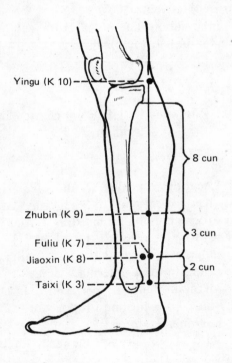

Fig. 91

11. Henggu (K 11)

Location: 5 cun below the umbilicus, on the superior border of symphysis pubis, 0.5 cun lateral to Qugu (Ren 2). (Col. Fig. 12)

Indications: Fullness and pain of the lower abdomen, dysuria, enuresis, nocturnal emission, impotence, pain of genitalia.

Method: Puncture perpendicularly 0.5-1.0 inch. Moxibustion is applicable.

Regional anatomy

Vasculature: The inferior epigastric artery and external pudendal artery.

Innervation: The branch of the iliohypogastric nerve.

12. Dahe (K 12)

Location: 4 cun below the umbilicus, 0.5 cun lateral to Zhongji (Ren 3). (See Fig. 92)

Indications: Nocturnal emission, impotence, morbid leukorrhea, pain in the external genitalia, prolapse of uterus.

Method: Puncture perpendicularly 0.5-1.0 inch. Moxibustion is applicable.

Regional anatomy

Vasculature: The muscular branches of the inferior epigastric artery and vein.

Innervation: The branches of subcostal nerve and the iliohypogastric nerve.

13. Qixue (K 13)

Location: 3 cun below the umbilicus, 0.5 cun lateral to Guanyuan (Ren 4). (See Col. Fig. 12)

Indications: Irregular menstruation, dysmenorrhea, dysuria, abdominal pain, diarrhea.

Method: Puncture perpendicularly 0.5-
1.0 inch. Moxibustion is applicable.
Regional anatomy
Vasculature: See Dahe (K 12).
Innervation: The subcostal nerve.

14.   Siman (K 14)

Location: 2 cun below the umbilicus, 0.5
cun lateral to Shimen (Ren 5). (Col. Fig. 12)
Indications: Abdominal pain and distension, diarrhea, nocturnal emission, irregular
menstruation, dysmenorrhea, postpartum
abdominal pain.
Method: Puncture perpendicularly 0.5-
1.0 inch. Moxibustion is applicable.
Regional anatomy
Vasculature: See Dahe (K 12).
Innervation: The eleventh intercostal
nerve.

15.   Zhongzhu (K 15)

Location: 1 cun below the umbilicus, 0.5
cun lateral to Yinjiao (Ren 7). (Col. Fig. 12)
Indications: Irregular menstruation, ab-
dominal pain, constipation.
Method: Puncture perpendicularly 0.5-
1.0 inch. Moxibustion is applicable.
Regional anatomy
Vasculature: See Dahe (K 12).
Innervation: The tenth intercostal nerve.

16.   Huangshu (K 16)

Location: 0.5 cun lateral to the umbilicus,
level with Shenque (Ren 8). (See Fig. 92)
Indications: Abdominal pain and distension, vomiting, constipation, diarrhea.
Method: Puncture perpendicularly 0.5-
1.0 inch. Moxibustion is applicable.

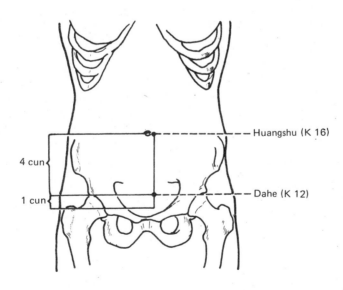

Fig. 92

Regional anatomy
Vasculature: See Dahe (K 12).
Innervation: The tenth intercostal nerve.

17.   Shangqu (K 17)

Location: 2 cun above the umbilicus, 0.5 cun lateral to Xiawan (Ren 10). (See Col. Fig. 12)
Indications: Abdominal pain, diarrhea, constipation.
Method: Puncture perpendicularly 0.5-1.0 inch. Moxibustion is applicable.
Regional anatomy
Vasculature: The branches of the superior and inferior epigastric arteries and veins.
Innervation: The ninth intercostal nerve.

18.   Shiguan (K 18)

Location: 3 cun above the umbilicus, 0.5 cun lateral to Jianli (Ren 11). (Col. Fig. 12)
Indications: Vomiting, abdominal pain, constipation, postpartum abdominal pain, sterility.
Method: Puncture perpendicularly 0.5-1.0 inch. Moxibustion is applicable.
Regional anatomy
Vasculature: The branches of the superior epigastric artery and vein.
Innervation: The eighth intercostal nerve.

19.   Yindu (K 19)

Location: 4 cun above the umbilicus, 0.5 cun lateral to Zhongwan (Ren 12). (See Col. Fig. 12)
Indications: Borborygmus, abdominal pain, epigastric pain, constipation, vomiting.

Method: Puncture perpendicularly 0.5-1.0 inch. Moxibustion is applicable.
Regional anatomy: See Shiguan (K 18).

20.   Futonggu (K 20)

Location: 5 cun above the umbilicus, 0.5 cun lateral to Shangwan (Ren 13). (See Col. Fig. 12)
Indications: Abdominal pain and distension, vomiting, indigestion.
Method: Puncture perpendicularly 0.5-1.0 inch. Moxibustion is applicable.
Regional anatomy: See Shiguan (K 18).

21.   Youmen (K 21)

Location: 6 cun above the umbilicus, 0.5 cun lateral to Juque (Ren 14). (Col. Fig. 12)
Indications: Abdominal pain and distension, indigestion, vomiting, diarrhea, nausea, morning sickness.
Method: Puncture perpendicularly 0.3-0.7 inch. To avoid injuring the liver, deep insertion is not advisable. Moxibustion is applicable.
Regional anatomy
Vasculature: See Shiguan (K 18).
Innervation: The seventh intercostal nerve.

22.   Bulang (K 22)

Location: In the fifth intercostal space, 2 cun lateral to the Ren Meridian. (See Col. Fig. 12)
Indications: Cough, asthma, distension and fullness in the chest and hypochondriac region, vomiting, anorexia.

Method: Puncture obliquely 0.3-0.5 inch. To avoid injuring the heart, deep insertion is not advisable. Moxibustion is applicable.

Regional anatomy

Vasculature: The fifth intercostal artery and vein.

Innervation: The anterior cutaneous branch of the fifth intercostal nerve; deeper, the fifth intercostal nerve.

23.   Shenfeng (K 23)

Location: In the fourth intercostal space, 2 cun lateral to the Ren Meridian. (See Col. Fig. 12)

Indications: Cough, asthma, fullness in the chest and hypochondriac region, mastitis.

Method: Puncture obliquely 0.3-0.5 inch. Moxibustion is applicable.

Regional anatomy

Vasculature: The fourth intercostal artery and vein.

Innervation: The anterior cutaneous branch of the fourth intercostal nerve; deeper, the fourth intercostal nerve.

24.   Lingxu (K 24)

Location: In the third intercostal space, 2 cun lateral to the Ren Meridian. (See Col. Fig. 12)

Indications: Cough, asthma, fullness in the chest and hypochondriac region, mastitis.

Method: Puncture obliquely 0.3-0.5 inch. Moxibustion is applicable.

Regional anatomy

Vasculature: The third intercostal artery and vein.

Innervation: The anterior cutaneous

branch of the third intercostal nerve; deeper, the third intercostal nerve.

25.   Shencang (K 25)

Location: In the second intercostal space, 2 cun lateral to the Ren Meridian. (See Col. Fig. 12)

Indications: Cough, asthma, chest pain.

Method: Puncture obliquely 0.3-0.5 inch. Moxibustion is applicable.

Regional anatomy

Vasculature: The second intercostal artery and vein.

Innervation: The anterior cutaneous branch of the second intercostal nerve; deeper, the second intercostal nerve.

26.   Yuzhong (K 26)

Location: In the first intercostal space, 2 cun lateral to the Ren Meridian. (See Col. Fig. 12)

Indications: Cough, asthma, accumulation of phlegm, fullness in the chest and hypochondriac region.

Method: Puncture obliquely 0.3-0.5 inch. Moxibustion is applicable.

Regional anatomy

Vasculature: The first intercostal artery and vein.

Innervation: The anterior cutaneous branch of the first intercostal nerve, the medial supraclavicular nerve; the first intercostal nerve.

27. Shufu (K 27)

Location: In the depression on the lower border of the clavicle, 2 cun lateral to the

Ren Meridian. (See Col. Fig. 12)

Indications: Cough, asthma, chest pain.

Method: Puncture obliquely 0.3-0.5 inch. Moxibustion is applicable.

Regional anatomy

Vasculature: The anterior perforating branches of the internal mammary artery and vein.

Innervation: The medial supraclavicular nerve.

Chapter 9

ACUPOINTS OF JUEYIN AND SHAOYANG MERIDIANS

The Pericardium Meridian of Hand Jueyin and the Sanjiao (Triple Energizer) Meridian of Hand Shaoyang are externally-internally related, the former runs from chest to hand and the latter goes from hand to head. The Gallbladder Meridian of Foot Shaoyang runs from head to foot, while the Liver Meridian of Foot Jueyin goes from foot to abdomen (chest). These two meridians are also externally-internally related. The above four meridians are mainly distributed in the lateral aspects of the trunk and the four limbs. The points of the four meridians are described as follows:

I. THE PERICARDIUM MERIDIAN OF HAND JUEYIN

1. Tianchi (P 1)

Location: In the fourth intercostal space, 1 cun lateral to the nipple (See Col. Fig. 13)

Indications: Suffocating sensation in the chest, pain in the hypochondriac region, swelling and pain of the axillary region.

Method: Puncture obliquely 0.2-0.4 inch. Deep puncture is not advisable. Moxibustion is applicable.

Regional anatomy
Vasculature: The thoracoepigastric vein, the branches of the lateral thoracic artery and vein.
Innervation: The muscular branch of the anterior thoracic nerve, the fourth intercostal nerve.

2. Tianquan (P 2)

Location: 2 cun below the level of the anterior axillary fold, between the two heads of m. biceps brachii. (See Col. Fig. 13)

Indications: Cardiac pain, distension of the hypochondriac region, cough, pain in the chest, back and the medial aspect of the arm.

Method: Puncture perpendicularly 0.5-0.7 inch. Moxibustion is applicable.

Regional anatomy
· Vasculature: The muscular branches of the brachial artery and vein.
Innervation: The medial brachial cutaneous nerve and the musculocutaneous nerve.

3. Quze (He-Sea Point, P 3)

Location: On the transverse cubital crease, at the ulnar side of the tendon of m.

biceps brachii. (See Fig. 93)

Indications: Cardiac pain, palpitation, febrile diseases, irritability, stomachache, vomiting, pain in the elbow and arm, tremor of the hand and arm.

Method: Puncture perpendicularly 0.5-0.7 inch, or prick with a three-edged needle to cause bleeding. Moxibustion is applicable.

Regional anatomy

Vasculature: On the pathway of the brachial artery and vein.

Innervation: The median nerve.

4. Ximen (Xi-Cleft Point, P 4)

Location: 5 cun above the transverse crease of the wrist, on the line connecting Quze (P 3) and Daling (P 7), between the

tendons of m. palmaris longus and m. flexor carpi radialis. (See Fig. 93)

Indications: Cardiac pain, palpitation, epistaxis, hematemesis, haemoptysis chest pain, furuncle, epilepsy.

Method: Puncture perpendicularly 0.5-1.0 inch. Moxibustion is applicable.

Regional anatomy

Vasculature: The median artery and vein; deeper, the anterior interosseous artery and vein.

Innervation: The medial antebrachial cutaneous nerve; deeper, the median nerve; deepest, the anterior interosseous nerve.

5. Jianshi (Jing-River Point, P 5)

Location: 3 cun above the transverse crease of the wrist, between the tendons of

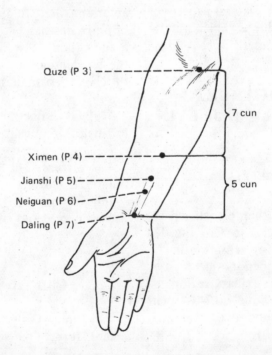

Fig. 93

m. palmaris longus and m. flexor carpi radialis. (See Fig. 93)

Indications: Cardiac pain, palpitation, stomachache, vomiting, febrile diseases, irritability, malaria, mental disorders, epilepsy, swelling of the axilla, contracture of the elbow and arm.

Method: Puncture perpendicularly 0.5-1.0 inch. Moxibustion is applicable.

Regional anatomy

Vasculature: The median artery and vein; deeper, the anterior interosseous artery and vein.

Innervation: The medial and lateral antebrachial cutaneous nerves, the palmar cutaneous branch of the median nerve; deeper, the anterior interosseous nerve.

6. Neiguan (Luo-Connecting Point, the Eight Confluent Point, P 6)

Location: 2 cun above the transverse crease of the wrist, between the tendons of m. palmaris longus and m. flexor radialis. (See Fig. 93)

Indications: Cardiac pain, palpitation, stuffy chest, pain in the hypochondriac region, stomachache, nausea, vomiting, hiccup, mental disorders, epilepsy, insomnia, febrile diseases, irritability, malaria, contracture and pain of the elbow and arm.

Method: Puncture perpendicularly 0.5-0.8 inch. Moxibustion is applicable.

Regional anatomy: See Jianshi (P 5).

7. Daling (Shu-Stream and Yuan-Primary Point, P 7)

Location: In the middle of the transverse crease of the wrist, between the tendons of

m. palmaris longus and m. flexor carpi radialis. (See Fig. 93)

Indications: Cardiac pain, palpitation, stomachache, vomiting, mental disorders, epilepsy, stuffy chest, pain in the hypochondriac region, convulsion, insomnia, irritability, foul breath.

Method: Puncture perpendicularly 0.3-0.5 inch. Moxibustion is applicable.

Regional anatomy

Vasculature: The palmar arterial and venous network of the wrist.

Innervation: Deeper, the median nerve.

8. Laogong (Ying-Spring Point, P 8)

Location: On the transverse crease of the palm, between the second and third metacarpal bones. When the fist is clenched, the point is just below the tip of the middle finger. (See Fig. 94)

Indications: Cardiac pain, mental disorder, epilepsy, gastritis, foul breath, fungus infection of the hand and foot, vomiting, nausea.

Method: Puncture perpendicularly 0.3-0.5 inch. Moxibustion is applicable.

Regional anatomy

Vasculature: The common palmar digital artery.

Innervation: The second common palmar digital nerve of the median nerve.

9. Zhongchong (Jing-Well Point, P 9)

Location: In the centre of the tip of the middle finger. (See Fig. 94)

Indications: Cardiac pain, palpitation, loss of consciousness, aphasia with stiffness and swelling of the tongue, febrile diseases,

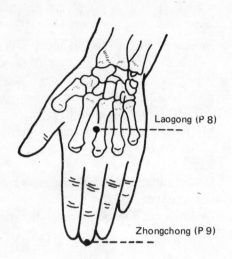

Fig 94

heat stroke, convulsion, feverish sensation in the palm.

Method: Puncture superficially 0.1 inch or prick with a three-edged needle to cause bleeding. Moxibustion is applicable.

Regional anatomy

Vasculature: The arterial and venous network formed by the palmar digital proprial artery and vein.

Innervation: The palmar digital proprial nerve of the median nerve.

II. SANJIAO MERIDIAN OF HAND-SHAOYANG

1. Guanchong (Jing-Well Point, S J 1)

Location: On the lateral side of the ring finger, about 0.1 cun posterior to the corner of the nail. (See Fig. 95)

Indications: Headache, redness of the eyes, sore throat, stiffness of the tongue, febrile diseases, irritability.

Method: Puncture superficially 0.1 inch, or prick with a three-edged needle to cause bleeding. Moxibustion is applicable.

Regional anatomy

Vasculature: The arterial and venous network formed by the palmar digital proprial artery and vein.

Innervation: The palmar digital proprial nerve derived from the ulnar nerve.

2. Yemen (Ying-Spring Point, S J 2)

Location: When the fist is clenched, the point is located in the depression proximal to the margin of the web between the ring and small fingers. (See Fig. 95)

Indications: Headache, redness of the eyes, sudden deafness, sore throat, malaria, pain in the arm.

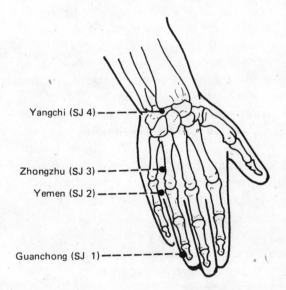

Fig. 95

Method: Puncture obliquely 0.3-0.5 inch towards the interspace of the metacarpal bones. Moxibustion is applicable.
Regional anatomy
Vasculature: The dorsal digital artery of the ulnar artery.
Innervation: The dorsal branch of the ulnar nerve.

3. Zhongzhu (Shu-Stream Point, S J 3)

Location: When the fist is clenched, the point is on the dorsum of the hand between the fourth and fifth metacarpal bones, in the depression proximal to the metacarpo-phalangeal joint. (See Fig. 95)
Indications: Headache, redness of the eyes, deafness, tinnitus, sore throat, febrile diseases, pain in the elbow and arm, motor impairment of fingers.
Method: Puncture perpendicularly 0.3-0.5 inch. Moxibustion is applicable.
Regional anatomy
Vasculature: The dorsal venous network of hand and the fourth dorsal metacarpal artery.
Innervation: The dorsal branch of the ulnar nerve.

4. Yangchi (Yuan-Primary Point, S J 4)

Location: On the transverse crease of the dorsum of wrist, in the depression lateral to the tendon of m. extensor digitorum communis. (See Fig. 95)
Indications: Pain in the arm, shoulder and wrist, malaria, deafness, thirst.
Method: Puncture perpendicularly 0.3-0.5 inch. Moxibustion is applicable.
Regional anatomy
Vasculature: The dorsal venous network

of the wrist and the posterior carpal artery.
Innervation: The terminal branch of the posterior antebrachial cutaneous nerve and the dorsal branch of the ulnar nerve.

5. Waiguan (Luo-Connecting Point, the Eight Confluent Point, S J 5)

Location: 2 cun above Yangchi (S J 4), between the radius and ulna. (See Fig. 96)
Indications: Febrile diseases, headache, pain in the cheek, strained neck, deafness, tinnitus, pain in the hypochondriac region, motor impairment of the elbow and arm, pain of the fingers, hand tremor.
Method: Puncture perpendicularly 0.5-1.0 inch. Moxibustion is applicable.
. Regional anatomy
Vasculature: Deeper, the posterior and anterior antebrachial interosseous arteries and veins.
Innervation: The posterior antebrachial cutaneous nerve; deeper, the posterior interosseous nerve and the anterior interosseous nerve.

6. Zhigou (Jing-River Point, S J 6)

Location: 3 cun above Yangchi (S J 4), between the radius and ulna, on the radial side of m. extensor digitorum. (See Fig. 96)
Indications: Tinnitus, deafness, pain in the hypochondriac region, vomiting, constipation, febrile diseases, aching and heavy sensation of the shoulder and back, sudden hoarseness of voice.
Method: Puncture perpendicularly 0.8-1.2 inches. Moxibustion is applicable.
Regional anatomy: See Waiguan (S J 5).

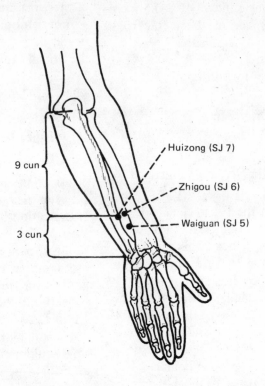

9 cun

3 cun

Huizong (SJ 7)

Zhigou (SJ 6)

Waiguan (SJ 5)

Fig. 96

7. Huizong (Xi-Cleft Point, S J 7)

Location: At the level with Zhigou (S J 6), about one finger-breadth lateral to Zhigou (S J 6), on the radial side of the ulna. (See Fig. 96)

Indications: Deafness, pain in the ear, epilepsy, pain of the arm.

Method: Puncture perpendicularly 0.5-1.0 inch. Moxibustion is applicable.

Regional anatomy

Vasculature: The posterior antebrachial interosseous artery and vein.

Innervation: The posterior and medial antebrachial cutaneous nerves; deeper, the posterior and anterior interosseous nerves.

8. Sanyangluo (S J 8)

Location: 4 cun above Yangchi (S J 4), between the radius and ulna. (See Col. Fig. 14)

Indications: Deafness, sudden hoarseness of voice, pain in the chest and hypochondriac region, pain in the hand and arm, toothache.

Method: Puncture perpendicularly 0.5-1.0 inch. Moxibustion is applicable.

Regional anatomy: See Huizong (S J 7).

9. Sidu (S J 9)

Location: On the lateral side of the fore-arm, 5 cun below the olecranon, between the radius and ulna. (See Col. Fig. 14)

Indications: Deafness, toothache, migraine, sudden hoarseness of voice, pain in the forearm.

Method: Puncture perpendicularly 0.5-1.0 inch. Moxibustion is applicable.

Regional anatomy: See Huizong (S J 7).

10.   Tianjing (He-Sea Point, S J 10)

Location: When the elbow is flexed, the point is in the depression about 1 cun superior to the olecranon. (See Fig. 97)

Indications: Migraine, pain in the neck, shoulder and arm, epilepsy, scrofula, goiter.

Method: Puncture perpendicularly 0.3-0.5 inch. Moxibustion is applicable.

Regional anatomy

Vasculature: The arterial and venous network of the elbow.

Innervation: The posterior brachial cutaneous nerve and the muscular branch of the radial nerve.

11.   Qinglengyuan (S J 11)

Location: 1 cun above Tianjing (S J 10) when the elbow is flexed.(See Col. Fig. 14)

Indications: Motor impairment and pain of the shoulder and arm, migraine.

Method: Puncture perpendicularly 0.3-0.5 inch. Moxibustion is applicable.

Regional anatomy

Vasculature: The terminal branches of the median collateral artery and vein.

Innervation: The posterior brachial cutaneous nerve and the muscular branch of the radial nerve.

12.   Xiaoluo (S J 12)

Location: On the line joining the olecranon and Jianliao (S J 14), midway between Qinglengyuan (S J 11) and Naohui (S J 13). (See Col. Fig. 14)

Indications: Headache, neck rigidity, motor impairment and pain of the arm.

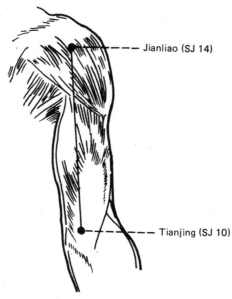

Fig. 97

Method: Puncture perpendicularly 0.5-0.7 inch. Moxibustion is applicable.
Regional anatomy
Vasculature: The median collateral artery and vein.
Innervation: The posterior brachial cutaneous nerve and the muscular branch of the radial nerve.

13.   Naohui (S J 13)

Location: On the line joining Jianliao (S J 14) and the olecranon, on the posterior border of m. deltoideus. (See Col. Fig. 14)
Indications: Goiter, pain in the shoulder and arm.
Method: Puncture perpendicularly 0.5-0.8 inch. Moxibustion is applicable.
Regional anatomy
Vasculature: The median collateral artery and vein.
Innervation: The posterior brachial cutaneous nerve, the muscular branch of the radial nerve; deeper, the radial nerve.

14.   Jianliao (S J 14)

Location: Posterior and inferior to the acromion, in the depression about 1 cun posterior to Jianyu (L I 15) when the arm is abducted. (See Fig. 97)
Indications: Pain and motor impairment of the shoulder and upper arm.
Method: Puncture perpendicularly 0.7-1.0 inch. Moxibustion is applicable.
Regional anatomy
Vasculature: The muscular branch of the posterior circumflex humeral artery.
Innervation: The muscular branch of the axillary nerve.

15.   Tianliao (S J 15)

Location: Midway between Jianjing (G 21) and Quyuan (S I 13), on the superior angle of the scapula. (See Col. Fig. 14)
Indications: Pain in the shoulder and elbow, stiffness of the neck.
Method: Puncture perpendicularly 0.3-0.5 inch. Moxibustion is applicable.
Regional anatomy
Vasculature: The descending branch of the transverse cervical artery; deeper, the muscular branch of the suprascapular artery.
Innervation: The accessory nerve and the branch of the suprascapular nerve.

16.   Tianyou (S J 16)

Location: Posterior and inferior to the mastoid process, on the posterior border of m. sternocleidomastoideus, almost level with Tianrong (S I 17) and Tianzhu (B 10). (See Col. Fig. 14)
Indications: Headache, neck rigidity, facial swelling, blurring of vision, sudden deafness.
Method: Puncture perpendicularly 0.3-0.5 inch. Moxibustion is applicable.
Regional anatomy
Vasculature: The posterior auricular artery.
Innervation: The lesser occipital nerve.

17.   Yifeng (S J 17)

Location: Posterior to the lobule of the ear, in the depression between the mandible and mastoid process. (See Fig. 98)
Indications: Tinnitus, deafness, otorrhea,

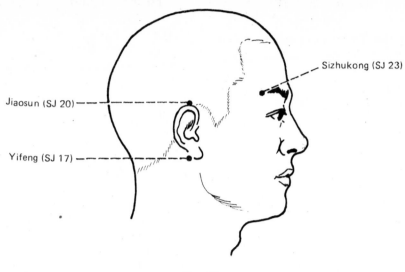

Fig. 98

facial paralysis, toothache, swelling of the cheek, scrofula, trismus.

Method: Puncture perpendicularly 0.5-1.0 inch. Moxibustion is applicable.

Regional anatomy

Vasculature: The posterior auricular artery and vein, the external jugular vein.

Innervation: The great auricular nerve; deeper, the site where the facial nerve perforates out of the stylomastoid foramen.

18.   Qimai (S J 18)

Location: In the centre of the mastoid process, at the junction of the middle and lower third of the curve formed by Yifeng (S J 17) and Jiaosun (S J 20) posterior to the helix. (See Col. Fig. 14)

Indications: Headache, tinnitus, deafness, infantile convulsion.

Method: Puncture subcutaneously 0.3-0.5 inch or prick with a three-edged needle to cause bleeding. Moxibustion is applicable.

Regional anatomy
Vasculature: The posterior auricular artery and vein.

Innervation: The posterior auricular branch of the great auricular nerve.

19.   Luxi (S J 19)

Location: Posterior to the ear, at the junction of the upper and middle third of the curve formed by Yifeng (S J 17) and Jiaosun (S J 20) behind the helix. (See Col. Fig. 14)

Indications: Headache, tinnitus, deafness, pain in the ear, infantile convulsion.

Method: Puncture obliquely 0.3-0.5 inch. Moxibustion is applicable.

Regional anatomy
Vasculature: The posterior auricular artery and vein.

Innervation: The anastomotic branch of the great auricular nerve and the lesser occipital nerve.

20　Jiaosun (S J 20)

Location: Directly above the ear apex, within the hair line. (See Fig. 98)

Indications: Tinnitus, redness, pain and swelling of the eye, swelling of the gum, toothache, parotitis.

Method: Puncture subcutaneously 0.3-0.5 inch. Moxibustion is applicable.

Regional anatomy

Vasculature: The branches of the superficial temporal artery and vein.

Innervation: The branches of the auriculotemporal nerve.

21.　Ermen (S J 21)

Location: In the depression anterior to the supratragic notch and slightly superior to the condyloid process of the mandible. The point is located with the mouth open. (See Col. Fig. 14)

Indications: Tinnitus, deafness, otorrhea, toothache, stiffness of the lip.

Method: Puncture perpendicularly 0.3-0.5 inch. Moxibustion is applicable.

Regional anatomy

Vasculature: The superficial temporal artery and vein.

Innervation: The branches of the auriculotemporal nerve and facial nerve.

22.　Erheliao (S J 22)

Location: Anterior and superior to Ermen (S J 21), at the level with the root of the auricle, on the posterior border of the hairline of the temple where the superficial temporal artery passes. (See Col. Fig. 14)

Indications: Migraine, tinnitus, lockjaw.

Method: Avoid puncturing the artery, puncture obliquely 0.1-0.3 inch. Moxibustion is applicable.

Regional anatomy

Vasculature: The superficial temporal artery and vein.

Innervation: The branch of the auriculotemporal nerve, on the course of the temporal branch of the facial nerve.

23.　Sizhukong (S J 23)

Location: In the depression at the lateral end of the eyebrow. (See Fig. 98)

Indications: Headache, redness and pain of the eye, blurring of vision, twitching of the eyelid, toothache, facial paralysis.

Method: Puncture subcutaneously 0.3-0.5 inch.

Regional anatomy

Vasculature: The frontal branches of the superficial temporal artery and vein.

Innervation: The zygomatic branch of the facial nerve and the branch of the auriculotemporal nerve.

III.　THE GALLBLADDER MERIDIAN OF FOOT-SHAOYANG

1.　Tongziliao (G 1)

Location: 0.5 cun lateral to the outer canthus, in the depression on the lateral side of the orbit. (See Fig. 99)

Indications: Headache, redness and pain of the eyes, failing of vision, lacrimation, deviation of the eye and mouth.

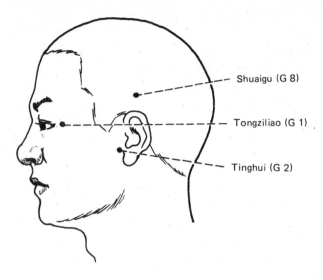

Shuaigu (G 8)

Tongziliao (G 1)

Tinghui (G 2)

Fig. 99

Method: Puncture subcutaneously 0.3-0.5 inch.

Regional anatomy

Vasculature: The zygomaticoorbital artery and vein.

Innervation: The zygomaticofacial and zygomaticotemporal nerves, the temporal branch of the facial nerve.

2.   Tinghui (G 2)

Location: Anterior to the intertragic notch, at the posterior border of the condyloid process of the mandible. The point is located with the mouth open. (See Fig. 99)

Indications: Deafness, tinnitus, toothache, motor impairment of the temporomandibular joint, mumps, deviation of the eye and mouth.

Method: Puncture perpendicularly 0.5-0.7 inch. Moxibustion is applicable.

Regional anatomy

Vasculature: The superficial temporal artery.

Innervation: The great auricular nerve and facial nerve.

3.   Shangguan (G 3)

Location: In the front of the ear, on the upper border of the zygomatic arch, in the depression directly above Xiaguan (S 7). (See Col. Fig. 15)

Indications: Headache, deafness, tinnitus, diplacusis, deviation of the eye and mouth, toothache.

Method: Puncture perpendicularly 0.3-0.5 inch. Deep puncture is not advisable. Moxibustion is applicable.

Regional anatomy

Vasculature: The zygomaticoorbital artery and vein.

Innervation: The zygomatic branch of the facial nerve and the zygomaticofacial nerve.

4. Hanyan (G 4)

Location: Within the hairline of the temporal region, at the junction of the upper 1/4 and lower 3/4 of the distance between Touwei (S 8) and Qubin (G 7).   (See Col. Fig. 15)

Indications: Migraine, vertigo, tinnitus, pain in the outer canthus, toothache, convulsion, epilepsy.

Method: Puncture subcutaneously 0.3-0.5 inch. Moxibustion is applicable.

Regional anatomy

Vasculature: The parietal branches of the superficial temporal artery and vein.

Innervation: The temporal branch of the auriculotemporal nerve.

5. Xuanlu (G 5)

Location: Within the hairline of the temporal region, midway of the border line connecting Touwei (S 8) and Qubin (G 7). (See Col. Fig. 15)

Indications: Migraine, pain in the outer canthus, facial swelling.

Method: Puncture subcutaneously 0.3-0.5 inch. Moxibustion is applicable.

Regional anatomy: See Hanyan (G 4).

6. Xuanli (G 6)

Location: Within the hairline, at the junction of the lower 1/4 and upper 3/4 of the distance between Touwei (S 8) and Qubin (G 7). (See Col. Fig. 15)

Indications: Migraine, pain in the outer canthus, tinnitus, frequent sneezing.

Method: Puncture subcutaneously 0.3-0.5 inch. Moxibustion is applicable.

Regional anatomy: See Hanyan (G 4).

7. Qubin (G 7)

Location: Directly above the posterior border of the pre-auricular hairline, about one finger-breadth anterior to Jiaosun (S J 20). (See Col. Fig. 15)

Indications: Headache, swelling of the cheek, trismus, pain in the temporal region, infantile convulsion.

Method: Puncture subcutaneously 0.3-0.5 inch. Moxibustion is applicable.

Regional anatomy: See Hanyan (G 4).

8. Shuaigu (G 8)

Location: Superior to the apex of the auricle, 1.5 cun within the hairline. (See Fig. 99)

Indications: Migraine, vertigo, vomiting, infantile convulsion.

Method: Puncture subcutaneously 0.3-0.5 inch. Moxibustion is applicable.

Regional anatomy

Vasculature: The parietal branches of the superficial temporal artery and vein.

Innervation: The anastomotic branch of the auriculotemporal nerve and great occipital nerve.

9. Tianchong (G 9)

Location: Directly above the posterior border of the auricle, 2 cun within the hairline, about 0.5 cun posterior to Shuaigu (G 8). (See Col. Fig. 15)

Indications: Headache, epilepsy, swelling and pain of the gums, convulsion.

Method: Puncture subcutaneously 0.3-0.5 inch.

Regional anatomy
Vasculature: The posterior auricular artery and vein.
Innervation: The branch of the great occipital nerve.

10.   Fubai (G 10)

Location: Posterior and superior to the mastoid process, midway of the curve line drawn from Tianchong (G 9) to Touqiaoyin (G 11). (See Col. Fig. 15)
Indications: Headache, tinnitus, deafness.
Method: Puncture subcutaneously 0.3-0.5 inch. Moxibustion is applicable.
Regional anatomy: See Tianchong (G 9).

11.   Touqiaoyin (G 11)

Location: Posterior and superior to the mastoid process, on the line connecting Fubai (G 10) and Wangu (G 12). (See Col. Fig. 15)
Indications: Pain of the head and neck, tinnitus, deafness, pain in the ears.
Method: Puncture subcutaneously 0.3-0.5 inch. Moxibustion is applicable.
Regional anatomy
Vasculature: The branches of the posterior auricular artery and vein.
Innervation: The anastomotic branch of the great and lesser occipital nerves.

12.   Wangu (G 12)

Location: In the depression posterior and inferior to the mastoid process. (See Col. Fig. 15)
Indications: Headache, insomnia, swelling of the cheek, retroauricular pain,

deviation of the eye and mouth, toothache.
Method: Puncture obliquely 0.3-0.5 inch. Moxibustion is applicable.
Regional anatomy
Vasculature: The posterior auricular artery and vein.
Innervation: The lesser occipital nerve.

13.   Benshen (G 13)

Location: 0.5 cun within the hairline of the forehead, 3 cun lateral to Shenting (Du 24). (See Col. Fig. 15)
Indications: Headache, insomnia, vertigo, epilepsy.
Method: Puncture subcutaneously 0.3-0.5 inch. Moxibustion is applicable.
Regional anatomy
Vasculature: The frontal branches of the superficial temporal artery and vein, and the lateral branches of the frontal artery and vein.
Innervation: The lateral branch of the frontal nerve.

14.   Yangbai (G 14)

Location: On the forehead, 1 cun directly above the midpoint of the eyebrow. (See Fig. 100)
Indications: Headache in the frontal region, pain of the orbital ridge, eye pain, vertigo, twitching of the eyelids, ptosis of the eyelids, lacrimation.
Method: Puncture subcutaneously 0.3-0.5 inch. Moxibustion is applicable.
Regional anatomy
Vasculature: The lateral branches of the frontal artery and vein.
Innervation: The lateral branch of the frontal nerve.

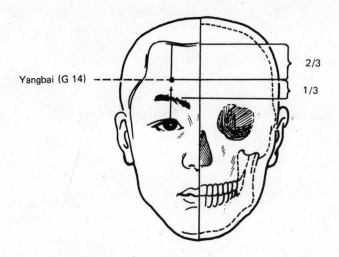

Yangbai (G 14)

2/3

1/3

Fig.100

15. Toulinqi (G 15)

Location: Directly above Yangbai (G 14), 0.5 cun within the hairline, midway between Shenting (Du 24) and Touwei (S 8). (See Col. Fig. 15)

Indications: Headache, vertigo, lacrimation, pain in the outer canthus, rhinorrhea, nasal obstruction.

Method: Puncture subcutaneously 0.3-0.5 inch. Moxibustion is applicable.

Regional anatomy

Vasculature: The frontal artery and vein.

Innervation: The anastomotic branch of the medial and lateral branches of the frontal nerve.

16. Muchuang (G 16)

Location: 1.5 cun posterior to Toulinqi (G 15), on the line connecting Toulinqi (G 15) and Fengchi (G 20). (See Col. Fig. 15)

Indications: Headache, vertigo, red and painful eyes, nasal obstruction.

Method: Puncture subcutaneously 0.3-0.5 inch. Moxibustion is applicable.

Regional anatomy

Vasculature: The frontal branches of the superficial temporal artery and vein.

Innervation: The anastomotic branch of the medial and lateral branches of the frontal nerve.

17. Zhengying (G 17)

Location: 1.5 cun posterior to Muchuang (G 16), on the line joining Toulinqi (G 15) and Fengchi (G 20). (See Col. Fig. 15)

Indications: Migraine, vertigo.

Method: Puncture subcutaneously 0.3-0.5 inch. Moxibustion is applicable.

Regional anatomy

Vasculature: The anastomotic plexus formed by the parietal branches of the superficial temporal artery and vein and the occipital artery and vein.

Innervation: The anastomotic branch of the frontal and great occipital nerves.

18.   Chengling (G 18)

Location: 1.5 cun posterior to Zhengying (G 17), on the line connecting Toulinqi (G 15) and Fengchi (G 20). (See Col. Fig. 15)
Indications: Headache, vertigo, epistaxis, rhinorrhea.
Method: Puncture subcutaneously 0.3-0.5 inch. Moxibustion is applicable.
Regional anatomy
Vasculature: The   branches   of   the occipital artery and vein.
Innervation: The branch of the great occipital nerve.

19.   Naokong (G 19)

Location: Directly above Fengchi (G 20), at the level with Naohu (Du 17), on the lateral side of the external occipital protuberance. (See Col. Fig. 15)
Indications: Headache, stiffness of the neck, vertigo, painful eyes, tinnitus, epilepsy.
Method: Puncture subcutaneously 0.3-0.5 inch. Moxibustion is applicable.
Regional anatomy: See Chengling (G 18).

20.   Fengchi (G 20)

Location: In the depression between the upper portion of m. sternocleidomastoideus and m. trapezius, on the same level with Fengfu (Du 16). (See Fig. 101)
Indications: Headache, vertigo, insomnia, pain and stiffness of the neck, blurred vision, glaucoma, red and painful eyes, tinnitus, convulsion, epilepsy, infantile convulsion, febrile diseases, common cold, nasal obstruction, rhinorrhea.
Method: Puncture 0.5-0.8 inch towards the tip of the nose. Moxibustion is applicable.
Regional anatomy
Vasculature: The   branches   of   the occipital artery and vein.
Innervation: The branch of the lesser occipital nerve.

21.   Jianjing (G 21)

Location: Midway between Dazhui (Du 14) and the acromion, at the highest point of the shoulder. (See Fig. 102)
Indications: Pain and rigidity of the neck, pain in the shoulder and back, motor impairment   of   the   arm,   insufficient lactation,   mastitis,   scrofula,   apoplexy, difficult labour.
Method: Puncture perpendicularly 0.3-0.5 inch. Moxibustion is applicable.
Regional anatomy
Vasculature: The   transverse   cervical artery and vein.
Innervation: The posterior branch of the supraclavicular nerve, the accessory nerve.

22.   Yuanye (G 22)

Location: On the mid-axillary line when the arm is raised, 3 cun below the axilla. (See Col. Fig. 15)
Indications: Fullness   of   the   chest, swelling of the axillary region, pain in the hypochondriac region, pain and motor impairment of the arm.
Method: Puncture obliquely 0.3-0.5 inch.
Regional anatomy
Vasculature: The thoracoepigastric vein,

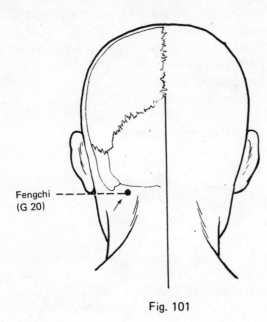

Fengchi
(G 20)

Fig. 101

the lateral thoracic artery and vein, the fifth intercostal artery and vein.

Innervation: The lateral cutaneous branch of the fifth intercostal nerve, the branch of the long thoracic nerve.

23.   Zhejin (G 23)

Location: 1 cun anterior to Yuanye (G 22), approximately at the level with the nipple. (See Col. Fig. 15)

Indications: Fullness of the chest, pain in the hypochondriac region, asthma.

Method: Puncture obliquely 0.3-0.5 inch. Moxibustion is applicable.

Regional anatomy

Vasculature: The lateral thoracic artery and vein, the fifth intercostal artery and vein.

Innervation: The lateral cutaneous branch of the fifth intercostal nerve.

24.   Riyue (Front-Mu Point of the Gallbladder, G 24)

Location: One rib below Qimen (Liv 14), directly below the nipple, in the seventh intercostal space. (See Fig. 103)

Indications: Pain in the hypochondriac region, vomiting, acid regurgitation, hiccup, jaundice, mastitis.

Method: Puncture obliquely 0.3-0.5 inch. Moxibustion is applicable.

Regional anatomy

Vasculature: The seventh intercostal artery and vein.

Innervation: The seventh intercostal nerve.

25.   Jingmen (Front-Mu Point of the Kidney, G 25)

Location: On the lateral side of the abdomen, on the lower border of the free

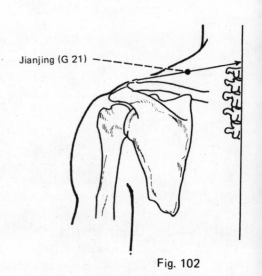

Jianjing (G 21)

Fig. 102

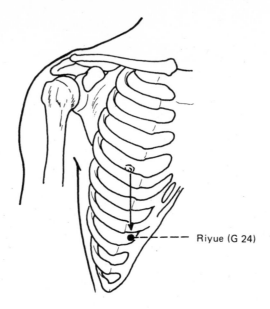

Fig. 103

end of the twelfth rib. (See Fig. 104)

Indications: Abdominal distention, borborygmus, diarrhea, pain in the lumbar and hypochondriac region.

Method: Puncture perpendicularly 0.3-0.5 inch. Moxibustion is applicable.

Regional anatomy

Vasculature: The eleventh intercostal artery and vein.

Innervation: The eleventh intercostal nerve.

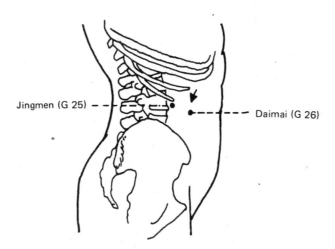

Fig. 104

26. Daimai (G 26)

Location: Directly below the free end of the eleventh rib where Zhangmen (Liv 13) is located, at the level with the umbilicus. (See Fig. 104)

Indications: Irregular menstruation, amenorrhea, leukorrhea, abdominal pain, hernia, pain in the lumbar and hypochondriac region.

Method: Puncture perpendicularly 0.5-0.8 inch. Moxibustion is applicable.

Regional anatomy

Vasculature: The subcostal artery and vein.

Innervation: The subcostal nerve.

27. Wushu (G 27)

Location: In the lateral side of the abdomen, anterior to the superior iliac spine, 3 cun below the level of the umbilicus. (See Col. Fig. 15)

Indications: Leukorrhea, lower abdominal pain, lumbar pain, hernia, constipation.

Method: Puncture perpendicularly 0.5-1.0 inch. Moxibustion is applicable.

Regional anatomy

Vasculature: The superficial and deep circumflex iliac arteries and veins.

Innervation: The iliohypogastric nerve.

28. Weidao (G 28)

Location: Anterior and inferior to the anterior superior iliac spine, 0.5 cun anterior and inferior to Wushu (G 27). (Col.Fig.15)

Indications: Leukorrhea, lower abdominal pain, hernia, prolapse of uterus.

Method: Puncture perpendicularly 0.5-1.0 inch. Moxibustion is applicable.

Regional anatomy

Vasculature: The superficial and deep circumflex iliac arteries and veins.

Innervation: The ilioinguinal nerve.

29. Juliao (G 29)

Location: In the depression of the midpoint between the anterosuperior iliac spine and the great trochanter.(Col.Fig.15)

Indications: Pain and numbness in the thigh and lumbar region, paralysis, muscular atrophy of the lower limbs.

Method: Puncture perpendicularly 0.5-1.0 inch. Moxibustion is applicable.

Regional anatomy

Vasculature: The branches of the superficial circumflex iliac artery and vein, the ascending branches of the lateral circumflex femoral artery and vein.

Innervation: The lateral femoral cutaneous nerve.

30. Huantiao (G 30)

Location: At the junction of the lateral 1/3 and medial 2/3 of the distance between the great trochanter and the hiatus of the sacrum (Yaoshu, Du 2). When locating the point, put the patient in lateral recumbent position with the thigh flexed. (Fig. 105)

Indications: Pain of the lumbar region and thigh, muscular atrophy of the lower limbs, hemiplegia.

Method: Puncture perpendicularly 1.5-2.5 inches. Moxibustion is applicable.

Regional anatomy

Vasculature: Medially, the inferior gluteal artery and vein.

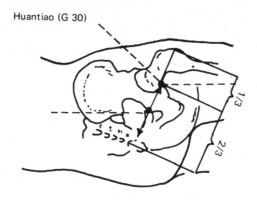

Huantiao (G 30)

Fig. 105

Innervation: The inferior gluteal cutaneous nerve, the inferior gluteal nerve; deeper, the sciatic nerve.

31.   Fengshi (G 31)

Location: On the midline of the lateral aspect of the thigh, 7 cun above the transverse popliteal crease. When the patient is standing erect with the hands close to the sides, the point is where the tip of the middle finger touches (See Fig. 106)

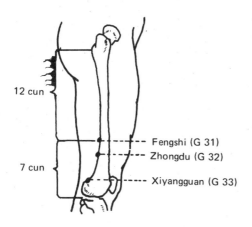

12 cun

7 cun

Fengshi (G 31)
Zhongdu (G 32)

Xiyangguan (G 33)

Fig. 106

Indications: Pain and soreness in the thigh and lumbar region, paralysis of the lower limbs, beriberi, general pruritus.

Method: Puncture perpendicularly 0.7-1.2 inches. Moxibustion is applicable.

Regional anatomy

Vasculature: The muscular branches of the lateral circumflex femoral artery and vein.

Innervation: The lateral femoral cutaneous nerve, the muscular branch of the femoral nerve.

32.   Zhongdu (G 32)

Location: On the lateral aspect of the thigh, 5 cun above the transverse popliteal crease, between m. vastus lateralis and m. biceps femoris. (See Fig. 106)

Indications: Pain and soreness of the thigh and knee, numbness and weakness of the lower limbs, hemiplegia.

Method: Puncture perpendicularly 0.7-1.0 inch. Moxibustion is applicable.

Regional anatomy: See Fengshi (G 31).

33. Xiyangguan (G. B. 33)

Location: 3 cun above Yanglingquan (G 34), lateral to the knee joint, between the tendon of m. biceps femoris and the femur. (See Fig. 106)

Indications: Swelling and pain of the knee, contracture of the tendons in popliteal fossa, numbness of the leg.

Method: Puncture perpendicularly 0.5-1.0 inch.

Regional anatomy

Vasculature: The superior lateral genicular artery and vein.

Innervation: The terminal branch of the lateral femoral cutaneous nerve.

34. Yanglingquan (He-Sea Point, Influential Point of Tendon, G 34)

Location: In the depression anterior and inferior to the head of the fibula. (Fig. 107)

Indications: Hemiplegia, weakness, numbness and pain of the lower extremities, swelling and pain of the knee, beriberi, hypochondriac pain, bitter taste in the mouth, vomiting, jaundice, infantile convulsion.

Method: Puncture perpendicularly 0.8-1.2 inches. Moxibustion is applicable.

Regional anatomy

Vasculature: The inferior lateral genicular artery and vein.

Innervation: Just where the common peroneal nerve bifurcates into the superficial and deep peroneal nerves.

35. Yangjiao (Xi-Cleft Point of the Yangwei Meridian, G 35)

Location: 7 cun above the tip of the external malleolus, on the posterior border of the fibula. (See Fig. 107)

Indications: Fullness of the chest and

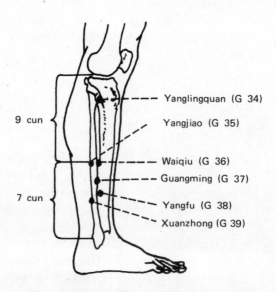

9 cun

7 cun

Yanglingquan (G 34)

Yangjiao (G 35)

Waiqiu (G 36)

Guangming (G 37)

Yangfu (G 38)

Xuanzhong (G 39)

Fig. 107

hypochondriac region, muscular atrophy and paralysis of the leg.

Method: Puncture perpendicularly 0.5-0.8 inch. Moxibustion is applicable.

Regional anatomy

Vasculature: The branches of the peroneal artery and vein.

Innervation: The lateral sural cutaneous nerve.

36.   Waiqiu (Xi-Cleft Point, G 36)

Location: 7 cun above the tip of the external malleolus, on the anterior border of the fibula. (See Fig. 107)

Indications: Pain in the neck, chest, thigh and hypochondriac region, rabies.

Method: Puncture perpendicularly 0.5-0.8 inch. Moxibustion is applicable.

Regional anatomy

Vasculature: The branches of the anterior tibial artery and vein.

Innervation: The superficial peroneal nerve.

37.   Guangming (Luo-Connecting Point, G 37)

Location: 5 cun directly above the tip of the external malleolus, on the anterior border of the fibula. (See Fig. 107)

Indications: Pain in the knee, muscular atrophy, motor impairment and pain of the lower extremities, blurring of vision, ophthalmalgia, night blindness, distending pain of the breast.

Method: Puncture perpendicularly 0.7-1.0 inch. Moxibustion is applicable.

Regional anatomy

Vasculature: The branches of the anterior tibial artery and vein.

Innervation: The superficial peroneal nerve.

38.   Yangfu (Jing-River Point, G 38)

Location: 4 cun above and slightly anterior to the tip of the external malleolus, on the anterior border of the fibula, between m. extensor digitorum longus and m. peronaeus brevis. (See Fig. 107)

Indications: Migraine, pain of the outer canthus, pain in the axillary region, scrofula, lumbar pain, pain in the chest, hypochondriac region and lateral aspect of the lower extremities, malaria.

Method: Puncture perpendicularly 0.5-0.7 inch. Moxibustion is applicable.

Regional anatomy: See Guangming (G 37)

39.   Xuanzhong (Influential Point of the Marrow, G 39)

Location: 3 cun above the tip of the external malleolus, in the depression between the posterior border of the fibula and the tendons of m. peronaeus longus and brevis. (See Fig. 107)

Indications: Apoplexy, hemiplegia, pain of the neck, abdominal distension, pain in the hypochondriac region, muscular atrophy of the lower limbs, spastic pain of the leg, beriberi.

Method: Puncture perpendicularly 0.3-0.5 inch. Moxibustion is applicable.

Regional anatomy: See Guangming (G 37).

40. Qiuxu (Yuan-Primary Point, G 40)

Location: Anterior and inferior to the external malleolus, in the depression on the lateral side of the tendon of m. extensor digitorum longus. (See Fig. 108)

Indications: Pain in the neck, swelling in the axillary region, pain in the hypochondriac region, vomiting, acid regurgitation, muscular atrophy of the lower limbs, pain and swelling of the external malleolus, malaria.

Method: Puncture perpendicularly 0.5-0.8 inch. Moxibustion is applicable.

Regional anatomy

Vasculature: The branch of the anterolateral malleolar artery.

Innervation: The branches of the intermediate dorsal cutaneous nerve and superficial peroneal nerve.

41. Zulinqi (Shu-Stream Point, the Eight Confluent Point, G 41)

Location: In the depression distal to the junction of the fourth and fifth metatarsal bones, on the lateral side of the tendon of m. extensor digiti minimi of the foot. (See Fig. 108)

Indications: Headache, vertigo, pain of the outer canthus, scrofula, pain in the hypochondriac region, distending pain of the breast, irregular menstruation, pain and swelling of the dorsum of foot, spastic pain of the foot and toe.

Method: Puncture perpendicularly 0.3-0.5 inch. Moxibustion is applicable.

Regional anatomy

Vasculature: The dorsal arterial and venous network of foot, the fourth dorsal metatarsal artery and vein.

Innervation: The branch of the intermediate dorsal cutaneous nerve of the foot.

42. Diwuhui (G 42)

Location: Between the fourth and fifth metatarsal bones, on the medial side of the tendon of m. extensor digiti minimi of foot. (See Fig. 108)

Indications: Pain of the canthus, tinnitus, distending pain of the breast, swelling and pain of the dorsum of foot.

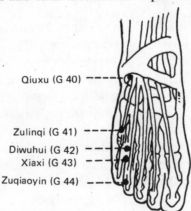

Qiuxu (G 40)

Zulinqi (G 41)
Diwuhui (G 42)
Xiaxi (G 43)
Zuqiaoyin (G 44)

Fig. 108

Method: Puncture perpendicularly 0.3-0.5 inch.

Regional anatomy: See Foot-Linqi (G 41).

43.   Xiaxi (Ying-Spring Point, G 43)

Location: On the dorsum of foot, between the fourth and fifth toe, proximal to the margin of the web. (See Fig. 108)

Indications: Headache, dizziness and vertigo, pain of the outer canthus, tinnitus, deafness, swelling of the cheek, pain in the hypochondriac region, distending pain of the breast, febrile diseases.

Method: Puncture perpendicularly 0.3-0.5 inch. Moxibustion is applicable.

Regional anatomy

Vasculature: The dorsal digital artery and vein.

Innervation: The dorsal digital nerve.

44.   Zuqiaoyin (Jing-Well Point, G 44)

Location: On the lateral side of the fourth toe, about 0.1 cun posterior to the corner of the nail. (See Fig. 108)

Indications: Migraine, deafness, tinnitus, ophthalmalgia, dream-disturbed sleep, febrile diseases.

Method: Puncture superficially about 0.1 inch. Moxibustion is applicable.

Regional anatomy

Vasculature: The arterial and venous network formed by the dorsal digital artery and vein and plantar digital artery and vein.

Innervation: The dorsal digital nerve.

IV. THE LIVER MERIDIAN OF FOOT-JUEYIN

1.   Dadun (Jing-Well Point, Liv 1)

Location: On the lateral side of the dorsum of the terminal phalanx of the great toe, between the lateral corner of the nail and the interphalangeal joint. (See Fig. 109)

Indications: Hernia, enuresis, uterine bleeding, prolapse of the uterus, epilepsy.

Method: Puncture subcutaneously 0.1-0.2 inch. Moxibustion is applicable.

Regional anatomy

Vasculature: The dorsal digital artery and vein.

Innervation: The dorsal digital nerve derived from the deep peroneal nerve.

2.   Xingjian (Ying-Spring Point, Liv 2)

Location: On the dorsum of the foot between the first and second toe, proximal to the margin of the web (See Fig. 109)

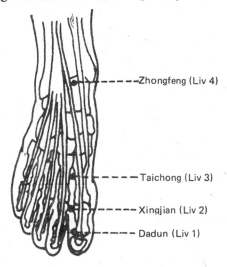

Fig. 109

Indications: Pain in the hypochondrium, abdominal distension, headache, dizziness and vertigo, congestion, swelling and pain of the eye, deviation of the mouth, hernia, painful urination, retention of urine, irregular menstruation, epilepsy, insomnia, convulsion.

Method: Puncture obliquely 0.3-0.5 inch. Moxibustion is applicable.

Regional anatomy

Vasculature: The dorsal venous network of the foot and the first dorsal digital artery and vein.

Innervation: The site where the dorsal digital nerves split from the lateral dorsal metatarsal nerve of the deep peroneal nerve.

3. Taichong (Shu-Stream and Yuan-Primary Point, Liv 3)

Location: On the dorsum of the foot, in the depression distal to the junction of the first and second metatarsal bones. (See Fig. 109)

Indications: Headache, dizziness and vertigo, insomnia, congestion, swelling and pain of the eye, depression, infantile convulsion, deviation of the mouth, pain in the hypochondriac region, uterine bleeding, hernia, enuresis, retention of urine, epilepsy, pain in the anterior aspect of the medial malleolus.

Method: Puncture perpendicularly 0.3-0.5 inch. Moxibustion is applicable.

Regional anatomy

Vasculature: The dorsal venous network of the foot, the first dorsal metatarsal artery.

Innervation: The branch of the deep peroneal nerve.

4. Zhongfeng (Jing-River Point, Liv 4)

Location: 1 cun anterior to the medial malleolus, midway between Shangqiu (Sp 5) and Jiexi (S 41), in the depression on the medial side of the tendon of m. tibialis anterior. (See Fig. 109)

Indications: Hernia, pain in the external genitalia, nocturnal emission, retention of urine, distending pain in the hypochondrium.

Method: Puncture perpendicularly 0.3-0.5 inch. Moxibustion is applicable.

Regional anatomy

Vasculature: The dorsal venous network of the foot and the anterior medial malleolar artery.

Innervation: The branch of the medial dorsal cutaneous nerve of the foot and the saphenous nerve.

5. Ligou (Luo-Connecting Point, Liv 5)

Location: 5 cun above the tip of the medial malleolus, on the medial aspect and near the medial border of the tibia. (See Fig. 110)

Indications: Retention of urine, enuresis, hernia, irregular menstruation, leukorrhea, pruritus valvae, weakness and atrophy of the leg.

Method: Puncture subcutaneously 0.3-0.5 inch. Moxibustion is applicable.

Regional anatomy

Vasculature: Posteriorly, the great saphenous vein.

Innervation: The branch of the saphenous nerve.

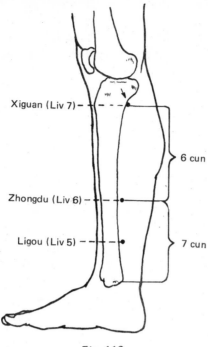

Xiguan (Liv 7)

6 cun

Zhongdu (Liv 6)

Ligou (Liv 5)

7 cun

Fig. 110

6.   Zhongdu (Xi-Cleft Point, Liv 6)

Location: 7 cun above the tip of the medial malleolus, on the medial aspect and near the medial border of the tibia. (See Fig. 110)

Indications: Abdominal pain, hypochondriac pain, diarrhea, hernia, uterine bleeding, prolonged lochia.

Method: Puncture subcutaneously 0.5-0.8 inch. Moxibustion is applicable.

Regional anatomy

Vasculature: The great saphenous vein.

Innervation: The branch of the saphenous nerve.

7.   Xiguan (Liv 7)

Location: Posterior and inferior to the medial condyle of the tibia, in the upper portion of the medial head of m. gastrocnemius, 1 cun posterior to Yinlingquan (Sp 9). (See Fig. 110)

Indication: Pain of the knee.

Method: Puncture perpendicularly 0.5-1.0 inch. Moxibustion is applicable.

Regional anatomy

Vasculature: Deeper, the posterior tibial artery.

Innervation: The branch of the medial sural cutaneous nerve; deeper, the tibial nerve.

8.   Ququan (He-Sea Point, Liv 8)

Location: When knee is flexed, the point is in the depression above the medial end of the transverse popliteal crease, posterior to the medial epicondyle of the femur, on the anterior part of the insertion of m.

semimembranosus and m. semitendinosus. (See Fig. 111)

Indications: Prolapse of uterus, lower abdominal pain, retention of urine, nocturnal emission, pain in the external genitalia, pruritus vulvae, pain in the medial aspect of the knee and thigh.

Method: Puncture perpendicularly 0.5-0.8 inch. Moxibustion is applicable.

Regional anatomy

Vasculature: Anteriorly, the great saphenous vein, on the pathway of the genu suprema artery.

Innervation: The saphenous.

9. Yinbao (Liv 9)

Location: 4 cun above the medial epicondyle of the femur, betweem m. vastus medialis and m. sartorius. (See Col. Fig. 17)

Indications: Pain in the lumbosacral region, lower abdominal pain, enuresis, retention of urine, irregular menstruation.

Method: Puncture perpendicularly 0.5-0.7 inch. Moxibustion is applicable.

Regional anatomy

Vasculature: Deeper, on the lateral side, the femoral artery and vein, the superficial branch of the medial circumflex femoral artery.

Innervation: The anterior femoral cutaneous nerve, on the pathway of the anterior branch of the obturator nerve.

10. Zuwuli (Liv 10)

Location: 3 cun directly below Qichong (S 30), on the lateral border of m. abductor longus. (See Col. Fig. 17)

Indications: Lower abdominal distention and fullness, retention of urine.

Method: Puncture perpendicularly 0.5-1.0 inch. Moxibustion is applicable.

Regional anatomy

Vasculature: The superficial branches of the medial circumflex femoral artery and vein.

Innervation: The genitofemoral nerve, the anterior femoral cutaneous nerve;

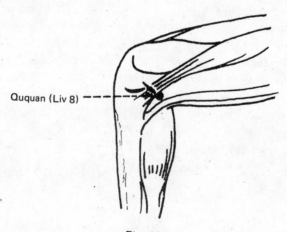

Ququan (Liv 8) ------

Fig. 111

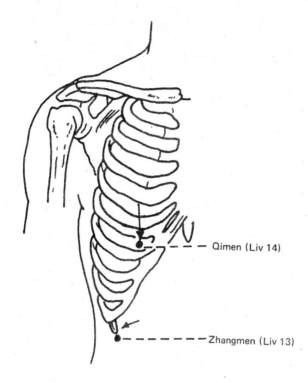

— Qimen (Liv 14)

—Zhangmen (Liv 13)

Fig. 112

deeper, the anterior branch of the obturator nerve.

nerve; deeper, the anterior branch of the obturator nerve.

11. Yinlian (Liv 11)

Location: 2 cun directly below Qichong (S 30), on the lateral border of m. abductor longus. (See Col. Fig. 17)

Indications: Irregular menstruation, leukorrhea, lower abdominal pain, pain in the thigh and leg.

Method: Puncture perpendicularly 0.5-1.0 inch. Moxibustion is applicable.

Regional anatomy

Vasculature: The branches of the medial circumflex femoral artery and vein.

Innervation: The genitofemoral nerve, the branch of the medial femoral cutaneous

12. Jimai (Liv 12)

Location: Inferior and lateral to the pubic spine, 2.5 cun lateral to the Ren Meridian, at the inguinal groove lateral and inferior to Qichong (S 30). (See Col. Fig. 18)

Indications: Lower abdominal pain, hernia, pain in the external genitalia.

Method: Moxibustion is applicable.

Regional anatomy

Vasculature: The branches of the external pudendal artery and vein, the pubic branches of the inferior epigastric artery and vein; laterally, the femoral vein.

Innervation: The ilioinguinal nerve;

deeper, in the inferior aspect, the anterior branch of the obturator nerve.

Innervation: Slightly inferiorly, the tenth intercostal nerve.

13. Zhangmen (Front-Mu Point of the Spleen, Influential Point of Zang Organs, Liv 13)

Location: On the lateral side of the abdomen, below the free end of the eleventh floating rib (See Fig. 112)

Indications: Abdominal distention, borborygmus, pain in the hypochondriac region, vomiting, diarrhea, indigestion.

Method: Puncture perpendicularly 0.5-0.8 inch. Moxibustion is applicable.

Regional anatomy

Vasculature: The terminal branch of the tenth intercostal artery.

14. Qimen (Front-Mu Point of the Liver, Liv 14)

Location: Directly below the nipple, in the sixth intercostal space (See Fig. 112)

Indications: Hypochondriac pain, abdominal distention, hiccup, acid regurgitation, mastitis, depression, febrile diseases.

Method: Puncture obliquely 0.3-0.5 inch. Moxibustion is applicable.

Regional anatomy

Vasculature: The sixth intercostal artery and vein.

Innervation: The sixth intercostal nerve.

Chapter 10

ACUPOINTS OF THE DU AND THE REN MERIDIANS AND THE EXTRAORDINARY POINTS

The Du (Governor Vessel) Meridian goes along the back midline, while the Ren (Conception Vessel) Meridian goes along the front midline. These two meridians and the twelve regular meridians are called the fourteen meridians. The experiential points which are not on the fourteen meridians are called the extraordinary points, which are introduced in this chapter.

I. THE DU MERIDIAN

1. Changqiang (Luo-Connecting Point, Du 1)

Location: Midway between the tip of the coccyx and the anus, locating the point in prone position. (See Figs. 113 and 114)

Indications: Diarrhea, bloody stools, hemorrhoids, prolapse of the rectum, constipation, pain in the lower back, epilepsy.

Method: Puncture perpendicularly 0.5-1.0 inch. Moxibustion is applicable.

Regional anatomy

Vasculature: The branches of the inferior hemorrhoid artery and vein.

Innervation: The posterior ramus of the coccygeal nerve, the hemorrhoid nerve.

2. Yaoshu (Du 2)

Location: In the hiatus of the sacrum. (See Col. Fig. 19)

Indications: Irregular menstruation, pain and stiffness of the lower back, hemorrhoids, muscular atrophy of the lower extremities, epilepsy.

Method: Puncture obliquely upward 0.5-1.0 inch. Moxibustion is applicable.

Regional anatomy

Vasculature: The branches of the median sacral artery and vein.

Innervation: The branch of the coccygeal nerve.

3. Yaoyangguan (Du 3)

Location: Below the spinous process of the fourth lumbar vertebra, at the level with the crista iliaca. (See Figs. 113 and 114)

Indications: Irregular menstruation, nocturnal emission, impotence, pain in the lumbosacral region, muscular atrophy, motor impairment, numbness and pain of the lower extremities.

Method: Puncture perpendicularly 0.5-1.0 inch. Moxibustion is applicable.

Regional anatomy

Vasculature: The posterior branch of the lumbar artery.

Innervation: The medial branch of the posterior ramus of the lumbar nerve.

4. Mingmen (Du 4)

Location: Below the spinous process of the second lumbar vertebra. (See Figs. 113 and 114)

Indications: Stiffness of the back, lumbago, impotence, nocturnal emission,

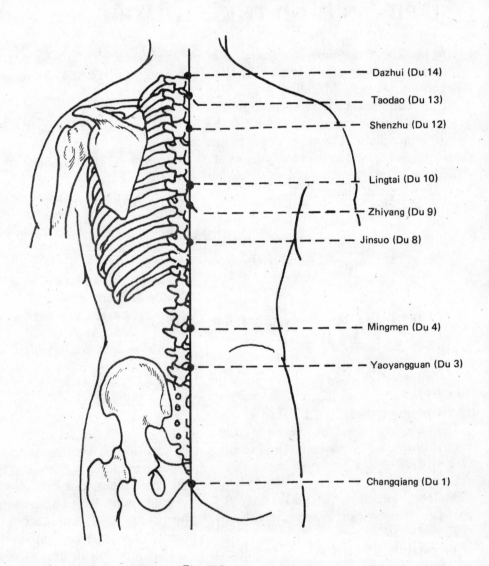

Dazhui (Du 14)

Taodao (Du 13)

Shenzhu (Du 12)

Lingtai (Du 10)

Zhiyang (Du 9)

Jinsuo (Du 8)

Mingmen (Du 4)

Yaoyangguan (Du 3)

Changqiang (Du 1)

Fig. 113

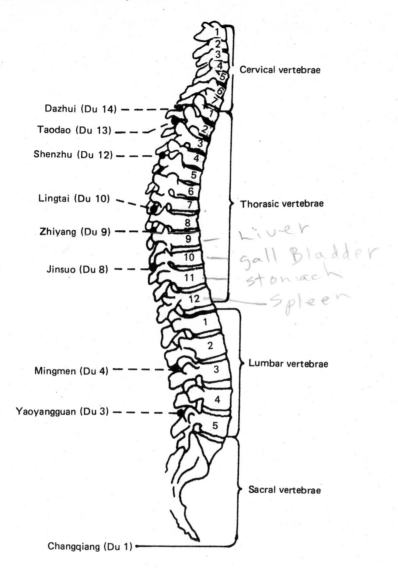

Cervical vertebrae

Dazhui (Du 14) — — — —

Taodao (Du 13) — — —

Shenzhu (Du 12) — — —

Lingtai (Du 10) — . —

Zhiyang (Du 9) — —

Thorasic vertebrae

Liver
gall Bladder
stomach
Spleen

Jinsuo (Du 8) — — —

Mingmen (Du 4) — — — —

Yaoyangguan (Du 3) — — — —

Lumbar vertebrae

Sacral vertebrae

Changqiang (Du 1) ————

Fig. 114

irregular menstruation, diarrhea, indigestion, leukorrhea.

Method: Puncture perpendicularly 0.5-1.0 inch. Moxibustion is applicable.

Regional anatomy: See Yaoyangguan (Du 3).

5.   Xuanshu (Du 5)

Location: Below the spinous process of the first lumbar vertebra. (See Col. Fig. 19)

Indications: Pain and stiffness of the lower back, diarrhea, indigestion.

Method: Puncture perpendicularly 0.5-1.0 inch. Moxibustion is applicable.

Regional anatomy: See Yaoyangguan (Du 3).

6. Jizhong (Du 6)

Location: Below the spinous process of the eleventh thoracic vertebra. (See Col. Fig. 19)

Indications: Pain in the epigastric region, diarrhea, jaundice, epilepsy, stiffness and pain of the back.

Method: Puncture perpendicularly 0.5-1.0 inch.

Regional anatomy

Vasculature: The posterior branch of the eleventh intercostal artery.

Innervation: The medial branch of the posterior ramus of the eleventh thoracic nerve.

7. Zhongshu (Du 7)

Location: Below the spinous process of the tenth thoracic vertebra. (See Col. Fig. 19)

Indications: Pain in the epigastric region, low back pain, stiffness of the back.

Method: Puncture perpendicularly 0.5-1.0 inch. Moxibustion is applicable.

Regional anatomy

Vasculature: The posterior branch of the tenth intercostal artery.

Innervation: The medial branch of the posterior ramus of the tenth thoracic nerve.

8. Jinsuo (Du 8)

Location: Below the spinous process of the ninth thoracic vertebra. (See Figs. 113 and 114)

Indications: Epilepsy, stiffness of the back, gastric pain.

Method: Puncture perpendicularly 0.5-1.0 inch. Moxibustion is applicable.

Regional anatomy

Vasculature: The posterior branch of the ninth intercostal artery.

Innervation: The medial branch of the posterior ramus of the ninth thoracic nerve.

9. Zhiyang (Du 9)

Location: Below the spinous process of the seventh thoracic vertebra, approximately at the level with the inferior angle of the scapula. (See Figs. 113 and 114)

Indications: Jaundice, cough, asthma, stiffness of the back, pain in the chest and back.

Method: Puncture obliquely upward 0.5-1.0 inch. Moxibustion is applicable.

Regional anatomy

Vasculature: The posterior branch of the seventh intercostal artery.

Innervation: The medial branch of the posterior ramus of the seventh thoracic nerve.

10. Lingtai (Du 10)

Location: Below the spinous process of the sixth thoracic vertebra. (See Figs. 113 and 114)

Indications: Cough, asthma, furuncles, back pain, neck rigidity.

Method: Puncture obliquely upward 0.5-1.0 inch. Moxibustion is applicable.

Regional anatomy

Vasculature: The posterior branch of the sixth intercostal artery.

Innervation: The medial branch of the posterior ramus of the thoracic nerve.

11.   Shendao (Du 11)

Location: Below the spinous process of the fifth thoracic vertebra. (See Col. Fig. 19)

Indications: Poor memory, anxiety, palpitation, pain and stiffness of the back, cough, cardiac pain.

Method: Puncture obliquely upward 0.5-1.0 inch. Moxibustion is applicable.

Regional anatomy

Vasculature: The posterior branch of the fifth intercostal artery.

Innervation: The medial branch of the posterior ramus of the fifth thoracic nerve.

12.   Shenzhu (Du 12)

Location: Below the spinous process of the third thoracic vertebra. (See Figs. 113 and 114)

Indications: Cough, asthma, epilepsy, pain and stiffness of the back, furuncles.

Method: Puncture obliquely upward 0.5-1.0 inch. Moxibustion is applicable.

Regional anatomy

Vasculature: The posterior branch of the third intercostal artery.

Innervation: The medial branch of the posterior ramus of the third thoracic nerve.

13.   Taodao (Du 13)

Location: Below the spinous process of the first thoracic vertebra. (See Figs. 113 and 114)

Indications: Stiffness of the back, headache, malaria, febrile diseases.

Method: Puncture obliquely upward 0.5-1.0 inch. Moxibustion is applicable.

Regional anatomy

Vasculature: The posterior branch of the first intercostal artery.

Innervation: The medial branch of the posterior ramus of the first thoracic nerve.

14.   Dazhui (Du 14)

Location: Below the spinous process of the seventh cervical vertebra, approximately at the level of the shoulders. (Figs. 113 & 114)

Indications: Neck pain and rigidity, malaria, febrile diseases, epilepsy, afternoon fever, cough, asthma, common cold, back stiffness.

Method: Puncture obliquely upward 0.5-1.0 inch. Moxibustion is applicable.

Regional anatomy

Vasculature: The branch of the transverse cervical artery.

Innervation: The posterior ramus of the eighth cervical nerve and the medial branch of the posterior ramus of the first thoracic nerve.

15.   Yamen (Du 15)

Location: 0.5 cun directly above the midpoint of the posterior hairline, in the depression below the spinous process of the first cervical vertebra (See Fig. 115)

Indications: Mental disorders, epilepsy, deafness and mute, sudden hoarseness of voice, apoplexy, stiffness of the tongue and aphasia, occipital headache, neck rigidity.

Method: Puncture perpendicularly 0.5-0.8 inch. Neither upward obliquely nor deep puncture is advisable. It is near the medullary bulb in the deep layer, and the depth and angle of the puncture should be paid strict attention to.

Regional anatomy

Vasculature: The branches of the occipital

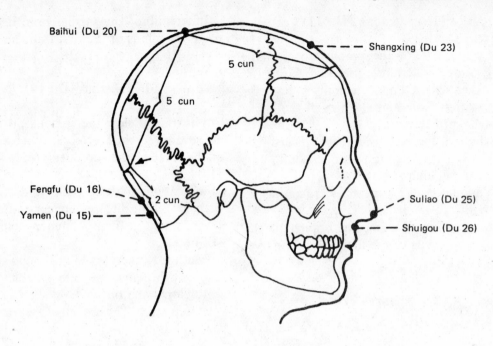

Fig. 115

artery and vein.

Innervation: The third occipital nerve.

16. Fengfu (Du 16)

Location: 1 cun directly above the midpoint of the posterior hairline, directly below the external occipital protuberance, in the depression between m. trapezius of both sides. (See Fig. 115)

Indications: Headache, neck rigidity, blurring of vision, epistaxis, sore throat, post-apoplexy aphasia, hemiplegia, mental disorders.

Method: Puncture perpendicularly 0.5-0.8 inch. Deep puncture is not advisable. Medullary bulb is in the deep layer, special attention should be paid in acupuncture.

Regional anatomy

Vasculature: The branch of the occipital artery.

Innervation: The branches of the third cervical nerve and the great occipital nerve.

17. Naohu (Du 17)

Location: On the midline of the head, 1.5 cun directly above Fengfu (Du 16), superior to the external occipital protuberance. (See Col. Fig. 19)

Indications: Epilepsy, dizziness, pain and stiffness of the neck.

Method: Puncture subcutaneously 0.3-0.5 inch. Moxibustion is applicable.

Regional anatomy

Vasculature: The branches of the occipital arteries and veins of both sides.

Innervation: The branch of the great occipital nerve.

18.   Qiangjian (Du 18)

Location: On the midline of the head, 1.5 cun directly above Naohu (Du 17), midway between Fengfu (Du 16) and Baihui (Du 20). (See Col. Fig. 19)

Indications: Headache, neck rigidity, blurring of vision, mania.

Method: Puncture subcutaneously 0.3-0.5 inch. Moxibustion is applicable.

Regional anatomy: See Naohu (Du 17).

19.   Houding (Du 19)

Location: On the midline of the head, 1.5 cun directly above Qiangjian (Du 18). (See Col. Fig. 19)

Indications: Headache, vertigo, mania, epilepsy.

Method: Puncture subcutaneously 0.3-0.5 inch. Moxibustion is applicable.

Regional anatomy: See Naohu (Du 17).

20.   Baihui (Du 20)

Location: On the midline of the head, 7 cun directly above the posterior hairline, approximately on the midpoint of the line connecting the apexes of the two auricles. (See Fig. 115)

Indications: Headache, vertigo, tinnitus, nasal obstruction, aphasia by apoplexy, coma, mental disorders, prolapse of the rectum and the uterus.

Method: Puncture subcutaneously 0.3-0.5 inch. Moxibustion is applicable.

Regional anatomy

Vasculature: The anastomotic network formed by the superficial temporal arteries and veins and the occipital arteries and veins on both sides.

Innervation: The branch of the great occipital nerve.

21.   Qianding (Du 21)

Location: On the midline of the head, 1.5 cun anterior to Baihui (Du 20).   (See Col. Fig. 19)

Indications: Epilepsy, dizziness, blurring of vision, vertical headache, rhinorrhea.

Method: Puncture subcutaneously 0.3-0.5 inch. Moxibustion is applicable.

Regional anatomy

Vasculature: The anastomotic network formed by the right and left superficial temporal arteries and veins.

Innervation: On the communicating site of the branch of the frontal nerve with the branch of the great occipital nerve.

22.   Xinhui (Du 22)

Location: 2 cun posterior to the midpoint of the anterior hairline, 3 cun anterior to Baihui (Du 20). (See Col. Fig. 19)

Indications: Headache, blurring of vision, rhinorrhea, infantile convulsion.

Method: Puncture subcutaneously 0.3-0.5 inch. This point is prohibited in infants with metopism. Moxibustion is applicable.

Regional anatomy

Vasculature: The anastomotic network formed by the right and left superficial temporal artery and vein and the frontal artery and vein.

Innervation: The branch of the frontal nerve.

23. Shangxing (Du 23)

Location: 1 cun directly above the midpoint of the anterior hairline. (Fig. 115)

Indications: Headache, ophthalmalgia, epistaxis, rhinorrhea, mental disorders.

Method: Puncture subcutaneously 0.3-0.5 inch or prick to cause bleeding. This point is prohibited in infants with metopism. Moxibustion is applicable.

Regional anatomy

Vasculature: The branches of the frontal artery and vein, and the branches of the superficial temporal artery and vein.

Innervation: The branch of the frontal nerve.

24. Shenting (Du 24)

Location: 0.5 cun directly above the midpoint of the anterior hairline. (See Col. Fig. 19)

Indications: Epilepsy, anxiety, palpitation, insomnia, headache, vertigo, rhinorrhea.

Method: Puncture subcutaneously 0.3-0.5 inch, or prick to cause bleeding. Moxibustion is applicable.

Regional anatomy

Vasculature: The branch of the frontal artery and vein.

Innervation: The branch of the frontal nerve.

25. Suliao (Du 25)

Location: On the tip of the nose. (See Fig. 115)

Indications: Loss of consciousness, nasal obstruction, epistaxis, rhinorrhea, rosacea.

Method: Puncture perpendicularly 0.2-0.3 inch, or prick to cause bleeding.

Regional anatomy

Vasculature: The lateral nasal branches of the facial artery and vein.

Innervation: The external nasal branch of the anterior ethmoidal nerve.

26. Shuigou (also known as Renzhong, Du 26)

Location: A little above the midpoint of the philtrum, near the nostrils. (See Fig. 115)

Indications: Mental disorders, epilepsy, hysteria, infantile convulsion, coma, apoplexy-faint, trismus, deviation of the mouth and eyes, puffiness of the face, pain and stiffness of the lower back.

Method: Puncture obliquely upward 0.3-0.5 inch.

Regional anatomy

Vasculature: The superior labial artery and vein.

Innervation: The buccal branch of the facial nerve, and the branch of the intraorbital nerve.

27. Duiduan (Du 27)

Location: On the median tubercle of the upper lip, at the junction of the skin and upper lip (See Col. Fig. 19)

Indications: Mental disorders, lip twitching, lip stiffness, pain and swelling of the gums.

Method: Puncture obliquely upward 0.2-0.3 inch.

Regional anatomy

Vasculature: The superior labial artery and vein.

Innervation: The buccal branch of the facial nerve, and the branch of the infraorbital nerve.

28. Yinjiao (Du 28)

Location: At the junction of the gum and the frenulum of the upper lip. (See Col. Fig. 19)

Indications: Mental disorders, pain and swelling of the gums, rhinorrhea.

Method: Puncture obliquely upward 0.1-0.2 inch, or prick to cause bleeding.

Regional anatomy

Vasculature: The superior labial artery and vein.

Innervation: The branch of the superior alveolar nerve.

II. THE REN MERIDIAN

1. Huiyin (Ren 1)

Location: Between the anus and the root of the scrotum in males and between the anus and the posterior labial commissure in females. (See Col. Fig. 20)

Indications: Vaginitis, retention of urine, hemorrhoids, nocturnal emission, enuresis, irregular menstruation, mental disorders.

Method: Puncture perpendicularly 0.5-1.0 inch. Moxibustion is applicable.

Regional anatomy

Vasculature: The branches of the perineal artery and vein.

Innervation: The branch of the perineal nerve.

2. Qugu (Ren 2)

Location: On the midpoint of the upper border of the symphysis pubis. (See Col. Fig. 20)

Indications: Retention and dribbling of

urine, enuresis, nocturnal emission, impotence, morbid leukorrhea, irregular menstruation, dysmenorrhea, hernia.

Method: Puncture perpendicularly 0.5-1.0 inch. Great care should be taken to puncture the points from Qugu (Ren 2) to Shangwan (Ren 13) of this meridian in pregnent women. Moxibustion is applicable.

Regional anatomy

Vasculature: The branches of the inferior epigastric artery and the obturator artery.

Innervation: The branch of the iliohypogastric nerve.

3. Zhongji (Front-Mu Point of the Bladder, Ren 3)

Location: On the midline of the abdomen, 4 cun below the umbilicus. (See Fig. 116)

Indications: Enuresis, nocturnal emission, impotence, hernia, uterine bleeding, irregular menstruation, dysmenorrhea, morbid leukorrhea, frequency of urination, retention of urine, pain in the lower abdomen, prolapse of the uterus, vaginitis.

Method: Puncture perpendicularly 0.5-1.0 inch. Moxibustion is applicable.

Regional anatomy

Vasculature: The branches of superficial epigastric artery and vein, and the branches of inferior epigastric artery and vein.

Innervation: The branch of the iliohypogastric nerve.

4. Guanyuan (Front-Mu Point of the Small Intestine, Ren 4)

Location: On the midline of the abdomen, 3 cun below the umbilicus. (See Fig. 116)

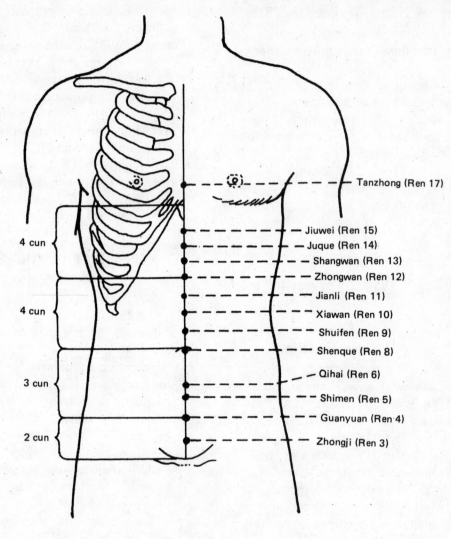

Fig. 116

Indications: Enuresis, nocturnal emission, frequency of urination, retention of urine, hernia, irregular menstruation, morbid leukorrhea, dysmenorrhea, uterine bleeding, postpartum hemorrhage, lower abdominal pain, indigestion, diarrhea, prolapse of the rectum, flaccid type of apoplexy.

Method: Puncture perpendicularly 0.8-

1.2 inches. This is one of the important points for tonification. Moxibustion is applicable.

Regional anatomy

Vasculature: See Zhongji (Ren 3).

Innervation: The medial branch of the anterior cutaneous branch of the twelfth intercostal nerve.

5.   Shimen (Front-Mu Point of Sanjiao, Ren 5)

Location: On the midline of the abdomen, 2 cun below the umbilicus. (See Fig. 116)

Indications: Abdominal pain, diarrhea, edema, hernia, anuria, enuresis, amenorrhea, morbid leukorrhea, uterine bleeding, postpartum hemorrhage.

Method: Puncture perpendicularly 0.5-1.0 inch. Moxibustion is applicable.

Regional anatomy

Vasculature: See Zhongji (Ren 3).

Innervation: The anterior cutaneous branch of the eleventh intercostal nerve.

6.   Qihai (Ren 6)

Location: On the midline of the abdomen, 1.5 cun below the umbilicus. (See Fig. 116)

Indications: Abdominal pain, enuresis, nocturnal emission, impotence, hernia, edema, diarrhea, dysentery, uterine bleeding, irregular menstruation, dysmenorrhea, amenorrhea, morbid leukorrhea, postpartum hemorrhage, constipation, flaccid type of apoplexy, asthma.

Method: Puncture perpendicularly 0.8-1.2 inches. This is one of the important points for tonification. Moxibustion is applicable.

Regional anatomy: See Shimen (Ren 5).

7.   Yinjiao (Ren 7)

Location: On the midline of the abdomen, 1 cun below the umbilicus. (See Col. Fig. 20)

Indications: Abdominal distention, edema, hernia, irregular menstruation, uterine bleeding, morbid leukorrhea, pruritus vulvae, postpartum hemorrhage, abdominal pain around the umbilicus.

Method: Puncture perpendicularly 0.8-1.2 inches. Moxibustion is applicable.

Regional anatomy

Vasculature: See Zhongji (Ren 3).

Innervation: The anterior cutaneous branch of the tenth intercostal nerve.

8.   Shenque (Ren 8)

Location: In the centre of the umbilicus. (See Fig. 116)

Indications: Abdominal pain, borborygmus, flaccid type of apoplexy, prolapse of the rectum, unchecked diarrhea.

Method: Puncture is prohibited. Moxibustion is applicable.

Regional anatomy

Vasculature: The inferior epigastric artery and vein.

Innervation: The anterior cutaneous branch of the tenth intercostal nerve.

9.   Shuifen (Ren 9)

Location: On the midline of the abdomen, 1 cun above the umbilicus. (See Fig. 116)

Indications: Abdominal pain, borborygmus, edema, retention of the urine, diarrhea.

Method: Puncture perpendicularly 0.5-1.0 inch. Moxibustion is applicable.

Regional anatomy

Vasculature: See Shenque (Ren 8).

Innervation: The anterior cutaneous

branch of the eighth and ninth intercostal nerves.

10. Xiawan (Ren 10)

Location: On the midline of the abdomen, 2 cun above the umbilicus. (See Fig. 116)

Indications: Epigastric pain, abdominal pain, borborygmus, indigestion, vomiting, diarrhea.

Method: Puncture perpendicularly 0.5-1.2 inches. Moxibustion is applicable.

Regional anatomy

Vasculature: See Shenque (Ren 8).

Innervation: The anterior cutaneous branch of the eighth intercostal nerve.

11. Jianli (Ren 11)

Location: On the midline of the abdomen, 3 cun above the umbilicus. (See Fig. 116)

Indications: Stomachache, vomiting, abdominal distention, borborygmus, edema, anorexia.

Method: Puncture perpendicularly 0.5-1.2 inches. Moxibustion is applicable.

Regional anatomy

Vasculature: The branches of the superior and inferior epigastric arteries.

Innervation: The anterior cutaneous branch of the eighth intercostal nerve.

12. Zhongwan (Front-Mu Point of the Stomach, Influential Point of the Fu Organs, Ren 12)

Location: On the midline of the abdomen, 4 cun above the umbilicus. (See Fig. 116)

Indications: Stomach ache, abdominal distention, borborygmus, nausea, vomiting, acid regurgitation, diarrhea, dysentery, jaundice, indigestion, insomnia.

Method: Puncture perpendicularly 0.5-1.2 inches. Moxibustion is applicable.

Regional anatomy

Vasculature: The superior epigastric artery and vein.

Innervation: The anterior cutaneous branch of the seventh intercostal nerve.

13. Shangwan (Ren 13)

Location: On the midline of the abdomen, 5 cun above the umbilicus. (See Fig. 116)

Indications: Stomach ache, abdominal distention, nausea, vomiting, epilepsy, insomnia.

Method: Puncture perpendicularly 0.5-1.2 inches. Moxibustion is applicable.

Regional anatomy: See Zhongwan (Ren 12).

14. Juque (Front-Mu Point of the Heart, Ren 14)

Location: On the midline of the abdomen, 6 cun above the umbilicus. (See Fig. 116)

Indications: Pain in the cardiac region and the chest, nausea, acid regurgitation, difficulty in swallowing, vomiting, mental disorders, epilepsy, palpitation.

Method: Puncture perpendicularly 0.3-0.8 inch. Moxibustion is applicable.

Regional anatomy: See Zhongwan (Ren 12).

15.   Jiuwei (Luo-Connecting Point, Ren 15)

Location: Below the xiphoid process, 7 cun above the umbilicus; locate the point in supine position with the arms uplifted. (See Fig. 116)

Indications: Pain in the cardiac region and the chest, nausea, mental disorders, epilepsy.

Method: Puncture obliquely downward 0.4-0.6 inch. Moxibustion is applicable.

Regional anatomy: See Zhongwan (Ren 12).

16.   Zhongting (Ren 16)

Location: On the midline of the sternum, at the level with the fifth intercostal space. (See Col. Fig. 20)

Indications: Distension and fullness in the chest and intercostal region, hiccup, nausea, anorexia.

Method: Puncture subcutaneously 0.3-0.5 inch. Moxibustion is applicable.

Regional anatomy

Vasculature: The anterior perforating branches of the internal mammary artery and vein.

Innervation: The medial branch of the anterior cutaneous branch of the sixth intercostal nerve.

17.   Tanzhong (Front-Mu Point of the Pericardium, Influential Point of Qi, Ren 17)

Location: On the anterior midline, at the level with the fourth intercostal space, midway between the nipples. (See Fig. 116)

Indications: Asthma, pain in the chest, fullness in the chest, palpitation, insufficient lactation, hiccup, difficulty in swallowing.

Method: Puncture subcutaneously 0.3-0.5 inch. Moxibustion is applicable.

Regional anatomy

Vasculature: See Zhongting (Ren 16).

Innervation: The anterior cutaneous branch of the fourth intercostal nerve.

18.   Yutang (Ren 18)

Location: On the anterior midline, at the level with the third intercostal space. (See Col. Fig. 20)

Indications: Pain in the chest, cough, asthma, vomiting.

Method: Puncture subcutaneously 0.3-0.5 inch. Moxibustion is applicable.

Regional anatomy

Vasculature: See Zhongting (Ren 16).

Innervation: The anterior cutaneous branch of the third intercostal nerve.

19.   Zigong (Ren 19)

Location: On the anterior midline, at the level with the second intercostal space. (See Col. Fig. 20)

Indications: Pain in the chest, asthma, cough.

Method: Puncture subcutaneously 0.3-0.5 inch. Moxibustion is applicable.

Regional anatomy

Vasculature: See Zhongting (Ren 16).

Innervation: The anterior cutaneous branch of the second intercostal nerve.

20. Huagai (Ren 20)

Location: On the the anterior midline, at the midpoint of the sternal angle, at the level with the first intercostal space. (See Col. Fig. 20)
and intercostal region, asthma, cough.

Method: Puncture subcutaneously 0.3-0.5 inch. Moxibustion is applicable.

Regional anatomy

Vasculature: See Zhongting (Ren 16).

Innervation: The anterior cutaneous branch of the first intercostal nerve.

21. Xuanji (Ren 21)

Location: On the anterior midline, in the centre of the sternal manubrium, 1 cun below Tiantu (Ren 22). (See Col. Fig. 20)

Indications: Pain in the chest, cough, asthma.

Method: Puncture subcutaneously 0.3-0.5 inch. Moxibustion is applicable.

Regional anatomy

Vasculature: See Zhongting (Ren 16).

Innervation: The anterior branch of the supraclavicular nerve and the anterior cutaneous branch of the first intercostal nerve.

22. Tiantu (Ren 22)

Location: In the centre of the suprasternal fossa. (See Fig. 117)

Indications: Asthma, cough, sore throat, dry throat, hiccup, sudden hoarseness of the voice, difficulty in swallowing, goiter.

Method: First puncture perpendicularly 0.2 inch and then insert the needle tip downward along the posterior aspect of the sternum 0.5-1.0 inch. Moxibustion is applicable.

Regional anatomy

Vasculature: Superficially, the jugular arch and the branch of the inferior thyroid artery; deeper, the trachea; inferiorly, at the posterior aspect of the sternum, the inominate vein and aortic arch.

Innervation: The anterior branch of the supraclavicular nerve.

23. Lianquan (Ren 23)

Location: Above the Adam's apple, in the depression of the upper border of the hyoid bone. (See Fig. 117)

Indications: Swelling and pain of the subglossal region, salivation with glosso-plegia, aphasia with stiffness of tongue by apoplexy, sudden hoarseness of the voice, difficulty in swallowing.

Method: Puncture obliquely 0.5-1.0 inch toward the tongue root. Moxibustion is applicable.

Regional anatomy

Vasculature: The anterior jugular vein.

Innervation: The branch of the cutaneous cervical nerve, the hypoglossal nerve, and the branch of the glossopharyngeal nerve.

24. Chengjiang (Ren 24)

Location: In the depression in the centre of the mentolabial groove. (See Fig. 117)

Indications: Facial puffiness, swelling of the gums, toothache, salivation, mental disorders, deviation of the eyes and mouth.

Method: Puncture obliquely upward 0.2-0.3 inch. Moxibustion is applicable.

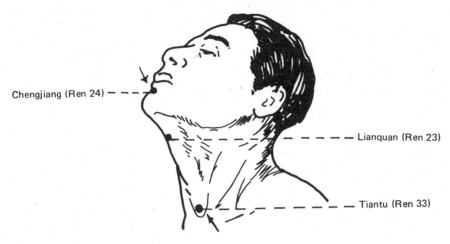

Chengjiang (Ren 24)

Lianquan (Ren 23)

Tiantu (Ren 33)

Fig. 117

Regional anatomy

Vasculature: The branches of the inferior labial artery and vein.

Innervation: The branch of the facial nerve.

III.   THE   EXTRAORDINARY POINTS

1.   Taiyang

Location: In the depression about 1 cun posterior to the midpoint between the lateral end of the eyebrow and the outer canthus. (See Fig. 118)

Indications: Headache, eye diseases, deviation of the eyes and mouth.

Method: Puncture perpendicularly 0.3-0.5 inch, or prick to cause bleeding.

2.   Yintang

Location: Midway between the medial ends of the two eyebrows. (See Fig. 118)

Indications: Headache, head heaviness, epistaxis, rhinorrhea, infantile convulsion, frontal headache, insomnia.

Method: Puncture subcutaneously 0.3-0.5 inch. Moxibustion is applicable.

3.   Shanglianquan

Location: 1 cun below the midpoint of the lower jaw, in the depression between the hyoid bone and the lower border of the jaw. (See Fig. 118)

Indications: Alalia, salivation with stiff tongue, sore throat, difficulty in swallowing, loss of voice.

Method: Puncture   obliquely   0.8-1.2 inches toward the tongue root.

4.   Erjian

Location: Fold the auricle, the point is at the apex of the auricle. (See Fig. 118)

Indications: Redness, swelling and pain of the eyes, febrile disease, nebula.

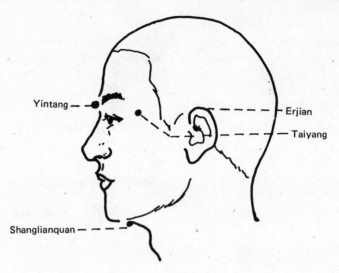

Fig. 118

Method: Puncture perpendicularly 0.1-0.2 inch or prick to cause bleeding. Moxibustion is applicable.

5. Yuyao

Location: At the midpoint of the eyebrow. (See Fig. 119)

Indications: Pain in the supraorbital region, twitching of the eyelids, ptosis cloudiness of the cornea, redness, swellin and pain of the eyes.

Method: Puncture subcutaneously 0.3-0.5 inch.

6. Sishencong

Location: A group of 4 points, at the

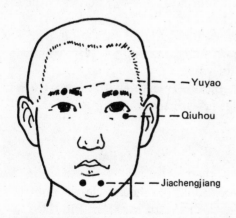

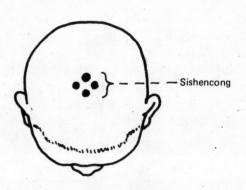

Fig. 119

vertex, 1 cun respectively posterior, anterior and lateral to Baihui (Du 20). (See Fig. 119)

Indications: Headache, vertigo, insomnia, poor memory, epilepsy.

Method: Puncture subcutaneously 0.5-1.0 inch. Moxibustion is applicable.

7.   Qiuhou

Location: At the junction of the lateral 1/4 and the medial 3/4 of the infraorbital margin. (See Fig. 119)

Indications: Eye diseases.

Method: Push the eyeball upward gently, then puncture perpendicularly 0.5-1.2 inches along the orbital margin slowly without movements of lifting, thrusting, twisting and rotating.

8.   Jiachengjiang

Location: 1 cun lateral to Chengjiang (Ren 24). (See Fig. 119)

Indications: Pain in the face, deviation of the eyes and mouth, spasm of facial muscle.

Method: Puncture obliquely 0.5-1.0 inch.

9.   Jinjin, Yuye

Location: On the veins on both sides of the frenulum of the tongue, Jinjin is on the left, Yuye, on the right. (See Fig. 120)

Indications: Swelling of the tongue, vomiting, aphasia with stiffness of tongue.

Method: Prick to cause bleeding.

10.   Bitong

Location: At the highest point of the nasolabial groove. (See Fig. 121)

Indications: Rhinitis, nasal obstruction, nasal boils.

Method: Puncture subcutaneously upward 0.3-0.5 inch.

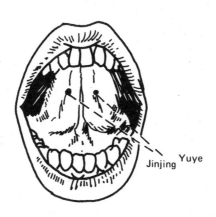

Fig. 120

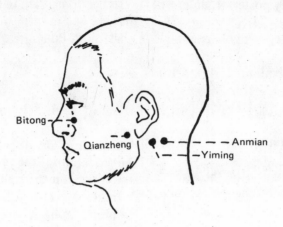

Fig. 121

11. Qianzheng

Location: 0.5-1.0 cun anterior to the auricular lobe. (See Fig. 121)

Indications: Deviation of the eyes and mouth, ulceration on tongue and mouth.

Method: Puncture obliquely 0.5-1.0 inch.

12. Yiming

Location: 1 cun posterior to Yifeng (S J 17). (See Fig. 121)

Indications: Eye diseases, tinnitus, insomnia.

Method: Puncture perpendicularly 0.5-0.8 inch.

13. Anmian

Location: Midpoint between Yifeng (S J 17) and Fengchi (G 20). (See Fig. 121)

Indications: Insomnia, vertigo, headache, palpitation, mental disorders.

Method: Puncture perpendicularly 0.5-0.8 inch.

14. Dingchuan

Location: 0.5 cun lateral to Dazhui (Du 14). (See Fig. 122)

Indications: Asthma, cough, neck rigidity, pain in the shoulder and back, rubella.

Method: Puncture perpendicularly 0.5-0.8 inch. Moxibustion is applicable.

15. Huatuojiaji

Location: A group of 34 points on both sides of the spinal column, 0.5 cun lateral to the lower border of each spinous process from the first thoracic vertebra to the fifth lumbar vertebra. (See Fig. 122)

Indications: See the following table.

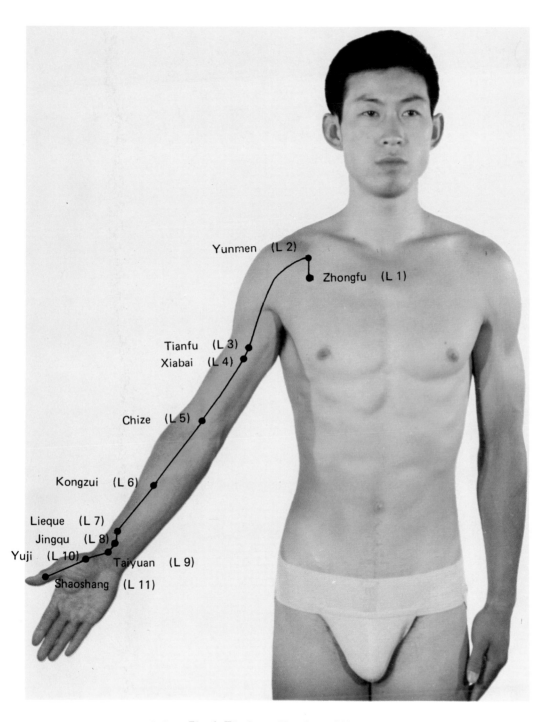

Yunmen (L 2)

Zhongfu (L 1)

Tianfu (L 3)
Xiabai (L 4)

Chize (L 5)

Kongzui (L 6)

Lieque (L 7)
Jingqu (L 8)
Yuji (L 10)
Taiyuan (L 9)
Shaoshang (L 11)

Colour Fig. 1 The Lung Meridian of Hand-Taiyin

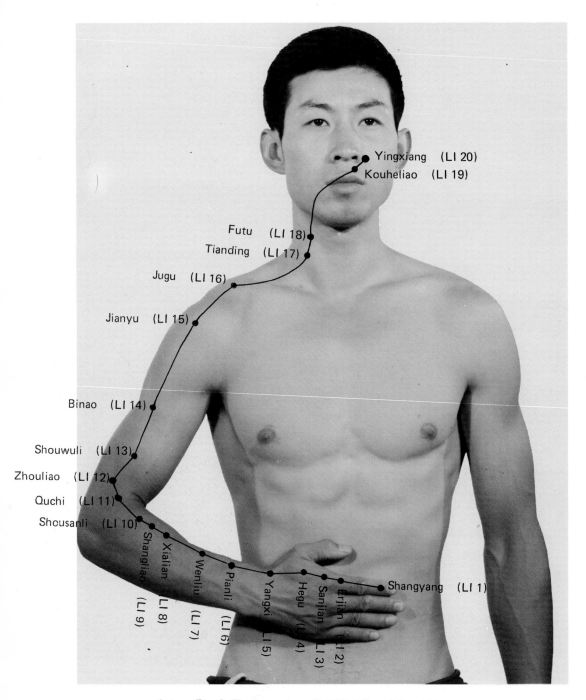

Colour Fig. 2 The Large Intestine Meridian of Hand-Yangming

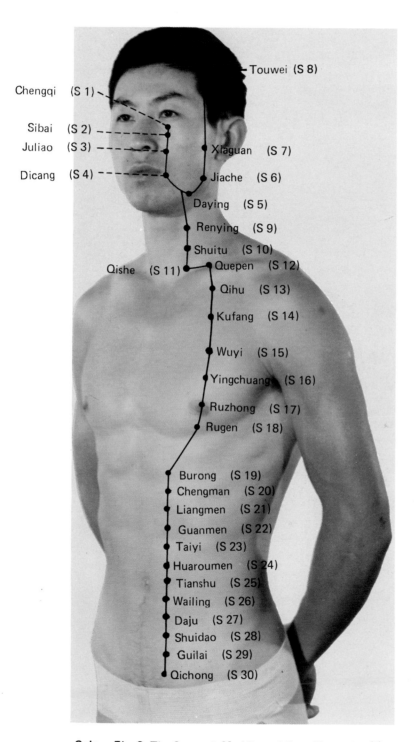

Colour Fig. 3 The Stomach Meridian of Foot-Yangming (I)

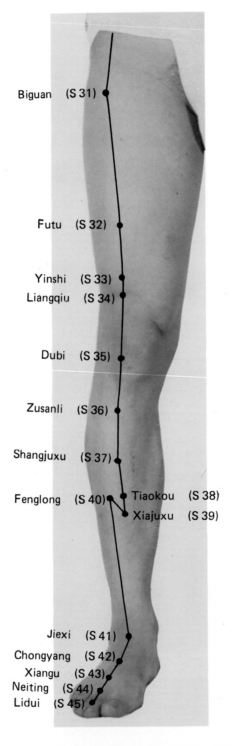

Biguan (S 31)

Futu (S 32)

Yinshi (S 33)
Liangqiu (S 34)

Dubi (S 35)

Zusanli (S 36)

Shangjuxu (S 37)

Fenglong (S 40) Tiaokou (S 38)
                 Xiajuxu (S 39)

Jiexi (S 41)
Chongyang (S 42)
Xiangu (S 43)
Neiting (S 44)
Lidui (S 45)

Colour Fig. 4 The Stomach Meridian of Foot-Yangming (II)

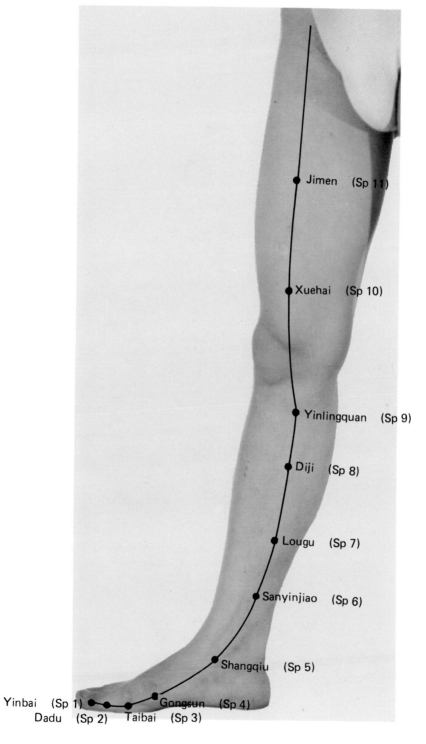

Jimen   (Sp 11)

Xuehai   (Sp 10)

Yinlingquan   (Sp 9)

Diji   (Sp 8)

Lougu   (Sp 7)

Sanyinjiao   (Sp 6)

Shangqiu   (Sp 5)

Yinbai   (Sp 1)
Dadu   (Sp 2)   Taibai   (Sp 3)   Gongsun   (Sp 4)

Colour Fig. 5 The Spleen Meridian of Foot-Taiyin (I)

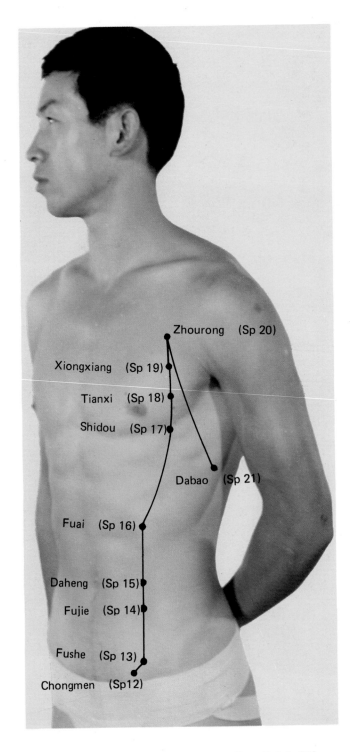

Colour Fig. 6 The Spleen Meridian of Foot-Taiyin (II)

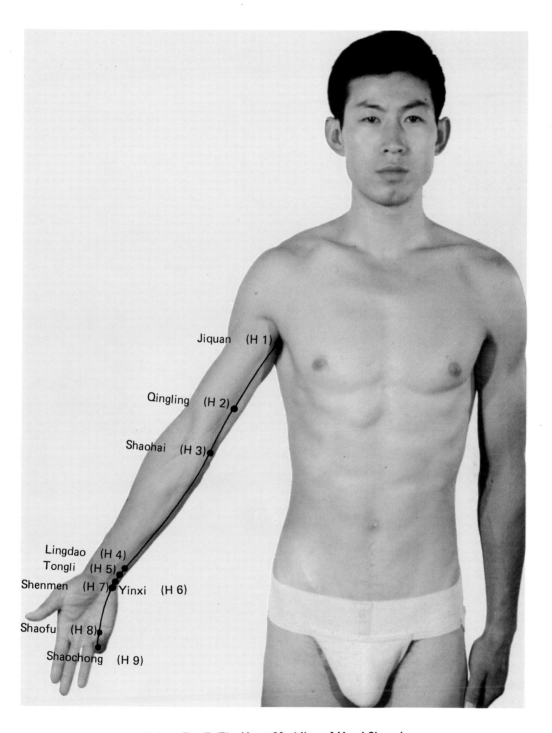

Jiquan (H 1)

Qingling (H 2)

Shaohai (H 3)

Lingdao (H 4)
Tongli (H 5)
Shenmen (H 7) Yinxi (H 6)

Shaofu (H 8)
Shaochong (H 9)

Colour Fig. 7 The Heart Meridian of Hand-Shaoyin

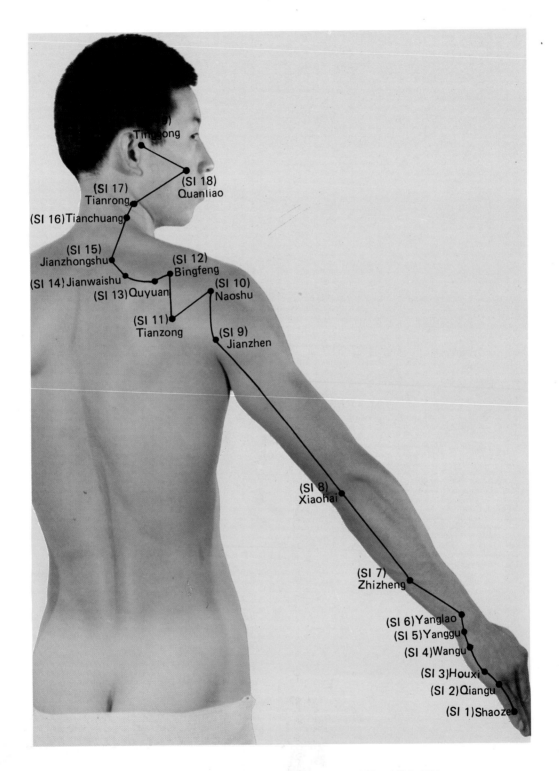

Colour Fig. 8 The Small Intestine Meridian of Hand-Taiyang

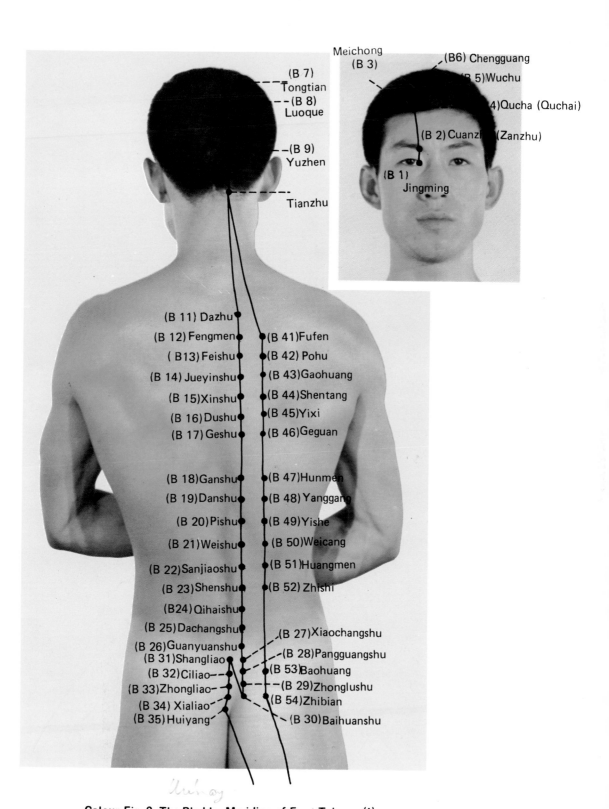

Colour Fig. 9 The Bladder Meridian of Foot-Taiyang (I)

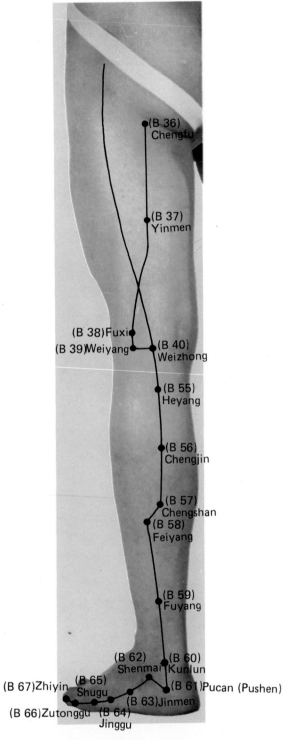

Colour Fig. 10 The Bladder Meridian of Foot-Taiyang (II)

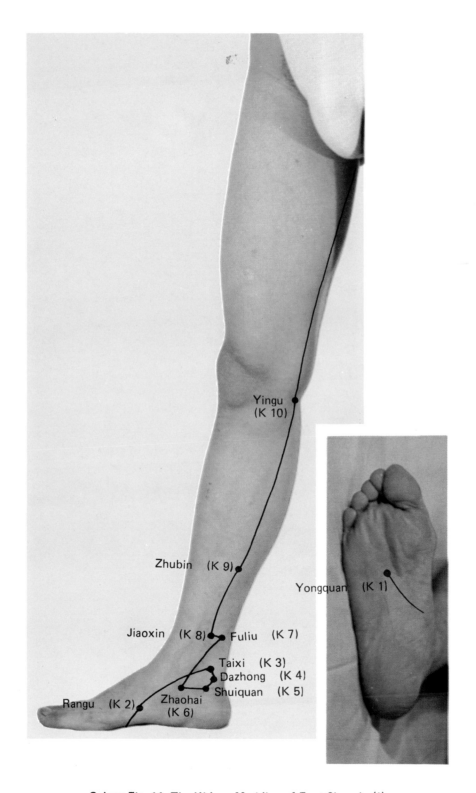

Colour Fig. 11 The Kidney Meridian of Foot-Shaoyin (I)

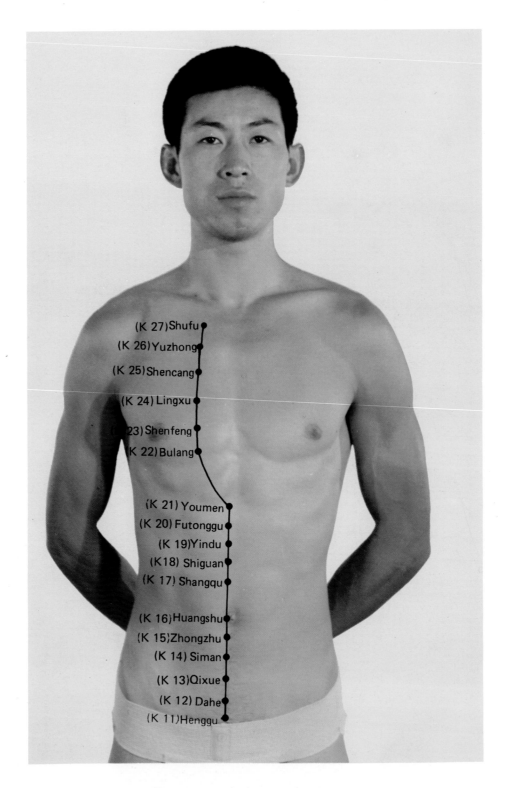

Colour Fig. 12 The Kidney Meridian of Foot-Shaoyin (II)

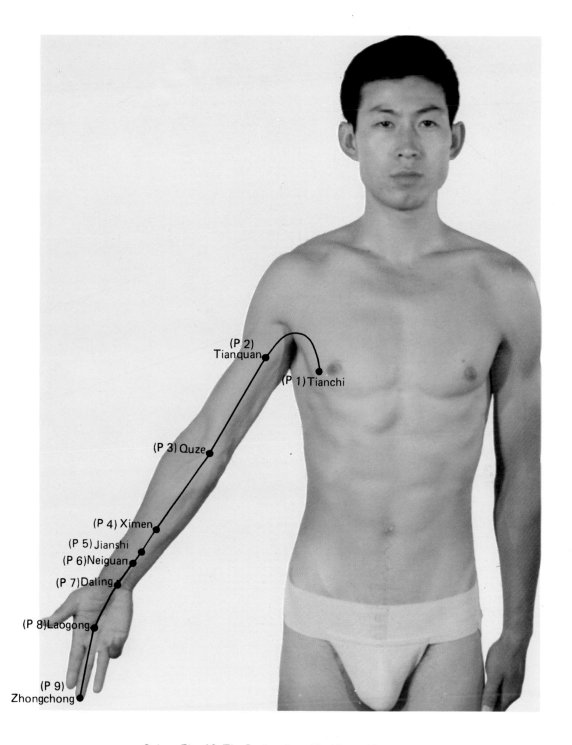

Colour Fig. 13 The Pericardium Meridian of Hand-Jueyin

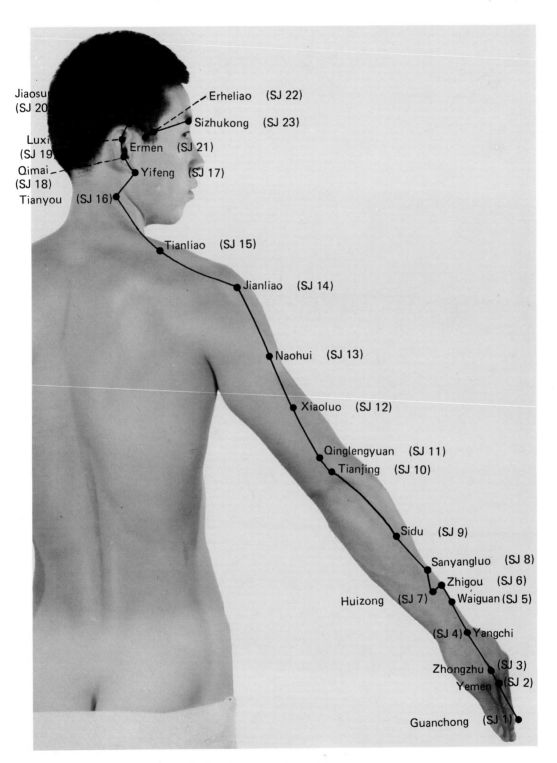

Jiaosun (SJ 20)

Erheliao (SJ 22)

Sizhukong (SJ 23)

Luxi (SJ 19)

Ermen (SJ 21)

Qimai (SJ 18)

Yifeng (SJ 17)

Tianyou (SJ 16)

Tianliao (SJ 15)

Jianliao (SJ 14)

Naohui (SJ 13)

Xiaoluo (SJ 12)

Qinglengyuan (SJ 11)

Tianjing (SJ 10)

Sidu (SJ 9)

Sanyangluo (SJ 8)

Zhigou (SJ 6)

Huizong (SJ 7)

Waiguan (SJ 5)

(SJ 4) Yangchi

Zhongzhu (SJ 3)

Yemen (SJ 2)

Guanchong (SJ 1)

Colour Fig. 14 The Sanjiao Meridian of Hand-Shaoyang

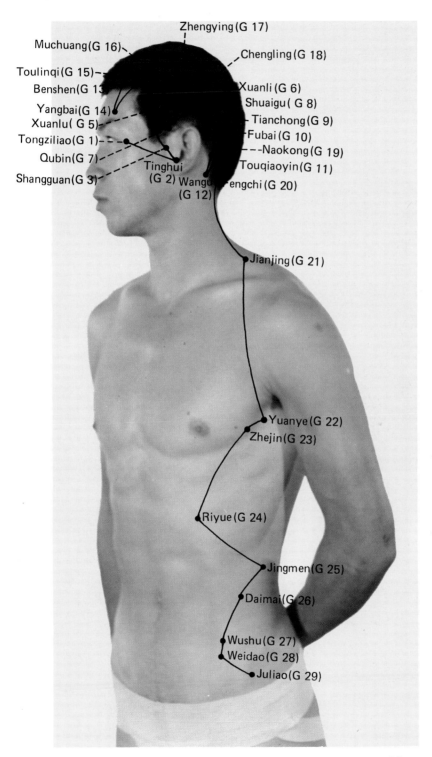

Zhengying(G 17)

Muchuang(G 16)

Toulinqi(G 15)

Benshen(G 13)

Yangbai(G 14)

Xuanlu(G 5)

Tongziliao(G 1)

Qubin(G 7)

Shangguan(G 3)

Tinghui
(G 2)

Wangu
(G 12)

Chengling(G 18)

Xuanli(G 6)

Shuaigu(G 8)

Tianchong(G 9)

Fubai(G 10)

Naokong(G 19)

Touqiaoyin(G 11)

Fengchi(G 20)

Jianjing(G 21)

Yuanye(G 22)

Zhejin(G 23)

Riyue(G 24)

Jingmen(G 25)

Daimai(G 26)

Wushu(G 27)

Weidao(G 28)

Juliao(G 29)

Colour Fig. 15 The Gallbladder Meridian of Foot-Shaoyang (I)

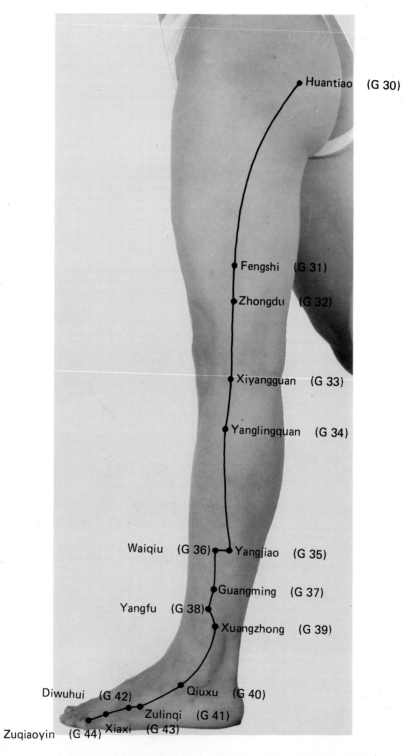

Huantiao (G 30)

Fengshi (G 31)

Zhongdu (G 32)

Xiyangguan (G 33)

Yanglingquan (G 34)

Waiqiu (G 36) Yangjiao (G 35)

Guangming (G 37)

Yangfu (G 38)

Xuangzhong (G 39)

Diwuhui (G 42) Qiuxu (G 40)

Zulinqi (G 41)

Zuqiaoyin (G 44) Xiaxi (G 43)

Colour Fig. 16 The Gallbladder Meridian of Foot-Shaoyang (II)

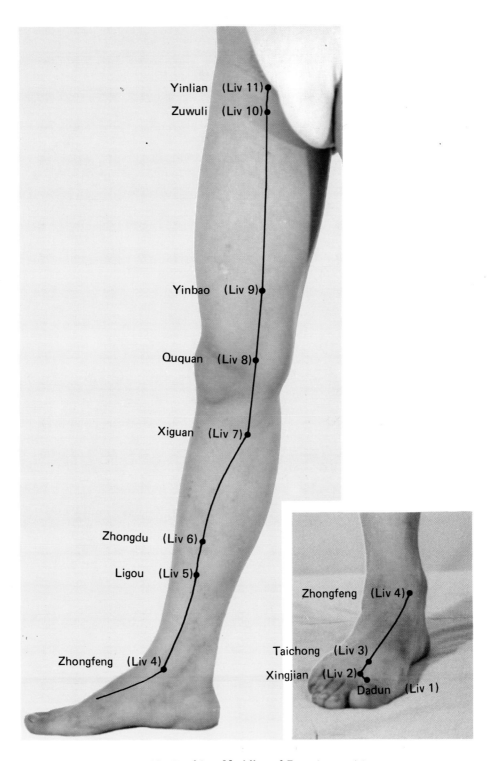

Colour Fig. 17 The Liver Meridian of Foot-Jueyin (I)

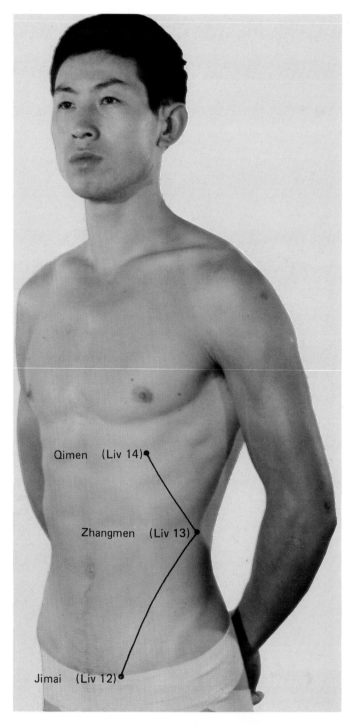

Qimen (Liv 14)

Zhangmen (Liv 13)

Jimai (Liv 12)

Colour Fig. 18 The Liver Meridian of Foot-Jueyin (II)

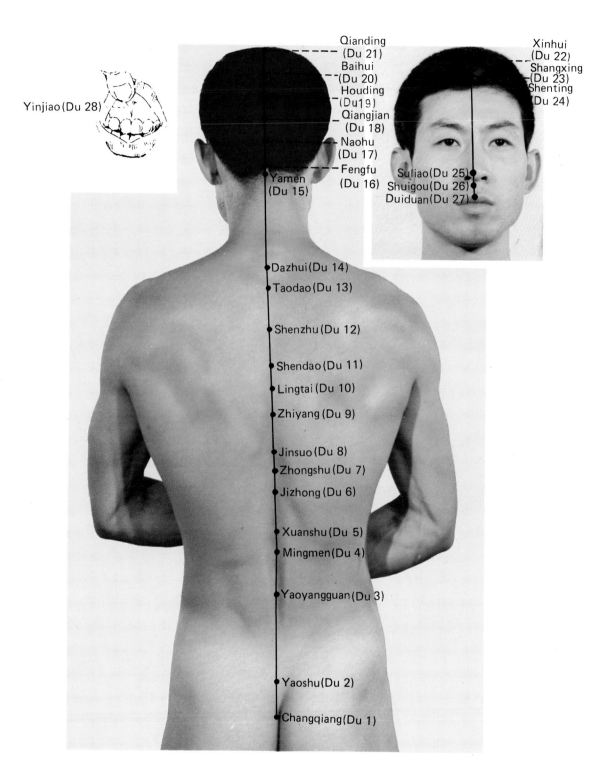

Yinjiao(Du 28)

Qianding
(Du 21)
Baihui
(Du 20)
Houding
(Du 19)
Qiangjian
(Du 18)
Naohu
(Du 17)
Fengfu
(Du 16)
Yamen
(Du 15)

Xinhui
(Du 22)
Shangxing
(Du 23)
Shenting
(Du 24)

Suliao(Du 25)
Shuigou(Du 26)
Duiduan(Du 27)

Dazhui(Du 14)
Taodao(Du 13)
Shenzhu(Du 12)
Shendao(Du 11)
Lingtai(Du 10)
Zhiyang(Du 9)
Jinsuo(Du 8)
Zhongshu(Du 7)
Jizhong(Du 6)
Xuanshu(Du 5)
Mingmen(Du 4)
Yaoyangguan(Du 3)
Yaoshu(Du 2)
Changqiang(Du 1)

Colour Fig. 19 The Du Meridian

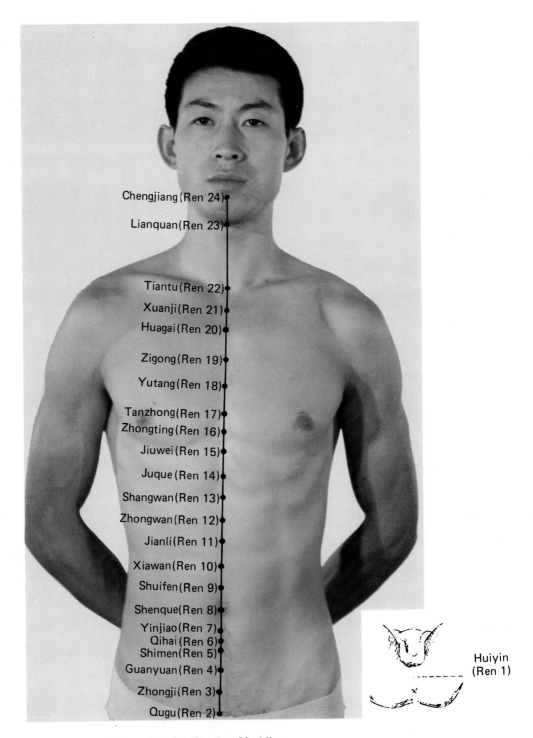

Chengjiang(Ren 24)
Lianquan(Ren 23)

Tiantu(Ren 22)
Xuanji(Ren 21)
Huagai(Ren 20)

Zigong(Ren 19)
Yutang(Ren 18)

Tanzhong(Ren 17)
Zhongting(Ren 16)
Jiuwei(Ren 15)
Juque(Ren 14)
Shangwan(Ren 13)
Zhongwan(Ren 12)
Jianli(Ren 11)
Xiawan(Ren 10)
Shuifen(Ren 9)
Shenque(Ren 8)
Yinjiao(Ren 7)
Qihai(Ren 6)
Shimen(Ren 5)
Guanyuan(Ren 4)
Zhongji(Ren 3)
Qugu(Ren 2)

Huiyin
(Ren 1)

Colour Fig. 20 The Ren Meridian

Conception

Huatuojiaji Points   Indications

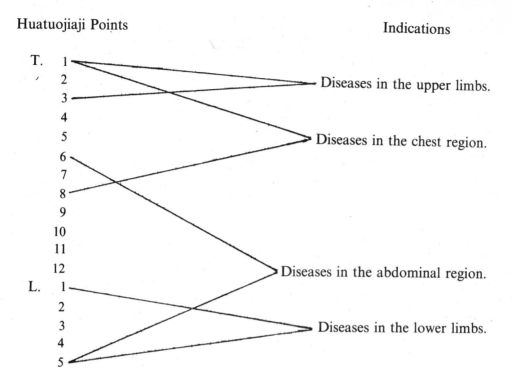

Method: Puncture perpendicularly 0.5-1.0 inch in the cervical and chest region, puncture perpendicularly 1.0-1.5 inches in the lumbar region. Moxibustion is applicable.

16.   Bailao

Location: 2 cun above Dazhui (Du 14), 1 cun lateral to the midline. (See Fig. 123)

Indications: Scrofula, cough, asthma, whooping cough, neck rigidity.

Method: Puncture perpendicularly 0.3-0.5 inch. Moxibustion is applicable.

17.   Weiguanxiashu

Location: 1.5 cun lateral to the lower border of the spinous process of the eighth thoracic vertebra. (See Fig. 123)

Indications: Diabetes, vomiting, abdominal pain, pain in the chest and hypochondriac region.

Method: Puncture obliquely 0.5-0.7 inch. Moxibustion is applicable.

18.   Shiqizhui

Location: Below the spinous process of the fifth lumbar vertebra. (See Fig. 123)

Indications: Lumbar pain, thigh pain, paralysis of the lower extremities, irregular menstruation, dysmenorrhea.

Method: Puncture perpendicularly 0.8-1.2 inches. Moxibustion is applicable.

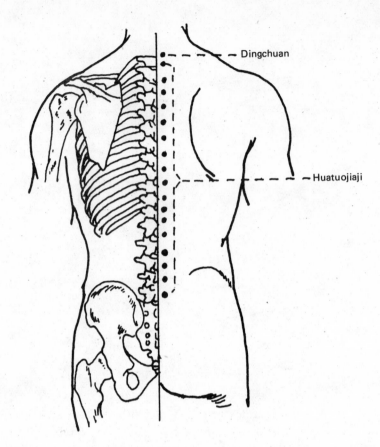

Fig. 122

19. Yaoqi

Location: 2 cun directly above the tip of the coccyx. (See Fig. 123)

Indications: Epilepsy, headache, insomnia, constipation.

Method: Puncture subcutaneously upward 1.0-2.0 inches. Moxibustion is applicable.

20. Pigen

Location: 3.5 cun lateral to the lower border of the spinous process of the first lumbar vertebra. (See Fig. 123)

Indications: Hepatosplenomegaly, lumbar pain.

Method: Puncture perpendicularly 0.5-0.8 inch. Moxibustion is applicable.

21. Yaoyan

Location: About 3.5 cun lateral to the lower border of the spinous process of the fourth lumbar vertebra. The point is in the depression appearing in prone position. (See Fig. 123)

Indications: Lumbar pain, frequency of

urine, irregular menstruation.

Method: Puncture perpendicularly 0.8-1.2 inches. Moxibustion is applicable.

irregular menstruation.

Method: Puncture perpendicularly 0.8-1.2 inches. Moxibustion is applicable.

22. Zigongxue

Location: 3 cun lateral to Zhongji (Ren 3). (See Fig. 124)

Indications: Prolapse of the uterus,

23. Jianqian (also known as Jianneiling)

Location: Midway between the end of the

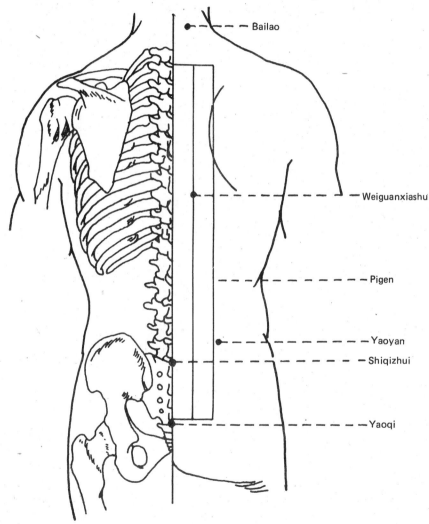

Fig. 123

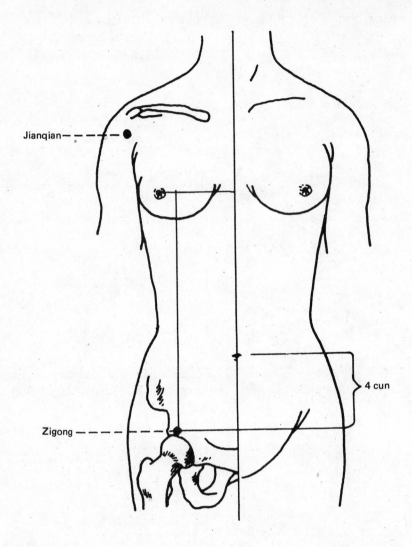

Fig. 124

anterior axillary fold and Jianyu (L I 15).
(See Fig. 124)

Indications: Pain in the shoulder and arm,
paralysis of the upper extremities.

Method: Puncture perpendicularly 0.8-
1.2 inches. Moxibustion is applicable.

24. Shixuan

Location: On the tips of the ten fingers,
about 0.1 cun distal to the nails. (See Fig.125)

Indications: Apoplexy, coma, epilepsy,
high fever, acute tonsillitis, infantile

convulsion, numbness of the finger tips.

Method: Puncture 0.1-0.2 inch superficially, or prick to cause bleeding.

25. Sifeng

Location: On the palmar surface, in the midpoint of the transverse creases of the proximal interphalangeal joints of the index, middle, ring and little fingers. (See Fig. 125)

Indications: Malnutrition and indigestion syndrome in children, whooping cough.

Method: Prick to cause bleeding, or squeeze out a small amount of yellowish viscous fluid locally.

26. Zhongkui

Location: On the midpoint of the proximal interphalangeal joint of the middle finger at dorsum aspect. (See Fig. 125)

Indications: Nausea, vomiting, hiccup.

Method: Moxibustion is applied with three moxa cones.

27. Baxie

Location: On the dorsum of the hand, at the junction of the white and red skin of the hand webs, eight in all, making a loose fist to locate the points. (See Fig. 125)

Indications: Excessive heat, finger numbness, spasm and contracture of the fingers, redness and swelling of the dorsum of the hand.

Method: Puncture obliquely 0.3-0.5 inch, or prick to cause bleeding. Moxibustion is applicable.

28. Luozhen

Location: On the dorsum of the hand, between the second and third metacarpal

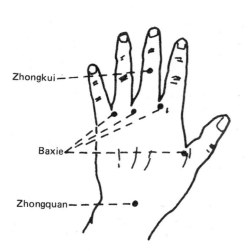
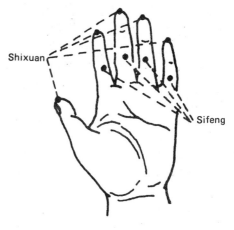

Fig. 125

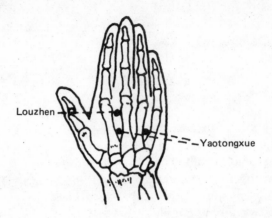

Fig. 126

bones, about 0.5 cun posterior to metacarpophalangeal joint. (See Fig. 126)

Indications: Sore neck, pain in the shoulder and arm.

Method: Puncture perpendicularly 0.5-0.8 inch.

29.   Yaotongxue

Location: On the dorsum of the hand, midway between the transverse wrist crease and metacarpophalangeal joint, between the second and third metacarpal bones, and between the fourth and fifth metacarpal bones, four points in all on both hands. (See Fig. 126)

Indication: Acute lumbar sprain.

Method: Puncture obliquely 0.5-1.0 inch toward the centre of metacarpus from both sides.

30.   Zhongquan

Location: In the depression between

Yangxi (L I 5) and Yangchi (S J 4). (See Fig. 125)

Indications: Stuffy chest, gastric pain, spitting of blood.

Method: Puncture perpendicularly 0.3-0.5 inch. Moxibustion is applicable.

31.   Erbai

Location: On the metacarpal aspect of the forearm, 4 cun above the transverse wrist crease, on the both sides of the tendon of m. flexor carpi radialis, two points on one hand. (See Fig. 127)

Indications: Hemorrhoids, prolapse of the rectum.

Method: Puncture perpendicularly 0.5-1.0 inch. Moxibustion is applicable.

32.   Bizhong

Location: On the lateral aspect of the forearm, midway between the transverse wrist crease and elbow crease, between the radius and the ulna. (See Fig. 127)

Indications: Paralysis, spasm and contracture of the upper extremities, pain of the forearm.

Method: Puncture perpendicularly 1.0-1.2 inches. Moxibustion is applicable.

33.   Zhoujian

Location: On the tip of the ulnar olecranon when the elbow is flexed. (See Fig. 128)

Indication: Scrofula

Method: Moxibustion is applied with seven to fourteen moxa cones.

34.   Huanzhong

Location: Midway between Huantiao (G 30) and Yaoshu (Du 2). (See Fig. 129)

Indications: Lumbar pain, thigh pain.

Method: Puncture perpendicularly 1.5-2.0 inches. Moxibustion is applicable.

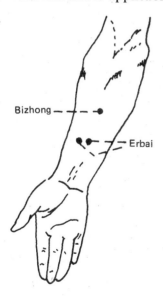

Fig. 127

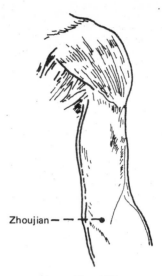

Fig. 128

35.   Baichongwo

Location: 1 cun above Xuehai (Sp 10). (See Fig. 130)

Indications: Rubella, eczema, gastro-intestinal parasitic diseases.

Method: Puncture perpendicularly 1.0-1.2 inches. Moxibustion is applicable.

36.   Xiyan

Location: A pair of points in the two depressions, medial and lateral to the patellar ligament, locating the point with the knee flexed. These two points are also termed medial and lateral Xiyan respectively. Lateral Xiyan overlaps with Dubi (S 35). (See Fig. 131)

Indications: Knee pain, weakness of the lower extremities.

Method: Puncture perpendicularly 0.5-1.0 inch. Moxibustion is applicable.

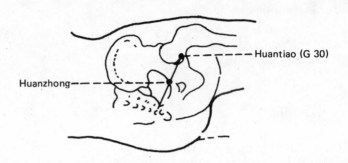

Fig. 129

37. Lanweixue

Location: The tender spot about 2 cun below Zusanli (S 36). (See Fig. 131)

Indications: Acute and chronic appendicitis, indigestion, paralysis of the lower extremities.

Method: Puncture perpendicularly 1.0-1.2 inches.

38. Heding

Location: In the depression of the midpoint of the superior patellar border. (See Fig. 131)

Indications: Knee pain, weakness of the foot and leg, paralysis.

Method: Puncture perpendicularly 0.3-0.5 inch. Moxibustion is applicable.

39. Dannangxue

Location: The tender spot 1-2 cun below Yanglingquan (G 34). (See Fig. 132)

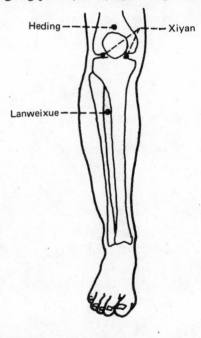

Fig. 131

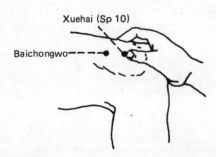

Fig. 130

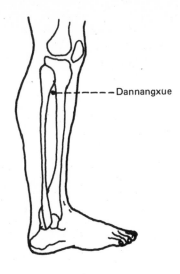

Fig. 132

Indications: Acute and chronic cholecystitis, cholelithiasis, biliary ascariasis, muscular atrophy and numbness of the lower extremities.

Method: Puncture perpendicularly 0.8-1.2 inches.

40.   Bafeng

Location: On the dorsum of foot, in the depressions on the webs between toes, proximal to the margins of the webs, eight points in all. (See Fig. 133)

Indications: Beriberi, toe pain, redness and swelling of the dorsum of the foot.

Method: Puncture obliquely 0.5-0.8 inch. Moxibustion is applicable.

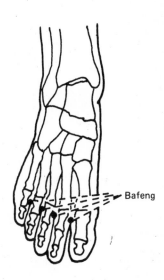

Fig. 133

Chapter 11

AETIOLOGY AND PATHOGENESIS

The subject of aetiology is the study of the causative factors of disease, whilst the study of pathogenesis concerns the actual bodily processes whereby disease occurs, develops and changes. Traditional Chinese medicine holds that there is normally a state of relative equilibrium between the human body and the external environment on the one hand, and among the zang-fu organs within the body on the other hand. This equilibrium is not static, but is in a state of constant self-adjustment, and in this way the normal physiological activities of the body are maintained. If external influences exceed the powers of adaptibility of the organism, or if the body itself is unable to adjust to changing conditions, then this relative equilibrium will be lost, and disease will develop. Whether a disease occurs or not, whilst associated with the presence of the various causative factors, is primarily determined by the physiological adaptibility of the body to the natural environment. This is the basic viewpoint of traditional Chinese medicine regarding pathogenesis.

I. AETIOLOGY

Numerous factors can cause disease, and these include the six exogenous factors, the seven emotions, improper diet, over strain, lack of physical exercise, traumatic injuries, bites by insects or wild animals, as well as stagnated blood and phlegm fluid. The symptoms and signs of any disease reflect the pathological reactions of the affected body to certain causative factors. The causative factors, therefore, are studied both as the objective causes of disease, and in the specific ways they affect the body. On the basis of this understanding, traditional Chinese medicine is able to identify the causative factors of disease by analysing the clinical manifestations. This is known as "seeking the causative factors by differentiating symptoms and signs." The study of aetiology, therefore, is based on developing a profound understanding of the characteristic clinical manifestations produced by each causative factor.

1. The Six Exogenous Factors

Wind, cold, summer heat, damp, dryness and fire (mild heat and heat) are the six climatic changes found in nature. Under normal conditions, they do not produce pathological changes in the body and are thus known as the "six types of qi" in the natural environment. These six types of qi

244

will only cause disease if either the climatic changes are extreme or sudden, or if the body's resistance is low. When responsible for inducing disease, these six types of qi are known as "the six exogenous pathogenic factors."

All the six pathogenic factors, when affecting the body, invade from the exterior via the skin, mouth or nose. For this reason, the pathological reactions they induce are known as "exogenous diseases."

Diseases due to the six exogenous factors are closely related to seasonal changes in the weather and to living environment. For example, heat syndromes mostly occur in summer, cold syndromes in winter, and damp syndromes are usually caused by prolonged exposure to damp. Another term for these syndromes is "seasonal diseases."

Each of the six exogenous pathogenic factors may affect the body singly or in combination. Examples are common cold due to pathogenic wind and cold, or *bi* syndrome due to pathogenic wind, cold and damp, etc. In the process of causing disease, the six exogenous factors may influence each other, and may also, under certain conditions, transform into each other. For example, pathogenic cold may transform into heat in the interior of the body, and prolonged summer heat may result in dryness by consuming the yin of the body, etc. The properties of the six exogenous factors and their specific pathological influences on the body are described as follows:

1) Wind   Wind is the predominant qi of spring but may also occur in any of the four seasons. Wind may easily invade the body after sweating, or whilst sleeping.

a) Wind is the primary exogenous pathogenic factor in causing disease, since cold, damp, dryness and heat all depend on wind to invade the body, it is stated in the forty-second chapter of *Plain Questions*: "Wind is the leading causative factor of many diseases."

Pathogenic wind can not only combine with the other five exogenous factors, but also with phlegm to form wind phlegm. Facial paralysis, for example, is mostly seen as a consequence of the obstruction of wind phlegm in the meridians.

b) Wind is a yang pathogenic factor and is characterized by "upward and outward dispersion." It can therefore easily invade the upper part of the body, i.e. the head and face, and the exterior portion of the body, leading to impairment of the opening and closing of the pores. Clinical manifestations are headache, nasal obstruction, itching or pain in the throat, facial puffiness, aversion to wind and sweating.

c) Wind in nature blows in gusts and is characterized by rapid changes. Disorders caused by pathogenic wind, therefore, are marked by migratory symptoms, rapid changes and abrupt onset of disease. The migratory joint pain of wandering *bi*, for example, which is caused by pathogenic wind, is known as wind *bi*. Urticaria caused by pathogenic wind is characterized by itching of the skin and wheals which appear and disappear from place to place.

d) Wind is characterized by constant movement. Moving pathogenic wind in the body can cause dizziness, vertigo, fremitus, convulsions and opisthotonos. Examples are tetanus and deviation of the mouth and eyes with spasm of the facial muscles.

2) Cold   Cold, the predominant qi of winter, may occur in other seasons but not as severely. Thin clothing, exposure to cold after sweating, being caught in rain, and wading in water in cold winter can give rise to invasion of pathogenic cold.

a) Cold is a yin pathogenic factor which consumes the yang qi of the body. As a result the warming function of the body will be impaired, resulting in symptoms such as cold limbs, cold pain in the epigastric and abdominal regions, diarrhoea containing undigested food, increased flow of clear urine, etc.

b) Cold is characterized by contraction and stagnation, resulting in impairment of the opening and closing of the pores, spasmodic contraction of tendons and meridians, and impaired circulation of qi and blood. Accompanying symptoms include pain, aversion to cold, lack of sweating and restricted movement of the limbs.

3) Summer Heat Summer heat is the predominant qi of summer, and unlike the other exogenous factors, is only seen in its own season. Summer heat diseases are induced by excessively high temperatures, overexposure to the blazing sun whilst working, and working or staying for too long in poorly ventilated places.

a) Summer heat, characterized by extreme heat, is a yang pathogenic factor which is transformed from fire. Clinical manifestations characterized by yang heat include high fever, restlessness, thirst, profuse sweating and a surging pulse.

b) Summer heat is characterized by upward direction, dispersion and consumption of body fluid. It usually affects the head and eyes, causing dizziness and blurred vision. Due to its dispersing function, pathogenic summer heat may cause the pores to stay open. The excessive sweating that causes may consume body fluid resulting in thirst with a strong desire to drink, dry mouth and tongue, scanty deep-yellow urine. In addition, there will be symptoms of qi deficiency such as reluctance to speak and lassitude.

Severe invasion of summer heat may disturb the mind, resulting in sunstroke with the symptoms of sudden collapse and coma.

c) Since summer is often characterized by high humidity, pathogenic summer heat is frequently combined with pathogenic damp. Clinical manifestations of summer heat and damp include dizziness, heaviness in the head, suffocating sensation in the chest, nausea, poor appetite, loose stools and general lassitude, in addition to fever, restlessness and thirst.

4) Damp Damp is the predominant qi of late summer — the period between summer and autumn — which in China is a hot, rainy season with abundant damp everywhere. Many diseases related to invasion by pathogenic damp occur at this time. Damp diseases may also be induced by living in damp conditions and places, wearing clothes made damp by sweat or rain, frequent exposure to water, and periods of prolonged rain.

a) Damp is characterized by heaviness and turbidity. Patients often complain of dizziness, a heavy sensation in the head as though it had been wrapped in a piece of cloth, heaviness of the body as though it were carrying a heavy load, and soreness, pain and heavy sensations in the joints. There may be turbid discharges from the body, such as suppurating sores, weeping eczema, profuse purulent leukorrhoea with a foul odour, turbid urine and stools containing mucus and even blood.

b) Damp is characterized by viscosity and stagnation. Patients affected by pathogenic damp usually have a stubborn sticky tongue coating, a viscous stool that is difficult to excrete, and obstructed urination. Diseases due to pathogenic damp tend to be prolonged and intractable, such as fixed *bi* syndrome, damp fever (intestinal typhoid) and eczema.

c) Damp is a yin pathogenic factor which impairs yang and easily obstructs qi circulation. Clinical manifestations include a full sensation in the chest, epigastric distention, difficult and scanty urination and hesitant bowel movements with viscous stools. Since the spleen "likes dryness and dislikes damp," pathogenic damp is likely to impair spleen yang, leading to distention and fullness in the epigastrium and abdomen, poor appetite, loose stools, reduced urination and oedema, due to poor transportation and transformation and inadequate dispersion of body fluids.

5) Dryness Dryness is the predominant qi of autumn, and in China often occurs in this season which is usually very dry.

a) Dryness consumes body fluid resulting in dryness of the nose and throat, dry mouth with thirst, chapped skin, withered body hair, constipation and reduced urination.

b) Pathogenic dryness often impairs the function of the lung, the "delicate" zang, which has the function of dispersing, descending and moistening. Dryness invades the lung through the nose or mouth. When lack of moisture impairs the dispersing and descending functions of the lung, there may be a dry cough with scanty sticky or bloody sputum.

6) Fire (mild heat and heat) Fire, caused by excess of yang qi, often occurs in summer, but may be seen in other seasons. Fire, mild heat and heat vary in degree. Of the three, fire is the most severe and mild heat the least severe, yet they all share similar characteristics. The terms of fire heat and mild-heat heat, therefore, are often used to describe their common features.

a) Fire is a yang pathogenic factor characterized by burning and upward direction. Clinical manifestations include high fever, restlessness, thirst, sweating, mouth and tongue ulcers, swollen and painful gums, headache and congestion of the eyes. Restlessness, insomnia, mania, emotional excitement and coma or delirium may occur if pathogenic fire disturbs the mind.

b) Pathogenic fire often consumes yin fluid. Burning pathogenic fire heat can consume yin fluid and force it to the exterior of the body, leading to insufficiency of body fluid. Clinically, apart from high fever, there may be thirst with desire to drink, dry lips and throat, constipation and deep-yellow scanty urine.

c) Invasion by fire stirs up wind and causes disturbance of blood. Excess of fire heat affects the Liver Meridian and deprives the tendons and meridian of nourishment, thus stirring up the liver wind. Clinical manifestations include high fever, coma, convulsion of the four limbs, neck rigidity, opisthotonos and upward staring of the eyes. These symptoms are known as "extreme heat stirring up wind."

When pathogenic fire heat disturbs blood, it speeds up blood circulation and gives rise to very rapid pulse. In severe cases, blood is forced out of the vessels, leading to epistaxis, spitting of blood, bloody stool, haematuria, uterine bleeding and menorrhagia. Pathogenic fire heat may stay in and rot the blood and flesh, thus creating carbuncle, furuncle, boil and ulcer.

In addition to the six exogenous pathogenic factors occurring in nature, there also exist some extremely infectious noxious epidemic factors. Although the characteristics of these are similar to those of mild-heat heat, they are severely toxic and can result in the sudden onset of severe diseases such as plague. The medical literature of traditional Chinese medicine describes epidemics of many diseases recognised by modern medicine, such as smallpox, cholera, diphtheria and toxic dysentery.

In addition to diseases caused by the six exogenous pathogenic factors, there are many diseases caused by functional disturbances of the zang-fu organs which nevertheless share similar clinical manifestations. These pathological changes are therefore referred to as endogenous wind, cold, damp, dryness and fire (heat) in order to avoid ambiguity. Descriptions of these pathogenic factors are ignored here and are covered in the chapter on the differentiation of syndromes of the zang-fu organs.

2.   The Seven Emotional Factors

The seven emotional factors in traditional Chinese medicine are joy, anger, melancholy, worry, grief, fear and fright. These are normal emotional responses of the body to external stimuli, and do not normally cause disease. Severe, continuous or abruptly occurring emotional stimuli, however, which surpass the regulative adaptability of the organism, will affect the physiological functions of the human body, especially when there is a preexisting oversensitivity to them. The qi and blood of the zang-fu organs will be disrupted leading to disease. The seven emotional factors differ from the six exogenous factors in that they directly affect the zang-fu organs, qi and blood. For this reason, they are considered to be the main causative factors of endogenous diseases.

Ancient doctors believed that different emotional factors tend to affect the circulation of qi and blood of specific internal organs, resulting in the following clinical manifestations and pathology: "Anger injures the liver, joy injures the heart, grief and melancholy injure the lung, worry injures the spleen, and fear and fright injure the kidney."

"Anger causes the qi to rise up; joy causes it to move slowly; grief drastically consumes it; fear causes it to decline; fright causes it to be deranged, and worry causes it to stagnate."

Many of these relationships are validated by clinical observation, but a concrete analysis of each individual case is necessary to confirm which internal organ is impaired and what pathological changes in the qi have developed.

The heart, liver and spleen are most closely involved with pathological changes resulting from the seven emotional factors, although any of the five zang organs may be affected. For example, excessive joy or fear may cause mental disturbance and dysfunction of the heart in dominating mental activities. Clinical manifestations include palpitations, insomnia, dream-disturbed sleep and mental confusion, and in severe cases, abnormal laughing and crying and mania. Prolonged anger or depression can impair the liver's function of maintaining the free flow of qi. Clinical manifestations include distention and pain in the hypochondriac region, irascibility, belching, sighing, the sensation of a foreign body in the throat, and irregular menstruation. In severe cases, bleeding due to impairment of the blood vessels may occur. Worry, grief and melancholy often affect the transporting and transforming function of the spleen, causing epigastric and abdominal distention, anorexia, etc.

The seven emotional factors may cause functional derangement of the heart, liver or spleen individually, or may impair the function of more than one of these zang organs. For example, worry can injure both heart and spleen, whilst prolonged depression and anger may cause disharmony between the liver and spleen.

3. Improper Diet, Overstrain, Stress and Lack of Physical Exercise

1) Improper diet Although food is of course necessary for maintaining life, improper diet may be one of the causative factors of disease, and may affect the body in the following three ways:

a) Overeating and malnutrition The quantity of food consumed should be appropriate to the requirements of the body. Either voracious eating or insufficient food intake may result in disease. If more food is eaten than the digestive system can properly digest, the function of the spleen and stomach will be impaired. Clinical manifestations include foul belching, sour regurgitation, distention and pain of the epigastric and abdominal regions, loss of desire to eat, vomiting and diarrhoea. The forty-third chapter of *Plain Questions* states: "Overeating will inevitably impair the gastro-intestinal function." Insufficient food intake will fail to provide the basis for the manufacture of qi and blood. In the long run, there will be loss of weight and weakness of antipathogenic qi.

b) Overindulgence in particular foods The human body can only obtain its nutritional needs when food intake is balanced. Overindulgence in one particular food may result in various forms of malnutrition or other diseases. For example, continuous intake of polished rice may result in beriberi. The inhabitants of inland plateaus run a greater risk of suffering from simple goiter through drinking only "Shashui" (drinking water lacking in iodine). Overindulgence in cold or raw food can easily injure spleen yang leading to the development of interior cold and damp with the symptoms of abdominal pain and diarrhea. Overindulgence in alcoholic drink or greasy, sweet and highly flavoured food may produce damp heat, phlegm and stagnation of qi and blood. When the functions of the spleen and stomach are impaired, there may be pathological changes such as full sensation in the chest with profuse sputum, dizziness, vertigo, bleeding haemorrhoids and carbuncles.

c) Intake of unclean food If unclean, decayed or poisonous food is eaten, the functions of the spleen and stomach will be impaired, resulting in pain and distention in the epigastric and abdominal regions, nausea, vomiting, borborygmus and diarrhoea. Unclean food may also cause parasitic diseases or food poisoning.

2) Overstrain, stress or lack of physical exercise Normal physical exertion and rest do not cause disease, and indeed form the basic conditions for building up the constitution and preventing disease. Overstrain and stress or lack of physical exertion, however, may cause disease, the thirty-nineth chapter of *Plain Questions* says: "Overstrain or stress consume the vital energy of the body." Prolonged overstrain or stress will weaken the antipathogenic qi and result in clinical manifestations such as loss of weight, lassitude, disinclination to speak, palpitations, insomnia, dizziness and blurred vision.

Excessive sexual activity will injure the kidney qi, resulting in symptoms of deficiency such as soreness and weakness of the lumbar region and knee joints, dizziness, tinnitus, impotence, ejaculatio praecox, lassitude and irregular menstruation.

An excessively comfortable life and lack of physical exercise can impair the circulation of qi and blood, weaken the function of the spleen and stomach, and sap body resistance. Clinical manifestations include softening of the bones and tendons, poor energy, poor appetite, lassitude, obesity, and shortness of breath on exertion. They may also induce other diseases.

4. Traumatic Injury and Insect or Animal Bites

Traumatic injuries include gunshots, incisions, contusions, scalds, burns, and sudden contracture or sprain due to carrying heavy loads. These can result in muscular swelling and pain, stagnation of blood, bleeding, injury to the tendons, fracture of the bones, dislocation of the joints, etc. Invasion of exogenous pathogenic qi into the affected areas, profuse bleeding, or injury to the internal organs can even cause coma or convulsions.

Insect or animal bites including the bites of poisonous snakes, wild beasts and rabid dogs may result in bleeding, pain and broken skin in mild cases, and toxicosis or even death in severe cases.

5. Phlegm Fluid and Stagnant Blood

Phlegm fluid and stagnant blood are the pathological products of dysfunction of the zang-fu organs. Both of them, however, having been produced, further affect the zang-fu organs and tissues — either directly or indirectly — and cause numerous diseases. Phlegm fluid and stagnant blood are therefore considered to be a kind of pathogenic factor.

1) Phlegm fluid Phlegm fluid results from accumulation of body fluid due to dysfunction of the lung, spleen and kidney and impairment of water metabolism. Phlegm is turbid and thick, whilst retained fluid is clear and dilute. The term phlegm fluid is the short form of the combination of the two.

Diseases caused by phlegm fluid include numerous syndromes involving either substantial or non-substantial phlegm fluid. Clinical manifestations vary according to the area of the body affected. Retention of phlegm in the lung, for example, may cause cough with profuse sputum and asthmatic breathing; phlegm afflicting the heart may lead to palpitations, coma and depressive and manic psychosis; obstruction of the meridians, bones and tendons by phlegm may cause tuberculosis of the cervical lymph nodes, subcutaneous nodules, suppurative inflammation of deep tissues, numbness of the limbs and body, and hemiplegia; phlegm fluid affecting the head and eyes may cause dizziness, vertigo, and blurred vision. Accumulation of phlegm and qi in the throat may lead to a "foreign body sensation." Retained fluid attacking the skin and muscles may cause oedema, general aching and a heavy sensation of the body; retention of fluid in the chest and hypochondrium may cause cough, asthmatic breathing, distention and pain there; retained fluid spreading to the stomach and intestines may lead to nausea, vomiting of sticky fluid, discomfort in the epigastrium and abdomen, and borborygmus.

Diseases caused by phlegm fluid cover a wide range, referring not only to those with such symptoms as visible sputum, but also to those with clinical manifestations characterized by phlegm fluid. General clinical manifestations include spitting of profuse sputum or sticky fluid, a rattling sound in the throat, a full sensation in the epigastric and abdominal regions, vomiting, dizziness and vertigo, palpitations, a sticky tongue coating and a string-taut rolling pulse.

2) Stagnant blood Stagnant blood is

mainly caused by impaired blood circulation due to either coldness or deficiency or stagnation of qi. Traumatic injuries may cause internal bleeding which accumulates and is not dispelled, leading to stagnant blood.

The clinical manifestations of stagnant blood vary according to the area affected. Stagnant blood in the heart, for example, may result in a suffocating sensation in the chest, cardiac pain and green purplish lips. Stagnant blood in the lung can cause chest pain and haemoptysis. Stagnant blood in the gastro-intestinal tract can lead to haematemesis and bloody stool. Stagnant blood in the liver may cause hypochondriac pain and palpable masses in the abdomen. Stagnant blood in the uterus can cause dysmenorrhoea, irregular menstruation, and a dark red menstrual flow with clots. Stagnant blood on the body surface may cause a purplish or green colour of the skin and subcutaneous haematoma.

Diseases due to stagnant blood, although they can be varied, share certain common characteristics:

a) Pain which is worse with pressure and stabbing in nature.

b) Bleeding which is deep or dark purple in colour containing clots.

c) Ecchymoses or petechiae, accompanied by pain in the affected parts, indicate stagnant blood retained in the superficial portion of the body. The tongue may be deep purple in colour or show purple spots.

d) There may be fixed purplish masses accompanied by pain.

II.   PATHOGENESIS

The onset of disease can be generalized as being due to disharmony of yin and yang and conflict between pathogenic qi and antipathogenic qi. Antipathogenic qi, known as *zheng* qi, refers to the functional activities of the human body as well as to its ability to resist disease. Pathogenic qi, known as *xie* qi, refers to all the various causative factors of disease. For disease to occur, there must be present both a relative weakness of antipathogenic qi and the presence of pathogenic qi. Whilst both together constitute the two major factors underlying the occurrence of disease, however, antipathogenic qi is primary, being the internal factor that allows the invasion of the external factor i.e. pathogenic qi. The seventy-second chapter of *Plain Questions* states: "Pathogenic qi cannot invade the body if the antipathogenic qi remains strong." The thirty-third chapter of the same book further states: "The antipathogenic qi must be weak if invasion of pathogenic qi takes place."

This dialectical approach, which pays attention to both internal and external conditions, in particular, the former, has played a major role in traditional Chinese medicine in understanding the nature of disease and guiding clinical practice.

Although diseases may be very complicated and varied, they can be generalized and understood in terms of pathological processes in the following three ways: disharmony of yin and yang, conflict between antipathogenic qi and pathogenic qi, and abnormal descending and ascending of qi. These three aspects of the development of disease are closely interconnected.

1.   Disharmony of Yin and Yang

Disharmony of yin and yang refers to

pathological changes involving either excess or deficiency of yin or yang, occurring when the body is invaded by pathogenic qi. Disease will not occur unless the body is invaded by pathogenic factors which cause derangement of yin and yang in the interior. Yin-yang disharmony, i.e. excess or deficiency of either yin or yang, is mainly manifested in the form of cold and heat, and excess and deficiency syndromes. In general, heat syndromes of excess type will occur in cases of excess of yang, and cold syndromes of excess type in cases of excess of yin. Cold syndromes of deficiency type will occur in cases of deficiency of yang, and heat syndromes of deficiency type in cases of deficiency of yin. In addition, in the course of the progression of disease, cold syndromes may manifest some false heat symptoms, in which excess of yin walls off yang, and heat syndromes some false cold symptoms in which excess of yang walls off yin.

All the contradictions and changes accurring in the disease process can be generalized in terms of yin and yang. Thus all the zang-fu organs and meridians are classified in terms of yin and yang; and qi and blood, nutrient qi and defensive qi, exterior and interior, ascending and descending of qi reflect yin and yang contradictions. Functional disturbance, derangement between qi and blood and between nutrient and defensive qi all belong to disharmony of yin and yang, which underlies the whole disease process and is the decisive factor in the occurrence and development of disease.

2. Conflict Between Antipathogenic Qi and Pathogenic Qi

The conflict between antipathogenic qi and pathogenic qi refers to the struggle between the body's powers of resistance and any pathogenic factors. This struggle has significance not only in relation to the onset of disease, but also to its progression and transformations. To some extent this struggle can be described as the main focus for the onset, progression and transfomation of disease. Invasion of pathogenic qi results in conflict between the antipathogenic qi and the pathogenic qi which destroys the yin-yang harmony of the body and causes functional disturbance of the zang-fu organs and meridians, derangement of qi and blood and abnormal ascending and descending of qi, leading to various pathological changes. These mainly manifest as excess or deficiency syndromes. Syndromes of excess type are likely to occur if there is both hyperactivity of pathogenic qi and sufficiency of antipathogenic qi. Syndromes of deficiency type, or syndromes of deficiency mixed with excess, are likely to occur if there is excess of pathogenic qi and deficiency of antipathogenic qi. The twenty-eight chapter of *Plain Questions* states: "Hyperactivity of pathogenic qi causes syndromes of excess type and consumption of essential qi will lead to syndromes of deficiency type." Excess here mainly refers to hyperactivity of pathogenic qi, i.e. the pathological reaction dominated by excess of pathogenic qi. It is commonly seen in the early and middle stages of diseases due to invasion of the exogenous pathogenic factors, and diseases caused by retention of phlegm fluid, stagnant blood and water damp as well as retention of food. Deficiency mainly refers to insufficiency of antipathogenic qi which is the pathological reaction dominated by decline of antipathogenic qi. It is commonly seen in diseases resulting from prolonged weakness of body constitution, poor function of the zang-fu organs, and deficiency of qi, blood and body fluid due to a lingering disease.

3.   Abnormal Descending or Ascending of Qi

Ascending, descending, outward and inward movement are the basic forms of the transmission of qi in its circulation through the body. Abnormal ascending and descending refers to pathological states of the zang-fu organs, meridians, yin and yang, qi and blood in which they fail to maintain their normal state of governing ascent and descent of qi.

The functional activities of the zang-fu organs and meridians, and the relationships between the zang-fu organs, meridians, qi, blood, yin and yang are maintained by the ascending, descending, outward and inward movement of qi circulation. Examples of this are the descending and dispersing function of lung qi; the spleen's function of sending up clear essence of food to the lung; the stomach's function of sending down partially digested food; the harmony between the heart and kidney and between fire (heart) and water (kidney). Abnormal ascending or descending of qi may affect the five zang and six fu organs, the interior and the exterior of the body, the four limbs and the nine openings, leading to a variety of pathological changes. Common examples include cough, asthmatic breathing, and a suffocating sensation in the chest caused by failure of lung qi to descend and disperse; belching and nausea caused by abnormal ascent of stomach qi; loose stools and diarrhoea caused by dysfunction of the spleen in transportation and transformation

and failure of its normal ascending function; insomnia and palpitations caused by disharmony between heart and kidney; and syncope due to derangement of qi, blood, yin and yang. Other examples are inability of the kidney to receive qi, upward floating of yang, failure of clear yang to ascend, and sinking of the qi of the middle jiao. All of these can be generalized as pathological changes caused by abnormal ascending and descending of qi.

Whilst all the zang-fu organs are involved in the ascending and descending of qi, the spleen and stomach qi plays an especially important role. This is because spleen and stomach provide the material basis for the acquired constitution. The spleen and stomach lie in middle jiao which connects with the other zang-fu organs in the upper and lower jiaos, and form the pivot of the mechanism for ascending and descending of qi. The physiological functions of the human body can be maintained only when both the ascending function of spleen qi and the descending function of stomach qi are normal. Harmonious functioning of the spleen and stomach is therefore essential to the ascending, descending, outward and inward movement of the qi of the whole body. Neither aspect exists in isolation, however, the ascending of spleen qi and descending of stomach qi must cooperate with the ascending and descending movement of the qi of the other zang-fu organs. If the ascending and descending functions of spleen and stomach fail, the clear yang will not be disseminated, acquired essence cannot be stored, the clean qi in the atmosphere and food cannot be received, and substances such as turbid phlegm will not be dispelled from the body. Numerous diseases will result. An understanding of the influence of the ascending and descending functions of spleen and stomach on the physiological activities of the whole body is therefore essential in clinical practice when regulating the functions of these two organs.

Chapter 12

DIAGNOSTIC METHODS

There are four diagnostic methods, namely, inspection, auscultation and olfaction, inquiring and palpation.

Inspection refers to the process in which the doctor observes with his eyes the systemic and regional changes in the patient's vitality, colour and appearance. Auscultation and olfaction determine the pathological changes by listening and smelling. Inquiring means to ask the patient or the patient's companion about the onset and progression of the disease, present symptoms and signs, and other conditions related to the disease. Palpation is a method of diagnosis in which the pathological condition is detected by feeling the pulse and palpating the skin, epigastrium, abdomen, hand, foot and other parts of the body.

As human body is an organic entity, its regional pathological changes may affect the whole body, and the pathological changes of the internal organs may manifest themselves on the body surface. *The Medical Book by Master of Danxi* says: "One should observe and analyse the external manifestations of the patient in order to know what is happening inside the body, for the disease of internal organs must have its manifestations on the body surface." By making analysis and synthesis of the pathological conditions ...ned by applying the four diagnostic methods, the doctor, therefore, can determine the causative factors and nature of the disease, thus providing basis for further differentiation and treatment.

Inspection, auscultation and olfaction, inquiring and palpation are the four approaches to understand the pathological conditions. They can not be separated, but relate to and supplement one another. In the clinical situation, only by combining the four can a comprehensive and systematic understanding of the condition of the disease be gained and a correct diagnosis made. Any inclination to one aspect while neglecting the other three is one-sided, therefore, is not suggested.

I. INSPECTION

Inspection is a method of diagnosis in which the doctor understands and predicts the pathological changes of internal organs by observing abnormal changes in the patient's vitality, colour, appearance, secretions and excretions. In their long-term medical practice, the Chinese physicians realized the close relationship between the external part of the body, especially the face and tongue, and the zang-fu organs. Any slight changes appearing in these areas can tell pathological conditions in various parts of the body.

Inspection of the exterior of the body, therefore, is of much help indiagnosis.

1. Observation of the Vitality

Vitality is the general manifestation of the vital activities of the human body, and the outward sign of relative strength of qi and blood of the zang-fu organs, which take essential qi as the basis. By observing vitality, one may get a rough idea of the strength of the antipathogenic qi of the human body and severity of the disease; this is highly significant for the prognosis.

If the patient is fully conscious and in fairly good spirits, responds keenly with a sparkle in the eyes, the patient is vigorous and the disease is mild. If the patient is spiritless with dull eyes and sluggish response or even mental disturbance, the patient lacks vigour and the disease is severe.

2. Observation of the Colour

Both the colour and lustre of the face are observed. There are five discolorations, namely, blue, yellow, red, pale and dark grey. Observation of the lustre of the face is to distinguish whether the complexion is bright and moist or dark and haggard.

People of different races have different skin colours, and there is wide variation among people of the same race. However, a lustrous skin with natural colour is considered normal.

The colour and lustre of the face are the outward manifestations of the relative strength of qi and blood of the zang-fu organs. Their changes often suggest various pathological conditions. Observation of these changes is valuable for diagnosing disease.

Here are the descriptions of the indications of the five discolorations.

A red colour often indicates heat syndromes, which may be of deficiency type or of excess type. When the entire face is red, it is a sign of a heat syndrome of excess type resulting from either exposure to exogenous pathogenic factors with the symptom of fever, or hyperactivity of yang of zang-fu organs. The presence of malar flush accompanied by tidal fever and night sweating suggests an interior heat syndrome due to yin deficiency.

A pale colour indicates cold syndromes of deficiency type and loss of blood. A pale complexion is often due to yin excess or yang deficiency. A bright white face with a puffy, bloated appearance is a sign of deficiency of yang qi. If the pale face is withered, it signifies blood deficiency.

A yellow colour indicates syndromes of deficiency type and damp syndromes. When the entire body, including the face, eyes and skin, is yellow, it is jaundice. If the yellowness tends toward bright orange, it is called yang jaundice resulting from damp heat. If the yellow is smoky dark, it is called yin jaundice resulting from either cold damp or long-term stagnation of blood. A pale yellow complexion without brightness is a sign of deficiency of both qi and blood.

A blue colour indicates cold syndromes, painful syndromes, stagnation of blood and convulsion. A pale complexion with a blue tinge is seen in a syndrome of excessive yin and cold with the symptom of severe pain in the epigasrium and abdomen. Blue purplish face and lips with the intermittent pain in the precordial region or behind the sternum are due to stagnation of the heart blood. Blue purplish face and lips accompanied by high fever and violent movement of the limbs in children are signs of infantile convulsion.

A dark grey colour indicates deficiency of the kidney and stagnation of blood. A pale and dark complexion accompanied with lumbar soreness and cold feet suggests insufficiency of the kidney yang. A dark complexion without brightness, accompanied by scaly skin signifies prolonged stagnation of blood.

Generally speaking, a lustrous and moist complexion indicates that the disease is mild, qi and blood are not deficient, and the prognosis is good; whilst a dark and haggard complexion suggests that the disease is severe, essential qi is already injured, and the prognosis is poor.

As to the clinical significance of the colour of secretions and excretions, such as nasal discharge, sputum, urine and vaginal discharge, those clear and white in colour generally denote deficiency and cold, while those turbid and yellow in colour indicate excess and heat.

3. Observation of the Appearance

Appearance refers to the body shape which can be described as strong, weak, heavy or skinny; and to the movement and posture related to disease.

Overweight with mental depression mostly suggests deficiency of qi and excess of phlegm damp. A thin person with dry skin indicates insufficiency of blood. Great loss of weight in the course of a long illness indicates the exhaustion of the essential qi.

The patient's movement and posture are outward manifestations of the pathological changes. There is a variation of movement and posture in different diseases. But on the whole, an active patient is usually manifesting a yang syndrome, whilst a passive manner is usually yin. For instance, a patient suffering from the lung syndrome of excess type with excessive phlegm is likely to sit there with the extended neck, whilst a patient with deficiency of qi manifesting as shortness of breath and dislike of speaking tends to sit there facing downward. Violent movement of the four limbs is mostly present in wind diseases such as tetanus, acute and chronic infantile convulsion. The occurrence of weakness, motor impairment and muscular atrophy of the limbs suggests *wei* syndromes. The presence of pain, soreness, heaviness and numbness in the tendons, bones and muscles accompanied by swelling and restricted movement of the joints points to *bi* syndromes. The appearance of numbness and impaired movement of the limbs on one side of the body indicates hemiplegia or wind stroke.

4. Observation of the Five Sense Organs

1) Observation of the eye   The liver opens into the eye, and the essential qi of the five zang and six fu organs all goes up into the eye. Therefore, abnormal changes in the eye are not only associated with the liver, but also reflect the pathological changes of other zang-fu organs. Apart from the expression of the eye, attention should also be paid to the appearance, colour and movement of the eye. For instance, redness and swelling of the eye are often due to wind heat or liver fire. Yellow sclera suggests jaundice. Ulceration of the canthus denotes damp heat. Upward, straight forward or sideways staring of the eye is mostly caused by disturbance of liver wind.

2) Observation of the nose   This is to

observe the appearance and discharge of the nose. The flapping of the ala nasi is often present in asthmatic breathing due to either heat in the lung or deficiency of qi of both the lung and kidney. Clear nasal discharge is due to exposure to wind cold, whilst turbid nasal discharge to wind heat. Prolonged turbid nasal discharge with stinking smell suggests chronic rhinitis or chronic sinusitis.

3) Observation of the ear Due attention is paid to the colour of the ear and conditions of the internal ear. Dry and withered auricles, burnt black in colour, present in the patient with a prolonged or severe illness, are due to consumption of the kidney essence not allowing it to nourish upwards. Purulent discharge in the ear, known as "Tin Er" (suppurative infection of the ear), is mostly caused by damp heat of the liver and gallbladder.

4) Observation of the gums Pale gums indicate deficiency of blood. Redness and swelling of the gums are due to flaring up of the stomach fire. If redness and swelling of the gums are accompanied by bleeding, it is due to injury of the vessels by the stomach fire.

5) Observation of the lips and mouth This is to observe the changes of the lips and mouth in colour, moisture and appearance. Pale lips denote deficiency of blood. Blue purplish lips suggest either retention of cold or stagnation of blood. Dry lips, deep red in colour, indicate excessive heat. Sudden collapse with open mouth is deficiency, whilst sudden collapse with lock jaw is excess.

6) Observation of the throat The focus is on abnormal changes of the throat in colour and appearance. Redness and swelling of the throat with soreness denote accumulation of heat in the lung and stomach. Redness and swelling of the throat with yellow or white

ulcer spots are due to excessive toxic heat in the lung and stomach. A bright red throat with a mild soreness suggests yin deficiency leading to hyperactivity of fire. If there occurs a false membrane over the throat, which is greyish white in colour, hard to remove, bleeds following forceful rubbing and regrows immediately, it indicates diphtheria resulting from heat in the lung consuming yin.

5. Observation of the Tongue

Observation of the tongue, also known as tongue diagnosis, is an important procedure in diagnosis by inspection. It provides primary information for the Chinese physicians to make diagnosis.

1) Physiology of the tongue The tongue directly or indirectly connects with many zang-fu organs through the meridians and collaterals. The deep branch of Heart Meridian of Hand-Shaoyin goes to the root of the tongue; the Spleen Meridian of Foot-Taiyin traverses the root of the tongue and spreads over its lower surface; the Kidney Meridian of Foot-Shaoyin terminates at the root of the tongue. So the essential qi of the zang-fu organs can go upward to nourish the tongue, and pathological changes of the zang-fu organs can be reflected by changes in tongue conditions. This is why the observation of the tongue can determine the pathological changes of the internal organs.

Observation of the tongue includes the tongue proper and its coating. The tongue proper refers to the muscular tissue of the tongue, which is also known as the tongue body. The tongue coating refers to a layer of "moss" over the tongue surface, which is produced by the stomach qi.

A normal tongue is of proper size, soft in

quality, free in motion, slightly red in colour and with a thin layer of white coating which is neither dry nor over moist.

The tongue is divided into four areas, namely, tip, central part, root and border. The tip of the tongue often reveals the pathological changes of the heart and lung; its border reveals those of the liver and gallbladder; its central part reveals those of the spleen and stomach; and its root reveals those of the kidney. This method of diagnosing the pathological changes of the zang-fu organs by dividing the tongue into corresponding areas is clinically significant.

2) Tongue diagnosis

a) Tongue proper   This is to observe the colour and form of the tongue proper.

i) Colour of the tongue proper

Pale tongue: A pale tongue is less red than a normal tongue, and indicates syndromes of deficiency type and cold syndromes caused by deficiency of yang qi or insufficiency of qi and blood.

Red tongue: A red tongue is bright red and redder than a normal tongue. It indicates various heat syndromes including interior heat syndromes of excess type and interior heat syndromes of deficiency type due to yin deficiency.

Deep red tongue: A deep red tongue indicates an extreme heat condition. In exogenous febrile diseases, it indicates invasion of the ying and xue (blood) systems by pathogenic heat. In endogenous diseases, it indicates yin deficiency leading to hyperactivity of fire.

Purple tongue: A blue purple tongue indicates stagnation of blood which is related to either cold or heat. A deep blue purplish tongue, dry and lustreless, is related to heat, whilst a pale purplish and moist tongue is related to cold. The presence of purplish spots on the tongue surface also indicates stagnation of blood.

ii) Form of the tongue proper

Swollen tongue: A swollen tongue is larger than normal. If a swollen tongue is delicate in quality and pale in colour, and with tooth prints on the border, it indicates yang deficiency of the spleen and kidney. The condition is due to impaired circulation of body fluid producing harmful water, retained fluid, phlegm and damp. If a swollen tongue is deep red in colour occupying the entire space of the mouth, it indicates excessive heat in the heart and spleen. If a swollen tongue is blue purplish and dark, it indicates toxicosis.

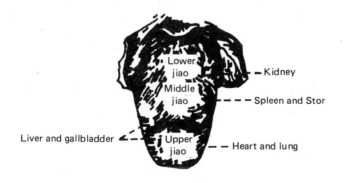

Fig. 134

Thin tongue: A thin tongue is smaller and thinner than normal. A thin and pale tongue indicates deficiency of qi and blood. A thin, dry and deep red tongue indicates hyperactivity of fire due to deficiency of yin in which body fluid is consumed.

Cracked tongue: Irregular streaks or cracks on the tongue indicate excessive heat consuming body fluid if the tongue is deep red in colour, and indicate deficiency of blood if the tongue is pale. A cracked tongue may be present in a normal person. If so, the cracks are not deep, and remain there all the time unchanged. This is considered normal.

Thorny tongue: The papillary buds over the surface of the tongue swell up like thorns. A thorny and red tongue indicates accumulation of pathogenic heat in the interior. The more severe the pathogenic heat is, the more enlarged and profuse the thorns will be.

Deviated tongue: A deviated tongue indicates windstroke or early threatening signs of windstroke.

Rigid tongue: A rigid tongue lacks flexibility and is difficult to protrude, retract or roll. A rigid tongue seen in exogenous febrile diseases often indicates invasion of the pericardium by heat, retention of turbid phlegm in the interior, or excessive pathogenic heat consuming body fluid. A rigid tongue present in endogenous diseases indicates wind stroke or early threatening signs of windstroke.

Flaccid tongue: A flaccid tongue is weak in motion, and often indicates extreme deficiency of qi and blood or consumption of yin fluid depriving the tongue of the nourishment. If a flaccid tongue is pale, it indicates deficiency of qi and blood. If it is deep red, it indicates collapse of yin.

b) Tongue coating:

i) Quality of the tongue coating

Thick coating and thin coating: The tongue coating is considered thin if the tongue proper can indistinctly be seen through it, and considered thick if the tongue proper can not be seen through it. One can understand the severity of the pathogenic factors and progression of the pathological conditions by distinguishing the thickness and thinness of the tongue coating. Generally speaking, a thin tongue coating is present if the superficial portion of the body is affected in a disease, or if the disease is due to deficiency of the anti-pathogenic qi. Retention of damp, phlegm or food in the interior, or inward transmission of the pathogenic factor from the exterior may produce a thick tongue coating. Thickening coating indicates inward transmission of the pathogenic factor from the exterior, and is a sign of aggravation of the disease. Thinning coating points to gradual elimination of the pathogenic factor, and is a sign of alleviation of the pathological conditions.

Moist coating and dry coating: One can understand the condition of the body fluid by distinguishing the moisture and dryness of the tongue coating. A normal tongue coating is moist and lustrous, which is the manifestation of normal dissemination of the body fluid. A dry tongue coating, which looks coarse and feels lacking moisture indicates consumption of body fluid due to excessive heat or consumption of yin fluid not allowing it to nourish upwards. If there is excessive moisture over the tongue surface, and the saliva dribbles when the tongue is stuck out in a severe case, it is a slippery tongue coating. The condition is caused by upward flooding of harmful water and damp.

Sticky coating and granular coating: Both sticky and granular tongue coating help deduce the turbid damp in the intestines and stomach. It is a sticky coating if the tongue is covered by a turbid layer of fine greasy substance which is hard to be scrubbed. A sticky tongue coating is often seen in syndromes resulting from retention of turbid damp and phlegm or retention of food. It will be a granular coating if the granules on the tongue surface are coarse, loose and thick like residue of making soy bean curds, and easily scrubbed. A pasty tongue coating often results from excessive yang heat bringing the turbid qi in the stomach upwards. It is also seen in syndromes caused by retention of turbid phlegm or retention of food.

Peeled coating: The tongue with a part of its coating peeling off is known as "geographic tongue." It is a sign of consumption of qi and yin of the stomach. If the entire coating peels off leaving the surface mirror smooth, the condition is known as glossy tongue. It is a sign of exhaustion of the stomach yin and severe damage of the stomach qi.

ii) Colour of the tongue coating

White coating: A thin and white coating is normal. Yet a white coating may appear in an illness. If so, it indicates exterior syndromes and cold syndromes. A thin and white coating is present in exterior cold syndromes, whilst a thick and white coating is seen in interior cold syndromes.

Yellow coating: A yellow coating indicates interior syndromes and heat syndromes. The deeper yellow the coating is, the more severe pathogenic heat it indicates. A light yellow coating points to mild heat; a deep yellow coating to severe heat; a burnt yellow coating to accumulation of heat.

Grey coating: A grey coating indicates interior syndromes, and may be seen in interior heat syndromes or syndromes resulting from cold and damp. If a grey coating is yellowish and dry, it signifies consumption of body fluid due to excessive heat. If a grey coating is whitish and moist, it implies retention of cold damp in the interior or retention of phlegm and fluid. As a grey coating often develops into a black coating, a greyish black coating is seen.

Black coating: A black coating indicates interior syndromes due to extreme heat or excessive cold. A black coating is often the outcome of the further development of a yellow coating or a grey coating. It is present at the severe stage of an illness. If a black coating is yellowish and dry, possibly with thorns, it signifies consumption of body fluid due to extreme heat. A pale black and slippery coating implies excessive cold due to yang deficiency.

3) **Precautions in tongue diagnosis**

a) As each disease undergoes a complicated process, the conditions of the tongue proper and its coating are the manifestations of interior complicated pathological changes. The conditions of the tongue proper mainly reflect deficiency or excess of the zang-fu organs and relative strength of the essential qi. The conditions of the tongue coating reflects the depth and nature of the invading pathogenic factors. A comprehensive analysis of the conditions of both the tongue proper and its coating is required on the basis of their respective indications. The condition of the tongue proper and that of its coating are generally conformable; the disease to be indicated is often the outcome of combining the two. For instance, retention of heat of excess type in the interior produces a red tongue with a dry and yellow coating; a pale tongue with a moist and white coating is often present in cold syndromes of deficiency type. But such situations as the condition of the tongue proper does not agree with the condition of its coating may occur. Only by a comprehensive analysis can reliable information be provided for furthur differentiation of syndromes.

b) It is desirable to observe the tongue in direct natural light. The patient is required to protrude the tongue naturally.

c) Some food and drugs may colour the tongue coating, and the thickness and moisture of the tongue coating may change after eating or scraping the tongue. Attention should be paid to the exclusion of false phenomena induced by such factors in the clinical situation.

II.   AUSCULTATION AND OLFACTION

Auscultation and olfaction refer to listening and smelling.

1.   Listening

a) Listening to the speech In general, speaking lustily indicates syndromes of excess type, while speaking feebly and in low tones indicates those of deficiency type. A hoarse voice or loss of voice in a severe case may be of deficiency type or of excess type. If they are present in exogenous diseases with a sudden onset, they are of excess type. Chronic or recurrent onset in endogenous diseases are of deficiency type.

Incoherent speech in loud voice accompanied by impaired consciousness indicates a syndrome of excess type due to disturbance of the mind by heat. Repeated speech in feeble voice accompanied by listlessness suggests a syndrome of deficiency type of the heart resulting from severe damage of the heart qi.

b) Listening to the respiration Feeble breathing indicates deficiency of qi. Forceful and coarse breathing accompanied by a loud voice suggests a syndrome of excess type due to excessive pathogenic heat in the interior.

Feeble asthmatic breathing accompanied by shortness of breath indicates deficiency of the qi of the lung and kidney, pertaining to deficiency type asthma. Coarse asthmatic breathing in loud tones with the preference for exhalation suggests retention of pathogenic factor in the lung impairing the functions of qi. This belongs to asthma of excess type.

c) Listening to the cough Cough is the manifestation of dysfunction of the lung in dispersing and descending leading to upward perversion of qi. Cough in a coarse voice indicates a syndrome of excess type, cough in a feeble voice suggests a syndrome of deficiency type. Unproductive cough or cough with a small amount of thick sputum implies injury of the lung by pathogenic dryness or dryness of the lung due to yin deficiency.

2.   Smelling

Stench smell of a secretion or excretion usually indicates heat syndromes of excess type; less stinking smell suggests cold syndromes of deficiency type; foul and sour smell implies retention of food. Different odours should be identified in order to deduce the nature of the disease. The source of the odour should also be traced for determining the locality of the disease.

III. INQUIRING

Inquiring is asking the patient or the patient's companion about the disease condition in order to understand the pathological process.

Inquiries are made systematically with questions focused on the chief complaint of the patient according to the knowledge necessary in differentiating a syndrome.

Inquiring covers a wide range of topics. Here is a brief introduction to inquiring about the present illness.

1. Chills and Fever

Apart from confirming the presence of chills and fever, we need to ask such questions as which is more severe, when they occur and what symptoms and signs accompany them, for this information is necessary for further differentiation of syndromes;

1) Chills accompanied by fever Simultaneous occurrence of chills and fever at the beginning of the disease indicates exogenous exterior syndrome. It is the manifestation of invasion of the body surface by the pathogenic factor and its contending with the antipathogenic qi. Exterior syndromes resulting from exposure to pathogenic wind cold usually manifest as severe chills and mild fever with the accompanying symptoms and signs such as absence of sweating, headache and general aching, and a superficial, and tense pulse. Exterior syndromes due to invasion by pathogenic wind heat are characterized by mild chills and severe fever; the patient also reveals thirst, sweating and a superficial and rapid pulse.

2) Alternate chills and fever The patient may notice alternate attacks of chills and fever. This is the representative symptom of intermediate syndromes. The patient may also complain of a bitter taste in the mouth, thirst and fullness and stuffiness in the chest and hypochondrium.

High fever following chills occurring at a definite time of the day suggests malaria.

3) Fever without chills Fever may occur without chills. Persistent high fever with aversion to heat instead suggests interior heat syndromes of excess type due to transmission of the pathogenic factors from the exterior to the interior with excessive heat in the interior. The accompanying symptoms and signs are profuse sweating, severe thirst and a surging pulse. If fever occurs or becomes worse at a fixed hour of the day just like the sea waves, it is known as tidal fever. Tidal fever in the afternoon or evening, accompanied by night sweating and a red tongue with little moisture indicates deficiency of yin; afternoon fever with constipation and fullness and pain in the abdomen suggests excess heat of the Yangming Meridian.

4) Chills without fever The subjective feeling of chills without fever indicates interior cold syndrome of deficiency type. The patient may also have chilled appearance, cold limbs and a deep, slow and weak pulse.

2. Perspiration

The patient should, first of all, be asked whether sweating is present or not. Further inquiring deals with the feature of sweating and its accompanying symptoms and signs.

Absence of sweating in exterior

syndromes indicates invasion by pathogenic cold; presence of sweating in exterior syndromes suggests either exterior syndromes of deficiency type resulting from exposure to pathogenic wind, or exterior heat syndromes due to invasion by pathogenic wind heat. The accompanying symptoms and signs are considered in differentiation.

Sweating that occurs during sleep and stops upon wakening is known as night sweating. It usually indicates deficiency of yin with hyperactivity of yang heat. The patient may also present tidal fever and a red tongue with little coating.

Frequent sweating which is worse on slight exertion is known as spontaneous sweating. It is a sign of deficiency of qi and deficiency of yang. The patient may also exhibit chills, listlessness and lassitude.

Profuse sweating accompanied by high fever, mental restlessness, thirst with preference for cold drinks and a surging pulse indicates interior heat syndromes of excess type resulting from excessive yang heat in the interior expelling the sweat out. Profuse sweating accompanied by listlessness, feeble energy, cold limbs and a deep and thready pulse in a severe case is a critical sign indicating total exhaustion of yang qi.

3. Appetite, Thirst and Taste

Poor appetite present in the patient with a prolonged illness manifesting as emaciation, loose stools, lassitude and a pale tongue with a thin white coating indicates weakness of the spleen and stomach; poor appetite accompanied by stuffiness in the chest, fullness in the abdomen and a thick, sticky tongue coating suggests stagnation of qi of

the spleen and stomach caused by retention of food or retention of pathogenic damp.

Excessive appetite and getting hungry easily in a skinny patient indicate excessive stomach fire.

Hunger with no desire to eat or eating a small amount of food suggests impairment of the stomach yin producing internal heat of deficiency type.

Lack of thirst during an illness suggests that body fluid is not consumed. It is present in cold syndromes or syndromes in which pathogenic heat is not noticeable. The presence of thirst indicates consumption of body fluid or retention of phlegm damp in the interior preventing body fluid from ascending. Further analysis is based on features of thirst, amount of drinks to be taken and the accompanying symptoms and signs.

A bitter taste in the mouth usually indicates hyperactivity of the fire of the liver and gallbladder. A sweetish taste and stickiness in the mouth imply damp heat in the spleen and stomach. Sour regurgitation means retention of heat in the liver and stomach. Tastelessness points to deficiency of the spleen with its impaired function of transportation.

4. Defecation and Urination

As the doctor does not observe the change in defecation and urination of the patient directly, it is necessary to make inquiries.

Constipation due to dryness of stool usually indicates accumulation of heat or consumption of body fluid. Loose stool suggests deficiency of the spleen or retention of damp in the spleen. Watery stool with undigested food implies deficiency of yang of the spleen and kidney. Bloody stool with mucus and tenesmus results from damp heat in the intestines and stagnation of qi in the intestinal tract.

Yellow urine generally indicates heat syndromes, while clear and profuse urine indicates absence of the pathogenic heat in an illness, or cold syndromes. Turbid urine suggests downward infusion of damp heat or downward leakage of turbid essence. Red urine implies injury of the vessels by heat. Clear urine increased in volume means infirmity of the kidney qi and dysfunction of the bladder in controlling urine, while scanty yellow urine with urgent and painful urination means downward infusion of damp heat into the bladder. Dribbling urination or retention of urine in a severe case is present not only in syndromes of deficiency type due to exhaustion of the kidney qi with its impaired function of controlling urine, but also in syndromes of excess type caused by obstructed qi activities of the bladder due to downward infusion of damp heat, stagnant blood or stones.

5. Pain

Pain is one of the most common symptoms complained of by the patient. Apart from a thorough understanding of the history and accompanying symptoms and signs, the nature and locality of pain must be asked. Differentiation of the nature of the pain is significant for deducing its etiology and pathology, while identification of the locality of the pain helps determine diseased zang-fu organs and meridians.

1) Nature of the pain

Distending pain: Distending pain manifesting as severe distension, mild pain and moving from place to place is a typical sign of qi stagnation. It often occurs in the chest, epigastric, hypochondriac and abdominal regions. But headache with a distending sensation in the head is due to upward disturbance by fire and heat.

Pricking pain: Pricking pain, sharp in nature and fixed in location, is a sign of stagnation of blood. It usually occurs in the chest, epigastric, hypochondriac and lower abdominal regions.

Weighty pain: Pain with a heavy sensation is a sign of damp blocking qi and blood, as damp is characterized by heaviness. It is often present in the head, four limbs and lumbar region.

Colicky pain: Colicky pain is a sign of abrupt obstruction of the qi by substantial pathogenic factors.

Pulling pain: Pulling pain which is spasmodic in nature and short in duration often relates to the disorders of the liver. It is caused by liver wind.

Burning pain: Pain with a burning sensation and preference for coolness often occurs in the hypochondriac regions on both sides and epigastric region. It results from invasion of the collaterals by pathogenic fire and heat or from excessive yang heat due to yin deficiency.

Cold pain: Pain with a cold sensation and preference for warmth often occurs in the head, lumbar, epigastric and abdominal regions. It is caused by pathogenic cold blocking the collaterals or lack of warmth and nourishment in the zang-fu organs and meridians due to deficiency of yang qi.

Dull pain: Dull pain is not severe. It is bearable lingering and may last for a long time. It is usually present in cold syndromes of deficiency type.

Hollow pain: Pain with a hollow sensation is caused by deficiency of blood leading to emptiness of vessels and retardation of blood circulation.

2) Locality of the pain Headache: Head is the meeting place of all the yang meridians and brain is the sea of marrow. Qi and blood of the five zang and six fu organs all go up into the head. If the pathogenic factors invade the head and block the clear yang, or if stagnation of qi and blood in endogenous diseases blocks the meridians and deprives the brain of the nourishment, headache will ensure. In cases of deficiency of qi and blood, head fails to be nourished, and the sea of marrow becomes empty; headache due to this is of deficiency type. Headache due to disturbance of the clear yang by the pathogenic factor is mostly of excess type.

Chest pain: As the heart and lung reside in the chest, chest pain indicates the pathological changes of the heart and lung.

Hypochondriac pain: The hypochondriac region is traversed by the Liver and Gallbladder Meridians. Obstruction or undernourishment of these meridians may produce hypochondriac pain.

Epigastric pain: Epigastrium (wan) refers to the upper abdomen in which the stomach situates. It is divided into three regions, namely, Shangwan, Zhongwan and Xiawan (upper, middle and lower wan respectively). Epigastric pain may result from invasion of the stomach by pathogenic cold, retention of food in the stomach or invasion of the stomach by the liver qi.

Abdominal pain: Abdomen is divided into upper abdomen, lower abdomen and sides of the lower abdomen. The upper abdomen refers to the area above the umbilicus and pertains to the spleen. The area below the umbilicus is the lower abdomen and pertains to the kidney, bladder, large and small intestines and uterus. Both sides of the lower abdomen is traversed by the Liver Meridian of Foot-

Jueyin. So according to the locality of the pain, the diseased zang-fu organs and meridians can be identified.

Abdominal pain caused by retention of cold, accumulation of heat, stagnation of qi, stagnation of blood, retention of food or parasitic diseases is excess in nature, while that caused by deficiency of qi, deficiency of blood or deficiency of cold is deficiency in nature.

Lumbago: The kidney resides in the lumbar region. Lumbago may result from obstruction of the meridians in the local area; besides, deficiency of the kidney failing to nourish the lumbar region is often the cause.

Pain in the four limbs: Pain in the four limbs may involve joints, muscles or meridians. It is casued by retardation of qi and blood circulation due to invasion of the exogenous pathogenic factors.

Besides, the duration of pain and its response to pressure should also be asked. Generally, persistent pain in a recent disease or pain which is aggravated by pressure indicates syndromes of excess type. Intermittent pain in a prolonged illness or pain which is alleviated by pressure often occurs in syndromes of deficiency type.

6.   Sleep

Insomnia means either difficulty in falling asleep, or inability to sleep soundly, waking easily and being unable to fall asleep again. Insomnia accompanied by dizziness and palpitations usually indicates failure of blood to nourish the heart due to deficiency of both the heart and spleen. Insomnia accompanied by restlessness in mind and dream-disturbed sleep suggests hyperactivity of the fire of the heart. Difficulty in falling asleep due to an uncomfortable and empty sensation in the stomach or gastric discomfort after a full meal implies derangement of the stomach qi leading to mental restlessness.

If lethargy is accompanied by dizziness, it indicates accumulation of phlegm damp in the interior. A situation of being half asleep with general lassitude suggests deficiency of the yang of the heart and kidney.

7. Menses and Leukorrhea

Women patients are also asked about the menses and leukorrhea, and for married women the obstetric history.

1) Menses Inquiring in this aspect covers menstrual cycle and period, amount, colour and quality of flow and the accompanying symptoms and signs. If it is necessary, questions concerning the date of the last menstrual period and age of menopause should be asked.

Menses of a shortened cycle, excessive in amount, deep red in colour and thick in quality relates mainly to excessive heat in the blood; light coloured menstrual flow profuse in amount and thin in quality indicates failure of qi to command blood. A prolonged cycle with scanty purplish dark discharge or blood clots suggests stagnation of blood due to cold; thin scanty and light-coloured flow implies deficiency of blood. Irregular menstrual cycle is a sign of disharmony of the Chong and Ren (Conception Vessel) Meridians due to obstruction of the liver qi.

Pre-menstrual or menstrual distending pain in the breasts and lower abdomen which intensifies on pressure means stagnation of qi and blood; cold pain in the lower abdomen during the period points to stagnation of blood due to cold; dull pain in the lower abdomen during or after the period which is alleviated by pressure is due to deficiency of qi and blood.

2) Leukorrhea Attention is paid to the colour, amount, quality and smell of leukorrhea.

Watery leukorrhea whitish in colour and profuse in amount indicates deficiency syndromes and cold syndromes; thick leukorrhea yellow or red in colour with offensive smell suggests excess syndromes and heat syndromes.

IV. PALPATION

Palpation is a method of diagnosis in which the pathological condition is detected by palpating, feeling and pressing certain areas of the body. It is discussed under the headings of feeling the pulse and palpation of different parts of the body.

1. Feeling the Pulse

The location for feeling the pulse at the present time is above the wrist where the radial artery throbs. It is divided into three regions: *cun*, *guan* and *chi* (Fig.135) The region opposite to the styloid process of the radius (the bony eminence behind the palm) is known as guan, that distal to guan (i.e. between guan and the wrist joint) is cun and that proximal to guan is chi. There have been in different ages various descriptions concerning the relationship between these three regions and their corresponding zang-fu organs. They are fundamentally conformable. It is generally acknowledged that the three regions of cun, guan and chi of

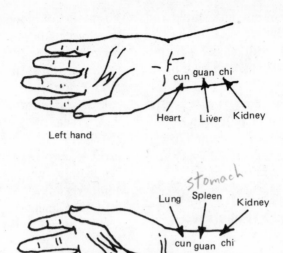

Left hand

Right hand

Fig. 135

the left hand reflect respectively the conditions of the heart, liver and kidney; and those of the right hand reflect the conditions of the lung, spleen and kidney.

In feeling the pulse, let the patient take either sitting or supine position with the arm placed approximately on a level with the heart, wrist extended and palm facing upward. This position facilitates smooth circulation of qi and blood. The doctor, by the side of the patient, first locates the guan region with the middle finger, then the cun and chi regions with the index and ring fingers. The three fingers are slightly flexed, presenting the shape of an arch. The finger tips are kept on the same horizontal level and the pulse is felt with the palmar side of the fingers. The space between each two fingers depends upon the height of the patient. If the patient is tall and has long arms, it is desirable to separate the fingers accordingly. If the patient is short and has

short arms, the three fingers are placed more closely. The method of "feeling the pulse in the guan region with one finger" is adopted in infantile cases, for a baby's pulse is not divided into these three regions.

The pulse is palpated by exerting three different finger forces, first lightly (superficial palpation), then moderately (middle palpation) and finally heavily (deep palpation). Generally the finger force of the same strength is exerted on the three regions at the same time and then feel the three regions separately according to the actual pathological conditions.

The pulse is differentiated in terms of depth (superficial or deep), speed (rapid or slow), strength (forceful or weak), shape (thick or thready, soft or hard) and rhythm. Different conditions of the pulse indicate different syndromes.

A normal pulse is smooth, even and forceful with the frequency of four beats per breath. However, the pulse may vary due to age, sex, body constitution, emotional state and climatic changes. Due attention should be paid to distinguishing it from an abnormal pulse.

Abnormal pulse readings and their clinical significance are as follows.

1) Superficial pulse (fu mai)   A superficial pulse can be easily felt with gentle touch. It indicates exterior syndromes, and is present at the early stage of exogenous diseases. Invasion of the body surface by the exogenous pathogenic factor creates its contending with wei qi. The pulsation is superficially situated, hence the superficial pulse. A superficial pulse may also be present in prolonged endogenous diseases. In this case, the pulse is superficial, large and weak, indicating outward floating of yang qi. This is a critical sign of the disease.

2) Deep pulse (chen mai)   A deep pulse is felt only on heavy pressure. It indicates interior syndromes. If the pulse is deep and forceful, it indicates interior syndromes of excess type. When the pathogenic factor invades the interior of the body, qi and blood circulation is blocked, presenting a deep and forceful pulse. If the pulse is deep and weak, it indicates interior syndromes of deficiency type.

3) Slow pulse (chi mai)   The rate is slow, with less than four beats per breath (less than sixty beats per minute). A slow pulse indicates cold syndromes. Qi contracts and blood flow stagnates on exposure to cold. The retarded circulation of qi and blood produces a slow pulse. If the slow pulse is forceful, it indicates an interior syndrome of excess type caused by retention of yin cold in the interior. If the slow pulse is weak, it indicates an interior syndrome of deficiency type due to deficiency of yang qi.

4) Rapid pulse (shu mai)   The rate is quick, with more than five beats per breath (more than ninety beats per minute). A rapid pulse indicates heat syndromes. Induced by pathogenic heat, the blood circulation is accelerated, the result being a rapid pulse. If excess heat is retained in the interior and the antipathogenic qi is still strong, their struggle will induce a rapid and forceful pulse. Deficiency of yin in a prolonged illness produces deficiency-heat in the interior, presenting a rapid and weak pulse. A rapid pulse may also be induced by outward floating of deficiency-yang. In this case, the pulse feels rapid, large, weak and empty.

5) Pulse of deficiency type (xu mai)   It is the general term for all the forceless pulses felt on the three regions at the three levels of pressure.

The pulse indicates syndromes of deficiency type due to deficiency of qi and blood. Deficiency of qi and blood implies weakness in activating blood circulation, thus producing a pulse of deficiency type.

6) Pulse of excess type (shi mai)   It is the general term for all the forceful pulses felt on the three regions at the three levels of pressure.

The pulse indicates syndromes of excess type. The struggle waged by the strong antipathogenic qi against the hyperactive pathogenic factor brings on excessive qi and blood, thus creating a pulse of excess type.

7) Surging pulse (hong mai)   A surging pulse is broad, large and forceful like roaring waves which come on powerfully and fade away. If a surging pulse lacks the momentum of roaring waves, it is called large pulse.

A surging pulse indicates excessive heat, and often occurs together with a rapid pulse.

Excessive heat in the interior dilates the blood vessels and accelerates qi and blood circulation, thus producing a surging pulse.

8) Thready pulse (xi mai) A thready pulse feels like a fine thread but is very distinct and clear. It indicates deficiency due to overstrain and stress or deficiency of qi and blood. It is often present in patients with weak body constitution in a prolonged illness manifesting as yin deficiency and blood deficiency. Deficiency of yin and blood means the inability to fill the vessels. Qi is also deficient and unable to activate the blood circulation, hence the thready pulse.

9) Rolling pulse (hua mai) A rolling pulse feels smooth and flowing like pearls rolling on a dish. It indicates phlegm and retained fluid, retention of food and excess heat. When excess type pathogenic factor is retained in the interior, the qi and blood circulation is activated, resulting in a smooth and flowing pulse. This pulse often occurs in women during pregnancy, indicating sufficient and harmonious qi and blood.

10) Hesitant pulse (se mai) A hesitant pulse feels rough and uneven. It indicates stagnation of qi, stagnation of blood, impairment of essence and deficiency of blood. Stagnation of qi and blood means blockage of vessels and impaired circulation of blood. This condition produces a hesitant and forceful pulse. When the essence is impaired and blood is insufficient, the vessels are not filled and blood circulation is retarded. This condition creates a hesitant and weak pulse.

11) String-taut pulse (xuan mai) A string-taut pulse feels taut, straight and long, giving the feeling of a string of a violin. It indicates disorders of the liver and gallbladder, painful syndromes, and phlegm and retained fluid.

A string-taut pulse in disorders of the liver and gallbladder is due to disturbance of the liver qi tightening the vessels; that in painful syndrome is due to tightness of the meridians and vessels; that in retention of phlegm and fluid in the interior is due to dysfunction of qi in transportation.

12) Tense pulse (jin mai) A tense pulse feels tight and forceful like a stretched rope. It indicates cold, pain and retention of food.

As cold is characterized by contraction, the vessels contract on exposure to cold, thus producing a tense pulse. The pulse is also present in painful syndromes, for painful syndromes are usually caused by pathogenic cold.

13) Soft pulse (ru mai) A soft pulse is superficial and thready, and hits the fingers without strength. It indicates damp disorders.

Pathogenic damp is characteristically viscous and stagnant, its invasion of the vessels blocks qi and blood and gives rise to a superficial, thready and forceless pulse.

14) Weak pulse (ruo mai) A weak pulse is deep and thready, and hits the fingers without strength. It indicates various syndromes due to deficiency of both qi and blood.

When blood is deficient, it fails to fill the vessels: when qi is deficient, the pulse is deprived of strength. So the pulse feels deep, thready and forceless.

15) Abrupt pulse (cu mai) An abrupt pulse feels hurried and rapid with irregular missed beats. It indicates excessive yang heat, stagnation of qi and blood, and retention of phlegm or food.

Excessive yang heat means failure of yin to restrain yang and thus produces an abrupt pulse. If this pulse is present in heat syndromes of excess type due to stagnation of qi and blood, retention of phlegm or food, or swelling and pain, it is abrupt and forceful. An abrupt and weak pulse is a sign of prostration.

Knotted pulse (jie mai) A knotted pulse is ... with irregular missed beats. It indicates exc... ...n, accumulation of qi, retention of co... ...n and stagnant blood.

Cold phlegm and stagn... 'ood block the vessels, while excessive yin n... s failure of yang to arrive. Hence the knotte... pulse.

17) Regularly intermittent pulse (dai m... i) A regularly intermittent pulse is slow and weak with missed beats at regular intervals. It is associated with declining zang qi; it also indicates wind syndromes, painful syndromes and disorders due to emotional fear and fright, or traumatic contusions and sprains.

The declining of the qi of the zang means insufficiency of qi and blood and may create discontinuation of qi flowing in the vessels. Therefore the pulse is slow and weak with regular missed beats at long intervals. The presence of a regularly intermittent pulse in wind syndromes, painful syndromes and disorders due to emotional fear and fright or traumatic contusions and sprains is due to disturbance of the heart qi leading to discontinuation of the qi flowing in the vessels.

As the process of a disease is complex, the above described abnormal pulses do not often appear in their pure form, the combination of two pulses or more is often present. The condition of a number of pulses present at the same time is called complicated pulse. The indication of a complicated pulse is the combination of indications of each single pulse. For instance, a superficial pulse indicates exterior syndromes, and a tense pulse indicates cold syndromes, a superficial and a tense pulse, therefore, indicates exterior cold syndromes. As a rapid pulse indicates heat syndromes, a superficial and rapid pulse indicates exterior heat syndromes.

2.   Palpation of Different Parts of the Body

Included is palpation of the epigastrium, abdomen, hand, foot and acupuncture points.

1) Palpation of the epigastrium Epigastrium refers to the upper abdomen, is also known as "below the heart." If this area feels hard and pain is aggravated on pressure, it indicates syndromes of excess type; when there is fullness in this area with a painless reaction to pressure, and the area feels soft, it indicates syndromes of deficiency type.

2) Palpation of the abdomen Abdominal pain which is alleviated by pressure is associated with deficiency, while that aggravated by pressure is related to excess. Abdominal distension and fullness with tympanic note on percussion indicate stagnation of qi if the abdomen does not feel hard on pressure and the urination is normal. If the abdomen feels like a rubber bag containing water, and dysurine is present, it suggests accumulation of fluid. Immovable hard masses in the abdomen with pain at a definite site indicate stagnation of blood. Unfixed soft masses or the intermittent feeling of an indefinite mass in the abdomen with unfixed painful areas indicate stagnation of qi.

3) Palpation of acupuncture points This method of palpation can be traced back to the early medical book *The Internal Classic*. One of its parts *Miraculous Pivot* says: "In order to see if the Back-Shu Point is located with accuracy, one may press the region to see if the patient feels sore or if the patient's original soreness gets relieved, in which case, the point has been located with accuracy. The fifteenth chapter of the same book also states, "When the five zang organs are diseased, the symptoms will manifest themselves in the conditions of the twelve Yuan-Primary Points with which they are connected. If we fully grasp the connections between the zang organs and their corresponding Yuan-Primary Points as well as the latter's external manifestations, there will be no difficulty for us to understand the nature of the diseases of the five zang organs."

Clinical practice in the recent years has demonstrated that during an illness tenderness or sensative reactions may occur along the courses of the involved meridians or at certain points where the qi of the meridian is converged. In gastralgia, for instance, tenderness may occur at Weishu (B 21) and Zusanli (S 36); in disorders of the liver there may be tenderness at Ganshu (B 18) and Qimen (Liv 14): while in appendicitis, it may occur at Shangjuxu (S 37) the lower He-Sea Point of the large intestine. These signs may assist in making dignosis for disorders of internal organs.

Chapter 13

DIFFERENTIATION OF SYNDROMES

Differentiation of syndromes is the method in traditional Chinese medicine of recognizing and diagnosing diseases. In accordance with the basic knowledge of traditional Chinese medicine, this method entails making a comprehensive analysis of the symptoms and signs obtained by applying the four diagnostic methods, in order to clarify their internal relationships, and ascertain their causes and nature as well as the relative strength of the antipathogenic qi and pathogenic factor, and the direction of the pathological development.

Differentiation of syndromes and determination of treatment are inseparable, one relating to the other. The former is the premise and foundation of the later. The methods of treatment, so determined, may in turn test the validity of the differentiation. Correct differentiation is a prerequisite for applying appropriate methods and attaining anticipated results.

There are a number of methods in traditional Chinese medicine for differentiating syndromes, including differentiation according to eight principles, differentiation according to the theory of qi and blood, differentiation according to the theory of zang-fu organs and differentiation according to the theory of meridians and collaterals, etc. Of these, differentiation according to eight principles is the general method. Differentiation according to the theory of qi and blood and that according to the theory of zang-fu organs are mainly concerned with endogenous diseases, while differentiation according to the theory of meridians and collaterals is principally concerned with disorders of meridians and collaterals. Each method has its own features and lays stress on a particular aspect while connecting with and supplementing the others. It is essential to understand and possess a thorough knowledge, through clinical practice, of the basic contents and characteristics of each method.

I. DIFFERENTIATION OF SYNDROMES ACCORDING TO EIGHT PRINCIPLES

The eight principles refer to eight basic categories of syndromes, namely, yin and yang, exterior and interior, cold and heat, and deficiency and excess. In differentiation of syndromes according to eight principles, these eight categories are applied in analysing various pathological manifestations determined by applying the four diagnostic methods, indicating the location of the disease, its nature and the relative strength of the pathogenic factor and antipathogenic qi.

The application of the eight principles forms the basis link, categorizing a variety of clinical manifestations in a general way. It is thus possible to understand and solve complicated problems systematically in the process of making diagnosis.

Although this method classifies pathological conditions into eight categories, they are inseparable and interconnected. Attention should be paid to this in the clinical situation in order to ensure a correct and comprehensive recognition of disease.

1.　Exterior and Interior

The categories of exterior and interior form two principles which are used to determine the depth of the diseased area and to generalize the direction of the development of a disease.

The skin, hair, muscles and their interspaces, and the superficial portion of meridians and collaterals of the human body belong to the exterior, while the five zang and six fu organs pertain to the interior.

1) Exterior syndromes Exterior syndromes refer to pathological conditions resulted from the invasion of the superficial portion of the body by exogenous pathogenic factors. They are marked by sudden onset of symptoms with short duration, and are often seen at the early stage of exogenous diseases. The chief manifestations are an intolerance to cold (or wind), fever, a thin tongue coating and a superficial pulse. The accompanying symptoms and signs are headache, general aching, nasal obstruction and cough. Clinical manifestations may vary according to the invading pathogenic factors and the body constitution of the patient. They are manifested as cold, heat, deficiency and excess. (Tab. 11)

Table 11. Differentiation of Cold, Heat, Deficiency and Excess in Exterior Syndromes

Syndromes	Symptoms and signs in common	Distinguishing symptoms and signs
Exterior cold		Severe chills, mild fever, no sweating, absence of thirst, thin, white and moist tongue coating, superficial and tense pulse.
Exterior heat	Chills, fever, headache, general aching, thin tongue coating, superficial pulse.	Mild chills, severe fever, no sweating or sweating, thirst, thin and yellow tongue coating, superficial and rapid pulse.
Exterior deficiency		Sweating.
Exterior excess		No sweating.

2) Interior syndromes Interior syndromes refer to pathological conditions resulted from the transmission of exogenous pathogenic factors to the interior of the body to affect zang-fu organs, or from the functional disturbances of zang-fu organs. Interior syndromes cover a wide range of pathological conditions and may occur in the following three conditions: transmission of persistent pathogenic factors from the exterior to the interior of the body to invade zang-fu organs; direct attack on zang-fu organs by exogenous pathogenic factors; drastic emotional changes, improper' diet and overstrain and stress, all of which affect zang-fu organs directly, leading to functional disturbances. For details of interior syndromes, refer to the differentiation of deficiency and excess, and to the differentiation of syndromes according to the theory of zang-fu organs.

3) Differentiation of exterior and interior syndromes The accompaniment of aversion to cold with fever, and changes in tongue coating and pulse are highly significant for differentiating exterior and interior syndromes in exogenous febrile diseases. Generally, fever accompanied by aversion to cold suggests exterior syndromes; fever with no aversion to cold, or aversion to cold with no fever indicates interior syndromes. A thin and white tongue coating, possible with red tongue borders, is often seen in exterior syndromes. The appearance of other abnormal qualities of tongue coating often indicates interior syndromes. A superficial pulse suggests exterior syndromes; a deep pulse suggests interior syndromes.

4) The relationship between exterior and interior syndromes In given conditions, exogenous pathogenic factors, if they are not expelled from the exterior of the body, may be transmitted to the interior, giving rise to interior syndromes. This is known as "transmission from the exterior to the interior." Pathogenic factors in some interior syndromes may be transmitted from the interior to the superficial portion of the body. This is known as "transmission from the interior to the exterior." The occurrence of the transmission mainly depends upon the relative strength of the pathogenic factor and antipathogenic qi. The transmission of pathogenic factors from the exterior to the interior is often due to weakened body resistance to disease, or to hyperactivity of the pathogenic factors, improper care, or incorrect or delayed treatment. The transmission of interior pathogenic factors to the interior is often the result of correct treatment and care, and strengthened body resistance to disease. Generally speaking, the inward transmission of pathogenic factors indicates an aggravation of the disease, while the outward transmission represents a tendency of pathogenic factors in the interior being expelled, thus indicating an alleviation of the disease.

In the process of the development of disease, there is a condition known as "the exterior and interior being diseased simultaneously." This may appear at the early stage of a disease, when both exterior and interior syndromes are seen at the same time. This also occurs when exogenous pathogenic factors are transmitted to the interior, while the exterior syndromes are still present. Prolonged endogenous diseases complicated with recent exogenous diseases, or exogenous diseases inducing acute attacks of chronic endogenous diseases may also be the causes. As exterior and interior syndromes are usually complicated with cold, heat, deficiency and excess, many different syndromes are exhibited in "the exterior and interior being diseased simultaneously," for example, exterior cold complicated with interior heat, exterior deficiency with interior excess, and exterior excess with interior deficiency.

5) Intermediate syndromes Intermediate syndromes refer to pathological conditions in which exogenous pathogenic factors fail to be transmitted completely to the interior, while the antipathogenic qi is not strong enough to expel the pathogenic factors to the body surface. The pathogenic factors thus remain between the exterior and interior. The chief clinical manifestations are alternate chills and fever, discomfort and fullness in the chest and hypochondrium, vomiting, anorexia, bitter taste in the mouth, dry throat, blurred vision and string-taut pulse. For details, refer to the Shaoyang Syndrome in the chapter "Differentiation of Syndromes According to the Theory of the Six Meridians."

2.   Cold and Heat

Cold and heat are the two principles used to differentiate the nature of a disease. According to the fifth chapter of *Plain Questions*: "Predominance of yang gives rise to heat, and predominance of yin gives rise to cold." Cold and heat syndromes are concrete manifestations of excess and deficiency of yin-yang. Distinguishing between cold and heat syndromes is important for guiding treatment.

1) Cold syndromes and heat syndromes Cold syndromes are pathological conditions resulted from exposure to exogenous pathogenic cold or from deficiency of yang in the interior of the body. Heat syndromes are pathological conditions caused by invasion of exogenous pathogenic heat or by

deficiency of yin in the interior of the body.

Since cold and heat syndromes are opposite in nature, the symptoms and signs they manifest are entirely different. Cold syndromes are revealed by aversion to cold, preference for warmth, tastelessness in the mouth, absence of thirst, pallor, cold limbs, lying with the body curled up, loose stools, clear urine which is increased in volume, pale tongue, white and moist coating, slow or tense pulse. Heat syndromes manifest as fever, preference for coolness, thirst with preference for cold drinks, redness of face and eyes, irritability, restlessness, constipation, deep-yellow and scanty urine, red tongue with yellow and dry coating, and rapid pulse.

Deciding whether a syndrome is of heat or cold nature cannot be based on one clinical manifestation alone. The correct conclusion is reached after careful observation of all the clinical manifestations. Of these, the presence of cold, heat and thirst and the conditions of complexion, four limbs, defecation, urination, tongue coating and pulse are the most important. Table 12 explains the differentiation of cold and heat conditions of excess type in interior syndromes.

2) The relationship between cold and heat syndromes Although cold syndromes and heat syndromes are opposite in nature, they have a close relationship. They can exist simultaneously, manifesting as complicated syndromes of cold and heat. In given conditions, they can also be transformed into each other, presenting either transformation of cold syndromes into heat, or of heat syndromes into cold. When the disease has developed to a very severe stage, syndromes of true heat and false cold or true cold and false heat may appear.

a) Complicated syndromes of cold and

Table 12. Differentiation of Cold and Heat Syndromes

Cold syndromes	Heat syndromes
Pallor, aversion to cold, absence of thirst or drinking a little hot drinks, loose stools, clear urine increased in volume	Red complexion, fever, thirst with preference for cold drinks, constipation, deep-yellow and scanty urine.
Pale tongue with white and moist coating.	Red tongue with yellow and dry coating.
Slow pulse.	Rapid pulse.

heat The patient may have simultaneous signs of heat in the upper half of the body, and of cold in the lower half. The syndrome like this is known as "heat above with cold below." This is one of the most frequently seen complicated syndromes of cold and heat. Clinically the "heat above" manifests as suffocation and heat sensation in the chest and a frequent desire to vomit, whilst the "cold below" presents abdominal pain which can be alleviated by warmth, and loose stools. The syndrome is often due to a complicated etiology involving both cold and heat. This leads to a pathological disharmony of yin and yang of various zang-fu organs, and manifests as excess of yang in the upper part of the body and excess of yin in the lower part.

Other frequently seen complicated syndromes are cold on the exterior with heat in the interior, and heat on the exterior with cold in the interior.

b) Transformation of cold and heat syndromes In transformation of a cold syndrome into heat, the cold syndrome occurs first and gradually changes into a heat syndrome. An example is exposure to exogenous pathogenic cold which may lead to an exterior cold syndrome and produce such symptoms and signs as fever, aversion to cold, general aching, no sweating, white tongue coating and superficial and tense pulse. If this pathogenic cold goes deep into the interior of the body and turns into heat, cold signs such as aversion to cold will subside, but fever persists and other heat signs such as irritability, thirst and yellow tongue coating will occur in succession. This indicates the transformation of exterior cold into interior heat.

In transformation of a heat syndrome into cold, the heat syndrome occurs first and gradually changes into a cold syndrome. An example is abrupt appearance of cold limbs, pallor, and a deep and slow pulse in the patient with high fever, profuse sweating, thirst, irritability, and a surging and rapid pulse. These are the manifestations of the transformation of a heat syndrome into a cold one.

The mutual transformation of cold and heat syndromes takes place in certain conditions, depending crucially on the relative strength of the pathogenic factor and antipathogenic qi. Generally speaking, transformation of cold into heat results from a strengthening of the antipathogenic qi and hyperactivity of yang qi. Constitutional deficiency of yang, or exhaustion of yang qi during the course of a disease, may lead to a failure of the antipathogenic qi in resisting the pathogenic factor, thus giving rise to transformation of a heat syndrome into a cold one.

c) True and false phenomena in cold and heat syndromes True heat with false cold refers to a syndrome in which there is heat in the interior of the body and false cold on the exterior. The syndrome is manifested as cold limbs, but a burning sensation in the chest and abdomen; no aversion to cold, but aversion to heat; and a deep but forceful pulse. In addition, there is thirst with preference for cold drinks, irritability, dry throat, foul breath, scanty, deep-yellow urine, constipation and a deep red tongue with yellow dry coating. In this syndrome, excessive internal heat hinders the yang qi from reaching the exterior.

True cold with false heat refers to a syndrome in which there is real cold in the interior and false heat on the exterior. Clinical manifestations are feverishness of the body, flushed face, thirst and a superficial pulse. However, the patient wants to cover up the body in spite of the feverishness, wants to take warm drinks to relieve the thirst, and has a superficial and weak pulse. In addition, there are other cold signs such as clear urine, loose stools and a pale tongue with white coating. In this syndrome, excessive yin cold in the interior forces the yang qi to the exterior.

It is clear that the appearance of a disease does not necessarily reflect its essential nature in these types of syndromes. Careful observation and analysis should be made, if the false and true phenomena are to be differentiated accurately. Attention should be paid to the following points: Whether the pulse is forceful or weak; whether the tongue is pale or red; whether the tongue coating is moist or dry; whether there is thirst or not;

whether the patient likes cold drinks or hot drinks; whether the chest and abdomen are warm or not; whether the urine is clear or yellow; and whether the patient wants to cover up the body or not.

3. Deficiency and Excess

Deficiency and excess are the two principles which are used to generalize and distinguish the relative strength of the antipathogenic qi and pathogenic factor. According to the twenty-eighth chapter of *Plain Questions*, "hyperactivity of the pathogenic factor causes excess; consumption of essential qi causes deficiency." Distinguishing whether a syndrome is of deficiency type or of excess type forms the basis for the determination of promoting the antipathogenic qi or eliminating the pathogenic factor in the treatment.

1) Syndromes of deficiency type and syndromes of excess type Deficiency refers to insufficiency of the antipathogenic qi, and therefore syndromes of deficiency type refer to pathological conditions resulted from deficiency of the antipathogenic qi. Excess refers to hyperactivity of the pathogenic factor, and therefore syndromes of excess type refer to pathological conditions in which the pathogenic factor is hyperactive, while the antipathogenic qi remains strong.

a) Syndromes of deficiency type Insufficiency of the antipathogenic qi of the human body may manifest as deficiency of yin, deficiency of yang, deficiency of qi or deficiency of blood, which may form different syndromes. For syndromes of qi deficiency and blood deficiency, refer to differentiation of syndromes according to the theory of qi and blood. The chief clinical manifestations of syndromes of yin deficiency and yang deficiency are described as follows:

b) Syndromes of yang deficiency and syndromes of yin deficiency   They general-

Table 13. Differentiation of Syndromes of Yin Deficiency and Yang Deficiency

Deficiency of yin	Deficiency of yang
Afternoon fever, malar flush, heat sensation in the palms and soles, night sweating, dryness of the throat and mouth, yellow urine, dry stools.	Chills, cold limbs, listlessness, lassitude, spontaneous sweating, absence of thirst, clear urine increased in volume, loose stools.
Red tongue with little coating.	Pale tongue with white coating.
Thready and rapid pulse.	Weak pulse.

ize pathological conditions resulted from deficiency of yang and yin of the body. According to the inter-consuming-supporting relationship of yin and yang, deficiency of yang leads to a relative excess of yin, and deficiency of yin leads to a relative excess of yang. In addition to the clinical manifestations of deficiency type, cold signs are seen in deficiency of yang, and heat signs are seen in deficiency of yin. However, they are essentially different from cold and heat syndromes caused respectively by excess of yin and excess of yang.

c) Syndromes of excess type   In syndromes of excess type, the clinical manifestations vary with the nature of the invading exogenous pathogenic factors and areas of the human body they invade. The following factors are mainly considered in distinguishing syndromes of deficiency type from those of excess type: Body shape, spirit, strength of voice and breath, response to pressure on painful areas, tongue coating and pulse. (Tab. 14)

Table 14. Differentiation of Syndromes of Deficiency Type and Syndromes of Excess Type

Syndromes of deficiency type	Syndromes of excess type
Emaciation, listlessness, lassitude, feeble breathing, dislike of speaking, pallor, palpitations, shortness of breath, insomnia, poor memory, spontaneous and night sweating, nocturnal emission, nocturnal enuresis, pain alleviated by pressure.	Sturdiness, agitation, sonorous voice, coarse breathing, distension and fullness in the chest and abdomen, pain aggravated by pressure, constipation or tenesmus, dysuria.
Dry tongue with no coating or little coating.	Thick and sticky tongue coating.
Pulse of deficiency type.	Pulse of excess type.

2) The relationship between syndromes of deficiency type and syndromes of excess type While syndromes of deficiency type and syndromes of excess type are essentially different, they are also interconnected, and one may affect the other. The clinical manifestations are described as follows.

a) Complication of deficiency and excess When deficiency of the antipathogenic qi and excess of the pathogenic factor manifest at the same time, this is known as a syndrome complicated with deficiency and excess.

Either deficiency of the antipathogenic qi or excess of the pathogenic factor may predominate in complicated syndromes. There are also complicated syndromes in which deficiency of the antipathogenic qi and excess of the pathogenic factor are on equal terms. Appropriate methods of treatment are determined on the basis of distinguishing which predominates and which is more urgent.

b) Transformation of deficiency and excess Although the pathogenic factor in syndromes of excess type may gradually subside, the antipathogenic qi is already injured due to delayed or incorrect treatment, thus transforming syndromes of excess type into syndromes of deficiency type. An example is a heat syndrome of excess type which manifests as high fever, thirst, sweating and superficial and rapid pulse. If the disease persists for a long time and consumes body fluid, this may transform into a syndrome of deficiency type showing emaciation, pallor, feebleness, little tongue coating or no coating, and thready and weak pulse.

In syndromes of deficiency type, insufficiency of the antipathogenic qi may impair the functions of certain zang-fu organs in distribution and transformation,

and produce endogenous pathogenic factors, thus eliciting various syndromes of excess type. Excess resulting from deficiency like this is also known as deficiency complicated with excess, or as deficiency of the root cause with excess of manifestations. In deficiency of qi of the spleen and lung, for example, dysfunction in transportation, transformation, dispersing and descending may produce endogenous pathogenic factors such as phlegm, retained fluid, harmful water or damp.

c) True and false phenomena in deficiency and excess False phenomena may appear in syndromes of deficiency type and those of excess type. Special care should be taken to distinguish them.

True excess with false deficiency refers to a syndrome of excess type which is accompanied by symptoms and signs similar to a syndrome of deficiency type. An example is accumulation of dryness and heat in the intestines and stomach, which hinders circulation of qi and blood, and elicits such symptoms and signs as indifference, a cold sensation of the body, cold limbs, and deep and slow pulse. But further examination of the patient will show a sonorous voice, coarse breathing, deep, slow but forceful pulse, distension and fullness in the abdomen, constipation, and red tongue with burnt-yellow coating. All this reveals that the accumulation of dryness and heat is the underlying cause of the pathological changes, while the symptoms and signs indicating the syndrome of deficiency type are false phenomena.

True deficiency with false excess refers to a syndrome of deficiency type which is accompanied by symptoms and signs similar to a syndrome of excess type. Deficiency of qi of the spleen and stomach, for example, may lead to weakness in transportation and transformation and give rise to distension, fullness and pain in the abdomen and string-taut pulse. However, the distension and fullness in the abdomen may be improved at times, while they usually persist in syndromes of excess type. In addition, the abdominal pain is not aggravated by pressure, and is sometimes alleviated by pressure. The pulse is string-taut, but it is also weak on heavy palpation. So deficiency of the middle jiao leading to dysfunction in transportation is the underlying cause of the pathological changes, while the distension, fullness and pain in the abdomen indicating a syndrome of excess type are false phenomena.

Distinguishing between true and false phenomena in deficiency and excess requires careful examination of the patient's pulse, tongue and other symptoms and signs. Factors such as the strength of the pulse, toughness of the tongue and response to pressure on the painful area must be assessed. In addition, the causative factors of the disease and medication taken before should be considered.

4.   Yin and Yang

Yin and yang form a pair of principles used to generalize categories of syndromes. Being the key link in the application of the eight principles, yin and yang are used to summerize the other three pairs of principles. Exterior, heat and excess fall into the category of yang, while interior, cold and deficiency fall into the category of yin. Yin and yang are also used to explain some of the pathological changes of the zang-fu organs and tissues, e.g. syndromes of collapse of vin, syndromes of collapse of yang,

syndromes of yin deficiency, syndromes of yang deficiency.

1) Yin syndromes and yang syndromes Yin syndromes refer to pathological conditions resulting from deficiency of yang qi in the body and retention of pathogenic cold. Yang syndromes refer to pathological conditions caused by hyperactivity of yang qi in the body and excess of pathogenic heat. Syndromes of deficiency type and cold syndromes come within yin syndromes; syndromes of excess type and heat syndromes come within yang syndromes. Generally speaking, so far as clinical manifestations are concerned, those characterized by excitation, fidgeting, hyperactivity and bright complexion fall into the category of yang syndromes, while those characterized by inhibition, quiescence, hyperactivity and sallow complexion fall into the category of yin syndromes.

2) Collapse of yin and collapse of yang Collapse of yin refers to pathological conditions resulting from massive consumption of yin fluid. Collapse of yang refers to pathological conditions caused by extreme exhaustion of yang qi in the body.

Both collapse of yin and collapse of yang are critical syndromes in the process of a disease. They may result from the further aggravation of yin deficiency and yang deficiency. They may also occur as a result of an abrupt aggravation in acute diseases, e.g. severe vomiting and diarrhoea or great loss of blood may elicit collapse of yin, and profuse sweating may cause collapse of yang.

As yin and yang depend upon each other, in the case of collapse of yin, the yang qi has nothing to depend upon, and therefore it dissipates from the body. In collapse of yang, yin fluid is also consumed. However, the predominating factors in the two syndromes are different, and corresponding methods of treatment must be adopted.

In addition to the various critical symptoms and signs of the disease which occur initially, sweating may be seen in the both syndromes. The distinguishing points are described as follows:

Table 15. Differentiation of Syndromes of Collapse of Yin and Collapse of Yang

Collapse of Yin	Collapse of Yang
Sticky sweat, feverishness of the body, warm hands and feet, shortness of breath, irritability, restlessness, thirst with preference for cold drinks.	Profuse cold sweat like pearls, coolness of the body, cold hands and feet, feeble breathing, listlessness, absence of thirst or preference for hot drinks.
Red and dry tongue.	Pale and moist tongue.
Thready, rapid and weak pulse.	Thready and fading pulse.

II. DIFFERENTIATION OF SYNDROMES ACCORDING TO THE THEORY OF QI AND BLOOD

This method of differentiation uses the theory of qi and blood to analyse and categorize the pathological changes of qi and blood into syndromes.

Although they form the material basis for the functional activities of zang-fu organs, at the same time, qi and blood depend upon zang-fu organs for their production and circulation. Therefore disorders of qi and blood may affect zang-fu organs, and disorders of zang-fu organs may affect qi and blood.

1. Syndromes of Qi

There are many pathological changes of qi, but they may generally be classified into four syndromes, namely, deficiency of qi, sinking of qi, stagnation of qi and perversion of qi.

1) Syndrome of deficiency of qi
The syndrome of deficiency of qi refers to pathological changes resulting from hypofunction of zang-fu organs.

Clinical manifestations: Dizziness, blurring of vision, dislike of speaking, lassitude, spontaneous sweating, all of which are worse on exertion; a pale tongue and a pulse of deficiency type.

Etiology and pathology: This syndrome is often due to weakness after long illness, feebleness in old age, improper diet, or excess of strain or stress. Insufficiency of the antipathogenic qi and hypofunction of zang-fu organs result in dislike of speaking and lassitude. Deficiency of qi also implies weakness of qi in propelling blood normally, hence qi and blood fail to go upward to nourish the head and eyes, the result being dizziness and blurring of vision. In case of weakness of defensive qi, it fails to control the opening and closing of pores, spontaneous sweating occurs. Because exertion further consumes qi, it will also cause aggravation of the above symptoms. The pale tongue is a consequence of the deficient nutrient qi which fails to go upward to nourish the tongue, and the deficient type pulse is due to weakness of qi in moving blood.

2) Syndrome of sinking of qi Sinking of qi is one of the pathological changes resulting from deficiency of qi. It is characterized by a weakness in holding ability within the category of qi deficiency. Since it often occurs in the middle jiao, it is also known as "sinking of qi of the middle jiao."

Clinical manifestations: Dizziness, blurring of vision, lassitude, a bearing-down distending sensation in the abdominal region, prolapse of the anus or uterus, gastroptosis and renal ptosis, a pale tongue, a pulse of the deficient type.

Etiology and pathology: The etiology of sinking of qi is the same as that of deficiency of qi. Dizziness, blurring of vision, lassitude, the pale tongue and pulse of the deficient type are common symptoms and signs in the syndrome of deficiency of qi. The bearing-down distending sensation in the abdominal region, prolapse of the anus or uterus, gastroptosis and renal ptosis are all possible outcomes of weakness in holding ability.

3) Syndrome of stagnation of qi The syndrome of stagnation of qi occurs when qi in a certain portion of the body or of a specific zang-fu organ is retarded and obstructed.

Clinical manifestations: Distension and pain.

Etiology and pathology: This syndrome is often due to mental depression, improper diet, invasion of exogenous pathogenic factors, or sprains and contusions. Hindrance of qi circulation is followed by obstruction of qi, which is the primary cause of distension and pain. These symptoms have the following features: Distension is more severe than pain; both distension and pain wax and wane with no fixed position; and the onset is often related to emotions and the symptoms may be alleviated temporarily by belching or flatus.

As stagnation of qi has varied causes and may involve different zang-fu organs, there exist, aside from distension, stuffiness and pain, separate clinical manifestations. For details, refer to the chapter dealing with differentiation of syndromes according to the theory of zang-fu organs.

4) Syndrome of perversion of qi In the syndrome of perversion of qi, there is a dysfunction of the qi in ascending and discending which leads to upward disturbance of the qi of zang-fu organs. This syndrome often refers to pathological changes resulting from upward disturbance of the qi of the lung and stomach, and from excessive ascending of the qi of the liver.

Clinical manifestations: Upward disturbance of the lung qi manifests as coughing and asthmatic breathing. Upward disturbance of the stomach qi gives rise to belching, hiccups, nausea and vomiting. Excessive ascending of the liver qi causes headache, dizziness and vertigo, coma, hemoptysis and hematemesis.

Etiology and pathology: Upward disturbance of the lung qi is often due to invasion of exogenous pathogenic factors or to retention of phlegm in the lung. In either case, the lung qi fails in its function to disperse and descend, but instead ascends and disturbs, giving rise to coughing and asthmatic breathing.

Retention of fluid, phlegm or food in the stomach, or invasion of the stomach by exogenous pathogenic factors may all block qi circulation and deprive the stomach qi of its function in descending. Upward disturbance of the stomach qi produces belching, hiccups, nausea and vomiting.

Injury of the liver by anger leads to excessive ascent of the liver qi and further, to upward disturbance of qi and fire of the liver, producing headache, dizziness and vertigo, and even coma, hemoptysis and hematemesis in severe cases.

2. Syndromes of Blood

There are three syndromes of blood, namely, deficiency of blood, stagnation of blood and heat in the blood.

1) Syndrome of deficiency of blood
The syndrome of deficiency of blood occurs when there is insufficient blood to nourish zang-fu organs and meridians.

- Clinical manifestations: Pallor or sallow complexion, pale lips, dizziness, blurring of vision, palpitations, insomnia, numbness of the hands and feet, a pale tongue and a thready pulse.

Etiology and pathology: This syndrome is often due to weakness of the spleen and stomach, hence qi and blood have an insufficient source, or due to excessive blood loss, or drastic emotional changes which consume yin blood. Deficiency of blood deprives the head, eyes and face of nourishment, causing dizziness, blurring of vision, pallor or sallow complexion and pale lips. Blood, failing to nourish the heart, may lead to disturbance of the mind, palpitations and insomnia appear. Numbness of the hands and feet originates from the lack of nourishment of meridians and collaterals. The pale tongue is a result of the deficiency of blood depriving the tongue of nourishment, whilst the thready pulse is a

consequence of insufficient blood in the vessels.

2) Syndrome of stagnation of blood
Stagnation of blood refers to the accumulation of blood in a local area due to hindrance of the blood circulation or to extravasated blood which has not been dispersed or immediately expelled from a fixed location in the body.

Clinical manifestations: Pain, mass tumours, hemorrhage, and ecchymoses or petechice.

Etiology and pathology: There are many causes of stagnation of blood, such as sprains and contusions, hemorrhage, retardation of qi circulation leading to retardation of blood circulation, deficiency of qi causing a weakness in the normal movement of blood, and invasion of the blood system by pathogenic cold or heat.

Pain, which is the main symptom, occurs as a consequence of obstruction by stagnant blood. The pain is fixed in location and stabbing in nature. Accumulation of stagnant blood in the local area forms mass tumours which have fixed positions and are firm on palpation. Obstruction of vessels by stagnant blood does not permit blood to circulate along the normal courses, and hence induces hemorrhage.

Hemorrhage of this sort occurs repeatedly and consists of purplish dark flow and may exhibit clots. Stagnation of blood may also manifest with purplish spots on the skin and tongue.

Cold, heat, excess and deficiency may all be causative factors of stagnation of blood, hence syndromes associated with these factors will be present along with the symptoms and signs listed above.

3) Syndrome of heat in the blood
Heat in the blood refers to the syndrome which results either from endogenous heat in

the blood system or from invasion of the blood system by exogenous pathogenic heat.

Clinical manifestations: Mental restlessness, or mania in severe cases, a dry mouth with no desire to drink, deep-red tongue, rapid pulse, possible occurrence of various hemorrhagic syndromes, profuse menstrual flow in women.

Etiology and pathology: This syndrome is often due to either invasion of exogenous pathogenic heat or to obstruction of liver qi turning into fire. Hyperactivity of heat in the blood disturbs the mind and results in mental restlessness or even mania in severe cases. Consumption of yin blood leads to a dry mouth, but since heat is not in the qi system, the patient does not want to drink. Excessive heat accelerates the blood circulation and hence a deep-red tongue and rapid pulse appear. Hyperactive heat in the blood system easily causes injury of the blood vessles, the result of which is epistaxis, hemoptysis, hematemesis, hematuria and profuse menstrual flow in women.

Acupuncture and moxibustion may regulate qi and blood. As stated in the first chapter of *Miraculous Pivot,* "Fine needles are applied to clear obstructions in meridians and collaterals and to regulate qi and blood." Another medical classic *Precious Supplementary Prescriptions* holds, "All diseases start from stagnation of qi and blood. Needling may promote smooth circulation of qi and blood...." In acupuncture clinics, suitable points are selected, and different techniques of needling and moxibustion are adopted to regulate qi and blood and to restore their harmonious states.

Appendix

Differentiation of syndromes according to the theory of wei (卫 defense), qi (气 vital energy), ying (营 nutrient) and xue (血 blood).

This method of differentiation of syndromes employs the theory of qi and blood with flexibility in the analysis of acute febrile diseases. Acute febrile diseases often occur when body resistance is weak and there is invasion of the human body by febrile pathogen or pestilential factors. They are characterized by abrupt onset of symptoms and are liable to injure yin and undergo frequent changes.

In the Qing Dynasty, Ye Tianshi attributed the occurrence of febrile diseases to the dysfunction of the wei, qi, ying and xue systems. Basically, he utilized the theory of wei, qi, ying and xue to analyse pathogenesis and differentiate syndromes, to identify the transmission and transformation of febrile diseases, and thus to determine treatment. Wei, qi, ying and xue not only generalize the pathological manifestations of febrile diseases, but also represent four different stages of pathological development in terms of the depth and severity of disease. The most superficial is the wei stage; the next in depth is the qi stage; deeper still is the ying stage, and the xue stage occurs when the disease lies deepest. Diseases of the wei and qi stages are mild and superficial, whilst diseases of the ying and xue stages are deep and severe.

1. Syndrome of the wei stage The syndromes of the wei stage refers to pathological changes resulting from dysfunction of defensive qi due to invasion of the muscles and body surface by exogenous febrile pathogen. The wei system is the exterior defense of the human body and includes the skin and muscles on the body surface. As it functions to readjust body temperature and resist exogenous pathogenic factors, it is closely related to defensive qi and the lung. Invasion by pathogenic factors may result in pathological changes of the lung and defensive qi.

Principal clinical manifestations are fever, mild aversion to wind and cold, headache, cough, absence of sweating or slight mild thirst, swelling and pain of the throat, red tongue tip and borders, a thin and white tongue coating, and a superficial and rapid pulse.

This syndrome is often seen at the early stage of acute febrile diseases. The retention of febrile pathogen at the body surface hinders defensive qi resulting in fever and slight aversion to wind and cold. Dysfunction of defensive qi in opening and closing the pores leads to either absence of or only slight sweating. Hindrance of defensive qi may also induce disturbance of the qi of the meridians, which may further cause headache. Furthermore, as the skin and body hair are related to the lung, hindrance of defensive qi may lead to dysfunction of the lung in dispersing, which manifests as coughing. The throat is the gateway of the lung, so invasion of the lung by febrile pathogen may give rise to swelling and pain of the throat. Slight thirst is a consequence of the consumption of body fluid by febrile pathogen. Red tongue borders and tip, thin and white tongue coating, and superficial and rapid pulse are signs of exterior heat.

The principle of treatment is to relieve the exterior syndromes with cool and pungent mild diaphoreties and to dissipate sweat through the wei system. The method of promoting lung qi in dispersing and descending is used in conjunction. If acupuncture is applied, points are mainly selected from the Lung Meridian of Hand-Taiyin, the Large Intestine Merid-

ian of Hand-Yangming, the Du Meridian and the Bladder Meridian of Foot-Taiyang.

2. Syndromes of the qi stage The syndromes of the qi stage are interior heat syndromes in which the febrile pathogen is transmitted inwards to affect zang-fu organs. In this stage there is fierce contension between the excessive pathogenic factor and the strong antipathogenic qi, which manifests in hyperactivity of yang and heat.

As invasion of the qi system by the pathogenic factor involves different zang-fu organs, various related pathological manifestations will occur. Frequently seen syndromes of the qi stage are retention of heat in the lung, retention of heat in the chest and diaphragm, retention of heat in the stomach, and retention of heat in the intestinal tract.

The main pathological manifestations of syndromes of the qi stage are fever, aversion to heat as opposed to aversion to cold, a red tongue with a yellow coating and a rapid pulse. These are often accompanied with mental restlessness, thirst and deep-yellow urine.

In retention of heat in the lung, cough, asthmatic breathing, chest pain, and expectoration of thick yellow sputum may be seen. Retention of heat in the chest and diaphragm may present mental restlessness and uneasiness. In retention of heat in the stomach, there may appear high fever, dysphoria, thirst with preference for cold drinks, profuse sweating, a dry and yellow tongue coating, a rapid and rolling pulse or superficial, large and forceful pulse. Retention of heat in the intestinal tract may exhibit tidal fever, constipation or faecal impaction with watery discharge, fullness, hardness and pain in the abdomen, a dry, yellow or even burnt-black tongue coating with thorns on the tongue, and a deep and forceful pulse of the excess type.

The common feature in syndromes of the qi stage is excessive heat. As febrile pathogen invades the qi system and causes a vigorous struggle between the antipathogenic qi and the pathogenic factor, excessive yang and heat appear in the form of fever with aversion to heat, deep-yellow urine, a red tongue with a yellow coating and a rapid pulse. Since the pathogenic factor has left the body surface, there is no aversion to cold. Consumption of body fluid by excessive heat leads to thirst. Disturbance of the mind by heat gives rise to mental restlessness. Retention of heat in the lung impairs the lung's function in descending, resulting in disorders of qi which manifest as coughing and chest pain. The heat in the lung condenses body fluid to phlegm, presenting profuse, thick and yellow sputum. Retention of heat in the chest and diaphragm hinders the passage of qi, and restlessness and uneasiness become apparent. When the exterior is affected by excessive heat, a persistent high fever occurs. Heat in the interior forces out the body fluid and profuse sweating results. Consumption of body fluid by excessive heat gives rise to dysphoria, thirst with preference for cold drinks, and dry, yellow tongue coating. Excessive movement of qi and blood due to hyperactive interior heat causes rolling and rapid pulse or superficial, large and forceful pulse. retention of heat in the intestinal tract combines with wastes and blocks the qi of fu organs, resulting in fullness, hardness and pain in the abdomen, constipation or faecal impaction with watery discharge. Excess of the Yangming fu organ with interior hyperactivity of heat and dryness manifests as afternoon fever, dry, yellow or even burnt

black tongue coating with thorns, and deep and forceful pulse of the excess type.

The principle of treatment is to clear heat from the qi system. Points are selected from the Du Meridian, Yangming Meridians of Hand and Foot, and meridians related to the diseased organs or areas. The method to treat excessive heat in the stomach and retention of heat in the intestinal tract is identical to that used from syndromes of the Yangming Meridian and Yangming fu organ in the differentiation of syndromes according to the theory of the six meridians.

In principle, points of the Lung Meridian of Hand-Taiyin and Large Intestine Meridian of Hand-Yangming are used for retention of heat in the lung. Points of the Pericardum Meridian of Hand-Jueyin, Heart Meridian of Hand-Shaoyin and Stomach Meridian of Foot-Yangming are usually selected for retention of heat in the chest and diaphragm.

3. Syndrome of the ying stage The syndrome of the ying stage is more severe and marked by further penetration of febrile pathogen. Ying refers to the qi in the blood, which flows internally to the heat. The syndrome of the ying stage is thus characterized by injury of ying yin and disturbance of the mind. Chief manifestations are feverishness of the body which is worse at night, dryness of the mouth without a strong desire to drink, mental restlessness, insomnia, deep-red tongue and thready, rapid pulse. In severe cases, faint skin rashes, delirium and cama may occur.

This syndrome is often a consequence of the inward transmission of diseases from the qi system, which has not been correctly treated. The further penetration of febrile pathogen injures the ying yin (nutrient yin), the outcome of which is feverishness of the body which is worse at night, and dry mouth without a strong desire to drink. As nutrient qi flows to the heart, heat in the ying system disturbs the heart, giving rise to mental restlessness and insomnia. Delirium is a sign of invasion of the pericardium by pathogenic heat, whilst faint skin rashes appear due to injury of the blood vessels by heat. The deep-red tongue and thready, rapid pulse are also signs of invasion of the ying system by heat.

The method of treatment is to clear off heat from the ying system. Acupuncture or bleeding by pricking the vessels may be adopted as auxiliary methods. Points are mainly used from the Heart Meridian of Hand-Shaoyin, the Pericardium Meridian of Hand-Jueyin and the Du (Governor Vessel) Meridian.

4) Syndrome of the xue stage The syndrome of the xue stage represents further development of the invasion of the ying system by the pathogenic factor. It arises from excessive heat stirring the blood and further disturbing the mind.

Chief manifestations are burning heat of the body, mania, delirium, obvious skin rashes; or hematemesis, hemoptysis, epistaxis, bloody stools and hematuria; dark deep-red tongue.

As the heart dominates the blood and houses the mind, injury of ying blood by heat leads to a burning sensation of the body and dark deep-red tongue. Excessive heat stirs the blood causing obvious skin rashes, hematemesis, hemoptysis, bloody stools and hematuria heat in the xue system also disturbs the mind, the result being mania and delirium.

The method of treatment is to cool the blood and to eliminate toxins. Acupuncture may assist by eliminating heat, promoting mental resuscitation, relieving convulsion and calming the mind. Points are selected

mainly from the Du (Governor Vessel) Meridian, Yangming Meridians of Hand and Foot, Shaoyin Meridian of Head and Jueyin Meridians of Hand and Foot.

III. DIFFERENTIATION OF SYNDROMES ACCORDING TO THE THEORY OF ZANG-FU ORGANS

The differentiation of syndromes according to the theory of zang-fu organs is used to analyze and synthesize the clinical data obtained by applying the four diagnostic methods. In this way the diseased zang-fu organs are identified, and the causes and nature of the disease are ascertained.

However diversified the types of diseases, and complex the clinical manifestations may be, their mechanisms are attributed to the dysfunction of zang-fu organs along with the impairment of the qi, blood or body fluid produced by the zang-fu organs. In making a differentiation clinically, the diseased organs should be identified first on the basis of their physiological functions and pathological characteristics, and then the nature of the disease such as cold or heat and deficiency or excess is distinguished according to the eight principles. Reliable information is thus provided for determining treatment. The differentiation of syndromes according to the theory of zang-fu organs is therefore closely combined, in clinical application, with the eight principles and the theory of qi and blood.

The zang-fu organs are interrelated and their diseases may affect one another. A disease may be confined to a single zang or fu organ, or two or more organs may be diseased at the same time. Proceeding from the concept of the unity of the organism, attention should be paid to the interrelation and mutual influence of zang-fu organs when making a differentiation. Only in this way can a comprehensive and correct diagnosis be made.

1. Syndromes of the Heart and Small Intestine

The physiological functions of the heart are dominating blood and vessels, and housing the mind. Pathological changes manifesting as disturbance of blood circulation and abnormal mental activities come within the diseases of the heart. Since the heart opens into the tongue, pathological changes of the tongue such as inflammation or ulceration of the tongue can be treated on the basis of differentiation of syndromes of the heart.

The physiological functions of the small intestine are dominating digestion and dividing the "clear" from the "turbid." Therefore the disorders of the small intestine are actually included in the disorders of the spleen. The syndrome of pain due to the disturbance of the qi of the small intestine is described here only.

1) Deficiency of the heart qi, deficiency of the heart yang Clinical manifestations: Both deficiency of the heart qi and deficiency of the heart yang may exhibit palpitations and shortness of breath, which become worse on exertion, spontaneous sweating and a thready, weak pulse or a missed-beat pulse. Deficiency of the heart qi also manifests as listlessness, lassitude and a pale tongue with white coating. The accompaniment of chills, cold limbs, cyanosis of lips and a pale, swollen and delicate tongue or a purplish dark tongue

indicates deficiency of the heart yang. Profuse sweating, cold limbs, feeble breathing, a feeble fading pulse and mental cloudiness or even coma are all critical signs of prostration of the heart yang.

Etiology and pathology: They are usually caused by gradual declining of the heart qi after a long illness, damage of yang qi by an abrupt severe disease or weakness of the qi of zang due to old age or to congenital deficiency. Insufficiency of the heart qi or heart yang implies weakness of the heart in propelling the blood, which explains palpitations and shortness of breath. As exertion consumes qi, they become worse on exertion. Insufficiency of blood in the vessels due to weakness of blood circulation leads to a thready and weak pulse. A missed-beat pulse is produced by discontinuation of the qi of vessels due to weakness of the heart in propelling the blood. In case of deficiency of qi and yang, the muscles and body surface fail to be controlled, spontaneous sweating results. Deficiency of qi leads to hypofunction of zang-fu organs, bringing on listlessness and lassitude. Deficiency of the heart yang deprives the blood of warmth and gives rise to retardation of blood circulation, the accompanying symptoms and signs being chills, cold limbs, cyanosis of lips and a purplish dark tongue. Extreme deficiency of yang creates an abrupt prostration and severe dissipation of zong (pectoral) qi from the body with critical signs of profuse sweating, cold limbs, feeble breathing, mental cloudiness or even coma, and a feeble fading pulse.

2) Deficiency of the heart blood, deficiency of the heart yin Clinical manifestations: Both deficiency of the heart blood and deficiency of the heart yin may manifest as palpitations, insomnia, dream-disturbed sleep and poor memory. If there are also pallor, pale lips, dizziness and vertigo, a pale tongue and a thready and weak pulse, this suggests deficiency of the heart blood. The accompaniment of mental restlessness, dryness of the mouth, heat sensation in the palms, and soles, tidal fever, night sweating, a red tongue and a thready and rapid pulse indicates deficiency of the heart yin.

Etiology and pathology: They often result from a weak body constitution, asthenia after a long illness or mental irritation which consumes the heart blood and heart yin. Insufficiency of yin blood deprives the heart of nourishment, leading to palpitations and poor memory. Disturbance of the mind results in insomnia and dream-disturbed sleep. Blood deficiency with inability to nourish upwards may produce dizziness and vertigo, pallor, pale lips, and a pale tongue. The insufficient blood in the vessels is the cause of a thready and weak pulse. Insufficiency of the heart yin produces deficiency type heat in the interior, which causes mental restlessness, dryness of the mouth, heat sensation in the palms and soles, malar flush, tidal fever, night sweating, a red tongue and a thready and rapid pulse.

3) Stagnation of the heart blood   Clinical manifestations: Palpitations, intermittent cardiac pain (stabbing or stuffy in nature in the precordial region or behind the sternum) which often refers to the shoulder and arm, a purplish dark tongue or purplish spots on the tongue and a thready and hesitant pulse or a missed-beat pulse. In severe cases there may occur cyanosis of face, lips and nails, cold limbs and spontaneous sweating.

Etiology and pathology: The syndrome often results from insufficiency of the heart qi and heart yang which causes retardation of blood circulation. The attack may be induced and the disease aggravated by mental irritation, exposure to cold after over strain and stress, or excessive indulgence in greasy food and alcoholic drinking, for all of which may elicit accumulation of phlegm and stagnation of blood. Stagnation of blood in the vessel of the heart creates palpitations and cardiac pain (stabbing pain if stagnation of blood predominates; stuffy pain if accumulation of phlegm predominates). As the Heart Meridian of Hand-Shaoyin traverses the shoulder region and the medial aspect of the arm, referred pain there occurs. Stagnation of the heart blood may cause retardation of general blood circulation, which is the cause of cyanosis of the face, lips and nails, a purplish dark tongue or purplish spots on the tongue and a thready and hesitant pulse or a missed-beat pulse. Deficiency of the heart yang and stagnation of the heart blood hinder yang qi from reaching the four limbs and body surface, and thus inducing cold limbs and spontaneous sweating.

4) Hyperactivity of the heart fire Clinical manifestations: Mental restlessness, insomnia, flushed face, thirst, ulceration and pain of the mouth and tongue, hot and deep yellow urine; hesitant and painful urination in severe cases; a red tongue and a rapid pulse.

Etiology and pathology: The syndrome is often due to mental depression which turns into fire in prolonged cases; to retention in the interior of the body of exogenous pathogenic factors turning into fire; or to excessive indulgence in pungent and hot food, cigarette smoking or alcoholic drinking, all of which produce heat and fire over a long period of time. The heart fire produced in the interior attacks the heart and results in disturbance of the mind, which is the cause of mental restlessness and insomnia. As the tongue is the sprout of the heart, the hyperactive heart fire flares upwards and causes ulceration and pain of the mouth and tongue. Consumption of body fluid by fire and heat gives rise to thirst, hot and deep yellow urine, and even hesitant and painful urination in severe cases. Flushed face, a red tongue and a rapid pulse are the outcomes of hyperactivity of pathogenic heat which accelerates the blood circulation.

5) Derangement of the mind ("phlegm misting the heart," "phlegm-fire disturbing the heart") Clinical manifestations: The syndrome of "phlegm misting the heart" often displays mental depression and dullness, or incoherent speech, weeping and laughing without an apparent reason, or sudden collapse, coma and gurgling with sputum in the throat. A white, sticky tongue coating and a string-taut and rolling pulse are present.

The syndrome of "phlegm-fire disturbing the heart" often exhibits derangement of the mind, mania, aggressive and violent behavior, insomnia, dream-disturbed sleep, flushed face, coarse breathing, constipation, deep-yellow urine, a yellow, sticky tongue coating and a rolling, rapid and forceful pulse.

Etiology and pathology: The syndrome of "phlegm misting the heart" is often due to mental depression which results in retardation of qi circulation and consequent inability of qi in distributing body fluid. The accumulation of body fluid forms phlegm, which mists the heart and produces the above symptoms and signs. Once the obstructed qi turns into fire, which changes body fluid to phlegm by condensation, the phlegm and fire intermingle and disturb the mind, the result would be the occurrence of excessive phlegm fire in the interior which manifests as mania, aggressive and violent

behaviour, insomnia, dream-disturbed sleep, a yellow, sticky tongue coating and a rolling, rapid and forceful pulse.

6) Pain due to disturbance of the qi of the small intestine Clinical manifestations: Acute pain of the lower abdomen, abdominal distension, borborygmus; or bearing-down pain in the testes referring to the lumbar region; a white tongue coating and a deep string-taut pulse.

Etiology and pathology: The syndrome is often due to improper diet, lack of care in wearing clothing appropriate to the weather, or carrying excessive weights. These may give rise to obstruction and sinking of the qi of the small intestine. Obstruction of the qi of the small intestine brings on acute pain of the lower abdomen, abdominal distension and borborygmus. Sinking of the qi of the small intestine effects bearing-down pain in the testes referring to the lumbar region. The white tongue coating and the deep, string-taut pulse are both signs of stagnation of qi.

Since the heart functions to dominate the blood and vessels and to house the mind, pathological changes with palpitations, insomnia and mental disorders as the main symptoms and signs are treated according to differentiation of syndromes of the heart. Points are mainly selected from the Heart Meridian of Hand-Shaoyin and the Pericardium Meridian of Hand-Jueyin. The corresponding Back-Shu Points are also used. The syndromes of the small intestine often manifest themselves in disturbance of the digestive function. The deficiency syndromes of the small intestine are included in the deficiency syndromes of the spleen. Their treatment is directed at the spleen and stomach. The heat syndrome of excess type of the small intestine is similar to hyperactivity of the heart fire. The painful syndrome due to disturbance of the qi of the small intestine may be included in the syndromes of accumulation of cold in the Liver Meridian. The suitable Back-Shu, Front-Mu and Lower He-Sea Points are generally selected as the main points and points of the Spleen, Stomach, Heart and Liver Meridians are used in combination, according to actual pathological conditions.

2. Syndromes of the Lung and Large Intestine

The lung is the hub of vital energy. It dominates qi, in particular, zong (pectoral) qi, which is formed in the lung; it controls respiration and takes charge of dispersing and descending; it relates externally to the skin and hair and opens into the nose. Pathological changes of the lung mainly manifest as insufficiency of zong (pectoral) qi and dysfunctions in respiration, dispersing and descending. As the lung is a delicate organ and most susceptible to cold or heat, and it relates to the skin and hair, it is often the first organ to be affected when exogenous pathogenic factors invade the body.

The large intestine functions to transmit the waste products and excrete them from the body. Pathological changes of the large intestine mainly manifest as dysfunctions in transmission.

1) Invasion of the lung by pathogenic wind Clinical manifestations: Invasion of the lung by wind cold displays such signs as cough with mucoid sputum, absence of thirst, nasal obstruction, watery nasal discharge; possible chills and fever; absence of sweating, headache, a thin, white tongue coating and a superficial, tense pulse. Invasion of the lung by wind heat generates cough with yellow purulent sputum, thirst, sore throat; possibly with heat sensation of the body and aversion to wind; headache, a thin, yellow tongue coating and a superficial, rapid pulse.

Etiology and pathology: The syndrome is due to invasion of the lung system by exogenous pathogenic wind complicated with either cold or heat. Invasion of the lung by wind cold impairs the lung's function in dispersing and descending and produces cough with mucoid sputum. As the lung opens into the nose, invasion of the lung by pathogenic cold affects the corresponding orifice and gives rise to nasal obstruction with watery nasal discharge. Since the lung is closely related to the skin and hair, invasion of the body surface by wind cold causes disharmony of ying (nutrient) qi and wei (defensive) qi, producing chills and fever, absence of sweating, and heat and body aches. A thin, white tongue coating and a superficial, tense pulse are both signs of wind cold affecting the body surface. Invasion of the lung by wind heat impairs the function of the lung in dispersing and descending, manifesting as cough with yellow purulent sputum. The consumption of body fluid by pathogenic heat is the cause of thirst. Upward disturbance of wind heat generates sore throat. The invasion of the body surface by wind heat impedes wei (defensive) qi, which explains heat sensation of the body, aversion to wind and headache. A thin, yellow tongue coating and a superficial, rapid pulse are both signs of wind heat affecting the body surface.

2) Retention of phlegm damp in the lung Clinical manifestations: Cough with much frothy or white, sticky sputum, fullness and stuffiness in the chest, gurgling with sputum in the throat, shortness of breath or asthmatic breathing; orthopnea in severe cases; a white, sticky tongue coating and a rolling pulse.

Etiology and pathology: This syndrome is often due to recurrent attacks of cough following exposure to exogenous pathogenic factors. This impairs the lung's function in disseminating body fluid, the accumulation the syndrome may result from the dysfunction of the spleen in transportation, which leads to the formation of phlegm damp. When this remains in the lung, the above symptoms will be induced or become above symtoms will be induced or become worse on exposure to pathogenic wind cold. Phlegm damp blocks the passage of qi and impairs the function of the lung qi, bringing on cough with much sputum, stuffiness in the chest, asthmatic breathing, gurgling with sputum in the throat, and in severe cases, orthopnea. Expectoration of frothy or white, sticky sputum, a white, sticky tongue coating and a rolling pulse are all signs of retention of phlegm damp in the interior.

3) Retention of phlegm heat in the lung Clinical manifestations: Cough, asthmatic and coarse breathing; flapping of ala nasi in severe cases; yellow, thick sputum or expectoration of foulsmelling bloody pus; chest pain on coughing, dryness of the mouth, yellow urine, constipation, a red tongue with yellow, sticky coating and a rooling, rapid pulse.

Etiology and pathology: This syndrome is often due to invasion of exogenous pathogenic wind heat, or invasion of wind cold which goes to the interior of the body and turns into heat after a period of retention. Heat in the lung changes body fluid into phlegm by condensation. The phlegm and heat intermingle and impair the descending function of the lung, the result being cough, asthmatic breating, chest pain and yellow, thick sputum. Phlegm heat

blocks the vessels of the lung, which leads to decomposition and thereby produces pus, effecting expectoration of bloody pus. Consumption of body fluid by pathogenic heat gives rise to dryness of the mouth and yellow urine. Failure of the lung qi in descending is the cause of constipation. A yellow, sticky tongue coating, a red tongue and a rolling, rapid pulse are all signs of retention of phlegm heat in the interior.

4) Deficiency of the lung qi Clinical manifestations: Feeble cough, shortness of breath which is worse on exertion, clear dilute sputum, lassitude, lack of desire to talk, low voice, aversion to wind, frigid appearance, spontaneous sweating, a pale tongue with thin, white coating and a weak pulse of the deficient type.

Etiology and pathology: This syndrome is often due to a prolonged cough which damages the qi and gradually leads to weakness of the lung qi. Or it may be due to overstrain and stress, or to weakness of yuan (primary) qi after a prolonged illness, either of which may cause insufficiency of lung qi and impairment of the lung's function in dominating qi. Feeble cough results from weakness of the lung qi and impairment of the lung's function in dominating qi and in descending. Shortness of breath and asthmatic breathing are the outcome of lack of qi following impairment of the lung's function in dominating qi. Insufficiency of the lung qi does not allow the qi to perform its function in distributing body fluid, the accumulation of which forms clear and dilute sputum. Weakness of wei (defensive) qi at the body surface produces aversion to wind, frigid appearance, spontaneous sweating. Lassitude, lack of desire to talk, low voice, a pale tongue with thin, white coating and a weak pulse of the deficient type are all signs of deficiency of qi.

5) Insufficiency of the lung yin
Clinical manifestations: Unproductive cough, cough with a small amount of sticky sputum, or cough with blood tinged sputum; dryness of the mouth and throat, afternoon fever, malar flush, night sweating, heat sensations in the palms and soles, a red tongue with a small amount of coating and a thre99, rapid pulse.

Etiology and pathology: This syndrome is often due to a prolonged cough which consumes the lung yin; to overstrain and stress; or to invasion of exogenous pathogenic dryness which causes insufficiency of the lung yin and, further, the production of deficiency type heat in the interior. Consumption of yin deprives the lung of moisture and allows upward disturbance of the lung qi, the result being cough with a small amount of sputum, dryness of the mouth and throat. Injury of the lung vessels by cough produces blood tinged sputum. Deficiency of yin leads to hyperactivity of fire, resulting in afternoon fever, malar flush, night sweating and heat sensations in the palms and soles. A red tongue with a small amount of coating, and a thready rapid pulse are both signs of heat due to deficiency of yin.

6) Damp heat in the large intestine
Clinical manifestations: Abdominal pain, tenesmus; blood and mucus in the stools, or, diarrhoea with yellow, watery stools; a burning sensation of the anus; scanty deep-yellow urine; possible fever and thirst; a yellow, sticky tongue coating and a rolling, rapid pulse or soft, rapid pulse.

Etiology and pathology: This syndrome often occurs in summer and autumn when pathogenic summer heat, damp and toxic heat invade the intestines and stomach. It may also be due to irregular food intake, excessive eating of raw and cold food, or intake of unclean food, all of which may injure the spleen, stomach and intestines. Abdominal pain is the outcome of retention of pathogenic damp heat in the intestines, which results in retardation of qi circulation. Damp heat injures the blood vessels of the intestinal tract and thus creates blood and mucus in the stools. Retention of damp heat in the large intestine impairs its function of transmission, eliciting diarrhoea with yellow, watery stools, burning sensation in the anus and scanty, deep yellow urine. Consumption of body fluid by excessive heat gives rise to fever and thirst. A yellow, sticky tongue coating and a rolling, rapid pulse or a soft, rapid pulse are all signs of retention of damp heat in the interior.

7) Consumption of the fluid of the large intestine Clinical manifestations: Dry stools, constipation, dryness of the mouth and throat, a red tongue with little moisture or with a dry yellow coating and a thready pulse.

Etiology and pathology: The syndrome often occurs to people in old age, to women after delivery, or in the late stage of a febrile disease when there is consumption of body fluid. Insufficiency of fluid in the large intestine leads to dryness, thus constipation ensues. Dryness of the mouth and throat, a red tongue with little moisture or with a dry yellow coating and a thready pulse are all signs of deficiency type heat due to consumption of fluids.

To treat syndromes of the lung, points of the Lung Meridian of Hand-Taiyin and its Back-Shu Point are often used as main points. To treat its syndromes of excess type, points of the Large Intestine Meridian of Hand-Yangming may be used in addition. Reducing manipulation method is applied; cupping or bleeding methods may also be used to promote smooth circulation of the qi of meridians and to restore the functions of the lung qi in dispersing and descending. The lung's syndromes of deficiency type are treated by combining points of the involved meridians, such as the Spleen Meridian of Foot-Taiyin and the Kidney Meridian of Foot-Shaoyin, with reinforcing or even-movement methods. The Back-Shu, Front-Mu and Lower He-Sea points are mainly used to treat syndromes of the large intestine. As the large intestine is closely related to the spleen and stomach in its physiological functions, the relevant points of the Stomach Meridian of Foot-Yangming and of the Spleen Meridian of Foot-Taiyin may be added according to the symptoms and signs.

3.   Syndromes of the Spleen and Stomach

The spleen functions to dominate transportation and transformation and control blood. When its qi ascends, its function is normal. So pathological changes of the spleen often manifest as dysfunction in transportation and transformation and in controlling blood and as sinking of the spleen qi.

The stomach functions to receive and digest food. When its qi descends, its function is normal. So pathological changes of the stomach often manifest as dysfunction of its qi in descending and as poor digestion.

The spleen and stomach dominate reception, digestion, transportation and transformation by sending the "clear" upwards and bringing down the "turbid." They serve as the source of qi and blood, which nourish the whole body. That is why the spleen and stomach are called the "source of acquired constitution."

1) Deficiency of the spleen qi Clinical manifestations: Sallow complexion, emaciation, lassitude, dislike of speaking, reduced appetite, abdominal distension, loose stools; or a bearing-down sensation in the abdominal region, viscera ptosis, prolapse of the anus; a pale tongue with a thin, white coating and a slowing-down, weak or soft, thready pulse.

Etiology and pathology: The syndrome is due to weakness after a prolonged illness, to overstrain and stress or to improper diet, all of which damage the spleen qi. Weakness of the spleen qi implies hypofunction in transportation and transformation, which gives rise to reduced appetite, abdominal distension and loose stools. Dysfunction of the spleen in transportation and transformation produces an insufficient source of qi and blood, the result being sallow complexion, emaciation, lassitude and dislike of speaking. Weakness after a prolonged illness hinders the spleen qi in ascending, and instead it sinks, resulting in bearing-down sensation in the abdominal region and possible prolapse of the uterus, prolapse of the anus, gastroptosis or renal ptosis. A pale tongue with thin, white coating, and a slowing-down, weak pulse or a soft thready pulse are all signs of deficiency of qi.

2) Dysfunction of the spleen in controlling blood Clinical manifestations: Pale complexion, lassitude, dislike of speaking, purpura, bloody stools, excessive menstrual flow, uterine bleeding, a pale tongue and a thready, weak pulse.

Etiology and pathology: This syndrome is due to weakness after a prolonged illness, or to overstrain and stress, either of which may weaken the spleen's function in controlling blood. Deficiency of the spleen implies impairment of its function in transportation and transformation, which produces an insufficient source of qi and blood, that explains pale complexion, lassitude and dislike of speaking. Weakness of the spleen qi indicates inability of the spleen to control blood, which leaks from the vessels and thus elicits purpura, bloody stools, excessive manstrual flow and uterine bleeding. A pale tongue and a thready, weak pulse are both signs of deficiency of qi and blood.

3) Deficiency of the spleen yang Clinical manifestations: Pallor, the four limbs being not warm; poor appetite; abdominal distension which is worse after eating or dull pain in the abdominal region which is better with warmth and pressure; loose stools; a pale and delicate tongue with white coating and a deep, slow pulse.

Etiology and pathology: This syndrome is a further development of deficiency of the spleen qi. It may also result from the intake of excessive raw and cold food or greasy and sweet food; or from excessive administration of herbs of cold nature, both of which damage the spleen yang. Deficiency of the spleen yang impairs the spleen's function in transportation and transformation, bringing on reduced appetite, abdominal distension and loose stools. Insufficiency of the spleen yang causes stagnation of yin cold and blockage of qi, the result being a dull pain in the abdominal region. The patient likes warmth and pressure in a cold syndrome of deficiency type. Deficiency of the spleen yang is unable to warm up the qi and blood and to promote their smooth circulation, thus pallor ensues and the four limbs are not warm. A pale and delicate tongue with white coating and a deep slow pulse are both signs of deficiency of the spleen yang.

4) Invasion of the spleen by cold damp Clinical manifestations: Fullness and distension in the epigastrium and abdomen, loss of appetite, sticky saliva, heaviness of the head and body, loose stools or diarrhoea, a white, sticky tongue coating and a soft pulse.

Etiology and pathology: This syndrome may be due to wading in water, being caught in the rain, sitting and sleeping in a damp place or excessive eating of raw and cold food. The syndrome may also result from excessive endogenous damp. In all these cases, the yang of the middle jiao may be strained and the function of the spleen in transportation and transformation impaired. Invasion of the spleen by cold damp impairs the spleen's function in transportation and transformation, resulting in fullness and distension in the epigastrium and abdomen, loss of appetite, loose stools or diarrhoea. As damp is characterized by heaviness and viscosity, blockage of the cold damp produces sticky saliva, and heaviness of the head and body. A white, sticky tongue coating and a soft pulse are both signs of excessive damp in the interior.

5) Damp heat in the spleen and stomach Clinical manifestations: Fullness and distension in the epigastrium and abdomen, loss of appetite, nausea, vomiting, bitter taste and stickiness in the mouth, heaviness of the body, lassitude; bright yellow face, eyes and skin; loose stools, scanty, yellow urine, a yellow, sticky tongue coating and a soft, rapid pulse.

Etiology and pathology: This syndrome is often due to invasion of exogenous pathogenic damp heat. It may also result from excessive indulgence in greasy and sweet food, or alcoholic drinking, all of which may produce damp heat in the interior. Retention of damp heat in the stomach and spleen impairs their functions in reception, digestion, transportation and transformation, causing fullness and distension in the epigastrium and abdomen, loss of appetite, nausea, vomiting and loose stools. Excessive damp heat gives rise to a sticky and bitter taste in the mouth and scanty yellow urine. As damp is characterized by heaviness and viscosity, blockage of the qi by damp leads to heaviness of the body and lassitude. Damp heat stirs up the bile which, therefore, permeats the muscles and skin, presenting bright yellow face, eyes and skin. A yellow sticky tongue coating and a soft rapid pulse are both signs of retention of damp heat in the interior.

6) Retention of food in the stomach Clinical manifestations: Distension, fullness and pain in the epigastrium and abdomen, foul belching sour regurgitation, and anorexia. There may be vomiting and hesitant bowel movements. The tongue coating is thick and sticky, and the pulse is rolling.

Etiology and pathology: This syndrome may be due to irregular food intake, voracious eating or eating of food which is difficult to digest. Retention of food in the stomach blocks the qi passage in the epigastrium and abdomen and thus causes distension, fullness and pain there. Dysfunction in digesting food brings the turbid qi upward, which is the cause of foul belching, sour regurgitation, anorexia and vomiting. Retention of the turbid part of the food blocks the large intestine and impairs its function in transmission, resulting in hesitant bowel movements. A thick, sticky tongue coating and a rolling pulse are both signs of retention of food.

7) Retention of fluid in the stomach due to cold Clinical manifestations: Epigastric fullness and pain which are worse on exposure to cold and better to warmth;

reflux of clear fluid or vomiting after eating; a white, slippery tongue coating and a slow pulse.

Etiology and pathology: This syndrome is often due to a constitutional deficiency of the stomach yang complicated by invasion of exogenous pathogenic cold; or to intake of excessive raw and cold food which causes retention of cold in the stomach. Retention of cold in the stomach blocks the stomach qi and produces epigastric fullness and pain, which are worse on exposure to cold but better to warmth, for exposure to cold may aggravate the retention while exposure to warmth may disperse cold and effect a smooth circulation of qi. Impairment of yang qi in a prolonged disease implies inability of yang qi to distribute body fluid. Thus the retained fluid is formed. If the retained fluid remains in the stomach and also disturbs upward, reflux of clear fluid and vomiting after eating follow. A white, slippery tongue coating and a slow pulse are both signs of deficient yang complicated with retention of cold and fluid in the interior.

8) Hyperactivity of fire in the stomach Clinical manifestations: Burning sensation and pain in the epigastric region; sour regurgitation and an empty and uncomfortable feeling in the stomach; thirst with preference for cold drinks; voracious appetite and getting hungry easily; vomiting, foul breath; swelling and pain or ulceration and bleeding of the gums; constipation, scanty yellow urine; a red tongue with yellow coating and a rapid pulse.

Etiology and pathology: This syndrome may result from excessive eating of hot and greasy food which turns into heat and fire, or from emotional depression which leads to invasion of the stomach by the liver fire.

Hyperactivity of fire in the stomach burns body fluid and thus produces burning pain in the epigastric region and thirst with preference for cold drinks. If obstruction of the liver qi turns into heat, it may impair the function of the stomach in descending, thus causing sour regurgitation and an empty and uncomfortable feeling in the stomach. Hyperactivity of heat in the stomach may result in hyperfunction of the stomach in digesting food, that is the reason for voracious appetite and getting hungry easily. Excessive heat in the stomach may make the stomach qi disturb upward, vomiting ensues. Since the Stomch Meridian traverses the gums, upward disturbance of the stomach fire along the meridian causes foul breath, swelling and pain or ulceration and bleeding of the gums. Constipation, scanty yellow urine, a red tongue with yellow coating, and a rapid pulse are all signs of hyperactivity of fire and heat in the interior.

9) Insufficiency of the stomach yin Clinical manifestations: Burning pain in the epigastric region, an empty and uncomfortable sensation in the stomach, hunger with no desire to eat; or dry vomiting and hiccups; dryness of the mouth and throat; constipation; a red tongue with little moisture and a thready rapid pulse.

Etiology and pathology: This syndrome may be due to hyperactivity of heat in the stomach which consumes the stomach yin or to consumption of the yin fluid by persistent pathogenic heat at the late stage of a febrile disease. Consumption of the stomach yin deprives the stomach of moisture and impairs its function of descending, the result being burning pain in the epigastric region, an empty and uncomfortable sensation in the stomach, dry vomiting and hiccups. Insufficiency of fluid in the stomach impairs the function of the stomach in receiving food, the consequence is hunger with no desire to eat. With deficiency of stomach yin the fluids fail to be sent upwards, creating dryness of the mouth and throat. Constipation, a red tongue with little moisture and thready rapid pulse are all signs of deficiency of yin producing interior heat.

Since the spleen and stomach are related externally and internally, disease of either of them often affect the other. The Back-Shu, Front-Mu, Yuan-Primary, Luo-Connecting and He-Sea Points of the Spleen Meridian of Foot-Taiyin and Stomach Meridian of Foot-Yangming are used as the main points. They are combined with points from the Liver Meridian of Foot-Jueyin and the Pericardium Meridian of Hand-Jueyin. Reinforcing or reducing needling technique, or moxibustion is applied according to actual conditions.

4.   Syndromes of the Liver and Gallbladder

The liver functions to promote the free flow of qi, dominate the tendons and open into the eye. Pathological changes of the liver mainly manifest themselves in dysfunctions of the liver in storing blood and in promoting the free flow of qi, and in disorders of the tendons.

The gallbladder functions to store and excrete the bile and thus assist in the digestion of food. The qi of the gallbladder is closely related to the human emotions. Since the gallbladder and liver are externally and internally related, the two organs are often diseased at the same time.

1) Stagnation of the liver qi Clinical manifestations: Mental depression; irritability; distending or wandering pain in the costal and hypochondriac regions; distension of the breasts; stuffiness in the chest; sighing; epigastric and abdominal distension and pain; poor appetite; belching; or possibly a foreign body sensation in the throat; irregular menstruation and dysmenorrhea in women; a thin, white tongue coating and a string-taut pulse. In prolonged cases, there may be pricking pain in the costal and hypochondriac regions or palpable mass may be present. The tongue is purplish dark in colour, or there are purplish spots on the tongue.

Etiology and pathology: The syndrome is often due to mental irritation which impairs the function of the liver in promoting the free flow of qi and results in stagnation of the liver qi, leading to retardation of the qi circulation, thus presenting mental depression, irritability, distending pain in the costal and hypochondriac regions and breasts, stuffiness in the chest and sighing. Transverse invasion of the spleen and stomach by the liver qi produces epigastric and abdominal distension and pain, poor appetite and belching. Retardation of the qi circulation allows damp to collect and phlegm may be formed; the phlegm and qi may accumulate in the throat, resulting in a foreign body sensation in the throat. Affected by dysfunction of qi, the circulation of both qi and blood is retarded and disharmony of the Chong and Ren (Conception Vessel) Meridians may result. This can cause irregular menstruation and dysmenorrhea. Long standing obstruction of the liver qi, leading to stagnation of qi and blood, may elicit palpable masses, accompanied by pricking pain in the costal and hypochondriac regions, a purple tougue or a tongue with purplish spots, and a string-taut pulse.

2) Flare-up of the liver fire Clinical manifestations: Distending pain in the head; dizziness and vertigo; redness, swelling and pain of the eyes; a bitter taste and dryness in the mouth; irritability; burning pain in the costal and hypochondriac regions; tinnitus like the sound of waves; yellow urine and constipation; hematemesis, hemoptysis or epistaxis; a red tongue with yellow coating and a string-taut, rapid pulse.

Etiology and pathology: This syndrome may be due to obstruction of the liver qi turning into fire with upward disturbance of the qi and fire or to excessive indulgence in cigarette smoking, alcoholic drinking or greasy food, which may lead to accumulation of heat and production of fire. Since fire is characterized by upward movement, the effect of the liver fire on the head and eyes may produce distending pain in the head, dizziness and vertigo, redness, swelling and pain of the eyes and a bitter taste and dryness in the mouth. The liver relates to the emotion of anger and irritability is the consequence of hyperactivity of the liver fire. Excessive liver fire burns the Liver Meridian and brings about a burning pain at the costal and hypochondriac region. When the liver fire attacks the ear along the Gallbladder Meridian, there may be tinnitus, which has abrupt onset, sounds like waves and is not alleviated by pressure. The injury of blood vessels by the liver fire may produce hematemesis, hemoptysis or epistaxis. Yellow urine, constipation, a red tongue with yellow coating and a string-taut, rapid pulse are all signs of hyperactivity of the liver fire in the interior.

3) Rising of the liver yang Clinical manifestations: Headache with distending sensation in the head, dizziness and vertigo, tinnitus, flushed face and red eyes, irritability, insomnia with dream-disturbed sleep, palpitations, poor memory, soreness and weakness of the low back and knees, a red tongue and a string-taut, thready and rapid pulse.

Etiology and pathology: This syndrome may be due to mental depression, anger and anxiety. They produce obstruction of the liver qi which later turns into fire. The fire consumes the yin blood in the interior and does not allow yin to restrain yang. The syndrome may also result from constitutional deficiency of the yin of the liver and kidney, in which case, the liver yang fails to be restrained. Excessive ascending of the yang and qi of the liver is the cause of headache with distending sensation in the head, dizziness and vertigo and tinnitus. Hyperactivity of the liver yang may produce redness of the face and eyes, and irritability. When there is deficiency of yin leading to excess of yang, the mind fails to be nourished and the harmonious state of yin and yang is broken. As a result, such symptoms as palpitations, poor memory, insomnia with dream-disturbed sleep ensue. Deficiency of the yin of the liver and kidney deprives the tendons and bones of nourishment and thus brings on soreness and weakness of the low back and knees. A red tongue and a string-taut, rapid pulse are both signs of deficiency of yin leading to hyperactivity of fire.

4) Stirring of the liver wind in the interior The occurrence of such symptoms and signs as dizziness and vertigo, convulsion, tremor and numbness, as a part of a process of pathological changes is referred to as liver wind, which may result from hyperactivity of the liver yang, extreme heat and deficiency of blood.

a) Liver yang turning into wind Clinical manifestations: Dizziness and vertigo, headache, numbness or tremor of the limbs,

dysphasia, a red and tremulous tongue and a string-taut, rapid pulse. In severe cases there may be sudden collapse, coma, stiffness of the tongue, aphasia, deviation of the mouth and eye, and hemiplegia.

Etiology and pathology: This syndrome often occurs to patients with a constitutional deficiency of yin and excess of yang. It may be induced by such factors as drastic emotional changes, overstrain and stress and excessive alcoholic drinking, all of which may further consume yin and give rise to abrupt rising of yang. Subsequently the liver wind is produced. The disturbance of the head and eyes by the liver yang produces dizziness, vertigo and headache. The tendons may be deprived of nourishment by either insufficiency of the liver yin or constitutional excess of phlegm leading to obstruction of qi and blood, and this may cause numbness or tremor of the limbs, and dysphasia. Sudden onset of rising liver yang may stir up wind and produce upward movement of qi and blood, which, in combination with phlegm fire, clouds the "clear cavity," and thus creating sudden collapse and coma. Invasion of the meridians by wind phlegm hinders the qi and blood circulation and brings on stiffness of the tongue with aphasia, deviation of the mouth and eye and hemiplegia. A red tongue and a string-taut, rapid pulse are both signs of hyperactivity of the liver yang.

b) Extreme heat stirring wind Clinical manifestations: High fever, convulsion, neck rigidity, upward staring of the eyes; in severe cases, opisthotonus, coma and lock jaw; a deep-red tongue and a string-taut, rapid pulse.

Etiology and pathology: This syndrome may occur in exogenous febrile diseases where excessive pathogenic heat stirs up the liver wind. If excessive pathogenic heat induces high fever, this may scorch the tendons, producing convulsion, neck rigidity, upward string of the eyes and opisthotonos. Disturbance of the mind by heat leads to coma. A deep-red tongue and a string-taut, rapid pulse are both signs of disorders of the liver with excessive heat.

c) Deficiency of blood producing wind Deficiency of the liver blood deprives the tendons of nourishment and thus stirs up deficiency type wind in the interior. For clinical manifestations, etiology and pathology refer to the syndrome of insufficiency of the liver blood.

5) Retention of cold in the Liver Meridian Clinical manifestations: Lower abdominal distending pain, with bearing-down sensation in the testes; the scrotum may be contracted; this pain can be aggravated by cold and alleviated by warmth; the tongue coating is white and slippery and the pulse deep and string-taut.

Etiology and pathology: This syndrome is due to invasion of the Liver Meridian by exogenous pathogenic cold which blocks the qi and blood circulation. The Liver Meridian curves around the external genitalia and passes through the lower abdominal region. As cold is characterized by contraction and stagnation, invasion of the meridian by cold may block the qi and blood circulation and thus leading to pain. Cold disperses with warmth and thus pain is relieved; when cold accumulates, the pain becomes worse. A white, slippery tongue coating and a deep, string-taut pulse are both signs of interior cold.

6) Insufficiency of the liver blood Clinical manifestations: Pallor, dizziness and vertigo, blurring of vision, dryness of the eyes, night blindness, numbness of the limbs, spasms of the tendons, scanty menstrual flow or amenorrhea, a pale tongue and a

thready pulse.

Etiology and pathology: This syndrome may be due to insufficient production of blood, to excessive loss of blood or to consumption of the liver blood by a prolonged illness. Deficiency of the liver blood deprives the heat and eyes of nourishment and may result in pallor, dizziness and vertigo, blurring of vision, dryness of the eyes and night blindness. When the liver blood fails to nourish the limbs and tendons, there may be numbness of the limbs and spasms of the tendons. Insufficiency of the liver blood empties the sea of blood, thus bringing on scanty menstrual flow and amenorrhea. A pale tongue and a thready pulse are the consequence of deficiency of blood.

7) Damp heat in the liver and gallbladder Clinical manifestations: Hypochondriac distension and pain, bitter taste in the mouth, poor appetite, nausea, vomiting, abdominal distension, scanty and yellow urine, a yellow, sticky tongue coating and a string-taut, rapid pulse. In addition there may be yellow sclera and skin of the entire body or fever. The occurrence of eczema of scrotum, swelling and burning pain in the testes or yellow foul leukorrhea with pruritus vulvae suggests damp heat in the Liver Meridian.

Etiology and pathology: This syndrome may be due to invasion of exogenous pathogenic damp heat or to excessive eating of greasy food which produces damp heat in the interior. In either case, damp heat accumulates in the liver and gallbladder. The accumulation of damp heat impairs the function of the liver and gallbladder in promoting the free flow of qi, causing hypochondriac pain. The upward overflow of the qi of the gallbladder leads to a bitter taste in the mouth. The accumulation of damp heat also impairs the function of the spleen and stomach in ascending and descending, eliciting poor appetite, nausea, vomiting and abdominal distension. Downward infusion of damp heat into the bladder brings on scanty, yellow urine. A yellow, sticky tongue coating and a string-taut, rapid pulse are both signs of damp heat in the liver and gallbladder. Once the function of the liver and gallbladder in promoting the free flow of qi is impaired, the bile, instead of circulating along its normal route, spreads to the exterior and results in yellow sclera and skin of the entire body. The presence of damp heat induces the qi to stagnate and fever may appear. Since the Liver Meridian curves around the external genitalia, downward infusion of damp heat along the Liver Meridian may produce eczema of the scrotum, or swelling and pain of the testes; and in women, pruritus vulvae and yellow foul leukorrhea may result.

The pathological changes of the liver cover a wide range. Since the liver and gallbladder are externally and internally related, disorders of the liver may affect the gallbladder, and vice versa. The two organs may thus be diseased at the same time. Principally needling is applied to treat their disorders. Points of the Liver Meridian of Foot-Jueyin and Gallbladder Meridian of Foot-Shaoyang are often used, accompanied by relevant points of the Spleen, Stomach, Kidney, Ren (Conception Vessel) and Du (Governor Vessel) Meridians according to symptoms and signs.

Reducing method is used for syndromes of excess type; reinforcing method for syndromes of deficiency type; even-movement method for syndromes complicated between deficiency and excess or syndromes of deficiency of the root cause with excess of manifestations.

5. Syndromes of the Kidney and Bladder

The kidney functions to store essence, serving as the source of reproduction and development; to dominate water metabolism, thus maintaining the balance of the body's fluid; to dominate bones and produce marrow, thus keeping the bones healthy and strong; and to open into the ear, the urino-genital orifice and the anus. Therefore, the kidney is regarded as the congenital foundation of life. Pathological changes of the kidney most often manifest as dysfunction in storing essence, disturbance in water metabolism, abnormality in growth, development and reproduction.

The physiological function of the bladder is to store and discharge urine. So pathological changes of the bladder chiefly manifest as abnormal urination.

1) Deficiency of the Kidney qi

Clinical manifestations: Soreness and weakness of the lumbar region and knee joints, frequent urination with clear urine, dribbling of urine after urination or enuresis; incontinence of urine in severe cases; spermatorrhea and premature ejaculation in men; clear, cold leukorrhea in women; a pale tongue with white coating and a thready, weak pulse.

Etiology and pathology: This syndrome may be due to weakness of the kidney qi in old age or insufficiency of the kidney qi in childhood. It may also result from overstrain and stress, or prolonged illnesses, both of which may lead to weakness of the kidney qi. As the kidney resides in the lumbar region, when the kidney qi is deficient, it may fail to nourish this area and give rise to soreness and weakness of the lumbar region and knee joints. Weakness of the kidney qi implies an inability of the bladder to control urination, hence frequent urination with clear urine, dribbling after urination, enuresis and incontinence of urine. Deficiency of the kidney qi weakens its function of storage, and thus spermatorrhea, premature ejaculation, and clear, cold leukorrhea result. A pale tongue with white coating and a thready, weak pulse are both signs of deficiency of the kidney qi.

2) Insufficiency of the kidney yang Clinical manifestations: Pallor, cold limbs, soreness and weakness of the lumbar region and knee joints, impotence, infertility, dizziness, tinnitus, a pale tongue with white coating and a deep, weak pulse.

Etiology and pathology: This syndrome may be due to a constitutional deficiency of yang, or weakness of the kidney in old age. It may also be due to a prolonged illness, or to excessive sexual activity, both of which may injure the kidney and produce deficiency of the kidney yang. In yang deficiency, the warming function of yang is impaired, hence cold limbs and pallor. Deficiency of the kidney yang deprives the bones, ears, brain, marrow of nourishment and may cause soreness of the lumbar region and weakness of the knee joints, dizziness and tinnitus. When the kidney yang is insufficient, the reproductive function is impaired with impotence in men, and infertility (due to cold uterus) in women resulting. A pale tongue with white coating and a deep, weak pulse are both signs of insufficiency of the kidney yang.

3) Insufficiency of the kidney yin Clinical manifestations: Dizziness, tinnitus, insomnia, poor memory, soreness and weakness of the lumbar region and knee joints, nocturnal emission, dryness of the mouth, afternoon fever, malar flush, night sweating, yellow urine, constipation, a red tongue with little coating and a thready, rapid pulse.

Etiology and pathology: This syndrome may be due to a prolonged illness, or to excessive sexual activity. It may also occur in the late stage of febrile diseases. In these cases the kidney yin is consumed. Deficiency of the kidney yin weakens the kidney in its function of producing marrow, dominating bones and nourishing the brain; the result is dizziness, tinnitus, poor memory, soreness and weakness of the lumbar region and knee joints. Deficiency of yin produces endogenous heat, hence afternoon fever, malar flush, night sweating, dryness of the mouth, yellow urine and constipation. Disturbance in the interior by heat of the deficiency type is the cause of nocturnal emission. Disturbance of the mind by heat leads to insomnia. A red tongue with little coating and a thready, rapid pulse are both signs of deficiency of yin leading to endogenous heat.

4) Damp heat in the bladder Clinical manifestations: Frequency and urgency of urination, burning pain in the urethra, dribbling urination or discontinuation of urination in mid-stream; turbid urine, deep-yellow in colour, hematuria; or stones in the urine; possible lower abdominal distension and fullness or lumbago; a yellow, sticky tongue coating and a rapid pulse.

Etiology and pathology: This syndrome may be due to invasion of exogenous pathogenic damp-heat which accumulates in the bladder. It may also result from excessive eating of hot, greasy and sweet food, leading to downward infusion of damp heat to the bladder. Accumulation of damp heat impairs the function of the bladder, resulting in frequency and urgency of urination, burning pain in the urethra, dribbling urination and yellow urine. Condensed by heat, the impurities in the urine form stones, which cause sudden discontinuation of urination in mid-stream, turbid urine or stones in the urine. Damp heat may injure the vessels and thus hematuria occurs. Blockage of the bladder is the cause of lower abdominal distension and fullness. Since a disorder of a fu organ may affect its corresponding zang organ, lumbago appears. A yellow, sticky tongue coating and a rapid pulse are both signs of accumulation of damp heat in the interior.

When the kidney yin and kidney yang are properly stored and kept from leaking, the kidney functions effectively. Syndromes of the kidney are mostly of deficiency type; and this is reflected in treatment. The Back-Shu Point of the kidney and points of the Ren and Du Meridians and the Meridian of Foot-Shaoyin are mainly selected. Points of the Spleen Meridian of Foot-Taiyin, Stomach Meridian of Foot-Yangming, Liver Meridian of Foot-Jueyin and Lung Meridian of Hand-Taiyin are used in combination. Moxibustion and reinforcing needling technique are applied for deficiency of yang qi. Only needling with reinforcing or even-movement technique is applied for deficiency of yin. Since the syndromes of the bladder often involve the kidney, the two organs are often treated at the same time. The Back-Shu Point and Front-Mu Point of the bladder and points of the Ren Meridian, the Kidney Meridian of Foot-Shaoyin and Spleen Meridian of Foot-Taiyin are needled with even-movement or reducing method.

Complicated Syndromes of Zang-Fu Organs

Syndromes in which two organs or more are diseased at the same time, or in succession, are known as "complicated syndromes." The commonly seen com-

plicated syndromes of the zang-fu organs are described as follows.

1) Disharmony between the heart and kidney Clinical manifestation:Mental restlessness, insomnia, palpitations, poor memory, dizziness, tinnitus, dryness of the throat, soreness of the lumbar region, spermatorrhea in dreams, tidal fever, night sweating, a red tongue with little coating and a thready, rapid pulse.

Etiology and pathology: The syndrome is often due to prolonged illnesses, overstrain and stress, or excessive sexual activity, all of which may injure the yin of the heart and kidney. It may also result from drastic emotional changes leading to obstruction of qi which turns into fire. The heart fire may become hyperactive in the upper part of the body and fail to infuse downwards to harmonize the kidney. The resulting imbalance between the heart and kidney disturbs the regulation of water and fire. When the kidney yin is insufficient, it may fail to rise up to harmonize the heart. The resulting hyperactivity of the heart fire may disturb the mind and manifest as mental restlessness, insomnia and palpitations. Consumption of the kidney essence leads to emptiness of the sea of marrow and produces dizziness, tinnitus and poor memory. Undernourishment of the lumbar region causes soreness of the back. Disharmony between the heart and kidney leads to disturbance of deficiency type fire and produces weakness in controlling the release of sperm with the symptom of spermatorrhea in dreams. A dry throat, tidal fever, night sweating, a red tongue with little coating and a thready, rapid pulse are all signs of deficiency of yin leading to hyperactivity of fire.

2) Deficiency of the qi of the lung and kidney Clinical manifestations: Asthmatic breathing, shortness of breath, and more exhalation than inhalation, all of which become worse on exertion; low voice, cold limbs, blue complexion, spontaneous sweating, incontinence of urine due to severe cough; a pale tongue with thin coating and a weak pulse of deficiency type.

Etiology and pathology: This syndrome is often due to prolonged cough which affects the lung and kidney in succession, resulting in deficiency of qi of both organs. It may also be due to overstrain and stress which injures the kidney qi and impairs the kidney's function of receiving qi. The lung controls respiration and the kidney dominates the reception of qi. "The lung is the commander of qi and the kidney is the root of qi." With deficiency of the qi of the lung and kidney, there may be asthmatic breathing, shortness of breath, and more exhalation than inhalation, all of which become worse on exertion. Deficiency of the lung leads to weakness of zong (pectoral) qi, causing low voice. Yang qi, being deficient, fails to warm up the exterior, resulting in cold limbs and a blue complexion. Deficiency of qi may cause weakness of wei (defensive) yang, which explains spontaneous sweating. Weakness of the kidney qi may impair the function of the bladder in controlling urine, incontinence of urine in coughing appears. A pale tongue with thin coating and a weak pulse of deficiency type are both signs of deficiency of yang qi.

3) Deficiency of the yin of the lung and kidney Clinical manifestations: Cough with a small amount of sputum, or with blood-tinged sputum; dryness of the mouth and throat; soreness and weakness of the lumbar region and knee joints; tidal fever, malar flush, night sweating, nocturnal emission; a red tongue with little coating and a thready, rapid pulse.

Etiology and pathology: This syndrome is often due to prolonged cough which injures the lung, giving rise to insufficiency of the yin fluid, which spreads from the lung to the kidney. It may also result from overstrain and stress, which consumes the kidney yin and thus prevents the kidney yin from nourishing the lung. In either case, deficiency of the yin of both organs results. Insufficiency of the lung yin deprives the lung of moisture, resulting in cough with a small amount of sputum and dryness of the mouth and throat. Deficiency of yin produces endogenous heat eliciting tidal fever, malar flush and night sweating. Injury of the lung vessels by deficiency type heat may produce blood-tinged sputum. Insufficiency of the kidney yin brings on soreness and weakness of the lumbar region and knee joints, and nocturnal emission. A red tongue with little coating and a thready, rapid pulse are both signs of deficiency of yin producing endogenous heat.

4) Deficiency of the yin of the liver and kidney Clinical manifestations: Dizziness, blurring of vision, dryness of the throat, tinnitus; heat sensation in the chest, plams and soles; soreness and weakness of the lumbar region and knee joints; malar flush, night sweating; nocturnal emission; scanty menstrual flow; a red tongue with little coating and a thready, rapid pulse.

Etiology and pathology: This syndrome is often due to drastic emotional changes and overstrain and stress which injure yin blood; or to a prolonged illness which consumes the yin of the liver and kidney. Deficiency of the yin of the liver and kidney deprives the head and eyes of nourishment and thus produces dizziness, blurring of vision and tinnitus. Deficiency of yin produces endogenous heat and thus results in heat sensation in the chest, palms and soles, malar flush, night sweating, dryness of the throat, a red tongue with little coating and a thready, rapid pulse. Disturbance by deficiency type fire in the interior causes nocturnal emission. Deficiency of the yin of the liver and kidney leads to a disturbance of the regulation of the Chong and Ren Meridians, hence the scanty menstrual flow.

5) Deficiency of the yang of the spleen and kidney Clinical manifestations: Pallor, cold limbs; soreness and weakness of the lumbar region and knee joints; loose stools or diarrhoea at dawn; facial puffiness and edema of the limbs; a pale swollen delicate tongue with thin white coating and a deep weak pulse.

Etiology and pathology: This syndrome is often due to a prolonged illness which consumes qi and injures yang, the disease spreading from the spleen to the kidney. It may also result from deficiency of the kidney yang with the spleen yang failing to be warmed and thus producing injury of the yang qi of both organs. Dysfunction of the yang of the spleen and kidney in providing warmth causes pallor, cold limbs and soreness and weakness of the lumbar region and knee joints. Insufficiency of yang qi does not allow normal digestion, transportation and transformation of food; the result is loose stools or diarrhoea at dawn. Deficiency of yang qi implies inability to transport and transform body fluid; the result is accumulation of harmful water and damp on the body surface, which manifests as facial puffiness and edema of the limbs. A pale swollen and delicate tongue with thin white coating and a deep, weak pulse are both signs of deficiency of yang.

6) Deficiency of the qi of the lung and spleen Clinical manifestations: General lassitude; cough with profuse, dilute, white sputum; poor appetite, loose stools; in

severe cases, facial puffiness and edema of the feet; a pale tongue with white coating

Etiology and pathology: This syndrome is often due to prolonged cough which may cause deficiency of the lung and later affect the spleen; or the deficiency of the spleen which weakens the source of the lung qi. Deficiency of qi implies hypofunction of zang-fu organs; that is the reason for general lassitude. Deficiency of qi does not allow normal distribution of body fluid, the accumulation of which forms phlegm damp. The retention of phlegm damp in the lung impairs the lung's function in descending and thus produces cough with profuse, dilute and white sputum. Dysfunction of the spleen in transportation manifests as poor appetite and loose stools. Deficiency of both the lung and spleen impairs the function of qi in circulating fluid, resulting in accumulation of harmful water and damp and producing facial puffiness and edema of feet. A pale tongue with white coating and a weak pulse are both signs of deficiency of qi.

7) Imbalance between the liver and spleen Clinical manifestations: Distension, fullness and pain in the costal and hypochondriac regions; mental depression or irritability; poor appetite, abdominal distension, loose stools; a thin tongue coating and a string-taut pulse.

Etiology and pathology: This syndrome is often due to injury of the liver by mental depression or irritation, or to injury of the spleen by irregular food intake or overstrain and stress. In both cases, the liver qi invades the spleen transversely, resulting in an imbalance between the two organs. Dysfunction of the liver in promoting the free flow of qi produces distension, fullness and pain in the costal and hypochondriac regions, mental depression or irritability. Invasion of the spleen by the liver qi impairs the spleen's function of transportation; poor appetite, abdominal distension and loose stools result. A string-taut pulse is a sign of liver disorders.

8) Disharmony between the liver and stomach Clinical manifestations: Distension and pain in the costal, hypochondriac and epigastric regions; belching, acid regurgitation, an empty and uncomfortable sensation in the stomach; mental depression or irritability; a thin tongue coating and a string-taut pulse.

Etiology and pathology: This syndrome is often due to injury of the liver by mental depression or irritation, and injury of the stomach by irregular food intake or overstrain and stress. The resulting hyperactivity of the liver and weakness of the stomach, therefore, leads to disharmony between the liver and stomach. Dysfunction of the liver in promoting the free flow of qi produces mental depression or irritability, and distension, fullness and pain in the costal and hypochondriac regions. Invasion of the stomach by the liver qi impairs the descending function of the stomach, manifesting as distension and pain in the epigastric region, belching, acid regurgitation and an empty and uncomfortable sensation in the stomach. A string-taut pulse is a sign of disorders of the liver.

9) Deficiency of both the heart and spleen Clinical manifestations: Sallow complexion, general lassitude, palpitations, poor memory, insomnia, dream-disturbed sleep, reduced appetite, abdominal distension, loose stools; irregular menstruation in women; a pale tongue with thin, white coating and a thready weak pulse.

Etiology and pathology: This syndrome may be due to poor recuperation after an illness; chronic hemorrhage; or worry, overstrain and stress. In any case, the heart blood is consumed and the spleen qi is weakened. On the other hand, a weakness of the spleen qi may fail to provide a source for the production of qi and blood, and thus make the heart blood even more deficient. Deficiency of qi and blood causes sallow complexion, general lassitude, a pale tongue with thin, white coating and a thready, weak pulse. Deficiency of the heart blood deprives the heart and mind of nourishment, eliciting palpitations, poor memory, insomnia and dream-disturbed sleep. When deficiency of the spleen impairs its function of transportation, there may be reduced appetite, abdominal distension and loose stools. Deficiency of qi and blood may weaken the Chong Meridian, and manifest as scanty menstrual flow or even amenorrhea. Weakness of the spleen qi implies inability of the spleen in controlling blood, and thus results in profuse menstrual flow.

10) Invasion of the lung by the liver fire Clinical manifestations: Burning pain in the costal and hypochondriac regions; paroxysmal cough or even hemoptysis in severe cases; quick temper, irritability, restlessness, heat sensation in the chest, bitter taste in the mouth; dizziness, red eyes; a red tongue with thin yellow coating and a string-taut, rapid pulse.

Etiology and pathology: This syndrome is often due to mental depression leading to obstruction of the liver qi which turns into fire. The upward invasion of the lung by the liver fire results in this syndrome. Obstruction of qi turns into hyperactive fire and impairs the liver's function in promoting the free flow of qi, manifesting as burning pain in the costal and hypochondriac regions, quick temper and irritability. Upward invasion of the lung by the liver qi and fire impairs the lung's descending function, leading to paroxysmal cough. Injury of the vessels of the lung by fire and heat creates hemoptysis. Flaring up of the liver fire gives rise to restlessness, heat sensation in the chest, bitter taste in the mouth, dizziness and red eyes. A red tongue with thin, yellow coating and string-taut, rapid pulse are both signs of hyperactivity of the liver fire in the interior.

Appendix: Differentiation of syndromes according to the theory of sanjiao.

Differentiation of syndromes according to the theory of sanjiao.

This method of differentiation is based upon the method of differentiating syndromes according to the theory of wei, qi, ying and xue in conjunction with the principles governing transmission and transformation of acute febrile diseases.

Acute febrile diseases result from the invasion of different febrile pathogens in the four seasons of a year. There are various types of acute febrile diseases with different features, for the invading pathogenic factors in the four seasons are different and the patients' constitutional reaction to these pathogenic factors varies. So far as the nature of the disease is concerned, there are two categories, namely, febrile pathogens, and damp heat. Pathological changes resulting from febrile pathogens are analysed with the theory of wei, qi, ying and xue, while the differentiation of pathological changes due to damp heat is described below.

1) Damp heat in the upper jiao Damp heat in the upper jiao is the early stage of invasion of the organism by damp heat. The disease is often located in the lung, skin and hair. As damp is closely related to the spleen and stomach, damp heat in the upper jiao is

often accompanied by symptoms and signs of these two organs. The main clinical manifestations are severe aversion to cold, mild fever or absence of fever, a heavy sensation in the head as if it were tightly wrapped by a cloth, heaviness of the limbs and trunk, a stifling sensation in the chest, absence of thirst, dull facial expression, epigastric fullness and distension, poor appetite, borborygmus, loose stools, a white, sticky tongue coating and a soft, slowing-down pulse.

This syndrome is often due to invasion of pathogenic damp which remains in the muscles and body surface, and blocks the spleen qi internally. Invasion of the muscles and body surface by pathogenic damp hinders wei yang, resulting in severe aversion to cold, although accumulation of damp heat may also lead to fever. Heaviness of the head as if it were tightly wrapped by a cloth is found when damp is lodged in the head. Retention of damp in the muscles and body surface causes heaviness of the limbs and trunk. Obstruction by damp of yang qi in the chest produces a stifling sensation in the chest. Since excessive damp does not consume body fluids, no thirst appears. The turbid damp clouding the clear yang gives rise to dull facial expression. Retention of damp in the spleen and stomach impairs their functions of reception, digestion, transportation and transformation, manifesting as epigastric fullness and distension, poor appetite, borborygmus and loose stools. As this is still at the early stage of the disease, damp has not yet turned into heat. Damp obstructing qi circulation produces a sticky white tongue coating and a soft, slowing-down pulse.

If damp has not turned into heat, the method of treatment is to warm and disperse damp on the exterior and in the interior. If heat signs are already pronounced, the method of treatment is to disperse heat and resolve damp. In acupuncture treatment, points are mainly selected from the Yangming Meridians of Hand and Foot and the Taiyin Meridians of Hand and Foot according to symptoms and signs.

2) Damp heat in the middle jiao Damp heat in the middle jiao is the middle stage of a damp heat disease, which exhibits mainly symptoms and signs of invasion of the spleen and stomach by damp. Obstruction of the middle jiao may affect both the upper and lower jiao, thus manifesting as fever which is indistinct at the first touch of the skin, but becomes pronounced after being felt for a rather long time; or fever which recurs after reduced by sweating; or fever which is more pronounced in the afternoon. In addition there may be heaviness of the limbs and trunk, distension and fullness in the chest and epigastrium, nausea, vomiting, anorexia, thirst with desire to drink only a little, scanty and deep-yellow urine, losse but hesitant stools; and in severe cases, dull facial expression with few words said or mental cloudiness; a sticky white tongue coating with a yellow tinge and a soft, rapid pulse.

This syndrome may result from transmission of damp heat in the upper jiao, or from invasion of pathogenic summer heat and damp. In either case the spleen and stomach are injured. It may also be due to improper diet which produces damp heat. Excessive damp heat with heat wrapped in damp gives rise to fever which is indistinct at the first touch of the skin, and becomes pronounced after being felt for a rather long time; and to fever which is worse in the afternoon. Damp heat is lingering and difficult to be resolved, this is the cause of recurrent fever. Retention of damp heat

causes retardation of qi circulation and hence dysfunction in ascending and descending. This results in distension and fullness in the chest and epigastrium, nausea, vomiting and anorexia. Heat consumes body fluid, but as damp dominates over heat, there is a thirst with desire to drink only a little. Retention of damp heat in the middle jiao impairs the spleen's function in transportation. This aspect of retardation of qi circulation is evidenced in the scanty and deep-yellow urine and the loose but hesitant stools. Obstruction of the clear cavity by damp heat gives rise to a dull facial expression with few words said, or mental cloudiness, the sticky white tongue coating with a yellow tinge and the soft, rapid pulse are both signs of damp heat.

The method of treatment is to clear off heat, resolve damp and promote the smooth circulation of qi. In acupuncture treatment, the main points are selected from the Spleen Meridian of Foot-Taiyin and the Stomach Meridian of Foot-Yangming.

3) Damp heat in the lower jiao Damp heat lodged in the lower jiao mainly affects the large intestine and bladder and hence manifests as abnormal urination and defecation. The symptoms and signs are retention of urine, thirst with desire to drink only a little, constipation, hardness and fullness in the lower abdomen, a sticky yellow or white tongue coating and a soft rapid pulse.

Damp heat retained in the bladder impairs its function of controlling urine, this explains retention of urine. Accumulation of damp in the lower jiao prevents body fluid from rising and a thirst with desire to drink only small quantities ensues. Damp retained in the large intestine impairs its function of transmission, blocking the qi of the fu organ and causing constipation and hardness and fullness in the lower abdomen. The sticky yellow or white tongue coating and the soft, rapid pulse are both signs of damp heat.

The method of treatment is to conduct the turbid downwards and relieve accumulation. In acupuncture treatment, points are mainly selected from the Ren Meridian, Bladder, Spleen and Stomach Meridians.

IV. DIFFERENTIATION OF SYNDROMES ACCORDING TO THE THEORY OF MERIDIANS AND COLLATERALS

This method uses the theory of meridians and collaterals to identify pathological changes according to the areas traversed by them and according to their related zang-fu organs. As meridians are the main pathways in the system, their pathological manifestations may be used as primary evidence in making differentiation.

1. Pathological Manifestations of the Twelve Meridians

As each of the twelve meridians is identified by its specific pathway and its relation with the specific zang-fu organ, the pathological manifestations of disorders of the twelve meridians may be grouped under two headings:

Dysfunction of the zang-fu organ to which the diseased meridian is related.

Disorders of the area supplied by the meridian.

Hence, the pathological manifestations of the twelve meridians are described as follows.

a) The Lung Meridian of Hand-Taiyin Cough, asthmatic breathing, hemoptysis, congested and sore throat, a sensation of fullness in the chest; pain in the supraclavicular fossa, shoulder, back and anterior border of the medial aspect of the arm.

b) The Large Intestine Meridian of Hand-Yangming Epistaxis, watery nasal discharge, toothache, congested and sore throat; pain in the neck, anterior part of the shoulder and anterior border of the lateral aspect of the upper limb; borborygmus, abdominal pain, diarrhea and dysentery.

c) The Stomach Meridian of Foot-Yangming Borborygmus, abdominal distension, edema, epigastric pain, vomiting, hunger, epistaxis, deviation of the mouth, congested and sore throat; pain in the chest, abdomen and lateral aspect of the lower limbs; fever and mania.

d) The Spleen Meridian of Foot-Taiyin Belching, vomiting, epigastric pain, abdominal distension, loose stools, jaundice, heaviness of the body, lassitude, stiffness and pain in the root of the tongue, swelling and coldness in the medial aspect of the thigh and knee.

e) The Heart Meridian of Hand-Shaoyin Cardiac pain, palpitations, hypochondriac pain, insomnia, night sweating, dryness of the throat, thirst, pain in the medial aspect of the upper arm and heat sensation in the palms.

f) The Small Intestine Meridian of Hand-Taiyang Deafness, yellow sclera, sore throat, swelling of the cheeks, distension and pain in the lower abdomen and pain in the posterior border of the lateral aspect of the shoulder and arm.

g) The Bladder Meridian of Foot-

Taiyang Retention of urine, enuresis, manic and depressive mental disorders, malaria, pain of the eyes, lacrimation when exposed to wind, nasal obstruction, rhinorrhea, epistaxis, headache; and pain in the nape, back, low back, buttocks and posterior aspect of the lower limbs.

h) The Kidney Meridian of Foot-Shaoyin Enuresis, frequent urination, nocturnal emission, impotence, irregular menstruation, asthmatic breathing, hemoptysis, dryness of the tongue, congested and sore throat, edema, pain in the lumbar region and in the posteriomedial aspect of the thigh, weakness of the lower limbs and heat sensation in the soles.

i) The Pericardium Meridian of Hand-Jueyin Cardiac pain, palpitations, mental restlessness, stuffiness in the chest, flushed face, swelling in the axilla, depressive and manic mental disorders, spasm of the upper limbs and heat sensation in the palms.

j) The Sanjiao (Triple Energizer) Meridian of Hand-Shaoyang Abdominal distension, edema, enuresis, dysuria, deafness, tinnitus, pain in the outer canthus, swelling of the cheeks, congested and sore throat; and pain in the retroauricular region, shoulder, and lateral aspect of the arm and elbow.

k) The Gallbladder Meridian of Foot-Shaoyang Headache, pain in the outer canthus, pain in the jaw, blurring of vision, bitter taste in the mouth, swelling and pain in the supraclavicular fossa, pain in the axilla; and pain along the lateral aspect of the chest, hypochondrium, thigh and lower limbs.

l) The Liver Meridian of Foot-Jueyin Low back pain, fullness in the chest, pain in the lower abdomen, hernia, vertical headache, dryness of the throat, hiccups, enuresis, dysuria and mental disturbance.

2. Pathological Manifestations of the Eight Extra Meridians

The eight extra meridians function to strengthen the relationship between the twelve regular meridians and regulate their qi and blood. They are closely related to the liver and kidney as well as the extra ordinary organs such as the uterus, brain and marrow. On the basis of their physiological functions and the areas they traverse, the pathological manifestations of the eight extra meridians are briefly described below.

a) The Du (Governor Vessel) Meridian Stiffness and pain in the spinal column, opisthotonos, headache and epilepsy.

b) The Ren (Conception Vessel) Meridian Leukorrhea, irregular menstruation, infertility in both women and men, hernia, nocturnal emission, enuresis, retention of urine, pain in the epigastric region and lower abdomen, and pain in the genital region.

c) The Chong Meridian Spasm and pain in the abdomen, irregular menstruation, infertility in both women and men, and asthmatic breathing.

d) The Dai Meridian Distension and fullness in the abdomen, weakness of the lumbar region, leukorrhea, prolapse of the uterus; and muscular atrophy, weakness and motor impairment of the lower limbs.

e) The Yangqiao Meridian Epilepsy, insomnia, redness and pain in the inner canthus, pain in the back and lumbar region, eversion of the foot and spasm of the lower limbs.

f) The Yinqiao Meridian Epilepsy, lethargy, pain in the lower abdomen; pain in the lumbar and hip regions referring to the public region; spasm of the lower limbs and inversion of the foot.

g) The Yangwei Meridian Exterior syndromes such as chills and fever.

h) The Yinwei Meridian Interior syndromes such as chest pain, cardiac pain and stomachache.

3. Pathological Manifestations of the Fifteen Collaterals

Each of the fourteen meridians (i.e. the twelve regular meridians, the Ren Meridian and Du Meridian, has a collateral, and in addition there is the Major Collateral of the spleen. They branch off from their respective meridians on the four extremities and circulate over the body surface. They function to strengthen the relation between each pair of externally and internally related meridians and transport qi and blood to various tissues and organs of the human body. Supplementary to the pathological manifestations of the meridians, the pathological manifestations of the collaterals are listed below.

a) The Collateral of Hand-Taiyin Heat sensations in the wrist and palm, shortness of breath, enuresis and frequent urination.

b) The Collateral of Hand-Shaoyin Fullness in the chest and diaphragm and aphasia.

c) The Collateral of Hand-Jueyin Cardiac pain and mental restlessness.

d) The Collateral of Hand-Yangming Toothache, deafness, a cold sensation in the teeth, and a stifling sensation in the chest and diaphragm.

e) The Collateral of Hand-Taiyang Weakness of joints, muscular atrophy and motor impairment of the elbow, and warts on the skin.

f) The Collateral of Hand-Shaoyang Spastic or flaccid cubital joint.

g) The Collateral of Foot-Yangming Depressive and manic mental disorders, muscular atrophy and weakness in the lower leg, congested and sore throat, and sudden hoarseness of voice.

h) The Collateral of Foot-Taiyang Nasal obstruction, watery nasal discharge, headache, pain in the back and epistaxis.

i) The Collateral of Foot-Shaoyang Coldness in the foot, paralysis of the lower limbs and inability to stand erect.

j) The Collateral of Foot-Taiyin Abdominal spasm, and cholera with vomiting and diarrhoea.

k) The Collateral of Foot-Shaoyin Retention of urine, lumbago, mental restlessness and stifling sensation in the chest.

l) The Collateral of Foot-Jueyin Priapism, pruritus in the public region, swelling of the testes and hernia.

m) The Collateral of Ren Meridian Distending pain and pruritus of abdominal skin tissues.

n) The Collateral of the Du Meridian Stiffness of the spinal column, a heavy sensation in the head, and tremor of the head.

o) The Major Collateral of the Spleen General aching, and weakness of the joints of the four limbs.

Appendix: Differentiation of syndromes according to the theory of the six meridians

Differentiation of syndromes according to the theory of the six meridians and subsequent determination of treatment belong to the theoretical system expounded in the book *On Febrile Diseases Due to*

Invasion of Cold. It represents the development and application of the theory of meridians and collaterals from *The Internal Classic.* This method is mainly used in the differentiation of exogenous diseases. The pathological manifestations of these exogenous diseases at different stages of development are classified into six syndromes according to their characteristics. These are Taiyang, Yangming and Shaoyang syndromes, and Taiyin, Shaoyin and Jueyin syndromes. The former three are known as the three yang syndromes, while the latter three are referred to as the three yin syndromes.

Differentiation of syndromes according to the theory of six meridians is closely related to the meridians and zang-fu organs. In terms of the meridians, the Taiyang, Yangming and Shaoyang Meridians traverse the posterior, anterior and lateral aspects of the body respectively. Consequently Taiyang syndrome may exhibit neck rigidity and pain in the posterior aspect of the head and neck; Yangming syndrome may manifest as flushed face, and fullness and pain in the abdomen; and in Shaoyang syndrome, fullness and distension in the costal and hypochondriac regions are present. As for the three yin syndromes, the abdominal pain and diarrhoea of Taiyin syndrome, the dryness of the mouth and throat of Shaoyin syndrome, and the pain and heat sensation in the heart, and vertical pain of Jueyin syndrome all relate to areas the three yin meridians traverse. When correlated to the zang-fu organs, the three yang syndromes identify pathological changes of the six fu organs. The bladder, for example, is the fu organ of Taiyang. When pathogenic factors are transmitted from the meridian to the fu organ, hence affecting the function of the bladder, retention of harmful water and dysuria may appear. The downward transmission of dryness and heat of the stomach, the fu of Yangming, may lead to symptoms and signs of the gastrointestinal tract such as constipation, and abdominal pain which is aggravated by pressure. Pathogenic invasion of the gallbladder, the fu of Shaoyang, may give rise to a bitter taste in the mouth and hypochondriac pain. Similarly, differentiation of the three yin syndromes is based upon pathological changes of the five zang organs. Examples are deficiency of the spleen yang in Taiyin syndrome, deficiency of the heart and kidney is Shaoyin syndrome and disturbance of the liver qi in Jueyin syndrome. Thus, it can be seen that differentiation of syndromes according to the theory of the six meridians reflects pathological changes of the meridians and zang-fu organs. Integral to this method of differentiation is the analysis of the stages of pathological development, including rules governing the transmission and transformation of diseases that result from the invasion of exogenous pathogenic cold. In this context it cannot be equated with differentiation of syndromes according to the theories of meridians and collaterals, and zang-fu organs.

Differentiating syndromes according to the six meridians entails making an analysis and synthesis of various pathological manifestations of exogenous diseases and their development in terms of the strength of resistance to the disease, the virulence of the pathogenic factors and the depth of disease. In this way, the pathology is determined, which subsequently serves as a guide to treatment. In the three yang syndromes, the antipathogenic qi is strong and the pathogenic factor is hyperactive; the disease tends to be active, manifesting syndromes of heat and excess nature. Treatment is aimed at eliminating the pathogenic factors. In the three yin syndromes, the pathogenic factor is hyperactive, while resistance to the disease is weak; the disease tends to be inactive manifesting syndromes of cold and deficiency nature. In this case the emphasis of the treatment is laid on promoting the antipathogenic qi.

Although syndromes of the six meridians differ, they are interrelated. Generally, exogenous diseases develop from the exterior to the interior. However, there are exceptions such as concurrent diseases in which there is a simultaneous onset of disease in two or three meridians; overlapping of diseases in which another meridian is affected even before the previously affected meridian has been cured; direct invasion of one of the six meridians by exogenous pathogenic factors; and transmission of diseases between a pair of externally and internally related meridians. In order to arrive at a correct diagnosis and hence to obtain the anticipated results from treatment, a good command of the basic and complicated syndromes is required.

1) Taiyang syndrome The Taiyang syndrome is an exterior syndrome often seen at the initial stage of exogenous disease. The main pathological manifestations are fever, aversion to cold, stiffness and pain at the posterior aspect of the head and neck, and a superficial pulse.

Taiyang dominates the exterior of the body, serving as the screen to the six meridians. When pathogenic wind cold invades the body, Taiyang is the first to be affected. Hindrance of wei yang from dispersing induces fever and aversion to cold. Injury of the Taiyang Meridian by pathogenic factors leads to disorders of the qi of the meridian, which, by its pathway, manifests as stiffness and pain of the posterior aspect of the head and neck. A superficial pulse appears when the pathogenic factor invades the muscles and body surface, and the antipathogenic qi moves outwards to resist it. As patients have different body constitutions and the invading pathogenic factors may differ in nature and severity, pathological changes and clinical manifestations of the Taiyang syndrome will vary. Sweating with a superficial and slowing-down pulse suggests invasion of Taiyang by wind, while absence of sweating with a superficial and tense pulse points to invasion of Taiyang by cold. Acupuncture treatment is aimed at eliminating exterior syndromes and promoting smooth circulation of the qi of the meridian. Points are selected from the Du Meridian and the Taiyang Meridians of Hand and Foot.

2) Shaoyang syndrome The Shaoyang syndrome is an outcome of the transmission and transformation of the Taiyang syndrome. The pathogenic factors have left the exterior represented by Taiyang, but yet they have not reached the interior represented by Yangming. Since the pathogenic factors remain between the exterior and interior, the Shaoyang syndrome is actually an intermediate syndrome. Its main pathological manifestations are alternate chills and fever, fullness in the costal and hypochondriac regions, anorexia, mental restlessness, vomiting, a bitter taste in the mouth, dryness of the throat, blurring of vision and a string-taut pulse.

When the pathogenic factor invades Shaoyang, it contends with the antipathogenic qi between the exterior and the interior. Subsequently, the qi circulation is hindered and its ascending and descending function is impaired. Alternate chills and fever are the outcome of the struggle between the pathogenic factor and the antipathogenic qi. Pathogenic invasion of the Shaoyang Meridian specifically leads to disorders of the qi of the meridian, which, as determined by its pathway, manifests as fullness in the costal and hypochondriac regions. Anorexia and vomiting are due to upward disturbance of the stomach qi, when the pathogenic factor in Shaoyang has reached the stomach. Inward disturbance of Shaoyang fire results in mental restlessness. Upward attack of the fire of the gallbladder along the Shaoyang Meridian produces a bitter taste in the mouth, dryness of the throat and blurring of vision. Obstruction of the qi of the liver and gallbladder causes string-taut pulse. The method of treatment is to harmonize Shaoyang by selecting points from the Shaoyang and Jueyin meridians.

3) Yangming syndrome   The Yangming syndrome represents a stage of extreme struggle between the antipathogenic qi and the pathogenic factor. It is an interior heat syndrome of excess type. In terms of location and characteristics of pathological manifestations, the Yangming syndrome can be classified into two categories, namely, syndrome of the Yangming Meridian and syndrome of the Yangming fu organ. Insubstantial heat spreading all over the body suggests the syndrome of the Yangming Meridian; substantial heat accumulating in the fu organs indicates the syndrome of the Yangming fu organ.

a) The main pathological manifestations of the syndrome of the Yangming Meridian are high fever, profuse sweating, extreme thirst, flushed face, mental restlessness, a dry, yellow tongue coating and a superficial and forceful pulse.

Pathogenic invasion of Yangming leads to hyperactivity of endogenous heat, which results in high fever and flushed face. Heat expells and consumes body fluids, which results in profuse sweating, extreme thirst and a dry, yellow tongue coating. Excessive Yangming heat disturbs the mind, which is expressed as mental restlessness and irritability. The strength of both the antipathogenic qi and the pathogenic factor accompanied with vigorous endogenous heat causes the superficial and forceful pulse. The method of treatment is to clear off heat using points of the Yangming Meridians of Hand and Foot and the Du Meridian.

b) The syndrome of the Yangming fu organ exhibits pathological manifestations such as feverishness of the body which is more pronounced in the afternoon, constipation, fullness and pain in the abdomen aggravated by pressure, restlessness, delirium, a dry yellow tongue coating or burnt-yellow coating with thorns on the tongue, and a deep and forceful pulse of excess type.

When the interior heat of Yangming mingles with the dry faeces, the qi of the fu organ is obstructed producing constipation and a fullness, also pain in the abdomen which may be aggravated by pressure. The accumulation of heat in the interior and flourishing of the qi of the Yangming Meridian in the afternoon combine to exhibit feverishness of the body which is more pronounced in the afternoon. The upward attack of pathogenic dryness and heat mixed with turbid qi disturbs the mind, manifesting as restlessness and delirium. The dry yellow tongue coating or burnt-yellow coating with thorns on the tongue, and the deep, forceful pulse of excess type are the consequences of consumption of body fluid by excessive heat and accumulation of dry faeces in the interior. The method of purgation is used in the treatment. Principally, the Front-Mu Points and Lower He-Sea Points of the Yangming Meridians of Hand and Foot are selected. Points of the Spleen Meridian of Foot-Taiyin may be used in conjunction.

4) Taiyin syndrome The Taiyin syndrome refers to a cold syndrome of deficiency type resulting from deficiency of the spleen qi and retention of cold damp in the interior. Its main pathological manifestations are abdominal fullness, vomiting, poor appetite, diarrhoea, abdominal pain which is alleviated with warmth or pressure, absence of thirst, a pale tongue with a white coating, and a slow or slowing-down pulse.

This syndrome is often due to constitutional deficiency of the spleen yang, direct invasion by pathogenic cold or inappropriate treatment of the three yang syndromes.

Insufficiency of the yang of the middle jiao implies not only dysfunction of the spleen in transportation and transformation, hence resulting in retention of cold damp in the interior, but also abnormal ascent and descent of qi which is the cause of abdominal fullness and pain, diarrhoea, vomiting and a poor appetite. As it is a cold syndrome of deficiency type, the abdominal pain can be alleviated by warmth or pressure. This is also the cause of the absence of thirst, the pale tongue with white coating and the slow or slowing-down pulse.

The method of treatment is to warm up the middle jiao and to disperse cold. The Back-Shu, Front-Mu and He-Sea Points of the Spleen Meridian of Foot-Taiyin and the Stomach Meridian of Foot-Yangming are selected as well as points from the Ren Meridian. Both needling and moxibustion are used.

5) Shaoyin syndrome The Shaoyin syndrome refers to pathological changes of the heart and kidney. When Shaoyin is diseased, the antipathogenic qi is extremely deficient. That is why the Shaoyin syndrome is characterized by systemic weakness. In the Shaoyin syndrome, there is hypofunction of the heart and kidney, manifesting either as deficiency of yang leading to excess of yin or deficiency of yin leading to hyperactivity of fire. When yang is deficient and yin is excessive, the pathogenic factors, influenced by excessive yin, turn into cold. When yin is deficient leading to hyperactivity of fire, the pathogenic factors turn into heat.

a) The cold syndrome of Shaoyin This syndrome principally exhibits aversion to cold, lying in a curled up position, listlessness with desire to sleep, cold limbs, diarrhoea with undigested food, absence of thirst or preference for hot drinks, profuse, clear urine, a pale tongue with white coating and a deep, feeble and thready pulse.

This syndrome is often due to deficiency of yang of the heart and kidney complicated with direct invasion of Shaoyin by exogenous pathogenic cold.

Deficiency of yang implies failure to warm up the body, the consequences are aversion to cold, lying in a curled up position and cold limbs. Furthermore, insufficiency of *yang qi* leads to listlessness with a desire to sleep. Deficiency of yang of Shaoyin deprives the spleen of warmth, therefore impairing its function in transportation and transformation and causing diarrhoea with undigested food. Deficiency of yang leading to excess of cold may also manifest as absence of thirst. But thirst may appear if yang deficiency of the lower jiao does not allow upward distribution of body fluids, or if excessive diarrhoea consumes body fluids. In either case, the patient prefers hot drinks and does not drink large quantities. Copious, clear urine, a pale tongue with white coating and a deep, and thready pulse are all signs of yang deficiency resulting in yin excess.

The method of treatment is to recover yang and eliminate cold. Points are selected from the Ren Meridian, Kidney Meridian of Foot-Shaoyin and Spleen Meridian of Foot-Taiyin. Both acupuncture and moxibustion should be used with the emphasis placed on moxibustion.

b) The heat syndrome of Shaoyin The main pathological manifestations are mental restlessness, insomnia, dryness of the mouth and throat, deep-yellow urine, a red or deep-red tongue, and a rapid, thready pulse.

This syndrome is often due to persistence of pathogenic heat which consumes the kidney yin, or to constitutional deficiency of yin complicated with pathogenic invasion which subsequently turns into heat.

Deficiency of the kidney yin leads to hyperactivity of the heart fire and a disturbance of the balance between water and fire, this explains mental restlessness and insomnia. As heat consumes the kidney yin, dryness of the mouth and throat, a red or deep-red tongue ensue. Deficiency of yin and hyperactivity of fire give rise to a rapid, thready pulse.

The method of treatment is to nourish yin and clear off fire. Points are selected from the Heart Meridian of Hand-Shaoyin and Kidney Meridian of Foot-Shaoyin.

6) Jueyin syndrome Jueyin means that yin is on the verge of extinction, while yang is starting to grow, and that there is yang within yin. When Jueyin is diseased, the antipathogenic qi is exhausted, and there is derangement of the balance between yin and yang. Hence this manifests principally as a complicated syndrome of cold and heat. The main symptoms and signs are emaciation, thirst, feeling of a stream of air ascending to the chest region, a hot and painful sensation in the chest, hunger with no desire to eat, cold limbs, diarrhoea, and vomiting or vomiting of round worms.

In this syndrome, there is heat in the liver and gallbladder, and cold and deficiency in the stomach and intestine. The syndrome is characterized by complication of cold and heat, disturbance of qi and poor transportation and transformation of food. Consumption of body fluids by pathogenic heat induces emaciation and thirst. Upward movement of yang heat gives rise to a feeling of a stream of air ascending and a hot and painful sensation in the chest. Hyperfunction of the liver in promoting the free flow of qi results in hunger. But the stomach and intestines are cold and deficient which does not allow normal digestion and transmission of food; this explains hunger with no desire to eat. Disturbance of qi in the stomach and intestines may cause vomiting and diarrhoea. When yang qi fails to reach the four limbs, there will be cold.

The warming method is combined with the method of clearing off heat in the treatment; the method of simultaneous elimination and reinforcement is adopted. Points are selected from the Liver Meridian of Foot-Jueyin, Ren Meridian and Gallbladder Meridian of Foot-Shaoyang. Points of the Spleen Meridian of Foot-Taiyin are used in conjunction.

Chapter 14

ACUPUNCTURE TECHNIQUES

Acupuncture is a procedure by which diseases can be prevented and treated through proper insertion of needles into points accompanied by different manipulations. Today those commonly used are filiform needle, cutaneous needle, intradermal needle, and three-edged needle, in which the filiform needle is widely and mostly used. In this chapter the following information is given.

I. FILIFORM NEEDLE

1. The Structure and Specification

The filiform needles are widely used at present in clinic. It is made of gold, silver, alloy, etc., but most of them are made of stainless steel. A filiform needle may be divided into five parts:

1) **Handle** the part webbed with filigree either of copper or stainless steel;

2) **Tail** the part at the end of the handle;

3) **Tip** the sharp point of the needle;

4) **Body** the part between the handle and the tip; and

5) **Root** the demarcation line between the body and the handle.

The length and gauge refer to the dimension of the needle body.

The common filiform needles vary in length and diameter.

Needles from Nos. 26-32 in diameter and 1-3 cun in length are most frequently used in clinic. The needle tip, in general, should be as sharp as a pine needle, the body is round

Table 16. Length

cun	0.5	1	1.5	2	2.5	3	3.5	4	4.5	5
mm	15	25	40	50	65	75	90	100	115	125

Table 17. Gauge

No	26	28	30	32	34
Dia.(cm)	0.45	0.38	0.32	0.26	0.22

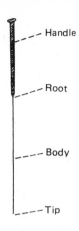

- - Handle

- - Root

- - Body

- - Tip

Fig. 136

and smooth, flexible and resilient, which is valued as the best quality. The filiform needles should be well stored to avoid damage. The damaged needles may cause discomfort to patient or bring about accidents. The needle tip should be preserved with special care by observing the following instructions.

1) Unused needles are suggested to store in a box with layers of gause or in a tube with dry cotton balls placed at the both ends to protect the needle tip.

2) On boiling water sterilization, needles should be bound steadily by gauze in case the needle tip hits against the wall of an autoclave.

3) On manipulation, insertion of the needle should be neither too forceful nor too fast to prevent it from getting bent. If the needle tip touches the bones, the needle should be withdrawn a little to avoid bending.

2.   Needling Practice

As the filiform needle is fine and flexible, it is very difficult to insert it into the skin without some strength exerted by the fingers and conduct manipulations. An appropriate finger force is the guarantee to minimize the pain and raise the therapeutic effects. The training of fingers may start with a short and thick filiform needle, progressing to a finer and longer one before clinical application.

1) Practise with sheets of paper Fold fine and soft tissues into a small packet about 5 x 8 cm in size and 1 cm in thickness, then bind the packet with gauze thread. Hold the paper packet in the left hand and the needle handle with the right hand. Insert the needle into the packet and rotate in and out clockwise and counter-clockwise. At the beginning, if you feel the needle stuck or difficult to rotate, take it easy and continue the exercise until you feel it easy to insert and rotate the needle. As your finger force grows stronger, the thickness of the paper packet may be increased. (See Fig. 137)

2) Practise with a cotton cushion Make a cotton cushion of about 5-6 cm. in diameter wrapped in gauze. Hold the cushion with the left hand and needle handle with the right hand. Insert the needle into it and practise a rotating lifting and thrusting procedure.

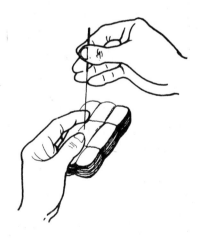

Fig. 137

According to the required postures during acupuncture and the reinforcing and reducing approach, practise the basic manipulation techniques. This purpose is to practise the different manipulations in acupuncture. (See Fig. 138)

3) Practise on your own body This may follow the manipulation methods on the paper packet and the cotton cushion so as to have personal experience of the needling sensation in clinical practice. Only by this can the practitioner really possess and produce beneficial results in acupuncture treatment.

3. Preparations Prior to Treatment

1) Inspection of the instruments Needles of various size, trays, forceps, moxe wool, jars, sterilized cotton ball, 75% alcohol or 1.5% iodine tincture, or 2% gentian violet, etc. should be carefully inspected and prepared before use.

2) Posture of the patient An appropriate posture of a patient is significant in correct location of points, manipulation for

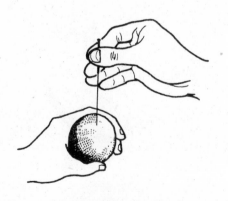

Fig. 138

acupuncture and moxibustion, prolonged retaining of the needle, and in prevention of fainting, bent needle, stuck needle or broken needle. The selection of a proper posture is therefore of importance clinically. Generally, the practitioner must be able to work without hindrance and the patient is relaxed and feels comfortable. The commonly-used postures adopted in the clinic are as follows:

a) Sitting in flexion: suitable for the points on the head, neck and back.

b) Sitting erect with elbows resting on a table: suitable for the points on the head, arm and shoulder. (See Fig. 140)

c) Lateral recumbent: suitable for the points at the lateral side of the body. (See Fig. 141)

d) Supine posture: suitable for the points on the head and face, chest and abdominal region, and areas of the four limbs. (See Fig. 142)

e) Prone posture: suitable for the points on the head, neck, back, lumbar and buttock regions, and the posterior region of the lower limbs. (See Fig. 143)

3) Sterilization:

a) Needle sterilization:

Autoclave sterilization:

Needles should be sterilized in an autoclave at 1.5 atmospheric pressure and 125°C for 30 minutes.

Boiling sterilization:

Needles and other instruments are boiled in water for 30 minutes. This method is easy and effective without any special equipment.

Medicinal sterilization:

Soak the needles in 75% alcohol from 30-60 minutes. Then take them out and wipe off the liquid from the needles with a piece of dry cloth. At the same time, the needle tray and forceps which have directly contacted with the filiform needles should also be sterilized in the same way. Besides, needles

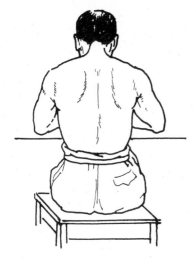

Fig. 139 Sitting in flexion

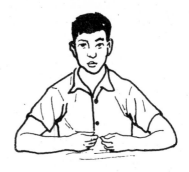

Fig. 140 Setting errect with elbows
resting on a table

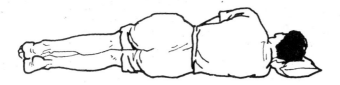

Fig. 141 Lateral recumbent

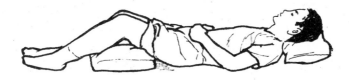

Fig. 142 Supine

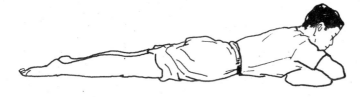

Fig. 143 Prone

used to treat some infectious cases should be sterilized and stored in separate place.

b) Skin disinfection:

The area on the body surface selected for needling must be sterilized. Generally, points on the local area must be sterilized with 75% alcohol, or first with 2.5% iodine, and then it is removed by a 70% alcohol cotton ball. If the disinfected area is accidently polluted, a second sterilization is imperative. The practitioner's fingers should be sterilized routinely.

II. NEEDLING METHODS

Various needling techniques and manipulations, which attach importance to insertion and withdrawal of the needle, have been summarized by practitioners based on their experience in the past dynasties.

1. Insertion

The needle should be inserted coordinately with the help of both hands. The posture for insertion should be correct so that the manipulation can be smoothly done. Generally the needle should be held with the right hand known as the puncturing hand. The left hand known as the pressing hand pushes firmly against the area close to the point. In the first chapter of *Miraculous Pivot,* it says: "Needle must be inserted into the body with the right hand assisted by the left hand." In the book *Classic on Medical Problems*, it is said that: "An experienced acupuncturist believes in the important function of the left hand, while an inexperienced believes in the important

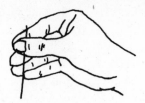

Fig. 144

function of the right hand." It is further stated in *Lyrics of Standard Profoundities* that: "Press heavily with the left hand to disperse qi and insert the needle gently and slowly to avoid pain." These explanations show the importance of the coordination of the right and left hands on insertion. According to the length of the needle and the location of the point, different methods of insertion are employed.

1) Inserting the needle aided by the pressure of the finger of the pressing hand Press beside the acupuncture point with the nail of the thumb or the index finger of the left hand, hold the needle with the right hand and keep the needle tip closely against the nail, and then insert the needle into the point. This method is suitable for puncturing with short needles such as for needling Neiguan (P 6), Zhaohai (K 6), etc.

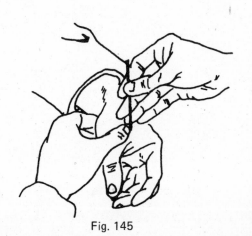

Fig. 145

2) Inserting the needle with the help of the puncturing and pressing hands Hold the needle tip with the thumb and the index finger of the left hand, leaving 0.2-0.3 cm. of its tip exposed, and hold the needle handle with the thumb and index finger of the right hand. As the needle tip is directly over the selected point, insert the needle swiftly into the skin with the left hand, meanwhile the right hand presses the needle downward to the required depth. This method is suitable for puncturing with long needles, such as those used in needling Huantiao (G 30), Zhibian (B 54), etc.

3) Inserting the needle with the fingers stretching the skin Stretch the skin where the point is located with the thumb and index finger of the left hand, hold the needle with the right hand and insert it into the point rapidly to a required depth. This method is suitable for the points on the abdomen where the skin is loose, such as Tianshu (S 25), Guanyuan (Ren 4), etc.

4) Inserting the needle by pinching the skin Pinch the skin up around the point with the thumb and index finger of the left hand, insert the needle rapidly into the point with the right hand. This method is suitable for puncturing the points on the head and face, where the muscle and skin are thin, such as Zanzhu (B 2), Dicang (S 4), Yintang (Extra), etc.

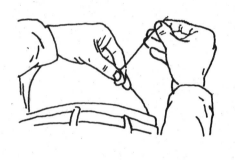

Fig. 146

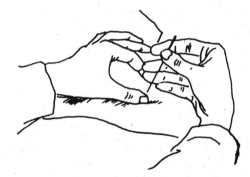

Fig. 147

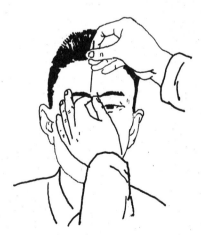

Fig. 148

2.   Angle and depth of insertion

In the process of insertion, angle and depth are especially important in acupuncture. Correct angle and depth help to induce the needling sensation, bring about the desired therapeutic results and guarantee safety. Different angles and depth at the same point punctured produce varied needling sensation and theapeutic effects. Appropriate angle and depth depends upon the location of the points, the therapeutic purpose, the patient's constitution and the type of figure, fat or thin.

1) The angle formed by the needle and the skin surface Generally, there are three kinds: perpendicular, oblique and horizontal.

a) Perpendicular:

Perpendicular, in which the needle is inserted perpendicularly, forming a 90° angle with the skin surface. Most points on the body can be punctured in this way.

b) Oblique:

This method is used for the points close to the important viscerae or where the muscle is thinner. Generally, the needle is inserted obliquely to form an angle of approximately 45° with the skin surface. Points such as Lieque (L 7) in the upper extremity, Jiuwei (Ren 15) of the abdominal region, Qimen (Liv 14) of the chest, and the points on the back, are often needled in this way.

c) Horizontal (also known as transverse insertion):

This method is commonly used in the areas where the muscle is thin, such as Baihui (Du 20), Touwei (S 8) on the head, Zanzhu (B 2), Yangbai (B 14) on the face, Tanzhong (Ren 17) on the chest, etc.

2) Depth of needle insertion Generally, a proper depth of needling induces better needling sensation without hurting the important viscerae. In clinic the depth of insertion mostly depends upon the constitution of the patient, the location of points and the pathological condition. For the elderly often suffering from deficiency of qi and blood, or for infants with delicate constitution, and such areas as the head, face and back region, shallow insertion is advisable. For the young and middle-aged with strong or fat constitutions, or for the points on the four extremities, buttocks and abdominal region, deep insertion is adopted.

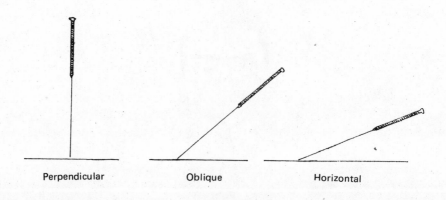

Perpendicular   Oblique   Horizontal

Fig. 149

3.   Manipulations and Arrival of Qi (Needling Reaction)

Manipulations: Needle manipulations may induce needling reaction, for which several methods should be applied.

The arrival of qi refers to soreness, numbness or a distending feeling around the point after the needle is inserted to a certain depth. At the same time the operator may feel tenseness around the needle.

1)The fundamental manipulation techniques

a) Lifting and thrusting:

After the needle tip penetrating the skin surface, the needle body is perpendicularly lifted and thrust in the point. This, known as lifting and thrusting, is applied only when the needle is inserted to a certain depth. But it is not appropriate to lift and thrust too much, otherwise, local pain or damage of the local tissues may take place.

b) Twirling or rotating:

After the needle has reached its desired depth, twirl and rotate the needle backward and forward continuously. Generally, the needle is rotated with an amplitude from 180° to 360°. Rotating clockwise or counter-clockwise alone may twine the muscle fibers and produce pain.

2) Waiting for and promoting qi

If qi fails to arrive after manipulation, some measures have to be taken, such as temporarily retaining the needle and then rotating again until qi is obtained. This is called "waiting for qi." If, after the insertion and manipulation of the needle, the patient does not feel or only has little needling sensation, the method of promoting qi should be used. The six auxiliary manipulations are seen below.

a) Pressing:

Slightly press the skin along the course of the meridian. It is described in *Compendium of Acupuncture and Moxibustion* that "the related meridian is pushed up and down to promote the circulation of qi and blood".

The main purpose of this method is to encourage the movement of qi through the related meridian and facilitate its sensation at the point. It is used in patients whose needling sensation is delayed.

b) Plucking:

Pluck the handle of the needle lightly, causing it to tremble and strengthening the stimulation to obtain qi. In *Compendium of Acupuncture and Moxibustion*, it says: "First, pluck the handle of the needle, after the arrival of qi, insert the needle a bit deeper. This is the reinforcing method." It is also pointed out in *Questions and Answers on Acupuncture and Moxibustion* that: "If qi does not flow smoothly, pluck the needle lightly and make qi travel faster."

The plucking method used to promote qi flow is for patients with retarded qi sensation due to qi deficiency.

c) Scraping:

When the needle is retained the thumb and index finger of the left hand support the body of the needle where it enters the skin, while the thumb of the right hand is placed on the tail end to hold the needle steady, then scrap the handle with the nail of the index or middle finger of the right hand upward from downward or vice versa. Scraping is used to spread the needling sensation.

d) Shaking:

Shaking of the needle can strengthen the needling sensation. In the book *Questions and Answers on Acupuncture and Moxibustion*, it is said that "shaking is an aid for qi flow." Moreover, shaking the needle may be used as an auxiliary method for reducing, i.e. before withdrawal of the needle, shake the needle to drive the pathogenic factors out. In

Compendium of Acupuncture and Moxibustion, it says, "First, shake the handle of the needle to cause arrival of qi. When qi arrives, withdraw the needle a little, which is known as the reducing method."

e) Flying:

In the book *Introduction to Medicine,* it says: "Twirling the needle quickly for three times is known as 'flying'." Twirl the needle and separate the thumb and index finger from it for several times until the needling sensation is strengthened.

f) Trembling:

Hold the needle with the fingers of the right hand and apply quick lift-thrust movement in small amplitude to cause vibration. It is stated in *Classic of Divine Resonance* that "hold the needle with the thumb and index finger of the right hand, lift and thrust it rapidly and lightly in a trembling way to promote qi." Therefore it is applied to strengthen the needling sensation and activate the flow of qi and blood.

3) Arrival of qi In the process of acupuncture, no matter what manipulation it is, the arrival of qi must be achieved. In the first chapter of *Miraculous Pivot,* it is described that "acupuncture therapy does not take effect until the arrival of qi." In *Ode of Golden Needle* it is said: "Quick arrival of qi suggests good effects in treatment; slow arrival of qi shows retarded effects in treatment." It indicates that the arrival of qi is especially important in acupuncture treatment.

a) Signs of the arrival of qi:

When the patient feels soreness, numbness, heaviness and distension around the point, or their transmission upward and downward along the meridians, it is a sign of the arrival of qi. Meanwhile, the operator should feel tenseness around the needle.

Lyrics of Standard Profoundities says: "It seems a fish bites on fishing pulling the line downward." This is a vivid description to whether the arrival of qi is obtained or not.

b) Factors influencing the arrival of qi:

i) Inaccurate location of the points:

It is very important to locate points correctly in acupuncture treatment. In case of inaccurate location, the required needling sensation will be affected.

ii) Improper depth of the needle insertion:

A given depth of insertion to each point is required. Either too deep or too shallow affects the arrival of qi.

iii) Imperfect manipulation:

The needle manipulation is requisite for the arrival of qi. The operator should practise it perfectly, otherwise, the expected effects can not be achieved.

iv) Weak constitution and dull sensation:

In chapter 67 of *Miraculous Pivot* it describes, "An individual with abundant yang qi may have a quick needling sensation; a healthy person responds with a normal rate to acupuncture, neither quick nor slow; and a man with excessive yin and deficient yang, (i.e. delicate constitution and dull sensation) may have a slow needling sensation." For severe cases there may not appear the needling sensation, and the therapeutic results are bad.

Acupuncturists in the past dynasties attached importance not only to the arrival of qi, but also to the activity of the "spirit qi" in the meridians. In *Compendium of Acupuncture and Moxibustion* it is said, "In case of arrival of the spirit qi, a tense feeling appears under the needle." The first chapter of *Miraculous Pivot* says, "A point is the place where the spirit qi enters and flows out." The function of acupuncture is to regulate the meridian qi. The arrival of qi is a manifestation of the normal activity of the spirit qi. Therefore, it is important in observation of the therapeutic effects.

4.   Retaining and Withdrawing the Needle

1) Retaining "Retaining" means to hold the needle in place after it is inserted to a given depth below the skin. Pathological conditions decide the retaining and its duration. In general, the needle is retained for fifteen to twenty minutes after the arrival of qi. But for some chronic, intractable, painful and spastic cases, the time for retaining of the needle may be appropriately prolonged. Meanwhile, manipulations may be given at intervals in order to strengthen the therapeutic effects. For some diseases the duration may last for several hours. For patients with a dull needling sensation, retaining the needle serves as a method to wait for qi to come.

2) Withdrawing On withdrawing the needle, press the skin around the point with the thumb and index finger of the pressing hand, rotate the needle gently and lift it slowly to the subcutaneous level, then, withdraw it quickly and press the punctured point for a while to prevent bleeding.

5.   Reinforcing and Reducing Methods

Reinforcing and reducing are two corresponding methods based on the guide line set in *Internal Classic*, i.e. reinforcing for the deficiency-syndrome and reducing for the excess-syndrome. The method which is able to invigorate the body resistance and to strengthen the weakened physiological function is called reinforcing, while that which is able to eliminate the pathogenic factors and to harmonize the hyperactive physiological functions is known as the reducing. Clinically, reinforcing or reducing method is applied according to the functional conditions of the patient.

Under different pathological conditions acupuncture may produce different regulating functions, or the effects of the reinforcing and reducing. If an individual is subject to a collapse condition, acupuncture functions to rescue yang from collapse; when an individual is under a condition of internal pathogenic heat, acupuncture functions to expel the heat outwards. Acupuncture can not only relieve the stomach and intestine spasms, but also strengthen the stomach and intestine peristalsis. This dual regulating function is closely related to the condition of anti-pathogenic factors of the human body. If it is vigorous, the meridian qi is easy to be activated and the regulating function is good. On the contrary, if it is lowered, the meridian qi is difficult to be excited and the regulating function is poor.

Acupuncture is an approach which can promote the transformation of the internal environment of the human body. For this purpose certain manipulations are created. Acupuncturists in past ages developed and summarized a lot of reinforcing and reducing methods which are still commonly used in clinic.

1) The basic reinforcing and reducing methods

a) Reinforcing and reducing by lifting and thrusting the needle:

In *Classic on Medical Problems*, it states,

"Heavy pressing of the needle to a deep region is known as reinforcing, while forceful lifting of the needle to the superficial region is known as reducing. It tells the reinforcing from the reducing by the force and speed used. After the needle is inserted to a given depth and the needling sensation appears, the reinforcing is obtained by lifting the needle gently and slowly, while thrusting the needle heavily and rapidly. The reducing is achieved by lifting the needle forcefully and rapidly while thrusting the needle gently and slowly.

b) Reinforcing and reducing by twirling and rotating the needle:

The reinforcing and reducing of this kind can be differentiated by the amplitude and speed used. When the needle is inserted to a certain depth, rotating the needle gently and slowly with small amplitude is called the reinforcing, on the contrary, rotating the needle rapidly with large amplitude is known as the reducing. In the seventy-third chapter of *Miraculous Pivot,* it says, "Twirling the needle slowly is the reinforcing and twirling the needle rapidly to promote the flow of qi is the reducing method." In addition, the reinforcing and reducing methods are distinguished by clockwise or counter-clockwise rotation of the needle. In other words, the right rotation is the reducing method, and the left rotation is the reinforcing method. In *Guide to Acupuncture* it describes, "Rotating the needle forward with the thumb means the reinforcing; rotating the needle backward with the thumb means the reducing." Of course, twirling of the needle doesn't follow on direction. There is a difference only between the speed of rotation and the force used. For example, in forth turning, the needle is rotated forcefully and rapidly by the thumb, however, in back turning, the needle is rotated gently and slowly by the thumb. The right rotation is just in the opposite way.

c) The reinforcing and reducing achieved by rapid and slow insertion and withdrawal of the needle:

This is another kind of reinforcing and reducing methods distinguished by the speed of insertion and withdrawal of the needle. In the first chapter of *Miracular Pivot*, it says that "inserting the needle slowly and withdrawing it rapidly is the reinforcing method, and inserting the needle rapidly and withdrawing it slowly is the reducing method." In the third chapter of *Miraculous Pivot* the same explanation is given. During manipulations the reinforcing method is performed by inserting the needle to a given depth slowly and lifting it rapidly just beneath the skin, and a moment later withdraw it. The reducing method is performed just in a opposite procedure.

d) The reinforcing and reducing achieved by keeping the hole open or close:

In Chapter 53 of *Plain Questions*, it says that "excess is due to the entrance of the pathogenic factor into the human body whereas deficiency is due to exit of the vital qi." On withdrawing of the needle, shake it to enlarge the hole and allow the pathogenic factor going out. This is called the reducing method. Conversely, pressing the hole quickly to close it and preventing the vital qi from escaping is called the reinforcing method.

e) The reinforcing and reducing achieved by the direction the needle tip pointing to:

In *Compendium of Acupuncture and Moxibustion*, it says, "The three yang meridians of hand run from the hand up to the head. The needle tip pointing downwards, i.e. against the meridian course, is known as the reducing method. The opposite direction of the needle tip pointing to, i.e. following the running course of the meridian, is known as the reinforcing method."

f) The reinforcing and reducing achieved by means of respiration:

In Chapter 27 of *Plain Questions*, it states, "The reinforcing is achieved by inserting the needle when the patient breathes in and withdrawing the needle when the patient breathes out. The reducing is achieved in an opposite way."

In addition to the above-mentioned methods, even reinforcing and reducing movement is also used in clinic. This method is used in treating diseases which are a typical to deficiency or excess nature. Lift, thrust and rotate the needle evenly and gently at moderate speed to cause a mild sensation and withdraw the needle at moderate speed as well.

2) Comprehensive reinforcing and reducing methods

a) Setting the mountain on fire:

This method is derived from the reinforcing procedures of slow and rapid insertion, lifting and thrusting and keeping the hole open or close. When it is applied, the patient feels warm at the punctured part. This method is often used to treat the diseases of deficiency-cold nature. During the operation, after the needle is inserted slowly beneath the skin the needle is repeatedly thrust thrice according to the superficial, medium and deep sequences, and lifted once. At a depth of 0.5 cun and the arrival of qi achieved the needle is lifted and thrust for nine times. Then the needle is inserted to a depth of 1 cun and lifted and thrust for another nine times. After that the needle is inserted to a depth of 1.5 cun, and lifted and thrust for nine times too. Repeated operations can be conducted for several times until a warm feeling is got. Quickly withdraw the needle and press the hole.

b) "Penetrating-heaven coolness":

This method is derived from the reducing procedures of slow and rapid insertion, lifting and thrusting and keeping the hole open or close. When this method is employed, the patient has a cool sensation at the punctured part. This method is usually applied to the excess syndrome and heat syndrome. After it is inserted quickly to a certain depth, the needle is repeatedly lifted thrice according to the deep, medium and superficial sequences and thrust once. At a depth of 1.5 cun and the arrival of qi achieved the needle is lifted quickly and thrust slowly for six times. After that the needle is lifted to a depth of 1 cun and given the same operation. Then the needle is further lifted to a depth of 0.5 cun and given the same operation too. Repeated operation can be conducted for several times until a cool feeling is got.

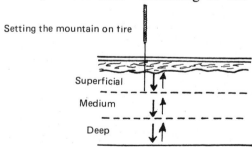

Setting the mountain on fire

Superficial

Medium

Deep

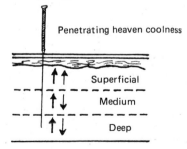

Penetrating heaven coolness

Superficial

Medium

Deep

Fig. 150

III. PRECAUTIONS, CONTRA-INDICATIONS AND MANAGEMENT OF POSSIBLE ACCIDENTS IN ACUPUNCTURE TREATMENT

1. Precautions and Contraindications in Acupuncture Treatment

1) It is advisable to apply few needles or to delay giving acupuncture treatment to the patients who are either famished or overeaten, intoxicated, overfatigued or very weak.

2) It is contraindicated to puncture points on the lower abdomen and lumbosacral region for women pregnant under three months. After three months pregnancy it is contraindicated to needle the points on the upper abdomen and lumbosacral region, and those points causing strong sensation such as Hegu (LI 4), Sanyinjiao (Sp 6), Kunlun (B 60) and Zhiyin (B 67).

3) Points on the vertax of infants should not be needled when the fontanel is not closed. In addition, retaining of needles is forbidden since the infants are unable to cooperate with the practitioner.

4) Needling should avoid the blood vessels to prevent bleeding. Points of the chest and back should be carefully needled to avoid injury of the vital organs. In Chapter 16 of *Plain Questions*, it says, "If you puncture the points at the chest and abdominal region, you should avoid hurting the five zang organs."

5) Historic medical literature of the past contraindicates certain points on the human body for puncture or deep puncture. Most of these points are located close to the vital organs or large blood vessels, such as

Chengqi (S 1) located below the eyeball, Jiuwei (Ren 15) near the important viscera, Jimen (Sp 11) near the femoral artery, etc. These points should generally be punctured obliquely or horizontally to avoid accidents.

2. Management of Possible Accidents

Although acupuncture is safe and free from side-effects, some accidents may take place owing to negligence of the contraindications, imperfect manipulations, or want of the knowledge of anatomy. If an accident really occurs, the practitioner should keep calm. As long as he solves the problem in time, serious consequences can be avoided. The possible accidents are seen as follows:

1) Fainting

Cause: This is often due to nervous tension, delicate constitution, hunger, fatigue, improper position or to the too forceful manipulation.

Manifestations: During acupuncture treatment, there may appear dizziness, vertigo, palpitation, short breath, fidgets, nausea, pallor, cold sweating, weak pulse. In severe cases, there may be cold extremities, drop of blood pressure, and loss of consciousness.

Management: When fainting aurae such as dizziness, vertigo, fidgets and nausea appear, stop needling immediately and withdraw all the needles. Then help the patient to lie down, and offer him some warm or sweet water. The symptoms will disappear after a short rest. In severe cases, in addition to the above management, press hard with the fingernail or needle Shuigou (Du 26), Zhongchong (P 9), Suliao (Du 25), Neiguan (P 6) and Zusanli (S 36), or apply moxibustion to Baihui (Du 20), Qihai (Ren

6) and Guanyuan (Ren 4). Generally, the patient will respond, but if not, other emergency measures should be taken.

2) Stuck needle

Cause: This may arise from nervousness, strong spasm of the local muscle after the insertion of the needle, twirling the needle with too large amplitude or in one direction only, causing muscle fibers to bind, or from a change of the position of the patient after the insertion of the needles.

Manifestations: After the needle is inserted, it is found at times difficult or impossible to rotate, lift and thrust the needles. This situation is known as stuck needle.

Management: Ask the patient to relax. If the needle is stuck due to excessive rotation in one direction, the condition will release when the needle is twirled in the opposite direction. If the stuck needle is caused by the tension of the muscle temporarily, leave the needle in place for a while, then withdraw it by rotating, or by massaging the skin near the point or by inserting another needle nearby to transfer the patient's attention.

If the stuck needle is caused by the changing of the position of the patient, the original posture should be resumed and then withdraw the needle.

Prevention: Sensitive patients should be encouraged to release their tensions. Avoid the muscle tendons during insertion. Twirling with too large amplitude or in one direction only shall in no case be allowed. In the process of manipulation, the posture of the patient should remain original.

3) Bent needle

Cause: This may result from unskillful manipulation or too forceful manipulation, or the needle striking the hard tissue, or a sudden change of the patient's posture for different reasons, or from an improper management of the stuck needle.

Manifestations: It is difficult to lift, thrust, rotate and withdraw the needle. At the same time, the patient feels pain.

Management: When the needle is bent, lifting, thrusting, and rotating shall in no case be applied. The needle may be removed slowly and withdrawn by following the course of bend. In case the bent needle is caused by the change of the patient's posture, move him to his original position, relax the local muscle and then remove the needle. Never try to withdraw the needle with force.

Prevention: Perfect insertion and gentle manipulation are required. The patient should have a proper and comfortable position. During the retaining period, change of the position is not allowed. The needling area shall in no case be impacted or pressed by an external force.

4) Broken needle

Cause: This may arise from the poor quality of the needle or eroded base of the needle, from too strong manipulation of the needle, from strong muscle spasm, or a sudden movement of the patient when the needle is in place, or from withdrawing a stuck needle.

Manifestations: The needle body is broken during manipulation and the broken part is below the skin surface.

Management: When it happens, the patient should be asked to keep calm to prevent the broken needle from going deeper into the body. If the broken part protrudes from the skin, remove it with forceps or fingers. If the broken part is at the same level of the skin, press the tissue around the site until the broken end is exposed, then remove it with forceps. If it is completely under the skin, surgery should be resorted to.

Prevention: To prevent accidents, careful

inspection of the quality of the needle should be made prior to the treatment to reject the needles which are not in conformity with the requirements specified. The needle body should not be inserted into the body completely, and a little part should be exposed outside the skin. On needle insertion, if it is bent, the needle should be withdrawn immediately. Never try to insert a needle with too much force.

5) Hematoma

Cause: This may result from injury of the blood vessels during insertion, or from absent pressing of the point after withdrawing the needle.

Manifestations: Local swelling, distension and pain after withdrawal of the needle.

Management: Generally, a mild hematoma will disappear by itself. If the local swelling and pain are serious, apply local pressing, or light massage, or warming moxibustion to help disperse the hematoma.

Prevention: Avoid injuring the blood vessels.

6) After-effect

Cause: It is mostly due to the unskilled manipulation and forceful stimulation.

Manifestations: After withdrawal of the needle, there may remain an uncomfortable feeling of soreness and pain, which may persist for a long period.

Management: For the mild cases, press the local area, and for severe cases, in addition to pressing, moxibustion is applied to the local area.

Prevention: Too forceful manipulation shall in no case be applied.

Appendix: Yang Jizhou's Twelve Manipulations

Yang Jizhou, an acupuncturist of the Ming Dynasty, summarized the twelve kinds of manipulations, of which all but the warming technique in the mouth are adopted in today's acupuncture treatment.

1) Needle insertion assisted by the thumb nail: Before the needle is inserted, press heavily on the point with the thumb nail to disperse qi and blood. In this way puncturing does not damage the defensive qi. This approach functions in four aspects: fixing the point to be needled; dispersing qi and blood to avoid injuring the defensive qi; distracting the patient's attention to reduce pain; avoiding bleeding.

2) Attentive insertion and manipulation Hold the needle handle with the right hand, thrust and rotate it deep into the muscles with force. After three breathings, lift the needle to the part just below the skin. After another three breathing, the needling sensation may appear. Then other manipulations may be followed.

3) Warming the needle in the mouth (omitted)

4) Entering of the needle a) Before needling, the patient and practitioner should keep even breath to calm the mind. b) The point should be located accurately, for example, points of the yang meridians on the four extremities should be located between the tendons and bones, while those of the yin meridians on the four extremities located at the place with the fingers responding to the arteries.

5) Pressing After the insertion and manipulation of the needle, but the patient does not feel the needling sensation, lightly press the skin with fingers along the course of the meridian on which the point is located, both above and below. The purpose is to make smooth flow of qi and blood and to facilitate the arrival of qi.

6) Scratching If an inserted needle is difficult to lift, thrust or even withdraw, the needle is stuck by the pathogenic factors. Scratch the needle with the thumb nail up and down along the course of the meridian to dispel the pathogenic factors from the meridians.

7) Withdrawing   On withdrawal of the needle, the practitioner should concentrate his mind and pull the needle slowly to the three levels. For reinforcing, heavy thrusting is applied, while for reducing, forceful withdrawal is used.

8) Twisting   A needle should not be twisted too tight, otherwise, it will be entangled by the muscles, causing sharp pain. In stagnation of qi twist the needle to promote smooth flow of qi and blood, and to disperse the defensive qi.

9) Turning   To treat the disease in the upper region, turn the needle forthward to make qi ascend, and to treat the disease in the lower region, turn the needle backward to make qi descend. Lifting the needle to the middle level, and turning the needle backward is the reinforcing method, and vice versa. The purpose is to promote smooth flow of qi.

10) Retaining   Before withdrawing the needle, keep the needle subcutaneously for a while, then withdraw it. The purpose is to keep the qi stable at the punctured part.

11) Shaking   When the needle is withdrawn in the level, shake the needle twice at each level to enlarge the punctured hole.

12) Pulling   On withdrawal of the needle, be sure that it is not stuck tightly. Then use the fingers to lift the needle out carefully — as if "pulling a tiger's tail."

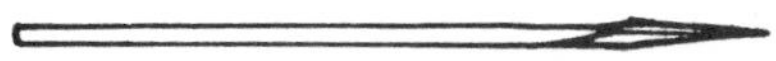

Fig. 151 The Three-edged Needle

IV.   THE THREE-EDGED NEEDLE

1.   Needle

The three-edged needle is developed from the sharp needle of the Nine Needles created in the ancient times. The needle is shaped in a round handle, a triangular head and a sharp tip. (See Fig. 151)

2.   Indications

The three-edged needle functions to promote the smooth flow of qi and blood in meridians, dispel blood stasis and eliminate the heat. It is advisable to treat blockage of the meridians, blood stasis, excess syndrome and heat syndrome, such as high fever, loss of consciousness, sore throat, local congestion or swelling.

3.   Manipulations

There are three kinds of manipulations.

1) Spot pricking: This is a method known as collateral pricking in ancient times used to treat disease by pricking the small vessels with a three-edged needle to obtain a little bloodletting. During the operation hold the handle of the three-edged needle with the right hand, prick swiftly about 0.05-0.1 cun deep at the area for bloodletting and withdraw the needle immediately. After pricking, press the punctured hole with a dry cotton ball until the bleeding stops. This is the most widely used method in clinics, for example, pricking Weizhong (B 40) to treat lumbago due to stagnation of blood, pricking Shaoshang (L 11) to treat sore throat, pricking Quze (P 3) and Weizhong (B 40) to treat acute vomiting, pricking Taiyang (Extra) or apex of the ear to treat acute conjunctivitis.

2) Clumpy pricking Prick around a small area or a reddened swelling, then press the skin to make the decayed blood escape. This method is mostly used for carbuncles, erysipelas, etc.

3) Pricking During the operation, pinch up the local skin with the left hand, prick the skin 0.5 cun deep with a three-edged needle to make bleed. If there is no bleeding, press the punctured part until bleeding occurs. This method is mostly used to treat multiple follicucitis. For multiple carbuncles of the neck, try to find the red spots at the both sides of the vertebra, and then prick them with a three-edged needle till bleeding.

4.   Precautions

1) Aseptic operation is applied to prevent infection.

2) For spot pricking, the operation should be slight, superficial, and rapid. Bleeding should not be excessive. Avoid injuring the deep large arteries.

3) Pricking shall in no case be applied for those with weak constitution, for pregnant women and those susceptible to bleeding.

V.   THE CUTANEOUS NEEDLE

1.   Needle

The cutaneous needle is also known as the plum-blossom needle and seven-star needle, which is made of five to seven stainless steel

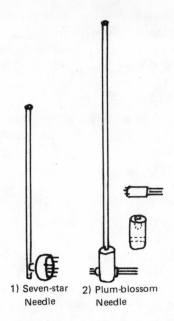

1) Seven-star   2) Plum-blossom
   Needle   Needle

Fig. 152 The Cutaneous Needle

needles inlaid onto the end of a handle. It is used to prick the skin superficially by tapping to promote the smooth flow of qi in the meridians and regulate the functions of the zang-fu organs.

1) The seven-star needle Composed of seven short stainless steel needles attached vertically to a handle five to six inches long.

2) The plum-blosom needle Composed of five stainless steel needles in a bundle and attached to a handle perpendicularly one foot long.

The tip of the needles should not be too sharp, but on the same level with equal space between them, otherwise, pain or bleeding may happen during tapping.

2.   Indications

This superficial tapping is particularly suitable to treat disorders of the nervous system and skin disease. It is used for headache, dizziness and vertigo, insomnia, gastrointestinal disease, gynecological disease, skin disease, painful joints and paralysis.

3.   Manipulation

After routine and local sterilization, hold the handle of the needle and tap vertically on the skin surface with a flexible movement of the wrist. (Fig. 153) The tapping may be light or heavy. Tap slightly until the skin becomes congested, or tap heavily until slight bleeding appears. The area to be tapped may be along the course of the meridians, or on the points selected, or on the affected area, or along the both sides of the spinal column.

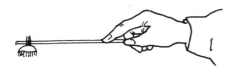

Fig. 153

4.   Precautions

1) The tips of the needles should be even and free from any hooks. On tapping, the tips of the needles should strike the skin at a right angle to the surface to reduce   pain.

2) Sterilize the needles and the local area to be treated. After heavy tapping, the local skin surface should be cleaned and sterilized to prevent infection.

3) Tapping is not allowed to apply to the local trauma and ulcers.

VI.   THE INTRADERMAL NEEDLE THERAPY

1.   Needle

The intradermal needle is a kind of short needle made of stainless steel wire, especially used for embedding in the skin. There are two types: the thumbtack type and grain-like type. The intradermal needle is also known as "embedding needle," developed from the ancient method of needle retaining. It can exert the continuous stimulation produced by the implanted needle.

1) The thumbtack-type needle, which is about 0.3 cm long with a head like a thumbtack; and

2) The grain-like needle, about 1 cm long with a head like a grain of wheat.

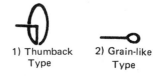

1) Thumback   2) Grain-like
   Type   Type

Fig. 154 The Intradermal Needle

2.   Indications

It is mostly used in clinic to treat some chronic or painful diseases which need long time retaining of the needle, such as headache, stomachache, asthma, insomnia, enuresis, abnormal menstruation, dysmenorrhen, etc.

3.   Manipulation

The grain-like needle is applied to points or tender spots on various parts of the body while the thumbtack-type needle is generally applied to the ear region. Embed the sterilized needle into the point, leaving its handle lying flat on the skin surface, and fixing it with a piece of adhesive tape.

4. Precautions

1) The duration of implantation depends on the pathological conditions in different seasons. In summer, the needles are generally retained for one to two days because of excessive sweating which is likely to cause infection. In autumn or winter, the retaining duration may be longer according to the need in specific cases.

2) Try to avoid embedding the intradermal needle at the joints to prevent pain on motion.

3) In the purulent infected area or skin ulcers it is not allowed to embed the needle.

4) During the embedding period, keep the area around the needle clean to prevent infection.

VII. THE NINE NEEDLES IN THE ANCIENT TIMES AND THE NEEDLING METHODS LISTED IN INTERNAL CLASSIC

1. The Nine Needles in the Ancient Times

The nine needles are those of different forms used in the ancient times. In Chapter 7 of *Miraculous Pivot*, it is stated that "each of the nine needles, long, short, big or small, has its specific usage."

1) The arrow-head needle, 1.6 inches long with a round head and sharp tip like an arrow, often used for superficial diseases.

2) Round needle, 1.6 inches long with a oval-rounded tip, used for disorders of the muscles or for massage treatment.

3) Blunt needle, 3.5 inches long with a round needle body and slightly sharp tip, used for blood vessels disease and pressing purpose.

4) Sharp-edged needle, 1.6 inches long with a triangle needle body and a sharp and pyramid tip, served as a scalpel for heat-toxin abscesses or for blood-letting.

5) Sword-shaped needle, 4 inches long, 0.25 inch wide, shaped as a sword, used for pain and drainage of pus.

6) Round-sharp needle, 1.6 inches long with a thin round body and a slightly large head, mainly used for sudden attack of rheumatic arthritis and pain.

7) Filiform needle, 1.6 inches long with a sharp tip and a thin body, used for cold, heat and painful conditions.

8) Long needle, 7 inches long with a round and sharp tip and big body, used to treat disorders of the deep tissue or persistent bi-syndrome.

9) Large needle, 4 inches long with a slightly round tip shaped as a stick, used to treat joint disorders due to the retention of water.

2. The Needling Methods Listed in Internal Classic

Many different needling methods are described in *Internal Classic*, in which the seventh chapter of *Miraculous Pivot* has concentrated a lot of needling methods including the location of the points.

1) The nine needling methods In Chapter 7 of *Miracular Pivot*, it says, "There are nine ways of needling applied to cope with nine different diseases."

a) Shu-point needling, used in treatment of disorders of the five zang organs, by which the needle is inserted at Ying-(Spring) Points of the yin meridians and the Shu-points. Strictly speaking, this is a combining method in selection of points.

b) Distant needling, used in treatment of disorders of the six fu organs, by which the needle is inserted at the points in the upper region distant from the affected regions located below. The Lower He-(Sea) Points of the six fu organs of the three yang meridians of foot are often selected. This is a combining method in selection of points.

c) Meridian needling, used to treat an affected meridian by needling along that meridian or the meridian related to the affected part.

d) Collateral needling, used to cause bleeding of the subcutaneous small vessels to eliminate blood stasis and treat the collateral diseases.

e) Crack needling, used to needle the space between two muscles to treat muscular pain.

f) Evacuation needling, used with a sword-shaped needle to perform surgical operation and remove purulent blood.

g) Shallow needling, used to treat superficial disorders. The cutaneous needle used is developed from this method.

h) Contralateral needling, indicating the needling applied to the points on the right side when the affected region is on the left or vice versa.

i) Heat needling, used with a red-hot needle to treat rheumatism. The fire puncture developed from this method is now used to treat scrofula and ulcers of yin nature.

2) The twelve needlings   In Chapter 7 of *Miraculous Pivot* it says, "There are twelve needlings in response to various diseases of the twelve regular meridians."

a) Coupled puncture, a method in which the needle is inserted at two corresponding points in the frontal and posterior regions of the body respectively in order to treat cardialgia and thoracodynia.

b) Trigger puncture, used to treat wandering pains. When pains are not localized in one definite area, perpendicular insertion of the needle into the affected regions should be applied with no immediate withdrawal, and the needle may be removed after a pressure has been applied to the affected region with the left hand.

c) Lateral puncture, a method to needling one side of the painful muscle, and shaking the needle forward and backward, anteriorly and posteriorly, right and left so as to expand the needle hole and relax the muscle. This method is used to treat rheumatic pains.

d) Triple puncture, a method in which the needles are inserted at three spots simultaneously, with one in the centre and two on both sides to treat rheumatism caused by cold pathogenic factor that attacks the body on a small scale but with a deep penetration.

e) Quintuple puncture, a method in which the needles are inserted at five spots with one in the centre and the four scattered around it. This method is applied to treat a relatively large area disorders caused by cold pathogenic factor.

f) Straight puncture across the skin, a method in which the skin in the region in which the points involved are located is pushed up with the fingers, and then the needle is inserted at the points and across the skin. This method is used to treat diseases caused by the cold pathogenic factor with the superficial invasion.

g) Shu-point puncture, a method in which the needle is perpendicularly inserted into a few points deeply and withdrawn rapidly to treat heat condition caused by excess of qi.

h) Short puncture, a method in which the needle is inserted with slight shaking down to the bone that suffers from rheumatism. And then the needle is gradually pushed further into the body until its tip reaches the region close to the affected bones. After that, the needle is moved up and down as if rubbing the bones. This method is applied to treat bone rheumatism caused by cold.

i) Superficial puncture, a method in which an oblique or shallow insertion is applied to treat muscular spasms caused by cold.

j) Yin puncture, a method in which the needling is applied to Taixi (K 3), a point of the Kidney Meridian of Foot-Shaoyin on both feet behind the medial malleolus to treat cold limbs and cold conditions.

k) Adjacent puncture, a method in which the needling is applied to the affected part vertically and laterally with one needle each to treat prolonged rheumatism.

l) Repeated shallow puncture, a method in which the needle is repeatedly inserted vertically and superficially and withdrawn rapidly to cause bleeding of the affected part in treating carbuncles and erysipelas.

3) The five needling techniques In the seventh chapter of *Miraculous Pivot,* it describes, "There are five needling techniques developed to treat various diseases associated with the five zang organs."

a) Extreme shallow puncture, a technique involving shallow insertion and immediate withdrawal of the needle without any injury of the muscles. This technique is developed in response to the diseases associated with the lungs, and it is a technique which functions to reduce the superficial pathogenic factors used in treatment of fever due to exogenous pathogenic factors, cough and asthma.

b) Leopard-spot puncture, a technique in which needles are used to pierce small blood vessels around the affected area to evacuate the points on the left, on the right, in the front, on sludged blood. This technique is developed in response to the disease associated with the heart by virtue of the fact that the heart is in control of the blood and blood vessels. This method may be used to treat swellings and pains.

c) Joint puncture, a technique in which the needle is inserted rapidly into the muscles around the joints of the extremities, but to avoid bleeding, to treat rheumatism of tendons. This technique is developed in response to the diseases associated with the liver by virtue of the fact that the liver is in control of tendons.

d) Hegu puncture, a technique in which the needle is inserted into the muscles of the affected area, obliquely right and left just like the claws of the chicken to cure rheumatic pain of the muscles. This technique is developed in response to the diseases associated with the spleen by virtue of the fact that the spleen is in control of the muscles.

e) Shu-point puncture, a technique in which the needle is thrust deeply to the bone to treat osteal pain. This technique is developed in response to the diseases associated with the kidney by virtue of the fact that the kidney is in control of the bones.

Chapter 15

MOXIBUSTION AND CUPPING

Moxibustion treats and prevents diseases by applying heat to points or certain locations of the human body. The material used is mainly "moxa-wool" in the form of a cone or stick. For centuries, moxibustion and acupuncture have been combined in clinical practice, thus they are usually termed together in Chinese. Chapter 73 of *Miraculous Pivot* states, "A disease that may not be treated by acupuncture may be treated by moxibustion." In *Introduction to Medicine* it says, "When a disease fails to respond to medication and acupuncture, moxibustion is suggested."

Cupping is a therapeutic approach by attaching small jars in which a vacuum is created. Cupping, sometimes used in combination with acupuncture, is elucidated herewith.

I. THE MATERIALS AND FUNCTIONS OF MOXIBUSTION

1. The Property of Artemisia Vulagaris Moxa

Artemisia Vulgaris is a species of chrysanthemum. The one produced in Qizhou is known as the best kind for moxa as the climate and soil is good for its growth. The leaves of the Qizhou Artemisia are thick with much more wool. Moxa cones and sticks made of this kind of Artemisia are thought the top quality used in moxibustion.

In *A New Edition of Materia Medica* appears the following description: "The moxa leaf is bitter and acrid, producing warmth when used in small amount and strong heat when used in large amount. It is of pure yang nature having the ability to restore the primary yang from collapse. It can open the twelve regular meridians, travelling through the three yin meridians to regulate qi and blood, expel cold and dampness, warm the uterus, stop bleeding, warm the spleen and stomach to remove stagnation, regulate menstruation and ease the fetus... When burned, it penetrates all the meridians, eliminating hundreds of diseases." Yang can be activated by the Artemisia leaf for its warm nature. The acrid odour of the leaf can travel through the meridians, regulate qi and blood, and expel cold from the meridians, and its bitter nature resolves dampness. As a result it is used as a necessary material in moxibustion treatment. In addition, the moxa wool can produce mild heat, which is able to penetrate deeply into the muscles. If it is replaced by other materials, an intolerable burning pain will result, and the effect is found poor than the moxa wool.

2.   Functions of Moxibustion

1) To warm meridians and expel cold Abnormal flow of qi and blood in the body is usually resulted from cold and heat. Cold causes slow flow or even stagnation of qi, and heat results in rapid flow of qi. "Normal heat activates blood circulation and cold impedes its smooth flow." Since stagnation of qi and blood is often relieved by warming up the qi, moxibustion is the right way to generate the smooth flow of qi with the help of the ignited moxa wool. In Chapter 75 of *Miraculous Pivot* it says, "If stagnation of blood in the vessels cannot be treated by warming-up with moxibustion, it cannot be treated by acupuncture." In Chapter 48 of *Miraculous Pivot* it states, "Depressed symptoms should be treated by moxibustion alone, because depression is due to blood stagnation caused by cold, which should be dispersed by moxibustion." It is easy to understand that moxibustion functions to warm up the meridians and promote blood circulation. Therefore, it is mostly used in clinic to treat diseases caused by cold-dampness and persistent diseases caused by pathogenic cold penetrating into the deep muscles.

2) To induce the smooth flow of qi and blood Another function of moxibustion is to induce qi and blood to flow upward or downward. For example, moxibustion is given to Yongquan (K 1) to treat the disorders caused by excess in the upper part and deficiency in the lower part of the body and liver yang symptoms due to upward

flowing of yang qi so as to lead the qi and blood to go downward. In Chapter 64 of *Miraculous Pivot*, it is pointed out that "when there is an excess of qi in the upper portion, the qi should be brought downward by needling the points in the lower portion." If the disorder is due to deficiency in the upper portion and excess in the lower portion of the body and due to sinking of qi caused by deficiency, such as prolapse of anus, prolapse of uterus, prolonged diarrheoa, etc, moxibustion to Baihui (Du 20) may lead yang qi to flow upward.

3) To strengthen yang from collapse Yang qi is the foundation of the human body. If it is in a sufficient condition, a man lives a long life; if it is lost, death occurs. Yang disorder is due to excess of yin, leading to cold, deficiency and exhaustion of the primary qi characterized by a fatal pulse. At this moment moxibustion applied can reinforce yang qi and prevent collapse. In Chapter 73 of *Miraculous Pivot it says,* "Deficiency of both yin and yang should be treated by moxibustion."

4) To prevent diseases and keep healthy In *Precious Prescriptions* appears the following description: "Anyone who travels in the southwest part of China, such as Yunnan and Sichuan provinces, should have moxibustion at two or three points to prevent sores or boils and to avoid

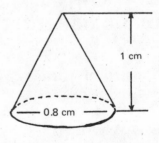

Fig. 155

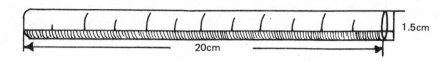

Fig. 156

pernicious malaria, epidemic diseases and pestilence." It is often said, "If one wants (S 36) to be healthy, you should often have moxibustion over the point Zusanli (S 36)". In *Notes on Bian Que's Moxibustion*, it says, "When a healthy man often has moxibustion to the points of Guangyuan (Ren 4), Qihai (Ren 6) Mingmen (Du 4) and Zhongwan (Ren 12), he would live a very long life, at least one hundred years' life." Clinical practice has proved that moxibustion is very much helpful in preventing disease and keeping healthy.

3. Materials for Moxibustion

Moxa wool, moxa cones, moxa sticks, matches and a tray should be ready beforehand.

1) Making of moxa cones Place a small amount of moxa wool on a board, knead and shape it into a cone with the thumb, index and middle fingers in three sizes. The smallest is as big as a grain of wheat; the medium size is about half a date stone, and the largest is the size of the upper part of the thumb. The two smaller cones are suitable for direct moxibustion, while the largest for indirect moxibustion. (See Fig. 155)

2) Making of moxa stick It is much more convenient to use moxa sticks than moxa cones. Simply roll moxa wool (other herbal medicine may be mixed in) into the shape of a cigar, using paper made of mulberry bark. (See Fig. 156)

II. CLASSIFICATION OF MOXIBUSTION

From the ancient times until now rich clinical experience has been gained in the moxibustion therapy. At first only the moxa cones were used. But now various approaches have been developed and used clinically, i.e. moxibustion with maxa cones, with moxa sticks, and with warming needle.

1. Moxibustion with Moxa Cone
Moxibustion with moxa cones may be direct

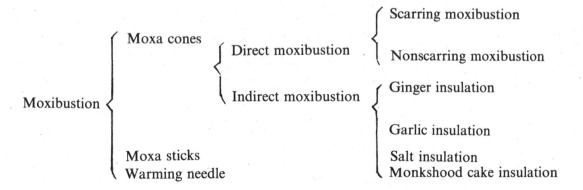

or indirect. Direct moxibustion is to place a moxa cone directly on the skin and ignite it, while indirect moxibustion is to place a moxa cone indirectly on the skin but insulated with some different medical substances. The names are nomenclatured according to the names of the different medical substances, for example, ginger used as the insulator is called moxibustion with ginger; salt used for insulation is called moxibustion with salt. One moxa cone used at one point is called one unit.

1) Direct moxibustion A moxa cone place directly on the point and ignited is called direct moxibustion, and is also known as "open moxibustion," which was widely used in the ancient times with better results. This type of moxibustion is subdivided into scarring moxibustion and nonscarring moxibustion according to whether the local scar is formed or not after moxibustion. (Fig. 157)

a) Scarring moxibustion (also known as "festering moxibustion"):

Prior to moxibustion, apply some onion or garlic juice to the site in order to increase the adhesion of the moxa cone to the skin, then put the moxa cone on the point and ignite it until it completely burns out. Repeat this procedure for five to ten units. This method may lead to a local burn, blister,

festering and scar after healing. Indications are certain chronic diseases such as asthma.

b) Nonscarring moxibustion:

A moxa cone is placed on a point and ignited. When half or two thirds of it is burnt or the patient feels a burning discomfort, remove the cone and place another one. No blister should be formed and there should be no festering and scar formation. Indications are diseases of chronic, deficient and cold nature such as asthma, chronic diarrhoea, indigestion, etc.

2) Indirect moxibustion

The ignited moxa cone does not rest on the skin directly but is insulated from the skin by one of four types of materials.

a) Moxibustion with ginger:

Cut a slice of ginger about 0.5 cm thick, punch numerous holes on it and place it on the point selected. On top of this piece of ginger, a large moxa cone is placed and ignited. When the patient feels it scorching, remove it and light another. This method is indicated in symptoms caused by weakness of the stomach and spleen such as diarrhoea, abdominal pain, painful joints and symptoms due to yang deficiency.

b) Moxibustion with garlic:

Cut a slice of garlic about 0.5 cm thick (a large single clove of garlic is desirable), punch holes in it, put it on the point with the

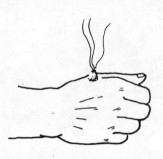

Fig. 157

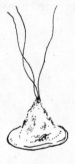

Fig. 158

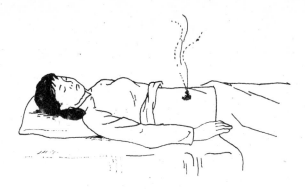

Fig. 159

ignited moxa cone above. Renew the cone when the patient feels it scorching. This method is indicated in scrofula, tuberculosis, the early stage of skin ulcer with boils, poisonous insect bite, etc.

c) Moxibustion with salt:

This is usually applied at the umbilicus, so it is also called "moxibustion at Shenque point." Fill the umbilicus with salt to the level of the skin, place a large moxa cone on the top of salt and then ignite it. (If the patient's umbilicus is not concave in shape, a piece of wet noodle can be put around the umbilicus then fill salt in it. The moxa cone can be placed and ignited on the top of it.) This method is effective in cases of abdominal pain, vomiting and diarrhoea, pain around the umbilicus, pain caused by hernia, prolonged dysentery, etc. In addition, moxibustion with salt has the function to restore yang from collapse, e.g. symptoms of excessive sweating, cold limbs and undetectable pulse. Large moxa cones may be used successively until sweating stops, pulse restores and the four extremities get warm. (Fig. 159)

d) Moxibustion with monkshood cake:

A coin-sized cake made of monkshood powder mixed with alcohol, is punched with numerous holes in it, and placed on the site for moxibustion with the moxa cone ignited and burnt on the top of it. Since it is of heat nature, the monkshood may warm yang and expel cold. This method is only suitable to treat deficient, and persistent yin-cold syndromes, such as impotence and ejaculatio precox caused by declination of the Mingmen fire.

2. Moxibustion with Moxa Sticks

Apply a lighted moxa stick over the selected point. It is easy to control heat and time during moxibustion, and the therapeutic effect is good, so it is often used today. This method includes two kinds: mild-warm moxibustion and sparrow-pecking moxibustion.

1) Mild-warm moxibustion

Apply an ignited moxa stick over the point to bring a mild warmth to the local area for five to ten minutes until the local area is red. (Fig. 160)

2) "Sparrow-pecking" moxibustion

When this method is applied, the ignited moxa stick is rapidly pecked over the point, paying attention not to burning the skin. In addition, the ignited moxa stick may be evenly moved from left to right or in circular

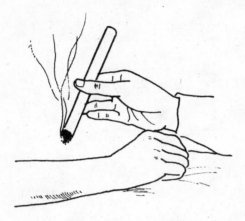

Fig. 160

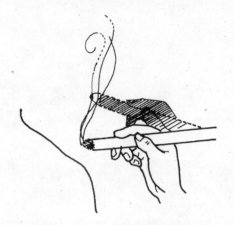

Fig. 161

movement. (Fig. 162)

3) Moxibustion with warming needle

Moxibustion with warming needle is a method of acupuncture combined with moxibustion, and is used for conditions in which both the retaining of the needle and moxibustion are needed. The manipulation is as follows:

After the arrival of qi and with the needle retained in the point, wrap the needle handle with a unit of moxa wool and ignite it to cause a mild heat sensation around the point. This method functions to warm the meridians and promote the free flow of qi and blood so as to treat painful joints caused by cold-damp, numbness with cold sensation and paralysis. (Fig. 162)

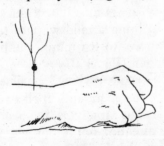

Fig. 162

Appendix: The Great Monad Herbal Moxa Stick and Thunder-Fire Herbal Moxa Stick

1) The Great Monad Herbal Moxa Stick

Compositions:

150 g of moxa wool,
 10 g of sulphur,
  5 g of musk,
  5 g of Resina Boswelliae Carterii,
  5 g of Myrrha,
  5 g of Colophonium,
  5 g of Cassia Twig,
  5 g of Eucommia Bark,
  5 g of Bitter Orange,
  5 g of Spina Gleditsiae,
  5 g of Herba Asari,
  5 g of Rhizoma Ligustici Chuanxiong,
  5 g of Radix Angelicae Pubescentis,
  5 g of Squama Manitis,
  5 g of Realgar,
  5 g of Radix Angelicae Dahuricae, and
  5 g of Scorpion.

These herbs are mixed together and ground into fine powders, put some powders on a piece of paper and cover it with another piece of paper. Several layers of fine powder covered with several layers of paper are made, then put a layer of clean moxa wool on the top and tightly roll them together like a fire cracker in shape, and naste the outside with a piece of white mulberry paper. The whole stick is fixed by the egg white, and dried in a cool place without sunshine. Leakage should be avoided.

Method: The area for moxibustion should be examined and marked. Burn one stick completely and rapidly put the ignited stick in a piece of dry cloth which has been folded into seven layers. Then direct the cloth with the ignited moxa stick in it to the skin to produce a heat sensation on the affected area and make it penetrate into the deep muscles. If the patient feels it scorching, the stick may be lifted a little. When the heat sensation becomes normal, press and iron the affected area until the heat on the ignited end extinguishes. Ignite another stick and go on ironing the affected area. In order to get good results and keep the heat on the affected area, it is better to prepare two sticks in turn for use. This method can warm and promote the free flow of qi and blood, dispel cold and dampness. It is, therefore, used for painful joints caused by wind, cold and dampness, and for prolonged diseases and pains such as abdominal pain, dysmenorrhea, hernia, etc.

2) Thunder-fire moxa stick Get two sheets of paper ready. One is thick, the other is thin. One sheet is paralleld with the other which has been already folded into double layers. On the top of the double-folded paper, place a layer of clean moxa wool. Slightly tap it with a wooden ruler or a rattan stick until it spreads squarely with even thickness. Then put some herbal powders on the moxa wool and roll them together like a fire cracker in shape. After

that it is wrapped up with a sheet of thin paper and fixed with egg white. The stick is dried in a cool place without sunshine. Avoid leakage of the roll.

Compositions:

100 g of moxa wool,
  15 g of Eagle Wood,
  15 g of Radix Inulae Helenii,
  15 g of Resina Boswelliae Carterii,
  15 g of Notopterygium,
  15 g of Dried ginger, and
  15 g of Squama Manitis.

These herbs should be ground into fine powder, and a little musk is added after sieving.

The method and indications are the same as those of the Great Monad Herbal moxa stick.

III. APPLICATION OF MOXIBUSTION

1. The Process and Volumn for Moxibustion

The Precious Prescriptions points out that "Moxibustion is generally applied to yang portion first, then yin portion; clinically it is applied to the upper part first and then the lower part." Treat the back first, the abdominal region second; the head and body first and the four extremities second. But the sequence should be given according to the pathological conditions.

The volume for moxibustion, including the size of moxa cone or duration of the moxa stick application should be in parallel to the patients' pathological conditions, general constitution, age and the site where moxibustion is to be applied. Generally, three to seven moxa cones are used for each point, and ten to fifteen minutes for the application of moxa stick.

2. Contraindications

1) Excess syndrome, and heat syndrome (including high fever caused by common cold or heat due to yin deficiency) are not allowed to be treated by moxibustion. It is stated in *Treatise on Febrile Diseases* that "a patient with feeble and rapid pulse should not be treated by moxibustion. Although the heat of moxibustion is weak, strong internal impact may produce," indicating that improper moxibustion may bring bad results.

2) Scarring moxibustion should not be applied to the face and head, and the area in the vicinity of the large blood vessels. According to the recordings of ancient literature, there are certain points which are advisable to acupuncture but not suitable for moxibustion, because most of them are close to the vital organs or arteries. Examples are Jingming (B 1), close to the eyeball, and Renying (S 9), above a large artery.

3) The abdominal region and lumbosacral region of the pregnant woman are not allowed to use moxibustion.

3. Management After Moxibustion

After moxibustion, different degrees of burns may remain in the local region, or there is only a slight red sign of burning which will disappear very soon. But sometimes, a few blisters result on the skin surface. Take care not to let small blisters break. They can be healed by themselves.

Large blisters should be punctured and drained. If pus is formed, the blister should be dressed to prevent further infection.

IV. CUPPING METHOD

Cupping is a therapy in which a jar is attached to the skin surface to cause local congestion through the negative pressure created by introducing heat in the form of an ignited material. In the ancient times in China, cupping method was called "horn method."

The animal horn was used to dispel pus. Along with continual development in clinical practice, the materials for making jars and the methods have been greatly improved. The range of indications has been expanded, since this method is simple and the therapeutic effect is good. This therapy was attracted with great attention and applied in a large scale by the broad masses, and also used as an auxillary method of acupuncture and moxibustion.

1. Types of Jars

There are a great variety of jars, but the commonly used clinically are as follows:

1) Bamboo jar Cut down a section of bamboo 3-7 cm in diameter and 8-10 cm in length, forming a cylinder shaped as a drum. One end is used as the bottom, and the other as the opening. The rim of the jar should be made smoothly. The bamboo jar is light, economical, easy to make and availabe in many places.

2) Glass cup Since the glass cup is transparent, the local congestion at the site for moxibustion can be seen so as to control the treatment.

2. Indications

The cupping method has the function of warming and promoting the free flow of qi and blood in the meridians, dispelling cold dampness, diminishing swellings and pains. In clinics, the cupping method is mainly used to treat *Bi* syndrome caused by wind dampness, such as pain of the low back, shoulders, and leg, gastrointestinal disorders such as stomachache, vomiting, and diarrhoea, and the lung disease such as cough and asthma.

The cupping method combined with bloodletting is suitable to treat acute sprains accompanied by blood stasis.

3. Manipulations

1) **Fire throwing method**   Throw a piece of ignited paper or an alcohol cotton ball into the cup, then rapidly place the mouth of the cup firmly against the skin on the desired location. This method is applied to the lateral side of the body, otherwise the burning paper or cotton ball may fall and hurt the skin.

2) **Fire twinkling method** Clamp a cotton ball soaked with 95% alcohol with the forceps or nippers, ignite it and put it into the cup, and immediately take it out and place the cup on the selected position.

Generally, the cup is sucked in place for ten minutes. The skin becomes congested with violet coloured blood stasis formation. On withdrawing the cup, hold the cup with the right hand, and press the skin around the rim of the cup with the left hand to let air in.

In addition, cupping may be combined with the bloodletting technique. First sterilize the area for cupping and prick a small vein with a triangular needle or intrademal needle, and the cupping follows.

4. Precautions

1) The patient should select a comfortable position. Cups in different sizes are used according to the cupping location. Generally, the areas where the muscle is abundant and elastic, free from hairs and bone ridges are selected.

2) The burning flame should be stronger enough to create a vacuum. Hold the cup with the rim close to the local area and cup it to the skin rapidly and deftly, otherwise, there will be no therapeutic effects.

3) It is not advisable to apply cupping to the patient with skin ulcer, edema, or on an area overlying large blood vessels, to the patient with high fever and convulsion; or to the abdominal and sacral regions of the pregnant women.

4) It is not suitable to apply cupping to the patient susceptible to spontaneous bleeding or endless bleeding after trauma.

5) After cupping, there is a blood stasis or bruise at the local area. Generally, it will disappear several days later. Small blisters occurring on the skin will absorb naturally several days later. If the blisters are severe, draw out the liquid by a sterile syringe, apply gentian violet and cover them with gause to prevent infection.

In case cupping is combined with bloodletting, remove the blood from the punctured hole with a dry cotton ball.

Chapter 16

A GENERAL INTRODUCTION TO ACUPUNCTURE TREATMENT

Acupuncture therapy takes the theories of traditional Chinese medicine as guidance to treat patients with acupuncture and moxibustion based upon differentiation of syndromes. This chapter deals mainly with the general laws of acupuncture therapy. The descriptions for the principles of treatment, the methods, the basic guidelines for prescription and selection of points are as follows:

I. GENERAL PRINCIPLES OF TREATMENT

The general principles of treatment are worked out under the guidance of the holistic concept and differentiation of syndromes. The general principles are of universal significance in decision of the treating methods and priscriptions.

1. Regulation of Yin and Yang

The occurrence of any diseases is, fundamentally speaking, due to the relative imbalance of yin and yang. Namely, the normal inter-consuming-supporting relationship between them is disturbed by either preponderance or discomfiture of yin and yang. Regulation of yin and yang is therefore a fundamental principle in clinical treatment. In the fifth chapter of *Miraculous Pivot*, it points out that "how to regulate yin and yang is most important in acupuncture treatment."

Yang in excess makes yin suffer and yin in excess makes yang suffer. Excessive heat (yang) is likely to injure yin essence, while excessive cold (yin) is likely to damage yang qi. In treatment, reduce excessive heat or expel cold through the methods of "removing the excess" and "reducing the preponderance." On regulating the preponderance of yin or yang, attention should be paid to the condition whether a corresponding yin or yang deficiency exists. If one is deficient, consideration should be given to both yang reduction and yin reinforcement, dispelling cold and warming yang simultaneously.

Yin in deficiency fails to control yang, manifested by deficiency heat syndrome and yang hyperactivity due to yin deficiency. Yang in deficiency fails to control yin, as shown in deficiency cold syndrome and excess of yin due to yang deficiency. In the fifth chapter of *Plain Questions*, it says, "Treat yin for yang problems and treat yang for yin problems," indicating that hyperactivity of yang due to yin deficiency should be treated by strengthening yin to control yang, while cold (yin) due to yang deficiency should be treated by reinforcing yang to control yin. If they are both deficient, yin and yang should be reinforced. In treating diseases marked by yin or yang deficiency, try to achieve yang from yin and achieve yin from yang, because they are interdependent. For example, the Front-Mu Points and Back-Shu Points are used respectively to regulate and replenish yin qi and yang qi of the zang-fu organs.

Yin and yang are considered the general principle for differentiation of syndromes. In a broad sense, "relieving deficiency by the tonifying method, reducing excess, dispelling cold by the warming method, nutrient and defensive qi regulation, and qi and blood promotion" all fall into the aspect of regulation of yin and yang. Acupuncture therapy is to apply different techniques of manipulations to points to treat diseases by means of regulating yin and yang.

2.   Strengthening the Body Resistance and Eliminating the Pathogenic Factors

The course of a disease is actually the process of struggle between the antipathogenic factors and pathogenic factors. Mobilizing the antipathogenic factors to defeat the pathogenic factors is the right way to cure the disease. Therefore, strengthening the body resistance and eliminating the pathogenic factors are also the important principles in clinical treatment.

To strengthen the body resistance is to reinforce the antipathogenic qi and build up health. Once the body resistance against disease is strengthened, the pathogenic factors are eliminated. Once the pathogenic factors are removed, the body resistance will be reinforced. Since they are closely related to each other, strengthening the body resistance is beneficial to dispelling the pathogenic factors and vice versa.

Clinically, the condition of the pathogenic factors and antipathogenic factors should be carefully observed, upon which, strengthening the body resistance first or dispelling the pathogenic factors first can be determined. For patients with weak body resistance but pathogenic factors not yet strong enough, the body resistance is strengthened first. For patients with excessive pathogenic factors but body resistance not yet damaged, the prime task is to eliminate the pathogenic factors. But for patients with weak body resistance and excessive pathogenic factors as well, both methods should be employed simultaneously. Try to distinguish what is primary from what is secondary. For those with weak body resistance priority should be placed on building body resistance and do something to get rid of the pathogenic factors, and vice versa. When the patient is in a relatively critical condition attacked by excessive pathogenic factors, and the body resistance is too weak, for which the pathogenic factors are not eliminated, strengthen the body resistance first and then remove the pathogenic factors. If the patient is in a very poor condition with excessive pathogenic factors, but with weak body resistance, eliminate the pathogenic factors first, and then strengthen the body resistance.

3.   Distinguishing the Primary from the Secondary

The conception of the primary and the secondary are relative to each other involving different meanings. In terms of the antipathogenic factors and pathogenic factors, the former is the primary, and the latter is the secondary. Judged by the etiology and manifestation, the etiology is the primary, and the manifestation is the secondary. As to the localization of a lesion, the internal portion is the primary, and the external is the secondary. As for the clinical course of a disease the original is the primary, while the complication is the secondary. This concept represents the two opposite aspects of one entity during the course of a disease. The symptom is generally the phenomenon and the secondary aspect, the root cause is generally the nature and the primary aspect.

Clinically, a disease should be assessed according to such different situations of the primary, the secondary, the root cause, the symptoms, the acute, and the chronic so as to ascertain the main aspect of the contradictions, and thus treated accordingly. Under general circumstances, the primary or root cause should be found first, but if the symptoms are acute, they should be treated first. If the symptoms and root cause are both serious, they should be taken into account at the same time.

Trying to find out the primary or root cause is of importance. In clinic, the nature and the primary aspect of a disease should be well commanded so as to treat the root cause. Some diseases, although their symptoms are different, the etiology and pathogenesis are the same, so they can be treated by the same method. For example, in case of sore throat due to yin deficiency of the kidney and low back pain due to yin deficiency of the kidney, the treatment to nourish the kidney yin is adopted. This is called "treating different diseases with the same method." For some other diseases,

although their symptoms are alike, the etiology and pathogenesis are different, different methods therefore should be used to treat the root cause. For instance, headache due to liver yang hyperactivity should be treated by nourishing yin to reduce yang, but headache caused by both qi and blood deficiency should be treated by reinforcing qi and blood. However headache caused by invasion of the meridians by wind cold must be treated by diminishing wind cold. This is called "treating the same disease with different methods."

Under certain circumstances, the symptoms are very critical, if not treated immediately, they shall affect the treatment of the root cause or perhaps cause death, in this case it is necessary to observe the principle of "treating the symptoms first when they are acute, and treating the root cause when these symptoms are relieved." For example, a patient with chronic cough and asthma caught a common cold, accompanied with fever and aversion to cold, common cold should be treated first because it is the acute aspect. After the common cold is relieved, treat chronic cough and asthma which are the primary aspect. But if the primary and secondary aspects are both serious, they must be treated at the same time.

Prevention is also an important aspect in treating the primary aspect. It includes prevention before the attack of a disease and prevention from deterioration after occurrence of a disease. China has long rich experience in health care, such as *Qigong, Taiji, Baduanjin*, etc. Acupuncture and moxibustion is also one of the traditional remedies to prevent diseases. Zusanli (S 36), for example, is an important tonifying point. Moxibustion to it is not only good for preserving health, but also good for preventing many kinds of diseases. Importance is attached to early diagnosis and treatment of disease for fear of its negative development. During the prevention and treatment of diseases, doctors are requested to know the laws of their occurrence and development and the ways of their transmission. It is recorded in *Treatise On Febrile Disease*, "If the illness is going to invade other meridians, needle Foot-Yangming Meridian to stop the development." The importance of preventing diseases from transmission is clearly stated here.

4. Treatment of Diseases According to Climatic and Seasonal Conditions, Geographical Locations and the Individual Condition

The climatic and seasonal conditions, geographical locations, patient's age, constitution and others must be taken into consideration to determine an appropriate method in acupuncture treatment.

1) Climatic and seasonal conditions In accordance with the characteristics of climate and seasons, appropriate therapeutic methods are used. It is said in Chapter 9 of *Miraculous Pivot,* "In spring, the pathogenic factors are most likely to attack the superficial layer; in summer, they are most likely to attack the skin; in autumn, they are most likely to attack the muscles; and in winter, they are most likely to attack the tendons and bones. In treatment of such disorders, the techniques should remain consistent with the seasons." Generally, in spring and summer, shallow acupuncture is applied, and in autumn and winter, the deep acupuncture is preferred.

In addition, the acupuncture time is also important. For instance, treatment of malaria is usually applied two to three hours before its attack, and dysmenorrhea is usually treated before the menstrual periods.

2) Geographical locations The appropriate therapeutic methods should be determined according to different geographical locations. Climate and life style vary in different regions, so do the physiological activities and pathological changes, therefore, the methods of treatment should be different. In Chapter 12 of *Plain Questions* it says, "In the north...people live in highlands and mountains, exposed to bitter wind and severe cold. People there prefer outdoor dwelling and milk, that's why they are susceptible to gastric distention due to accumulation of cold for which moxibustion is advisable." "In the south...it is damp, foggy and dewy, people there prefer to sour taste and preserved food, so they have tight muscles and red skin. People in this region are susceptible to cramps of tendons and rheumatism, for which acupuncture is advisable." The above shows that therapeutic methods are closely related to geographical locations, life style and nature of diseases.

3) Individual conditions Treatment is also based on age, sex and constitution. For example, men and women are different in physiology, women have menstruation, pregnancy and puerperal problems, so the points should be carefully selected when treatment is given. People of different ages are different in physiology and pathology. As to constitution, there are strong, weak, more heat, more cold. Besides, the sensitivity to acupuncture varies individually. In the Chapter 38 of *Miraculous Pivot,* it says, "A middle-aged strong person with sufficient qi and blood, and hard skin may, if being attacked by the pathogenic factors, be treated by a deep needling with the needle retained for some time." It says again, "Since an infant has weak muscles and less volume of blood and qi, acupuncture treatment is given twice a day with shallow needling and weak stimulation." It is further pointed out in Chapter 5 of *Miraculous Pivot* that "a deep needling with the needle retained for some time should be applied to physical labourers, whereas, slow insertion of the needle should be given to mental workers."

II. THERAPEUTIC METHOD

The therapeutic methods are worked out under the guidance of the treating principles and differentiation of syndromes, including selection of points and application of acupuncture and moxibustion. Acupuncture therapy concerns the theory, method, prescription and point. Clinically, the four are closely related to one another. According to *Internal Classic* and other medical literature as well as the clinical experiences, there are six kinds of therapeutic methods, namely, the reinforcing, reducing, warming, clearing, ascending and descending.

1. Reinforcing

The reinforcing method is used to strengthen the body resistance and the zang-fu organs and replenish yin, yang, qi, blood with acupuncture and moxibustion. It is indicated to the deficiency-syndrome. It is said in Chapter 10 of *Miraculous Pivot* that "reinforcing is applied in case of deficiency," and said again in Chapter 73 of *Miraculous*

Pivot that "yin and yang deficiency should be treated by moxibustion." The commonly-used reinforcing methods are as follows:

For reinforcing kidney qi, Shenshu (B 23), Guanyuan (Ren 4), Taixi (K 3), etc. are used either with the reinforcing method or moxibustion.

For reinforcing qi of the spleen and stomach, Zhongwan (Ren 12), Qihai (Ren 6), Zusanli (S 36), etc. are used either with the reinforcing method or moxibustion.

For replenishing qi and blood, Pishu (B 20), Geshu (B 17), Zusanli (S 36), Sanyinjiao (Sp 6), etc. are used either with the reinforcing method or moxibustion.

For nourishing kidney yin, Taixi (K 3), Zhaohai (K 6), Zhishi (B 52), etc. are used with the reinforcing method. But the reinforcing method shall in no case be used if the pathogenic factors are excessive and strong, or if the pathogenic factors are not yet completely eliminated, or if the deficiency syndrome is associated with excessive and strong pathogenic factors.

2. Reducing

The reducing method is to dispel the pathogenic factors and remove stagnation in order to help restore the body resistance, and is advisable to the excess syndrome. In the tenth chapter of *Miraculous Pivot,* it says that "excessive and strong pathogenic factors should be eliminated by the reducing method," and it says again in the first chapter of *Miraculous Pivot* that "in acupuncture therapy... the excessive and strong pathogenic factors must be dispelled" and "fullness should be relieved." It is stated in the fifth chapter of *Plain Questions* that "blood stagnation should be treated by bleeding."

The commonly used reducing methods are as follows:

For dispelling wind to relieve the exterior syndrome, Fengchi (G 20), Hegu (LI 4), etc. are needled with the reducing method.

For promoting defecation and reducing heat, Quchi (LI 11), Tianshu (S 25) and Fenlong (S 40) are needled with the reducing method.

For invigorating blood circulation and removing blood stasis, the corresponding points are pricked to bleed to treat blood stagnation.

For removing indigestion, Jianli (Ren 11), Zusanli (S 36) and Sifeng (Extra) are punctured with the reducing method.

But the reducing method shall not be applied to the deficiency syndrome or to cases of deficiency complicated with the excess syndrome.

3.   Warming

The warming method is used to warm the meridians and remove obstructions from them, warm and nourish yang qi, warm the middle *jiao* to dispel cold and restore yang from collapse, etc. It is applied for cold syndromes. In Chapter 74 of *Plain Questions*, it says, "Cold syndromes should be treated by the warming method," and says again in the tenth chapter of the same book that "retain needles for cold syndromes." In Chapter 73 of the same book it states that "if the regular meridians become tight, moxibustion is applied." In Chapter 64 of *Miraculous Pivot*, it points out that "in case of coagulation, give warmth and promote the free flow of qi," and further stated in Chapter 48 of the same book that "moxibustion is applied in case of cold in blood."

The commonly used warming methods are as follows:

Remove cold from the meridians by warmth. Acupuncture with needle retaining or moxibustion is applied to the points along the meridian affected by the pathogenic cold.

For warming the middle *jiao* to dispel cold, Zhongwan (Ren 12) and Zusanli (S 36) are punctured with needle retaining or moxibustion.

For restoring yang from collapse, moxibustion is applied to Guanyuan (Ren 4) and Shenque (Ren 8) to treat cold extremities due to the decline of yang qi.

But the warming method cannot be used for heat syndromes, and moxibustion should be carefully used for syndrome of yin deficiency.

4.   Clearing

The clearing method, known as a febrifugal approach, is used to clear off the pathogenic heat for resuscitation, or for heat syndromes. In Chapter 74 of *Plain Questions*, it states that "heat syndromes should be treated by swift needling." *Compendium of Acupuncture and Moxibustion* says that "the internal pathogenic heat must be cleared off."

The commonly used clearing methods are as follows:

For dispelling the pathogenic heat, Dazhui (Du 14), Quchi (LI 11) and Hegu (LI 4) are often needled with the reducing method.

For heat syndromes in the zang-fu organs, the Jing-(Well) Point and Ying-(Spring) Point of the affected meridians are often needled with the reducing method or blood-letting.

For clearing off heat and resuscitation, Renzhong (Du 26) and the twelve Jing-(Well) Points (L 11,H 9,P 9,LI 1, SJ 1, and SI 1 - on both sides) are needled with the reducing method or bloodletting.

5.   Ascending

The ascending method is used to raise yang qi and lift the zang-fu organs from sinking. It is for failure of ascending pure yang and sinking of the qi in the middle jiao. Chapter 74 of *Plain Questions* says that "prolapse must be treated by the ascending method."   In Chapter 10 of *Miraculous Pivot,* it says that "ptosis must be treated by moxibustion." The Chapter 74 of the same book points out "qi decending from the upper portion must be corrected by pushing it up."

Clinically, acupuncture with the reinforcing method and moxibustion is applied to the local points in combination with Baihui (Du 20), Qihai (Ren 6) Guanyuan (Ren 6), Zusanli (S 36), etc. to treat dizziness and vertigo due to failure of pure yang in ascending, sinking of qi from the middle jiao, visceroptosis, prolapse of rectum and prolonged dysentery.

But the ascending method shall not be used for patients with yin deficiency and yang hyperactivity.

6.   Descending

The descending method is used to make the upward perverted qi go down and to subdue yang. In Chapter 74 of *Plain Questions*, it says that "upward perverted flow of qi should be checked by the descending method." In Chapter 64 of *Miraculous Pivot,* it says, "Conduct the qi downward if it is excessive in the upper part," and says again in Chapter 19 of the same book, "Apply acupuncture to Zusanli (S 36) to make the perverted qi of the stomach descend." In clinics, the commonly used descending methods are as follows:

For regulation of the stomach by keeping its perverted qi to descend, Tanzhong (Ren 17), Zhongwan (Ren 12), Neiguan (P 6) and Zusanli (S 36) are needled with the even movement.

For soothing the liver and subduing liver yang. Fengchi (G 20), Taichong (Liv 3) and Yongquan (K 1) are needled with the reducing method.

But the descending method cannot be used for deficiency syndroms or deficiency syndrome in the upper part and excess in the lower part of the body. In addition, the descending method can be subdivided into many approaches, but they are not discussed in this section.

III.   THE BASIC PRINCIPLES FOR PRESCRIPTION AND SELECTION OF POINTS

Acupuncture and moxibustion is a therapy by needling or moxibustion to certain points of the human body. Therefore, proper prescription including selection and combination of points and the method of treatment employed are significant to the curative effects. In prescription, points should be selected according to their functions and the planned method should be decided on basis of differentiation of syndromes. The following is an brief introduction to the basic principles for prescription and selection of points.

1.   Acupuncture Prescription

1) What is an acupuncture prescription
Acupuncture prescription refers to the desired plan to be conducted in treating certain diseases. The selection of points and methods used are included. The prescription should list the combination of points, methods of manipulation — reinforcing or reducing, duration and frequency of treatment, etc. Generally, a list of points in the order from upper to lower portion of the body, from the back to the abdominal region, or from the most important ones to the secondary ones should be made. Then put down a particular point on one side or bilateral sides, methods of manipulation, duration of needle retaining and course of treatment, etc.

In the prescription, the following symbols are commonly used for methods of manipulation:

T or+stands for reinforcing;

⊥ or−stands for reducing;

I or± stands for even movement;

∴ stands for cutaneous needle;

o− stands for imbedding needle;

↓ stands for bleeding with a three-edged needle;

Δ stands for moxibustion;

X stands for moxibustion with moxa sticks;

φ stands for warming needle.

2) Number of points in a prescription

Diseases vary in their occurrence and development. Different prescriptions are used according to the different individuals and diseases. It is stated in Chapter 74 of *Plain Questions* that "diseases may appear in severity or mildness, treatment should be given according to individual conditions, and prescriptions may be large or small." In Chapter 59 of *Miraculous Pivot* it says that "diseases are changeable, thus there are countless methods of treatment to be considered by reference to the condition. A mild case should be treated by selecting a few points, while a severe case treated by selecting many points." Generally, there are five acupuncture prescriptions according to the number of points selected. They are "big prescription," "small prescription," "odd prescription," "even prescription," and "compound prescription." The big prescription refers to the selection of a great number of points, and is applied to a wide range of disorders in the zang-fu organs, meridians and collaterals. For intance, a prescription for hemiplegia caused by windstroke and epilepsy are often treated by selection of a large number of points. A small prescription refers to the selection of less points and is widely used in common ailments, such as malaria and epigastric pain.A compound prescription refers to the application of two or more than two groups of points with different functions for complicated cases which have two or over two symptoms simultaneously. For instance, when headache appears at the same time with diarrhoea, the prescriptions for both should be used. In addition, an "odd prescription" indicates only a point is used. For instance, Ximen (P 4) is prescribed to treat cardiac pain. Shuigou (Du 26) is for pain in the back and lumbar region. Moreover, an even prescription means a pair of points selected, e.g. the combination of Back-(Shu) Point with Front-(Mu) Point, Yuan-(Primary) Point with Luo-(Connecting) Point, and points in the upper part with the Eight Confluent Points in the lower part of the body.

2. Principles for Point Selection

Selection of points along the course of meridians is the basic principle in acupuncture treatment, which is performed according to the theory of that diseases are related to meridians. In application there are three methods of point selection, namely, selecting points from the affected meridian, selecting points from the related meridian, and selecting points from several meridians. The first refers to a selection of points on the diseased meridian to which one of the organs is related. The second refers to a selection of points not only from the affected meridian, but also from the meridian related to the affected meridian according to the relations between the zang-fu organs and meridians. Generally, points of the exteriorly-interiorly related meridians or points of the "mother-son" related meridians are selected according to the theory of Five Elements. The third is used for symptoms caused by several diseased meridians, i.e. when a patient does not respond to the selected points of one or two meridians, points of other meridians should be used too. Since point selection along the meridians is guided by the theory of the zang-fu organs and meridians it is essential to have a full understanding of physiology and pathology, the running course of the meridians, the

exterior and interior relationship of yin and yang and the function of points.

There are three categories of point selection:

1) Selection of nearby points   Nearby refers to the local area of the disease or the adjacent area of the disease.

a) Selection of local points   Local refers to the vicinity of the disease. For example, Jingming (B 1) and Zanzhu (B 2) are selected for eye disease; Juliao (S 3) and Yingxiang (LI 20) for nose disease; Tinggong (SI 19) and Tinghui (G 2) for ear disease; Zhongwan (Ren 12) for epigastric disease and Taiyang (Extra) for headache. When there is an ulcer, wound or scar in the local area, select adjacent points instead of the local.

b) Selection of adjacent points: Adjacent refers to the location close to the diseased area. For instance, Shangxing (Du 23) and Tongtian (B 7) are selected for nose disease; Fengchi (G 20) and Fengfu (Du 16) for headache; and Zhangmen (Liv 13) and Tianshu (S 25) for gastric pain. The adjacent points may be used independently or in combination with the local points. Points from the head and trunk selected for problems of the five sense organs and zang-fu organs are within this category.

2) Selection of distant points   Distant refers to a location far from the diseased area. Generally, these points are located below the elbows and knees. It is said in Chapter 70 of *Plain Questions*, "Points on the lower portion should be selected for the upper problems, points on the upper should be selected for the lower problems, and points on the side of the body should be selected for middle problems." For example, Zusanli (S 36) is selected to treat epigastric and abdominal disorders, Hegu (LI 4) is selected to treat facial disorders, Xingjian

(Liv 2) is selected to treat swelling and red eyes, and Baihui (Du 20) is selected to treat chronic dysentery (Table 19)

Table 19. Examples for Distant and Nearby Point Selection

Diseased area	Distant Points	Adjacent Points	Local Points
Forehead	Hegu (L I 4),	Baihui (Du 20)	Yangbai (G 14)
Temple head	Waiguan (S J 5), Zulinqi (G 41)	Fengchi (G 20)	Taiyang (Extra), Shuaigu (G 8)
Nape	Houxi (S I 3), Kunlun (B 60)	Dazhui (Du 14)	Tianzhu (B 10)
Eye	Yanglao (S I 6), Taichong (Liv 3)	Muchuang (G 16)	Jingming (B 1)
Nose	Lieque (L 7), Lidui (S 45)	Shangxing (Du 23)	Yingxiang (L I 20)
Mouth and cheek	Hegu (L I 4), Jiexi (S 41)	Quanliao (S I 18)	Dicang (S 4), Jiache (S 6)
Ear	Zhongzhu (S J 3), Xiaxi (G 43)	Fengchi (G 20)	Tinghui (G 2), Yifeng (S J 17)
Throat	Yuji (L 10), Zhaohai (K 6)	Tianzhu (B 10)	Lianquan (Ren 23), Tianrong (S I 17)
Chest	Neiguan (P 6), Fenglong (S 40)	Zhongfu (L 1)	Tanzhong (Ren 17)
Costal region	Zhigou (S J 6), Yanglingquan (G 34)	Zhangmen (Liv 13)	Qimen (Liv 14)
Upper abdomen	Neiguan (P 6), Zusanli (S 36)	Liangmen (S 21)	Zhongwan (Ren 12)
Lower abdomen	Sanyinjiao (Sp 6), Ququan (Liv 8)	Tianshu (S 25)	Guanyuan (Ren 4)
Lumbar region	Weizhong (B 40), Houxi (S I 3)	Ciliao (B 32)	Shenshu (B 23), Dachangshu (B 25)
Rectum	Chengshan (B 57),	Baihuanshu (B 30)	Changqiang (Du 1)

Selection of the distant points forms an important part in the point selection. For example, points on the four extremities are selected for disorders of the head, trunk and zang-fu organs. The system of meridians is a crisscross network running longitudinally and transversely, superficially and deeply. In combination of points, different approaches are conducted, such as combining the above with the below, combining the left with the right (or crossing combination), combining the exterior with the interior, and combining the local with the distant.

Selecting points on the left side to treat disorders on the right side and vice versa is known as the crossing combination of points. It is clearly analyzed in the fifth chapter of *Plain Questions* as the "contralateral puncture" (see Chapter 14).

3) Selection of symptomatic points: This refers to the selection of the corresponding points according to some prominent symptoms. For example, Dazhui (Du 14) and Quchi (LI 11) are selected to treat fever, and Shuigou (Du 26) and Yongquan (K 1) are selected to treat loss of consciousness in emergent cases.

Selection of the empirical points falls into this category. For example, Sifeng (Extra) is selected to treat infantile indigestion. Moxibustion applied to Erbai (Extra) is for hemorrhage of hemorrhoids (Table 20.)

IV. APPLICATION OF SPECIFIC POINTS

Specific points are those on the fourteen meridians with specific treating significance. They are indicated in various diseases. Clinically, they can be used flexibly according to the above-mentioned prin-

Table 20.   Example for Symptomatic Point Selection

Symptoms	Points	
Fever	Dazhui (Du 14),	Quchi (L I 11), Hegu (L I 4)
Coma	Shuigou (Du 26),	Shixuan (Extra)
Night sweating	Houxi (S I 3),	Yinxi (H 6)
Clenched jaws	Xiaguan (S 7),	Jiache (S 6), Hegu (L I 4)
Cough, asthma	Tiantu (Ren 22),	Dingchuan (Extra)
Suffocated chest	Tanzhong (Ren 17),	Neiguan (P 6)
Cardiac pain	Neiguan (P 6),	Ximen (P 4)
Hypochondriac pain	Zhigou (S J 6),	Yanglingquan (G 34)
Abdominal distention	Qihai (Ren 6),	Zusanli (S 36)
Constipation	Zhigou (S J 6),	Zhaohai (K 6)
Convulsion	Hegu (L I 4),	Taichong (Liv 3)
Epistaxis	Shangxing (Du 23),	Hegu (L I 4)

ciples in point selection. Specific points bear different names as mentioned in the chapter "General Introduction to Points." Here is a further exploration into their characteristics in the clinical application.

1. Specific Points on the Four Extremites

1) The Five-Shu Points   These are five points of the twelve regular meridians located below the elbow and knee, namely, Jing-(Well), Ying-(Spring), Shu-(Stream), Jing-(River) and He-(Sea). They are imaged by the ancients as the flowing water, representing the volume of qi in the meridians. They are located in an order from below to above and the qi in them increases one by one. It is described in the first chapter of *Miraculous Pivot*, "The points at which qi springs up are called well points; the points where qi flows copiously are called spring points; the points where qi flows like a stream are called stream points; the points where qi flows through are called river points; and the points where qi gathers are

called sea points." The sixty-eight problem in *Classic on Medical Problems* says that "Jing-(Well) Points are indicated in the fullness of the chest; Ying-(Spring) Points in the febrile diseases; Shu-(Stream) Points in the heavy sensation of the body and painful joints; Jing-(River) Points in cough and asthma due to pathogenic cold and heat; and He-(Sea) Points in diarrhea due to perversive flow of qi." Generally speaking, Jing-(Well) Points are indicated in mental illness related to the zang organs; Ying-(Spring); Shu-(Stream) and Jing-(River) Points are indicated in disorders along the outer course of the affected meridians. Points on the yin meridians are indicated in the disorders of the internal organs. The He-(Sea) Points are indicated in problems related to the fu organs, the Lower He-(Sea) Points are taken as the main points.

The Combination of Mother and Son Points for Reinforcing and Reducing

In addition to the selection of the Five Shu

Points according to their therapeutic properties, the Five Shu Points can be selected according to the interpromoting, interacting, overacting and counteracting relations of the Five Elements to which they are respectively attributed. The Jing-(Well), Ying-(Spring), Shu-(Stream), Jing-(River) and He-(Sea) Points of the yin meridians are attributed to the Five Elements in the order of wood, fire, earth, metal and water, but those of the yang meridians in the order of metal, water, wood, fire and earth. Based on the interpromoting relation of the Five Elements, each meridian has a "mother" point and a "son" point. For instance, the Lung Meridian relates to metal, the "mother" of metal is earth, then the "mother point" of the Lung Meridian is Taiyuan (L 9) which attributes to earth. The "son" of metal is water, so the "son point" of the Lung Meridian is Chize (L 5) which attributes to water. The "mother point" of a meridian has a reinforcing effect, while the "son point" has a reducing effect. Reinforce the mother for deficiency syndrome and reduce the son for excess syndrome when this principle is applied for treatment, but differentiation of syndromes should be done to see the affected meridian and organ, as well as the presentation of excess and deficiency before the selection of points. In practice the two methods are used: reinforcing or reducing the affected meridian and reinforcing or reducing the related meridian.

a) Reinforcing or reducing the affected meridian:

For example, when the Lung Meridian is involved in a deficiency syndrome with symptoms of chronic cough, asthma on exertion, weak voice, profuse sweating and thready weak pulse, the "mother point" of the Lung Meridian Taiyuan (L 9) is used with the reinforcing method. (Taiyuan attributes to earth. The lung pertains to metal, which is promoted by earth, so Taiyuan is the mother point of the Lung Meridian.) When the Lung Meridian is involved in an excess syndrome with abrupt onset of cough, dyspnea, coarse voice, stuffy sensation in the chest, failure to lie flat, and superficial slippery forceful pulse, Chize (L 5), the "son point" of the Lung Meridian is used with the reducing method. Chize attributes to water, which is promoted by metal, so Chize is the son point of the Lung Meridian.

b) Reinforcing or reducing the related meridian:

Reinforcing or reducing the related meridian is applied on the basis of the relations of the Five Elements of the zang-fu organs. For example, the deficiency syndromes of the Lung Meridian can be treated by reinforcing Taibai (Sp 3), the earth point of the Spleen Meridian, which relates to the Lung Meridian (the spleen pertains to earth; the lung pertains to metal, which is promoted by earth). In contrast, the excess syndrome of the Lung Meridian can be treated by reducing Yingu (K 10), the water point of the Kidney Meridian, which relates to the Lung Meridian. (The kidney pertains to water, the lung pertains to metal, which promotes water.) In addition, the mother and son points can be selected from the exteriorly-interiorly related meridians. For example, the deficiency syndrome of the Lung Meridian can be treated by reinforcing Quchi (L I 11), the mother point of the Large Intestine Meridian, but the excess syndrome of the Lung Meridian can be treated by reducing Erjian (L I 2), the son point of the Large Intestine Meridian. (The large intestine pertains to metal. Erjian attributes to water, which is promoted by metal.)

Table 21. The Five Shu Points of the Yin Meridians

Meridian	Five Shu Point	I (Wood) Jing-(Well)	II (Fire) Ying-(Spring)	III (Earth) Shu-(Stream)	IV (Metal) Jing-(River)	V (Water) He-(Sea)
The Three Yin Meridians of Hand	Lung Hand-Taiyin	Shaoshang (L 11)	Yuji (L 10)	Taiyuan (L 9)	Jingqu (L 8)	Chize (L 5)
	Pericardium Hand-Jueyin	Zhongchong (P 9)	Laogong (P 8)	Daling (P 7)	Jianshi (P 5)	Quze (P 3)
	Heart Hand-Shaoyin	Shaochong (H 9)	Shaofu (H 8)	Shenmen (H 7)	Lingdao (H 4)	Shaohai (H 3)
The Three Yin Meridians of Foot	Spleen Foot-Taiyin	Yinbai (Sp 1)	Dadu (Sp 2)	Taibai (Sp 3)	Shangqiu (Sp 5)	Yinlingquan (Sp 9)
	Liver Foot-Jueyin	Dadun (Liv 1)	Xingjian (Liv 2)	Taichong (Liv 3)	Zhongfeng (Liv 4)	Ququan (Liv 8)
	Kidney Foot-Shaoyin	Yongquan (K 1)	Rangu (K 2)	Taixi (K 3)	Fuliu (K 7)	Yingu (K 10)

Table 22. The Five Shu Points of the Yang Meridians

Meridian	Five Shu Point	I (Metal) Jing-(Well)	II (Water) Ying-(Spring)	III (Wood) Shu-(Stream)	IV (Fire) Jing-(River)	V (Earth) He-(Sea)
The Three Yang Meridians of Hand	Large Intestine Hand-Yangming	Shangyang (L I 1)	Erjian (L I 2)	Sanjian (L I 3)	Yangxi (L I 5)	Quchi (L I 11)
	Sanjiao Hand-Shaoyang	Guanchong (S J 1)	Yemen (S J 2)	Zhongzhu (S J 3)	Zhigou (S J 6)	Tianjing (S J 10)
	Small Intestine Hand-Taiyang	Shaoze (S I 1)	Qiangu (S I 2)	Houxi (S I 3)	Yanggu (S I 5)	Xiaohai (S I 8)
The Three Yang Meridians of Foot	Stomach Foot-Yangming	Lidui (S 45)	Neiting (S 44)	Xiangu (S 43)	Jiexi (S 41)	Zusanli (S 36)
	Gallbladder Foot-Shaoyang	Zuqiaoyin (G 44)	Xiaxi (G 43)	Zulinqi (G 41)	Yangfu (G 38)	Yanglingquan (G 34)
	Bladder Foot-Taiyang	Zhiyin (B 67)	Zutonggu (B 66)	Shugu (B 65)	Kunlun (B 60)	Weizhong (B 40)

Table 23. The "Mother" and "Son" Points for Reinforcing and Reducing

Meridian	Mother Point (Reinforcing)	Son Point (Reducing)
Lung Meridian of Hand-Taiyin	Taiyuan (L 9)	Chize (L 5)
Large Intestine Meridian of Hand-Yangming	Quchi (L I 11)	Erjian (L I 2)
Stomach Meridian of Foot-Yangming	Jiexi (S 4)	Lidui (S 45)
Spleen Meridian of Foot-Taiyin	Dadu (Sp 2)	Shangqiu (Sp 5)
Heart Meridian of Hand-Shaoyin	Shaochong (H 9)	Shenmen (H 7)
Small Intestine Meridian of Hand-Taiyang	Houxi (S I 3)	Xiaohai (S I 8)
Bladder Meridian of Foot-Taiyang	Zhiyin (B 67)	Shugu (B 65)
Kidney Meridian of Foot-Shaoyin	Fuliu (K 7)	Yongquan (K I)
Pericardium Meridian of Hand-Jueyin	Zhongchong (P 9)	Daling (P 7)
Sanjiao Meridian of Hand-Shaoyang	Zhongzhu (S J 3)	Tianjing (S J 10)
Gallbladder Meridian of Foot-Shaoyang	Xiaxi (G 43)	Yangfu (G 38)
Liver Meridian of Foot-Jueyin	Ququan (Liv 8)	Xingjian (Liv 2)

2) The Lower He-(Sea) Points of the Six Fu Organs The Lower He-(Sea) Points refer to the six He-(Sea) Points pertaining to the six fu organs along the three yang meridians of foot. In the fourth chapter of *Miraculous Pivot* it says, "The six fu organs, i.e. stomach, large intestine, small intestine, gallbladder, bladder and Sanjiao are closely related to the three yang meridians of foot on each of which there is a Lower He-(Sea) Point." At the same time, the three yang meridians of foot communicate with the three yang meridians of hand. The stomach, bladder and gallbladder pertain to the three yang meridians of foot, while the large intestine, small intestine and Sanjiao not only communicate with the three yang meridians of hand, but also closely connect with the three yang meridians of foot. The stomach communicates with Zusanli (S 36); the large intestine with Shangjuxu (S 37); the small intestine with Xiajuxu (S 39), all pertaining to the Stomach Meridian of Foot-Yangming. The large intestine and the small intestine pertain to the stomach. It means that their physiological activities work upward and downward. The bladder and Sanjiao communicating with Weizhong (B 40) and Weiyang (B 31) respectively pertain to the Bladder Meridian of Foot-Taiyang, owing to the water passage of Sanjiao connected with the bladder. The gallbladder communicates with Yanglingquan (G 34), a point of the Gallbladder Meridian of Foot-Shaoyang. As it is mentioned in the fourth chapter of *Miraculous Pivot*, "The disorders of the six fu organs can be treated by the He-(Sea) Points." For example, gastric pain and sour regurgitation are treated by Zusanli (S 36); dysentery or appendicitis is treated by Shangjuxu (S 37); biliary pain and vomiting are treated by Yanglingquan (G 34).

3) The Yuan-(Primary) Points The Yuan-(Primary) Points are located in the vicinity of the wrist and ankle. The twelve Yuan-(Primary) Points are closely related to the five zang and the six fu organs, and they are the points where the primary qi of the zang-fu organs is retained. Disorders of the zang-fu organs are usually relieved by needling the twelve Yuan-(Primary) Points. The first chapter of *Miraculous Pivot* says, "When the five zang organs are diseased, the symptoms will manifest themselves in the conditions of the twelve Yuan-(Primary) Points with which they are connected. Each of the five zang organs is connected with its own Yuan-(Primary) Point. For this reason, if we fully grasp the connections between zang organs and their corresponding Yuan-(Primary) Points as well as the latter's external manifestations, there will be no difficulty for us to understand the nature of the diseases of the five zang organs...The twelve Yuan-(Primary) Points are effective for treating the diseases of the five zang and six fu organs." Similar to the Shu-(Stream) Points there is a Yuan-(Primary) Point on the yang meridians. The Yuan-(Primary) Points are closely related to Sanjiao and primary qi.

The primary qi originates from the kidneys, distributing over the whole body and concerning the qi activities. It travels over each yang meridian through Sanjiao. The place where the primary qi is centred is the location of the Yuan-(Primary) Point. Therefore, they are indicated in deficiency and excess syndromes of their respective related organs.

4) The Luo-(Connecting) Points The Luo-(Connecting) Points are situated at the places where the meridians are distributed and the cross of the two exteriorly-interiorly

Table 24. The Lower He-(Sea) Points Pertaining to the Six Fu Organs

Six Fu-Organs	Lower He-(Sea) Point
Stomach	Zusanli (S 36)
Large intestine	Shangjuxu (S 37)
Small intestine	Xiajuxu (S 39)
Gallbladder	Yanglingquan (G 34)
Bladder	Weizhong (B 40)
Sanjiao	Weiyang (B 39)

Table 25. The Yuan-(Primary) Points

Meridian	Yuan-(Primary) Point
Lung Meridian of Hand-Taiyin	Taiyuan (L 9)
Large Intestine Meridian of Hand-Yangming	Hegu (L I 4)
Stomach Meridian of Foot-Yangming	Chongyang (S 42)
Spleen Meridian of Foot-Taiyin	Taibai (Sp 3)
Heart Meridian of Hand-Shaoyin	Shenmen (H 7)
Small Intestine Meridian of Hand-Taiyang	Wangu (S I 4)
Bladder Meridian of Foot-Taiyang	Jinggu (B 64)
Kidney Meridian of Foot-Shaoyin	Taixi (K 3)
Pericardium Meridian of Hand-Jueyin	Daling (P 7)
Sanjiao Meridian of Hand-Shaoyang	Yangchi (S J 4)
Gallbladder Meridian of Foot-Shaoyang	Qiuxu (G 40)
Liver Meridian of Foot-Jueyin	Taichong (Liv 3)

related meridians. On the limbs, each of the twelve regular meridians has a Luo-(Connecting) Point, which connects with its respective exteriorly-interiorly related meridians. That's why the Luo-(Connecting) Points are indicated in the syndromes of their respective exteriorly-interiorly related meridians. *Guide to the Classics of Acupuncture* states that "the Luo-(Connecting) Points are located between two meridians...If they are punctured, symptoms of the exteriorly-interiorly related meridians can be treated." For example, the spleen and stomach are exteriorly-interiorly related, Gongsun (Sp 4), the Luo-(Connecting) Point of the Spleen Meridian can treat not only the diseases of the Spleen Meridian, but also those of the Stomach Meridian. In addition, there are Luo-(Connecting) Points of the Ren and Du Meridians and a major Luo-(Connecting) Point of the Spleen on the trunk. Jiuwei (Ren 15) is the Luo-(Connecting) Point of the Ren Meridian, the collateral of which is distributed on the abdomen to connect the qi of the abdomen. Changqiang (Du 1) is the Luo-(Connecting) Point of the Du Meridian, with its collaterals ascending bilaterally along the spine, and is distributed on the head, joining the Bladder Meridian of Foot-Taiyang in the vicinity of scapula to connect the qi of the back. Dabao (Sp 21) is the Luo-(Connecting) Point of the Spleen Meridian, the collateral of which is distributed on the hypochondrium to connect the qi and blood of the body. Therefore, Jiuwei (Ren 15) can be used for abdominal disease; Changqiang (Du 1) for back disorders, and Dabao (Sp 21) for all the joint problems.

The Combination of the Yuan-(Primary) Points and the Luo-(Connecting) Points

The Yuan-(Primary) Points and Luo-(Connecting) Points may be used independently or in combination. The combination of them is called the "host and guest combination," which is applied according to the occurring order of the diseases on the exteriorly-interiorly related meridians. When a meridian is first affected, its Yuan-(Primary) Point is used, while for second affected meridian, its Luo-(Connecting) Point is used. For instance, both the Lung Meridian and the Large Intestine Meridian are diseased, but the former is affected first, Taiyuan (L 9), its Yuan-(Primary) Point is selected as a main point, and Pianli (LI 6), the Luo-(Connecting) Point of the Large Intestine Meridian is used as a combining point. On the contrary, if the Large Intestine Meridian is diseased first and then the Lung Meridian, Hegu (LI 4), the Yuan-(Primary) Point should be prescribed as a main point, while Lieque (L 7), the Luo-(Connecting) Point as a combining point. This method is adopted when the externally-internally related meridians are affected. And it is known as the combination of the exterior-interior points.

5) The Xi-(Cleft) Points The Xi-(Cleft) Points are those located at the sites where qi and blood in the meridians is converged and accumulated. There are sixteen Xi-(Cleft) Points in all of the twelve regular meridians. In addition, they can be found on each Yangqiao, Yinqiao, Yangwei and Yinwei Meridians. The Xi-(Cleft) Points are used primarily in treatment of the acute diseases

Table 26. The Luo-(Connecting) Points

Meridian	Luo-(Connecting) Point
Lung Meridian of Hand-Taiyin	Lieque (L 7)
Large Intestine Meridian of Hand-Yangming	Pianli (L I 6)
Stomach Meridian of Foot-Yangming	Fenglong (S 40)
Spleen Meridian of Foot-Taiyin	Gongsun (Sp 4)
Heart Meridian of Hand-Shaoyin	Tongli (H 5)
Small Intestine Meridian of Hand-Taiyang	Zhizheng (S I 7)
Bladder Meridian of Foot-Taiyang	Feiyang (B 58)
Kidney Meridian of Foot-Shaoyin	Dazhong (K 4)
Pericardium Meridian of Hand-Jueyin	Neiguan (P 6)
Sanjiao Meridian of Hand-Shaoyang	Waiguan (S J 5)
Liver Meridian of Foot-Jueyin	Guangming (G 37)
Gallbladder Meridian of Foot-Shaoyang	Ligou (Liv 5)
Ren Meridian	Jiuwei (Ren 15)
Du Meridian	Changqiang (Du 1)
The Major Luo-(Connecting) Point of the Spleen	Dabao (Sp 21)

appearing in their corresponding organs. For example, Kongzui (L 6), the Xi-(Cleft) Point of the Lung Meridian of Hand-Taiyin is effective to hemoptysis; Wenliu (LI 7) of the Large Intestine Meridian of Hand-Yangming is helpful to borborygmus and abdominal pain; Liangqiu (S 34) of the Stomach Meridian of Foot-Yangming works for epigastric pain, Ximen (P 4) of the Pericardium Meridian of Hand-Jueyin is effective to cardiac pain and fullness of the chest.

6) The Eight Confluent Points of the Eight Extra Meridians The Eight Confluent Points are those in the extremities connecting the eight extra meridians. Gongsun (Sp 4) of the Spleen Meridian connects with the Chong Meridian; and Neiguan (P 6) of the Pericardium Meridian links with the Yinwei Meridian. These two meridians are confluent in the chest, heart and stomach. Zulinqi (G 41) of the Gallbladder Meridian connects with the Dai Meridian, and Waiguan (S J 5) of the Sanjiao (Triple Energizer) Meridian connects with the Yangqiao Meridian. These two meridians are confluent at the outer canthus, retroauricle, cheek, shoulder and diaphragm. Houxi (S I 3) of the Small Intestine Meridian leads to the Du (Governor Vessel) Meridian, and Shenmai (B 62) of the Bladder Meridian connects with the Yangqiao Meridian. The two meridians are confluent at the inner canthus.

Table 27. The Xi-(Cleft) Points

	Meridian	Xi-(Cleft) Point
Three Yin Meridians of Hand	Lung Meridian of Hand-Taiyin Pericardium Meridian of Hand-Jueyin Heart Meridian of Hand-Shaoyin	Kongzui (L 6) Ximen (P 4) Yinxi (H 6)
Three Yang Meridians of Foot	Large Intestine Meridian of Hand-Yangming Sanjiao Meridian of Hand-Shaoyang Small Intestine Meridian of Hand-Taiyang	Wenliu (L I 7) Huizong (S J 7) Yanglao (S I 6)
Three Yin Meridians of Foot	Stomach Meridian of Foot-Yangming Gallbladder Meridian of Foot-Shaoyang Bladder Meridian of Foot-Taiyang	Liangqiu (S 34) Waiqiu (G 36) Jinmen (B 63)
Three Yang Meridians of Hand	Spleen Meridian of Foot-Taiyin Liver Meridian of Foot-Jueyin Kidney Meridian of Foot-Shaoyin	Điji (Sp 8) Zhongdu (Liv 6) Shuiquan (K 5)
Extra Meridians	Yangqiao Meridian Yinqiao Meridian Yangwei Meridian Yinwei Meridian	Fuyang (B 59) Jiaoxin (K 8) Yangjiao (G 35) Zhubin (K 9)

nape, ear, shoulder and back. Lieque (L 7) of the Lung Meridian leads to the Ren (Conception Vessel) Meridian, and Zhaohai (K 6) of the Kidney Meridian connects with the Yinqiao Meridian. The two meridians are confluent in the lung system, throat and diaphragm. The Eight Confluent Points are indicated in diseases of the extra meridians and their related regular meridians according to their connexions. *Introduction to Medicine* says that "among the 360 points on the whole body, 66 points located at the four extremities are important, and among these 66 points, the Eight Confluent points

are considered the most important." In practice, the Eight Confluent points may be used independently. For instance, problems of the Du Meridian are treated by Houxi (S I 3), disorders of the Chong Meridian are treated by Gongsun (Sp 4) or the Confluent Point on the upper limb can be combined with the Confluent Point on the lower limb. For example, Neiguan (P 6) is combined with Gongsun (Sp 4) to treat diseases of the heart, chest and stomach. Houxi (S I 3) is combined with Shenmai (B 62) for diseases of the neck, shoulder, back and inner canthus.

Table 28.   The Eight Confluent Points of the Eight Extra Meridians

Confluent Point	Regulate Meridian	Extra Meridian	Indications
Neiguan (P 6)	Pericardium	Yinwei	Heart, chest, stomach
Gongsun (Sp 4)	Spleen	Chong	
Houxi (S I 3)	Small Intestine	Du	Neck, shoulder, back inner canthus
Shenmai (B 62)	Bladder	Yangqiao	
Waiguan (S J 5)	Sanjiao	Yangwei	Retroauricle, cheek, outer canthus
Zulinqi (G 41)	Gallbladder	Dai	
Lieque (L 7)	Lung	Ren	Throat, chest, lung
Zhaohai (K 6)	Kidney	Yinqiao	

2. Specific Points on the Head and Trunk

1) **Back-Shu Points**   The specific points on the back are called the Back-Shu Points, where the qi of the zang-fu organs is infused. They are named in accordance with their corresponding zang-fu organs, such as the Back-Shu Point of the heart is called Xinshu (B 15); the Back-Shu Point of the lung is called Feishu (B 13); the Back-Shu Point of the liver is called Ganshu (B 18) and so on.

When the zang-fu organs are diseased, there appears a tenderness in the corresponding Back-Shu Point. In Chapter 51 of *Miraculous Pivot*, it says, "In order to make sure of the point located accurately, one may press the part to see if the patient's original pain gets relieved, if so, the point has been located correctly." The Back-Shu Points are indicated in diseases of the corresponding zang-fu organs. For instance, Feishu (B 13) may be used for the problems of the lung;

Ganshu (B 18) is used for the problems of the liver, etc. In addition, the Back-Shu Points can be used for the illness of the sense organs. For instance, Ganshu (B 18), the Back-Shu Point of the liver, may be chosen to treat eye troubles, as eye is the opening of the liver. Shenshu (B 23), the Back-Shu Point of the kidney, can be prescribed to treat ear disorders, as ear is the opening of the kidney.

2) The Front-(Mu) Points The Front-(Mu) Points are those located at the chest and abdomen, where the qi of the zang-fu organs is infused. Since they are situated closely to their respective related zang-fu organs, any problems of the zang-fu organs can be seen in the corresponding Front-(Mu) Points. For instance, a tenderness may appear in Riyue (G 24) or Qimen (Liv 14) if the gallbladder is affected, and if the stomach is diseased, there is a tenderness in Zhongwan (Ren 12). Therefore, the Front-(Mu) Points are mainly applied to treat disorders of the zang-fu organs and in the local areas. For example, liver disorders associated with hypochondriac pain may be treated by needling Qimen (Liv 14), and abdominal pain due to large intestine disorders may be relieved by needling Tianshu (S 25).

The Back-Shu Points and the Front-Mu Points work for diseases of the zang-fu organs. In addition, they are of different nature of yin and yang. The Back-Shu Points located on the back pertain to yang, while the Front-Mu Points located on the chest and abdomen pertain to yin. It is stated in the sixty-seventh problem of *Classic on Medical Problems*, "Diseases of the zang organs (yin) are manifested in the Back-Shu Points, and the diseases of fu organs (yang) are manifested in the Front-Mu Points." Therefore, the Back-Shu Points are mainly

used to treat the problems of five zang organs, and the Front-Mu Points are mainly effective to the problems of six fu organs. For example, Xinshu (B 15) is helpful to the heart diseases; Ganshu (B 18) works for the liver diseases; Zhongwan (Ren 12) is effective to the stomach diseases and Tianshu (S 25) is good for the large intestine diseases.

This is one of the methods to treat yang disease from yin and vice versa (Table 29)

The Combination of the Back-Shu Points and the Front-Mu Points:

The Back-Shu Points and the Front-Mu Points may be used independently or in combination. Whenever an internal organ is affected, the Back-Shu Point or the Front-Mu Point pertaining to that organ may be prescribed. The application of both may strengthen the therapeutic effects. For instance, Weishu (B 21) on the back and Zhongwan (Ren 12) on the abdomen may be selected for gastric disorders; or Pang-guangshu (B 28) in the sacral region and Zhongji (Ren 3) in the lower abdomen for disorders of the bladder.

3) The Eight Influential Points of the Eight Tissues The Eight Influential Points refer to the specific points which have particular effects in treatment of disorders relating to the zang, fu organs, qi, blood, tendon, pulse and vessels, bone and marrow. Each of the Eight Influential Points overlaps the other point. It is said in *Classic on Medical Problems*, "Zhongwan (Ren 12) is the Influential Point of the fu organs; Zhangmen (Liv 13) is the

Influential Point of the zang organs; Yanglingquan (G 34) is the Influential Point of tendons; Xuanzhong (G 39) is the Influential Point of marrow; Geshu (U 17) is the Influential Point of blood; Dazhu (B 11) is the Influential Point of bone; Taiyuan (L 9) is the Influential Point of pulse and vessels; and Tanzhong (Ren 17) is the Influential Point of qi. For interior heat syndrome, Tanzhong (Ren 17), the Influential Point of qi is applied." In clinics, they are used not only for heat syndromes, but also for all kinds of diseases of the eight tissues. For example, Zhangmen (Liv 13) may be selected for diseases of the zang organs and Geshu (B 17) may be used for disorders of blood.

Table 29. The Back-Shu Points and Front-(Mu) Points

Internal Organs	Back-Shu Point	Front-(Mu) Point
Lung	Feishu (B 13)	Zhongfu (L 1)
Pericardium	Jueyinshu (B 14)	Tanzhong (Ren 17)
Heart	Xinshu (B 15)	Juque (Ren 14)
Liver	Ganshu (B 18)	Qimen (Liv 14)
Gallbladder	Danshu (B 19)	Riyue (G 24)
Spleen	Pishu (B 20)	Zhangmen (Liv 13)
Stomach	Weishu (B 21)	Zhongwan (Ren 12)
Sanjiao	Sanjiaoshu (B 22)	Shimen (Ren 5)
Kidney	Shenshu (B 23)	Jingmen (G 25)
Large Intestine	Dachangshu (B 25)	Tianshu (S 25)
Small Intestine	Xiaochangshu (B 27)	Guanyuan (Ren 4)
Bladder	Pangguangshu (B 28)	Zhongji (Ren 3)

Table 30.   The Eight Influential Points

Tissue	Influential Point
Zang organs	Zhangmen (Liv 13)
Fu organs	Zhongwan (Ren 12)
Qi	Tanzhong (Ren 17)
Blood	Geshu (B 17)
Tendon	Yanglingquan (G 34)
Pulse, vessels	Taiyuan (L 9)
Bone	Dazhu (B 11)
Marrow	Xuanzhong (G 39)

4) The Crossing Points The Crossing Points refer to those located at the intersection of two or more meridians, including the twelve regular meridians and the eight extra meridians. There are about ninety crossing points and most of them are distributed on the trunk, the head and the face. They can be used to treat disorders of the pertaining meridians and the intersected meridians. Generally, they are often used to treat the diseases appearing simultaneously in meridians intersecting each other. For example, Guanyuan (Ren 4) and Zhongji (Ren 3) located at the intersection of three yin meridians and the Ren Meridian may be used to treat diseases of the three foot yin meridians. Sanyinjiao (Sp 6), a crossing point in the three foot yin meridians is used for diseases of the Liver, Spleen and Kidney Meridians.

The number of the Crossing Points increased after the publication of *Systematic Classic of Acupuncture, Plain Questions* edited by Wang Bing, *Medical Highlights, the Illustrated Manual of Acupoints on the New Bronze Figure, Compendium of Acupuncture*, and *Illustrated Supplement to the Classified Classics*. The following is made based on *Systematic Classic of Acupuncture*.

Table 31. The Crossing Points on the Yang Meridians

Point \ Meridian	Du Meridian	Foot-Taiyang	Hand-Taiyang	Foot-Shaoyang	Hand-Shaoyang	Foot-Yangming	Hand-Yangming	Yangwei	Yangqiao	Dai Meridian	Remarks
Shenting (Du 24)	0	✓				✓					
Shuigou (Du 26)	0					✓	✓				
Baihui (Du 20)	0	✓									
Naohu (Du 17)	0										
Fengfu (Du 16)	0							✓			
Yamen (Du 15)	0							✓			
Dazhui (Du 14)	0	✓		✓		✓					
Taodao (Du 13)	0										
Changqiang (Du 1)	0										Knotting at Shaoyin
Jingming (B 1)		0	✓			✓					
Dazhu (B 11)		0	✓								
Fengmen (B 12)	✓	0									
Fufen (B 41)		0	✓								
Fuyang (B 59)		0						✓	✓		Xi-(Cleft) of Yangqiao
Shenmai (B 62)		0						✓	✓		Promoted by Yangqiao
Pucan (B 61)		0						✓	✓		Root of Yangqiao
Jinmen (B 63)		0						✓	✓		Collateral of Yangwei
Naoshu (SI 10)			0					✓	✓		
Bingfeng (SI 12)			0	✓	✓	✓	✓				
Quanliao (SI 18)			0		✓						
Tinggong (SI 19)			0	✓	✓						
Tongziliao (G 1)			✓	0	✓						
Shangguan (G 3)				0	✓	✓					

											Remarks
Hanyan (G 4)				0	✓	✓					
Xuanli (G 6)		✓		0							
Qubin (G 7)		✓		0							
Shuaigu (G 8)		✓		0							
Fubai (G 10)		✓		0							
Touqiaoyin (G 11)		✓		0							
Wangu (G 12)		✓		0							
Benshen (G 13)				0				✓			
Yangbai (G 14)				0				✓			
Toulinqi (G 15)		✓		0				✓			
Muchuang (G 16)				0				✓			
Zhengying (G 17)				0				✓			
Chengling (G 18)				0				✓			
Naokong (G 19)				0				✓			
Fengchi (G 20)				0				✓			
Jianjing (G 21)				0				✓			
Riyue (G 24)				0							Meeting with Foot-Taiyin
Huantiao (G 30)		✓		0							
Daimai (G 26)				0						✓	
Wushu (G 27)				0						✓	
Weidao (G 28)				0						✓	
Juliao (G 29)				0							
Yangjiao (G 35)				0				✓			Xi-(Cleft) of Yangwei
Tianliao (SJ 15)					0						
Yifeng (SJ 17)				✓	0						
Jiaosun (SJ 20)				✓	0		✓				
Erheliao (SJ 22)			✓	✓	0						
Chengqi (S 1)						0			✓		Meeting with Ren Meridian
Juliao (S 3)						0			✓		
Dicang (S 4)						0	✓		✓		
Xiaguan (S 7)				✓		0					
Touwei (S 8)				✓		0		✓			
Qichong (S 39)						0					Starting point of Chong Meridian
Binao (LI 14)							0				Meeting with the collateral of Hand-Yangming
Jianyu (LI 15)							0		✓		
Jugu (LI 16)							0		✓		
Yingxiang (LI 20)						✓	0				

*"0" indicates the meridian of origin and "✓" the crossing meridian.

The Crossing Points on the Yin Meridians

Points \ Meridian	Ren	Foot-Taiyin	Hand-Taiyin	Foot-Jueyin	Hand-Jueyin	Foot-Shaoyin	Hand-Shaoyin	Yinwei	Yinqiao	Chong Meridian	Remarks
Chengjiang (Ren 24)	0										Meeting with Foot-Yangming
Lianquan (Ren 23)	0							✓			
Tiantu (Ren 22)	0							✓			
Shangwan (Ren 13)	0										Meeting with Foot-Yangming & Hand-Taiyin
Zhongwan (Ren 12)	0										Promoted by Hand-Taiyang, Shaoyang & Foot Yangming
Xiawan (Ren 10)	0	✓									
Yinjiao (Ren 7)	0									✓	
Guanyuan (Ren 4)	0	✓		✓		✓					
Zhongji (Ren 3)	0	✓		✓		✓					
Qugu (Ren 2)	0			✓							
Huiyin (Ren 1)	0									✓	Along with Du & Chong Meridians
Sanyinjiao (Sp 6)		0		✓		✓					
Chongmen (Sp 12)		0		✓							
Fushe (Sp 13)		0		✓				✓			
Daheng (Sp 15)		0						✓			
Fuai (Sp 16)		0						✓			
Zhongfu (L 1)		✓	0								
Zhangmen (Liv 13)				0							Meeting with Foot-Shaoyang
Qimen (Liv 14)		✓		0				✓			
Tianchi (P 1)					0						Meeting with Foot-Shaoyang
Henggu (K 11)						0				✓	
Dahe (K 12)						0				✓	
Qixue (K 13)						0				✓	
Siman (K 14)						0				✓	
Zhongzhu (K 15)						0				✓	
Huangshu (K 16)						0				✓	
Shangqu (K 17)						0				✓	
Shiguan (K 18)						0				✓	
Yindu (K 19)						0				✓	
Futonggu (K 20)						0				✓	
Youmen (K 21)						0				✓	

Zhaohai (K 6)					0			✓		Promoted by Yinqiao
Jiaoxin (K 8)					0			✓		Xi-(Cleft) of Yinqiao
Zhubin (K 9)					0		✓			Xi-(Cleft) of Yinwei

Chapter 17

INTERNAL DISEASES

I. EMERGENCY DISEASES AND SYNDROMES CAUSED BY EXOGENOUS PATHOGENIC FACTOR

1. Wind Stroke

Wind stroke is an emergency case manifested by falling down in a fit with loss of consciousness, or hemiplegia, slurred speech and deviated mouth. It is characterized by abrupt onset with pathological changes varying quickly like the wind, from which the term "wind stroke" comes.

Etiology and Pathogenesis

Wind stroke often occurs in the aged who are in poor health, with deficiency of qi and blood, or deficiency in the lower part of the body and excess in the upper part. It may be caused by deficiency of the kidney yin due to sexual indulgence, or by irregular food intake, which impedes the transportation and transformation function of the spleen, leading to production of phlegm from accumulated dampness and transformation into heat. Then there appears imbalance of yin and yang in the zang-fu organs. Other causative factors are exasperation, agitation, alcohol indulgence or overeating, over

strain and stress, or invasion of exogenous pathogenic wind, all leading to upsurge of liver yang and heart fire, which makes qi and blood go upward together with turbid phlegm, disturbing the mind and resulting in this disease. In mild cases there are only symptoms showing dysfunction of the meridians and collaterals, while in severe cases both dysfunction of zang-fu organs and that of the meridians and collaterals are manifested. The syndrome indicating the attack on the zang-fu organs may be subdivided into tense (excess) type and flaccid (deficiency) type.

Tense (excess) syndrome results from disturbance of the mind by the phlegm heat, or collection of excessive fire in the heart and liver, while flaccid (deficiency) syndrome results from deficiency of the primary qi or collapse of the kidney yang. In untreated or improperly treated cases, the tense syndrome tends to become flaccid and the prognosis is often poor.

Differentiation
a) Attack on the zang-fu organs:
i) Tense syndrome:
Main manifestations: Falling down in a fit with loss of consciousness, tightly closed hands and clenched jaws, flushed face, coarse breathing, rattling in the throat, retention of urine, constipation, red tongue

with thick yellow or dark grey coating, string-taut, rolling and forceful pulse.

Analysis: Wind stirred up by upsurge of liver yang sends qi and blood upwards, which together with the accumulated phlegm fire disturb the mind, leading to sudden loss of consciousness with tightly closed hands and clenched jaws, flushed face, coarse breathing, retention of urine and constipation. Excessive wind phlegm brings about rattling in the throat. Red tongue with thick yellow coating or dark grey coating, string-taut, rolling and forceful pulse are the signs of wind combined with phlegm fire.

ii) Flaccid syndrome:

Main manifestations: Falling down in a fit and sudden loss of consciousness with mouth agape and eyes closed, snoring but feeble breathing, flaccid paralysis of limbs, incontinence of urine, flaccid tongue, thready, weak pulse, and in severe cases cold limbs, or flushing of face as rouged, fading or big floating pulse.

Analysis: Severe weakness of primary qi, separation of yin and yang and exhaustion of qi in the zang organs are indicated in mouth agape, eyes closed, snoring but feeble breathing, flaccid paralysis, and incontinence of urine. Flaccid tongue and thready weak pulse suggest the deficiency of blood and prostration of the kidney yang. If complicated with cold limbs, flushed face, fading or big floating pulse, it is a critical case, indicating exhaustion of yin in the lower portion of the body and upward going of the isolated yang.

b) Attack on the meridians and collaterals

There are two categories. One is that only the meridians and collaterals are attacked without the zang-fu organs being involved. The other is that after wind stroke the functions of the affected zang-fu organs have been restored, yet there exists stagnation of qi and blood in the meridians and collaterals.

Main manifestations: Hemiplegia, numbness of the limbs, deviated mouth, slurring of speech, accompanied by headache, dizziness, vertigo, twitching of muscles, red eyes and flushed face, thirst, dryness of the throat, irritability, string taut and rolling pulse.

Analysis: Wind phlegm enters the meridians and collaterals due to imbalance of yin and yang, or after treatment the functions of the affected zang-fu organs have been restored, but wind phlegm still blocks the meridians and collaterals, causing retarded circulation of qi and blood. Hence appears hemiplegia, numbness of the limbs, deviated mouth and slurring of speech. If complicated with upsurging of liver yang, and upward disturbance of wind yang, the symptoms are headache, dizziness, vertigo and twitching of muscles. If there is excessive fire in the heart and liver, there may be red eyes and flushed face, thirst, dryness of the throat and irritability. Stagnation of wind phlegm in the meridians and collaterals leads to a string-taut and rolling pulse.

Treatment

a) Attack on the zang-fu organs:

i) Tense syndrome

Method: Points of the Du Meridian, the Liver Meridian of Foot-Jueyin and the twelve Jing-(Well) points are selected as the main points to promote resuscitation, reduce wind and fire and resolve phlegm. Either reducing method or pricking, to cause little bleeding, is applied.

Prescription: Baihui (Du 20), Shuigou (Du 26), Fenglong (S 40), Taichong (Liv 3), Yongquan (K 1), twelve Jing-(Well) points on both hands (L 11, H 9, P 9, LI 1, SJ 1, SI 1).

Supplementary Points:

Clenched Jaws: Xiaguan (S 7), Jiache (S 6), Hegu (L 14)

Aphasia and stiffness of tongue: Yamen (Du 15), Lianquan (Ren 23), and Tongli (H 5).

Explanation: As the condition is due to disturbance of the heart by phlegm fire associated with upsurging of liver yang and upward flowing of qi and blood, Baihui (Du 20) and Shuigou (Du 26) are selected to regulate qi of the Du Meridian, effecting resuscitation, Yongquan (K 1) is selected to conduct the heat downward, and Taichong (Liv 3) to subdue the upsurging of qi in the Liver Meridian and pacify the liver yang. Pricking the twelve Jing-(Well) points on both hands, where qi of the three yin and three yang meridians meet, may dispel heat and regain consciousness. The spleen and stomach are the source of phlegm production. Fenglong (S 40), the Luo-(Connecting) point of the Stomach Meridian can invigorate the functions of the spleen and stomach and help to resolve the turbid phlegm. Since the Yangming Meridians of Hand and Foot supply the cheeks, Xiaguan (S 7), Jiache (S 6) and Hegu (LI 4) are chosen to promote the circulation of qi and blood for relieving the clenched jaws. Yamen (Du 15) and Lianquan (Ren 23), being local and adjacent points of the tongue, and Tongli (H 5), the Luo-(Connecting) point of the Heart Meridian, may relieve stiffness of tongue.

ii) Flaccid syndrome

Method: Moxibustion is applied to points of the Ren Meridian to restore yang from collapse.

Prescription: Shenque (Ren 8), Qihai (Ren 6) (indirect moxibustion with salt), Guanyuan (Ren 4).

Explanation: Shenque (Ren 8), Qihai (Ren 6) and Guanyuan (Ren 4) are located on the lower abdomen along the Ren Meridian and are the main points effective for collapse. Heavy moxibustion applied on Guanyuan (Ren 4), a meeting point of the Ren Meridian and three yin meridians, can strengthen the primary qi, and restore yang from collapse.

b) Attack on the meridians and collaterals:

Method: Points along the Du Meridian and the yang meridians of the affected side are mainly used to regulate qi and blood, remove obstruction from the meridians and collaterals and reduce the wind. Needle with even movement first from the healthy side and then the affected side.

Prescription: Baihui (Du 20), Tongtian (B 7), Fengfu (Du 16).

Upper limbs: Jianyu (LI 15), Quchi (LI 11), Waiguan (SJ 5), Hegu (LI 4).

Lower limbs: Huantiao (G 30), Yanglingquan (G 34), Zusanli (S 36), Jiexi (S 41).

Supplementary points:

Upward disturbance of wind yang:

Reducing is applied to Fenchi (G 20) and Taichong (Liv. 3), and reinforcing to Taixi (K 3) and Sanyinjiao (Sp 6).

Excessive fire in the heart and liver:

Reducing is applied to Daling (P 7) and Xingjian (Liv 2), and reinforcing to Taixi (K 3).

Deviated mouth: Dicang (S 4), Jiache (S 6).

Explanation: Du Meridian is the sea of all yang meridians. Baihui (Du 20), Fengfu (Du 16) combined with Tongtian (B 7) can eliminate wind and remove obstruction from the meridians and collaterals. Since the yang meridians dominate the exterior of the body and qi, points of the yang meridians are selected to regulate qi and blood of the body and promote smooth circulation in the upper and lower portions of the body. For the upper disturbance of wind yang, Fengchi (G 20) and Taichong (Liv 3) are selected to reduce the wind and pacify the liver. Reinforcing applied to Taixi (K 3) promotes the production of the kidney yin to nourish the liver. Reinforcing applied to Sanyinjiao (Sp 6) nourishes yin and pacifies yang.

For excessive fire in the heart and liver, reducing Daling (P 7) and Xingjian (Liv 2) can eliminate the fire, while reinforcing to Taixi (K 3) nourishes yin to reduce the fire. Dicang (S 4) and Jiache (S 6) are selected for the purpose of promoting a free circulation of qi in the meridians and collaterals around the facial region.

Remarks

a) Wind stroke is referred to cerebral hemorrhage, thrombosis, embolism, subarachnoid hemorrhage, etc. When the acute stage is over, there may be sequelae, such as hemiplegia, monoplegia, aphasia, etc.

b) Prophylactic measures for wind stroke:

The old aged with deficiency of qi and excessive phlegm, or with manifestations of upsurging of liver yang marked by dizziness and palpitations, may have premonitory symptoms such as stiff tongue, slurred speech and numbness of the finger tips. Attention should be paid to diet and life style and avoid overstraining. Frequent moxibustion on Zusanli (S 36) and Xuanzhong (G 39) may prevent an attack of wind stroke.

2. Syncope

Syncope is manifested by sudden fainting, pallor, cold limbs and loss of consciousness, which are often resulted from emotional excitement, fright, or debilitation and overstraining.

Etiology and Pathogenesis

a) Deficiency type:

Syncope of this type is often caused by general deficiency of the primary qi and failure of clear yang in ascending due to over strain or grief and fright, or by exhaustion of qi after profuse bleeding.

b) Excess type:

It is due mainly to emotional disturbances, such as anger, fear and fright, leading to deranged flow of qi, which rushes upwards to the heart and chest, blocking the windpipe and disturbing the mind, or due to upsurging of liver yang, and upward flowing of qi followed by perversion of blood flow after a fit of anger, leading to disturbance of the mind, and resulting in loss of consciousness.

Differentiation

a) Deficiency syndrome:

Main manifestations: Feeble breathing with mouth agape, spontaneous sweating, pallor, cold limbs, deep and thready pulse.

Analysis: Dizziness, vertigo, loss of consciousness, feeble breathing are the symptoms caused by deficiency of primary qi with sudden perversion of its flow, sinking of qi in the spleen and stomach and failure of the clear yang in ascending. Cold limbs are caused by failure of yang qi to reach there. Weakness of primary qi and disabilities of vital qi in controlling the pores are shown in spontaneous sweating, and mouth agape. Deep thready pulse also suggests deficiency of vital qi.

b) Excess syndrome:

Main manifestations: Coarse breathing, rigid limbs, clenched jaws, deep and excess-type pulse.

Analysis: Perversion of qi after a fit of anger makes qi activity impeded and blood rushing upward together with qi to disturb the mind, and hence occur sudden collapse, loss of consciousness, clenched jaws and rigid limbs. Obstruction of qi in the lung gives rise to coarse breathing. Deep and excess-type pulse is a sign of excess syndrome.

Syncope manifestated by sudden loss of consciousness should be distinguished from wind stroke and epilepsy.

Wind stroke: Loss of consciousness is complicated by hemiplegia and deviated mouth. Usually there are sequelae after restoration to consciousness.

Epilepsy: Loss of consciousness is accompanied by convulsions, expectoration of frothy saliva or yelling. When the consciousness is regained the patient becomes as normal as usual.

Treatment
a) Deficiency syndrome:
Method: Points of the Du and Pericardium Meridians are selected as the main points to promote resuscitation, reinforce qi and invigorate yang. Reinforcing is applied in acupuncture, combined with moxibustion.

Prescription: Shuigou (Du 26), Baihui (Du 20), Neiguan (P 6), Qihai (Ren 6), Zusanli (S 36).

Explanation: Shuigou (Du 26), Baihui (Du 20) and Neiguan (P 6) are the points for resuscitation. Qihai (Ren 6) and Zusanli (S 36) are good for reinforcing qi and invigorating yang.

b) Excess syndrome:
Method:Reducing is applied to points of the Du and Pericardium Meridians to promote resuscitation and regulate the flow of qi.

Prescription: Shuigou (Du 26), Hegu (LI 4), Zhongchong (P 9), Laogong (P 8), Taichong (Liv 3), Yongquan (K 1).

Explanation: Shuigou (Du 26) and Zhongchong (P 9) are used to promote resuscitation. Hegu (LI 4) and Taichong (Liv 3) are the points for regulating the circulation of qi and blood. Laogong (P 8) and Yongquan (K 1) promote a clear mind and smooth flow of qi and blood.

Remarks
This condition includes simple fainting, postural hypotension, hypoglycemia, hysteria, etc.

3. Sunstroke

Sunstroke is an acute case occurring in summer, manifested by high fever, irritability, nausea, or even followed by collapse and loss of consciousness. The onset of this disease is due mostly to prolonged exposure to the sun, or to an environment with high temperature.

Etiology and Pathogenesis
Summer heat, a pathogenic factor, is prevalent in summer time when the weather is scorching. Long exposure to the sun and to an environment with high temperature damages qi. Invasion of pathogenic summer heat in a condition of lower resistance brings about sunstroke. Summer heat is a pathogenic factor of yang nature with a tendency to attack the human body quickly. Therefore the onset is abrupt and the changing of the pathological condition is rapid. Pathogenic summer heat is likely to damage the primary qi and consume the body fluid, leading to exhaustion of qi and yin. Furthermore, pathogenic summer heat may penetrate the pericardium and disturb the mind, followed by impairment of consciousness. Sunstroke, according to its clinical manifestations, may be classified into mild and severe types.

Differentiation

a) Mild type:

Main manifestations: Headache, dizziness, profuse sweating, hot skin, coarse breathing, dry mouth and tongue, dire thirst, superficial, large and rapid pulse.

Analysis: Pathogenic summer heat tends to attack the head and gives rise to headache and dizziness. Hot skin results from the accumulation of pathogenic summer heat in the body surface. Profuse sweating, coarse breathing, dry mouth and tongue, dire thirst are all due to evaporation of body fluid by the summer heat. Superficial, large and rapid pulse is a sign showing the presence of the pathogenic summer heat.

b) Severe type:

Main manifestations: Headache, dire thirst, and shortness of breath at first, and then collapse, loss of consciousness, sweating, deep and forceless pulse.

Analysis: This syndrome mostly occurs in those doing physical labour in the scorching summer sun. Overfatigue plus the attack of summer heat results in lowered body resistance and excessiveness of the pathogenic factor with consumption of qi and body fluid. So there are headache, dire thirst and shortness of breath at the very beginning. The pathogenic summer heat can rapidly penetrate into the interior, affecting the pericardium and disturbing the mind. Therefore loss of consciousness follows. Sweating and deep, forceless pulse indicate exhaustion of qi and body fluid.

Treatment

a) Mild type:

Method: Reducing is applied to the points of the Du, Pericardium and Large Intestine Meridians to eliminate the summer heat.

Prescription: Dazhui (Du 14), Neiguan (P 6), Quchi (LI 11), Weizhong (B 40).

Explanation: Dazhui (Du 14), the meeting point of the Du Meridian and all yang meridians, Weizhong (B 40), also named Xuexi, and Quchi (LI 11), an important point for eliminating heat, are used to dispel the summer heat. Neiguan (P 6), the Luo-(Connecting) point of Jueyin Meridian of Hand, is chosen to reduce the fire and to protect the heart.

b) Severe type:

Method: Reducing is applied to the points of the Du Meridian to promote resuscitation, and to dispel the summer heat.

Prescription: Shuigou (Du 26), Baihui (Du 20), Shixuan (Extra), Quze (P 3), Weizhong (B 40).

Explanation: Summer heat is a pathogenic factor of yang nature, which is apt to attack the pericardium and disturb the mind. Shuigou (Du 26) and Baihui (Du 20) are selected to promote resuscitation. Quze (P 6), the He-(Sea) point of Hand-Jueyin, Weizhong (B 40), the He-(Sea) point of Foot Taiyang are pricked superficially to remove the heat from the blood. Blood letting at Shixuan (Extra) can reduce heat and promote resuscitation.

Remarks

a) This illness includes thermoplegia, thermospasm, heliosis, etc.

b) Scraping therapy: It is a popular treatment for mild sunstroke. Dip a smooth spoon into water or vegetable oil and scrape the both sides of the spine, the neck, intercostal spaces, shoulder regions, cubital and axilla fossae until purplish red colour appears.

4. Common Cold

Common cold is an exogenous ailment with headache, nasal obstruction, aversion to wind and fever as its main manifestations. It often results from lowered superficial resistance and invasion of the exogenous pathogenic factors. It may occur in any season. According to the difference in weather, pathogenic factors and body constitution, the manifestations can be classified into two types: wind cold and wind heat.

Etiology and Pathogenesis

This disease is often due to delicate constitution and weakened body resistance which makes the body inadaptable to intense changes of the weather with abnormal cold or warmth. Then the exogenous pathogenic wind invades the body through the pores, skin, mouth and nose, leading to manifestations related to lung and the defensive function. Very often pathogenic wind combined with other pathogenic factors like pathogenic cold causes a wind cold syndrome, or with pathogenic heat causes a wind heat syndrome. Invasion of exogenous pathogenic wind and cold may retard the lung's dispersing function and block the pores, while invasion of exogenous pathogenic wind and heat may impair the lung's descending function by the evaporating heat, and lead to abnormal functioning of the pores. In addition, since the patient's body build is different and the internal and external causes are mutually influenced, the manifestations after invasion by the pathogenic factors must be varied. For patients with yang deficiency, wind cold syndrome is mostly seen, while for those with yin deficiency, wind heat syndrome is often found.

Differentiation

a) Wind cold:

Main manifestations: Chills, fever, anhidrosis, headache, soreness and pain of the limbs, nasal obstruction, running nose, itching of the throat, cough, hoarse voice, profuse thin sputum, thin white tongue coating, superficial and tense pulse.

Analysis: Invasion of the body surface by pathogenic wind and cold impairs the dispersing function of the lung and affects the nose, causing nasal obstruction and discharge. Pathogenic cold is of yin nature, which is likely to damage yang. Impairment of superficial yang is manifested by exterior symptoms such as chills, fever, anhidrosis, headache, even soreness and pain of the limbs. Thin white tongue coating and superficial tense pulse are the signs showing the invasion of the lung and the superficial defensive system by pathogenic wind and cold.

b) Wind heat:

Main manifestations: Fever, sweating, slight aversion to wind, pain and distending sensation of the head, cough with yellow, thick sputum, congested and sore throat, thirst, thin white or yellowish tongue coating, superficial and rapid pulse.

Analysis: Pathogenic wind heat often attacks the body through the nose and mouth. The lung is involved first. Pathogenic wind of yang nature is characterized by upward and outward dispersion. When a fight goes on between the pathogenic wind heat and the body resistance, fever, slight aversion to wind and sweating result. When the pathogenic wind heat attacks the head, symptoms like pain and distending sensation occur in the head. In case the lung fails in dispersing and descending, there appears cough with yellow, thick sputum. When the pathogenic wind heat stifles the air passage, there is congested sore throat with thirst. Thin, white or yellowish tongue coating, and superficial rapid pulse are the signs showing the lung and the defensive system being attacked by the pathogenic wind heat.

Treatment

a) Wind cold:

Method: Reducing is applied to the points of the Du, Taiyang and Shaoyang Meridians to eliminate wind cold and relieve exterior symptoms. Even movement combined with moxibustion is applied to patients with weakened constitutions.

Prescription: Fengfu (Du 16), Fengmen (B 12), Fengchi (G 20), Lieque (L 7), Hegu (LI 4).

Explanation: Fengfu (Du 16) is used to relieve the exterior symptoms, eliminate wind and check headache. Fengmen (B 12), a point of the Taiyang Meridian which dominates the surface of the whole body, is selected to regulate the circulation of qi in this meridian, to eliminate wind cold and to relieve chills and fever. As the pathogenic cold has attacked the surface of the body, and the lung is the organ related to the skin and hair, Lieque (L 7), the Luo-(Connecting) point of the Lung Meridian, is used to promote the dispersing function of the lung and to check cough. Fengchi (G 20), a point at the intersection of the Foot Shaoyang and Yangwei Meridians, of which the latter dominates yang and the exterior, is used to eliminate wind cold. Since the Taiyin and Yangming Meridians are externally and internally related, Hegu (LI 4), the Yuan-(Primary) point of the Yangming Meridian, is used to eliminate the pathogenic factors and relieve the exterior symptoms.

b) Wind heat:

Reducing is applied to the points of the Du, Shaoyang and Yangming Meridians to eliminate wind heat.

Prescription: Dazhui (Du 14), Quchi (LI 11), Waiguan (SJ 5), Hegu (LI 4), Yuji (L 10), Shaoshang (L 11).

Explanation: The Du Meridian is the sea of all the yang meridians. Dazhui (Du 14), a point where all the yang meridians meet, is used to eliminate heat and other pathogenic factors of yang nature. Hegu (LI 4) and Quchi (LI 11) are the Yuan-(Primary) point and the He-(Sea) point of the Yangming Meridian of Hand respectively. Since the Yangming and Taiyin Meridians of Hand are externally and internally related, reducing applied to these two points can clear lung qi and reduce heat. Yuji (L 10), the Ying-(Spring) point of the Lung Meridian, in combination with Shaoshang (L 11), can eliminate heat from the lung and ease the throat. Waiguan (SJ 5), the Luo-(Connecting) point of the Shaoyang Meridian of Hand connecting with the Yangwei Meridian, can dispel pathogenic factors of yang nature in the exterior of the body and eliminate heat.

Remarks

a) The above treatment can also be used for other viral and bacterial infections of the upper respiratory tract as well as influenza. However, common cold should be distinguished from other infectious diseases with similar symptoms at the early stage.

b) Prophylactic measures: Moxibustion is applied daily to Fengmen (B 12) or Zusanli (S 36) to prevent common cold during its prevalence.

5. Malaria

Malaria is a disease characterized by paroxysms of shivering chills and high fever occurring at regular intervals, mostly found in late summer and early autumn, but also sporadically occurring in other seasons. The causative factor is the malarial pestilential factor. The recurrence of chills and fever varying with the condition of yin and yang and body constitution, may be once every day, every second day or every third day, known respectively as quotidian malaria, tertian malaria and quartan malaria according to the interval between attacks. In chronic cases there may be a mass in the hypochondriac region, termed "malaria with splenomegaly."

Etiology and Pathogenesis

The disease is believed to be caused mainly by the malarial pestilential factor together with invasion of pathogenic wind, cold, summer heat and dampness. Improper food intake, overstrain and stress, and irregular daily life can predispose one to malaria by weakening the body resistance. Invasion of the Shaoyang Meridian by the pathogenic factors causes ying-wei disharmony, resulting in malaria.

a) The pestilential factor together with the pathogenic wind cold, summer heat, and dampness invades the body, resides in the portion between the exterior and interior, and moves outward and inward between ying and wei. When they move inward to struggle with yin, there are chills, and when they move outward to fight with yang, there is fever. It is clear that the paroxysm of chills and fever depends on the struggle between the antipathogenic factors and pathogenic factors. If the pathogenic factors and the antipathogenic factors are separated from each other, or if the pathogenic factors avoid fighting with the ying and wei, there appears an interval between the paroxysms.

b) Only when the body resistence is weak, the pestilential factor invades the body. Weakened body resistance may be due to abnormal daily life, overstrain, or deficiency of qi and blood caused by improper transportation and transformation function of the spleen and stomach as a result of irregular food intake. Zhang Jingyue once said: "Malaria is an exogenous disease.... Only in the condition of delicate health, or overstrain and stress, is one apt to be attacked by the malarial pathogenic factor."

In a word, the causative factor is the pestilential factor, but the condition of body resistance plays a very important role. One with the body resistance vigorous enough to prevent the invasion by pathogenic factors seldom suffers from malaria, whereas one with lowered body resistance is apt to be attacked.

Differentiation

Main manifestations: Paroxysms of shivering chills and high fever with general hot sensation, preceded by yawning and lassitude. There appear intolerable headache, flushed face and red lips, stifling feeling in the chest and hypochondriac region, bitter taste and dry mouth, and dire thirst. At the end of the paroxysm the patient breaks out in profuse perspiration and fever subsides with the body felt cool. Thin, sticky and yellow tongue coating, string-taut and rapid pulse. In chronic cases a mass in the hypochondriac region — splenomegaly is usually found.

Analysis: Occurrence of shivering chills and high fever is due to the fight of the pathogenic factors against ying and wei in the portion between the exterior and interior of the body. There appears an interval between paroxysms of chills and fever if the pathogenic factors avoid fighting with ying and wei. Yawning, lassitude and chills with shivering are caused by the invasion of pathogenic factors which suppress yang qi. General hot sensation, intolerable headache, flushed face and red lips indicate that the accumulated pathogenic cold has turned into heat. The stifling feeling in the chest and hypochondriac region, and bitter taste in the mouth suggest that the pathogenic factors in the Shaoyang Meridian and in the portion between the exterior and interior impair the circulation of qi and blood. Thirst results from the consumption of the body fluids by heat. Thin, sticky and yellow tongue coating, string-taut and rapid pulse are the signs related to the presence of cold and heat and the contradiction between the antipathogenic factors and pathogenic factors. The chronic case with a mass formed in the hypochondriac region is due to deficiency of qi and blood and stagnation of excessive phlegm in the meridians and collaterals.

Treatment

Method: Reducing is applied to the points of the Du and Shaoyang Meridians to regulate the Du Meridian and to harmonize the Shaoyang Meridians. Treatment is given two hours prior to the paroxysm. If chills are predominant during the paroxysm, acupuncture is advised to combine with moxibustion. If fever is the dominant symptom, acupuncture alone is employed.

Prescription: Dazhui (Du 14), Taodao (Du 13), Houxi (S I 3), Jianshi (P 5), Yemen (S J 2), Zulinqi (G 41).

Supplementary points:

High fever: Quchi (L I 11) with reducing method.

Malaria with splenomegaly: Needling of Zhangmen (Liv 13) and moxibustion at Pigen (Extra).

High fever with delirium and mental confusion:

Prick the twelve Jing-(Well) points (L 11, H 9, P 9, L I 1, S I 1, S I 1).

Explanation: Dazhui (Du 14), the meeting point of the three yang meridians and the Du Meridian, can promote the circulation of qi in the yang meridians and help to eliminate pathogenic factors, in combination with Taodao (Du 13), which can remove obstruction from the Du Meridian and regulate yin and yang. They are the chief points for malaria. Yemen (SJ 2) and Zulinqi (G 41), two points along the Shaoyang Meridians can harmonize qi of the Shaoyang Meridians. Houxi (SI 3), a point of Taiyang Meridian of Hand, can activate the circulation of qi in the Taiyang and the Du Meridians and drive pathogenic factors out. Jianshi (P 5), a point of Jueyin Meridian of Hand, is an empirical point for malaria. Combination of all the above mentioned points can promote the circulation of qi in the yang meridians, and help to eliminate pathogenic factors, relieve both the symptoms, harmonize ying and wei, and check malaria. Quchi (LI 11), a point of Yangming Meridian of Hand, combined with Dazhui (Du 14) can dispel heat. Zhangmen (Liv 13), the influential point dominating zang organs can regulate qi in the zang organs. Pigen, an extra point, is selected to treat the mass in the hypochondriac region.

Acupuncture treatment of tertian malaria has achieved better effects. Pernicious malaria should be treated by acupuncture in combination with medicine.

II. ZANG-FU SYNDROMES

1. Cough

Cough, a main symptom of the lung problems, may result either from attack by exogenous pathogenic factors disturbing the dispersion of qi of the lung, or from disorders of the lung itself or other diseased zang-fu organs affecting the lung.

Etiology and Pathogenesis

a)   Invasion by the exogenous pathogenic factors:

The lung dominates qi and is regarded as an umbrella protecting the five zang organs. Upward it connects the throat and has its opening in the nose, governing respiration. Externally it associates with the skin and hair. Once the lung is attacked by the exogenous pathogenic factors, the qi of the lung is blocked and fails to descend, thus resulting in cough.

Since the weather changes in different seasons, the exogenous pathogenic factors attacking the human body are various. Cough is therefore divided into two types: wind cold and wind heat.

b)   Internal injury:

Cough resulted from functional impairment of the zang-fu organs falls into the category of cough due to internal injury, such as cough caused by dryness of the lung with deficiency of yin leading to failure of the qi of the lung to descend, or by disorders of the other organs affecting the lung. For example, in case of weakened spleen yang, the accumulated dampness may be turned into phlegm which goes upward to the lung, affecting the normal activities of qi and leading to cough. Stagnation of liver qi may be turned into fire, which flares up and injures the lung fluid, also resulting in cough. As said in *Internal Classic:* "Cough can be caused by disturbance not only of the lung, but of any other zang-fu organs." No matter which zang-fu organ is dysfunctioned, cough may result if the lung is affected. The commonly seen cough caused by internal injury in clinic results from dryness of the lung with deficiency of yin, and blockage of the lung by phlegm.

Differentiation

a)   Invasion by the exogenous pathogenic factors:

i) Wind-cold type:

Main manifestations: Cough, itching of the throat, thin and white sputum, aversion to cold, fever, anhidrosis, headache, nasal obstruction and discharge, thin, white tongue coating and superficial pulse.

Analysis: Cough, itching of the throat, thin and white sputum, nasal obstruction and discharge result from the attack of the lung by pathogenic wind cold, which is stagnated in the respiratory tract, affecting the dispersion of the qi of the lung. Headache, aversion to cold, fever and anhidrosis are due to wind cold affecting the skin and hair, and residing on the body surface. Thin, white tongue coating and superficial pulse indicate the presence of the pathogenic factors staying in the lung and in the superficial part of the body.

ii) Wind-heat type:

Main manifestations: Cough with yellow, thick sputum, choking cough, thirst, sore throat, fever, or headache, aversion to wind, sweating, thin, yellow tongue coating, superficial and rapid pulse.

Analysis: In case of the attack of the lung by the pathogenic wind heat, the function of the lung in clarifying the passage and sending down the qi is impaired. The fluids are heated and turned into phlegm, and so cough with yellow, thick sputum or choking cough takes place. When the heat in the lung injures body fluid, thirst and sore throat occur. When the pathogenic factors stay in the skin and hair, their conflict with the body resistance gives rise to headache, aversion to wind, sweating and fever. Thin, yellow tongue coating, and superficial rapid pulse are the signs of wind heat staying in the lung and in the superficial part of the body.

b) Internal injury:

i) Blockage of the lung by phlegm:

Main manifestations: Cough with profuse, white and sticky sputum, stuffiness and depression of the chest, loss of appetite, white, sticky tongue coating and rolling pulse.

Analysis: "The spleen is considered as the source in the production of sputum and the lung as a container to store it." If the spleen fails in its transformation and transportation, the water dampness will no longer be transported and then gathered to form phlegm, which goes upward to the lung, affecting the qi of the lung and causing its failure in descending. The result is cough with profuse sputum or with white, sticky sputum. If water dampness stays in the middle jiao, impairing its activity, there may be stuffiness and depression of the chest and loss of appetite. White, sticky tongue coating and rolling pulse are due to internal obstruction by the phlegm.

ii) Dryness of the lung with deficiency of yin:

Main manifestations: Dry cough without sputum or with scanty sputum, dryness of the nose and throat, sore throat, spitting blood or even coughing blood, afternoon fever, malar flush, red tongue, thin coating, thready and rapid pulse.

Analysis: Dryness is easy to consume the body fluid. If the lung is injured by dryness, the function of the lung will be impaired, manifested by dry cough without sputum or with scanty sputum, dryness of the nose and throat, or sore throat. If the lung vessels are injured by dryness, blood in the sputum or hemoptysis results. If there is deficiency of yin of the lung with endogenous heat, afternoon fever and malar flush may be present. Red tongue, thin coating, and thready rapid pulse are the signs indicating deficiency of yin and dryness of the lung.

Treatment

a) Invasion by exogenous pathogenic factors:

Method: Select the points from the Taiyin and Yangming Meridians of Hand as the principal ones. Both acupuncture and moxibustion are applied in case of wind cold, while only acupuncture is used in case of wind heat to activate the dispersing function of the lung and to relieve the symptoms.

Prescription: Lieque (L 7), Hegu (LI 4), Feishu (B 13).

Supplementary points:

Pain and swelling of the throat: Shaoshang (L 11).

Fever and aversion to cold: Dazhui (Du 14), Waiguan (SJ 5).

Explanation: The Taiyin and Yangming Meridians of Hand are exteriorly-interiorly related. Lieque (L 7), the Luo-(Connecting) point, and Hegu (LI 4), the Yuan-(Primary) point, are selected in combination with Feishu (B 13) to strengthen the functional activities of the lung, to relieve symptoms and to eliminate the exogenous pathogenic factors, resulting in smooth flow of qi of the lung and the normal dispersing function of the lung.

b) Internal injury:

i) Blockage of the lung by phlegm:

Method: Select the Back-Shu point and the points of the Yangming Meridian of Foot as the principal points. Both reinforcing and reducing methods should be considered in acupuncture treatment, or combined with moxibustion to strengthen the function of the spleen and to resolve phlegm.

Prescription: Feishu (B 13), Zhongwan (Ren 12), Chize (L 5), Zusanli (S 36), Fenglong (S 40).

Explanation: The Back-Shu point and the Front-Mu point are the points where qi of the zang-fu organs converges. Feishu (B 13) and Zhongwan (Ren 12) are selected in combination with Zusanli (S 36), the He-(Sea) point of Yangming Meridian of Foot, to strengthen the function of the spleen and harmonize the stomach, remove dampness and resolve phlegm. Chize (L 5), the He-(Sea) point of the Lung Meridian, is able to reduce the pathogenic factors from the lung and relieve cough. Fenglong (S 40), the Luo-(Connecting) point of the Yangming Meridian of Foot, is selected to strengthen smooth transport of qi in the spleen and stomach. Thus the body fluids are normally distributed following the free flow of qi and phlegm is resolved.

ii) Deficiency of yin with dryness of the lung:

Method: Select the Back-Shu point and Front-Mu point of the Lung Meridian as the principal points. Even-movement is applied in acupuncture treatment to nourish yin, eliminate dryness and descend lung qi.

Prescription: Feishu (B 13), Zhongfu (L 1), Lieque (L 7), Zhaohai (K 6).

Supplementary points:

Kongzui (L 6) and Geshu (B 17) in case of coughing blood.

Explanation: The selection of Feishu (B 13) and Zhongfu (L 1) is a method of combining Back-Shu point and Front-Mu point. It is used to regulate the lung passage and descend lung qi. Lieque (L 7), the Luo-(Connecting) point of the Lung Meridian of Hand-Taiyin, is connected with the Ren Meridian. Zhaohai (K 6) is a point of the Kidney Meridian of Foot-Shaoyin curving around the genital organ. The two points located up and down are selected as a combination of the Eight Confluent points to nourish yin, eliminate dryness, clear the throat and descend the lung qi. Kongzui (L 6), the Xi-(Cleft) point of the lung, is indicated in acute cases of the lung. Geshu (B 17) is a blood point of the Eight Influential Points. The two points are used in combination to stop bleeding.

Remarks

a) If cough is accompanied by fever and asthma, see "Common Cold" and "Asthma."

b) Cough is often seen in common cold, acute and chronic bronchitis, pneumonia, bronchiectasis and pulmonary tuberculosis.

c) Cupping:

Fengmen (B 12), Feishu (B 13).

d) Cutaneous needle:

Tap along the Du Meridian and the Bladder Meridian on the upper part of the back till the skin becomes red or bleeds slightly.

2. Asthma

Asthma is a common illness characterized by repeated attacks of paroxysmal dyspnea with wheezing.

Generally speaking, it involves a variety of disorders resulting from disturbance of qi activities, and can be divided into two types: deficiency and excess.

Etiology and Pathogenesis

The causative factors are varied from the exogenous pathogenic factors to weakened body resistance. Asthma due to exogenous pathogenic factors is of excess type, and that due to weakened body resistance is of deficiency type.

a) Excess type:

Wind-cold type: It denotes asthma due to invasion of wind cold, which impairs the smooth flow of the lung qi, injures the skin and hair, and makes the pores closed. Since the lung and the superficial defensive system are weakened, the lung qi fails to disperse and descend, leading to cough.

Phlegm-heat type: It refers to asthma due to failure of the spleen in transformation and transportation, resulting in production of phlegm from the accumulated dampness. Long-standing retention of phlegm turns into heat, or excessive fire of the lung evaporates the fluids to phlegm. When the phlegm fire stays in the lung, the lung qi is stagnated and the normal activity of the lung is impaired. Failure of the lung qi in descending function results in asthma.

b) Deficiency type:

i) Lung deficiency: A prolonged and protracted cough can weaken and injure the lung qi. Overstrain and internal injury can also bring about deficiency of the lung qi. In either case, shortness of breath and dyspnea may occur.

ii) Kidney deficiency: Overwork and sexual indulgence can injure the kidney. A severe or chronic disease weakens the body resistance and damages the essential qi. Long-standing asthma also affects the kidney. In any of the above cases, failure of the kidney in receiving qi may give rise to asthma.

Differentiation

a) Excess type:

i) Wind-cold type:

Main manifestations: Cough with thin sputum, rapid breathing, accompanied by chills, fever, headache, and anhidrosis at the early stage, absence of thirst, white tongue coating, superficial and tense pulse.

Analysis: The lung is in charge of respiration and is associated with the skin and hair, which are first attacked by wind cold in the invasive procedure. If wind cold resides in the lung, stagnation of qi and failure of the lung qi in dispersing result in cough with thin sputum and rapid breathing. If wind cold still resides in the superficial part of the body to make the pores close, there appear chills, fever, headache and anhidrosis. Since the wind cold has not transformed into heat yet, thirst is absent. White tongue coating, superficial and tense pulse are the signs of wind cold staying in the lung and the defensive system.

ii) Phlegm-heat type:

Main manifestations: Rapid and short breathing, strong and coarse voice, cough with thick yellow sputum, sensation of chest stuffiness, fever, restlessness, dryness of the mouth, thick yellow or sticky coating, rolling and rapid pulse.

Analysis: Phlegm heat turned from dampness or long-standing phlegm fire gathered in the lung blocks the air passage, causing impairment of the lung qi, and thus presenting rapid and short breathing, strong and coarse voice, and cough with thick yellow sputum. When the phlegm stays in the lung, sensation of chest stuffiness appears. Fever, restlessness and dryness of the mouth are due to the presence of the fire heat. Thick yellow or sticky coating, rolling and rapid pulse are the signs of the phlegm heat.

b) Deficiency type:

i) Lung deficiency:

Main manifestations: Short and rapid breathing, feeble voice, weak and low sound of coughing, sweating on exertion, pale tongue, pulse of deficiency type.

Analysis: The lung dominates qi. When there is deficiency of the lung qi the function of the lung is impaired. There appear short and rapid breathing, feeble voice, weak and low sound of coughing. When the lung qi is weak, and the superficial defensive system is not strong, even mild exertion will induce sweating. Pale tongue and pulse of deficiency type are the signs of deficiency of the lung qi.

ii) Kidney deficiency:

Main manifestations: Dyspnea on exertion after longstanding asthma, severe wheezing, indrawing of the soft tissues of the neck, short breath, lassitude and weakness, sweating, cold limbs, pale tongue, deep and thready pulse.

Analysis: Long-standing asthma affects the kidney which is the source of qi. The kidney in lowered functioning fails to receive qi, and therefore dyspnea on exertion, severe wheezing and short breath appear. When there is deficiency of the kidney qi in a chronic case, emaciation and lassitude happen. Exhausted kidney yang may lead to weakening of the superficial defensive yang, and hence sweating. If the yang qi fails to warm up the body surface, cold limbs appear. Pale tongue, deep and thready pulse are the signs of weakened kidney yang.

Treatment

a) Wind cold:

Method: Points of the Hand-Taiyin and Hand-Yangming Meridians are selected as the principal points. Reducing method is applied in combination with moxibustion to eliminate wind cold and soothe asthma.

Prescription: Feishu (B 13), Fengmen (B 12), Dazhui (Du 14), Lieque (L 7), Hegu (LI 4).

Explanation: Feishu (B 13) and Fengmen (B 12) are the points of the Foot-Taiyang Meridian and located in the vicinity of the lung. They are able to clear the lung and eliminate wind. Dazhui (Du 14), Lieque (L 7) and Hegu (LI 4) are in function to eliminate wind and cold, clear the lung and soothe asthma.

b) Phlegm heat:

Method: Points of the Hand-Taiyin and Foot-Yangming Meridians are selected as the principal points with reducing method applied to resolve phlegm, reduce heat and soothe asthma.

Prescription: Feishu (B 13), Dingchuan (Extra), Tiantu (Ren 22) Chize (L 5), Fenglong (S 40).

Explanation: Chize (L 5), the He-(Sea) point of the Hand-Taiyin Meridian, is able to reduce phlegm heat and soothe asthma. Fenglong (S 40), a point of the Foot-Yangming Meridian, is able to strengthen the spleen function and resolve phlegm. Feishu (B 13) is applied to clear the lung and regulate the flow of qi. Tiantu (Ren 22) is in function to descend qi and resolve phlegm. Dingchuan (Extra) is an empirical point to pacify breathing.

c) Deficiency type:

i) Lung deficiency:

Method: Points of the Hand-Taiyin and Foot-Yangming Meridians are selected as the principal points with reinforcing method applied to strengthen the lung qi. Moxibustion is also advisable.

Prescription: Feishu (B 13), Taiyuan (L 9), Zusanli (S 36), Taibai (Sp 3).

Explanation: Taiyuan (L 9), the Yuan-(Primary) point of the Lung Meridian, is able to reinforce the lung qi. Feishu (B 13) used in acupuncture and moxibustion, can strengthen the lung qi. Zusanli (S 36) is the He-(Sea) point of the Stomach Meridian of Foot-Yangming. Taibai (Sp 3) is the Yuan-(Primary) point of the Spleen Meridian. The lung pertains to metal and the spleen to earth, which is able to promote metal. "Reinforce the mother in case of deficiency." Zusanli (S 36) and Taibai (Sp 3) are selected here to strengthen the lung through invigorating the spleen and stomach.

ii) Kidney deficiency:

Method: Points of the Foot-Shaoyin and Ren Meridians are selected as the principal points with reinforcing method applied to strengthen the kidney function in receiving qi. Moxibustion is also advisable.

Prescription: Taixi (K 3), Shenshu (B 23), Feishu (B 13), Tanzhong (Ren 17), Qihai (Ren 6).

Supplementary points:

Persistent asthma: Shenzhu (Du 12), Gaohuang (B 43)

Deficiency of the spleen: Zhongwan (Ren 12), Pishu (B 20).

Explanation: Taixi (K 3), the Yuan-(Primary) point of the Kidney Meridian, is able in combination with Shenshu (B 23) to strengthen the primary qi of the kidney. Tanzhong (Ren 17), the qi point of the Eight Influential Points, and Feishu (B 13), the Back-Shu point of the lung, are needled to reinforce qi and pacify breathing. Qihai (Ren 6), an important point to reinforce qi, is able to regulate qi in the lower jiao, reinforce the kidney, strengthen the primary qi, invigorate yang and control essence. Puncture on these points strengthens the kidney in receiving qi and pacify breathing. Moxibustion on Shenzhu (Du 12) and Gaohuang (B 43) may relieve chronic asthma, while moxibustion on Zhongwan (Ren 12) and Pishu (B 20) may strengthen the function of the spleen and reinforce qi.

Remarks

This condition includes bronchial asthma,

asthmatic bronchitis, obstructive pulmonary emphysema and dyspnea present in some other diseases. However, for symptomatic dyspnea, a combined treatment should be taken into account.

3. Epigastric Pain

Epigastric pain is a common symptom, often characterized by repeated recurrence. Since the pain is close to the cardia, it was also named "cardio-abdominal pain" or "cardiac pain" in ancient times.

Etiology and Pathogenesis

a) Irregular food intake, preference for raw and cold food and hunger injure the spleen and stomach, causing failure of the spleen in transportation and transformation and failure of the stomach qi in descending, then pain appears.

b) Anxiety, anger and mental depression damage the liver, causing failure of the liver in dominating free flow of qi, adversely attacking the stomach, impeding its activity and hindering its qi descending, then pain appears.

c) Generally lowered functioning of the spleen and stomach, due to invasion of pathogenic cold, which is stagnated in the stomach, causes failure of the stomach qi in descending, then pain occurs.

Differentiation

a) Retention of food:

Main manifestations: Distending pain in the epigastrium, aggravated on pressure or after meals, belching with fetid odour, anorexia, thick, sticky tongue coating, deep, forceful or rolling pulse.

Analysis: Retention of food in the stomach makes the stomach qi fail to descend, then distending pain in the epigastrium and belching with fetid odour occur. Retention of food is an excess condition, pain is therefore aggravated upon pressure. Since the stomach is injured by retention of food, pain becomes worse after meals and anorexia appears. Thick, sticky tongue coating, deep, forceful or rolling pulse are the signs of retention of food.

b) Attack of the stomach by the liver qi:

Main manifestations: Paroxysmal pain in the epigastrium, radiating to the hypochondriac regions, frequent belching accompanied by nausea, vomiting, acid regurgitation, abdominal distension, anorexia, thin, white tongue coating, deep, string-taut pulse.

Analysis: Stagnation of the liver qi makes the liver fail to dominate the free flow of qi. If the depressed liver qi attacks the stomach, pain in the epigastrium appears. As the Liver Meridian locates along both hypochondriac regions, the pain is wandering and may be referred to both hypochondriac regions. In case of stagnation of the qi, belching occurs, even symptoms like nausea, vomiting, acid regurgitation, abdominal distension and anorexia may appear. Thin, white tongue coating and deep string-taut pulse are the signs of attack of the stomach by the perversive liver qi.

c) Deficiency of the stomach with stagnation of cold:

Main manifestations: Dull pain in the epigastrium, which may be relieved by pressure and warmth, general lassitude, regurgitation of thin fluid, thin, white tongue coating, deep, slow pulse.

Analysis: Lowered function of the spleen and stomach with cold invasion retards transportation and transformation, so dull pain appears in the epigastrium. The spleen dominates the limbs. If the spleen yang is weak, general lassitude occurs, as well as the regurgitation of thin fluid. Since the condition is due to deficiency and cold, pain is relieved on pressure and by warming. Thin, white coating and deep slow pulse are the signs of lowered function of the spleen and stomach with cold stagnation.

Treatment

a) Retention of food:

Method: The Front-(Mu) point of the stomach and the points of the Yangming Meridian of Foot are selected with reducing method applied to remove retention, pacify the stomach and relieve pain.

Prescription: Jianli (Ren 11), Neiguan (P 6), Zusanli (S 36), Inner-Neiting (Extra).

Explanation: Zhongwan (Ren 12) is the Front-(Mu) point of stomach, Zusanli (S 36), the Lower He-(Sea) point of the Stomach and Neiguan (P 6), a Confluent Point. They are indicated in stomach, heart and chest disorders, and used in combination to pacify the stomach and relieve pain. Inner-Neiting (Extra) is an empirical point to treat retention of food.

b) Attack of the stomach by the liver qi:

Method: Points of Jueyin and Yangming Meridians of Foot are selected as the principal points with the reducing method applied to remove the stangnation of liver qi, to pacify the stomach and to relieve pain.

Prescription: Qimen (Liv 14), Zhongwan (Ren 12), Neiguan (P 6), Zusanli (S 36), Taichong (Liv 3).

Explanation: Qimen (Liv 14) is the Front-(Mu) point of the liver and Taichong is the Yuan-(Primary) point of the Liver Meridian. The two are used in combination to remove the stagnation of liver qi, regulate the flow of qi and relieve pain. Zusanli (S 36), Zhongwan (Ren 12) and Neiguan (P 6) are applied to pacify the stomach, relieve pain and check vomiting.

c) Deficiency of the stomach with stagnation of cold:

Method: The Back-Shu points and points of the Ren Meridian are selected as the principal points with both acupuncture and moxibustion to warm up the middle jiao, dispel cold and regulate the flow of qi and relieve pain.

Prescription: Zhongwan (Ren 12), Qihai (Ren 6), Pishu (B 20), Neiguan (P 6), Zusanli (S 36), Gongsun (Sp 4).

Explanation: Acupuncture and moxibustion at Zhongwan (Ren 12) and Zusanli (S 36) warm the middle jiao, dispel cold, regulate the flow of qi and relieve pain. Neiguan (P 6) and Gongsun (Sp 4), the Confluent Points, are indicated to treat stomach disorders. Moxibustion on Pishu (B 20) strengthens the spleen, pacifies the stomach, dispels cold and relieves pain. Indirect moxibustion with ginger on Qihai (Ren 6) is most desirable in the treatment of chronic gastric pain due to cold of deficiency type, as ginger and moxa together have the function of dispelling cold.

Remarks

a) Epigastric pain is a symptom found in peptic ulcer, gastritis, gastric neurosis and diseases of the liver, gallbladder and pancreas.

b) Cupping: Cupping is applied with large or medium-sized cups mainly to the upper abdomen or Back-Shu points for ten to fifteen minutes.

4. Vomiting

Vomiting is a common symptom in clinic, resulting from the failure of the stomach qi to descend, or from other disorders affecting the stomach. It may occur in many diseases, but the most common causes are retention of food, attack of the stomach by the liver qi and hypofunction of the spleen and stomach.

Etiology and Pathogenesis

Overeating of raw, cold and greasy food leads to upward perversion of the stomach qi, resulting in vomiting.

Emotional disturbance and depression of the liver qi harm the stomach, impairing the downward movement of the stomach qi, causing vomiting.

Weakness of the spleen and stomach or overstrain leads to hypofunction of the stomach in transportation and transformation, then causing retention of food. The stomach qi ascends instead of descends.

Differentiation

a) Retention of food:

Main manifestations: Acid fermented vomitus, epigastric and abdominal distension, belching, anorexia, loose stool or constipation, thick, granular tongue coating, rolling and forceful pulse.

Analysis: Retention of food impedes the function of the spleen and stomach in transportation and transformation. Since qi in the middle jiao is stagnated, there appear epigastric and abdominal distension, belching and anorexia. Retention of food leads to upward flowing of the turbid qi, so acid fermented vomitus, and loose stool or constipation occur. Thick, granular tongue coating and rolling, forceful pulse are the signs of retention of food.

b) Attack of the stomach by the liver qi:

Main manifestations: Vomiting, acid regurgitation, frequent belching, distending pain in the chest and hypochondriac regions, irritability with an oppressed feeling, thin, sticky tongue coating, string-taut pulse.

Analysis: Depressed liver qi attacks the stomach, causing upward perversion of the stomach qi, so there occur vomiting, acid regurgitation, frequent belching, distending pain in the chest and hypochondriac regions. In case of stagnation of the liver qi, irritability with an oppressed feeling occurs. Thin, sticky tongue coating and string-taut pulse are the signs of the stagnation of the liver qi.

c) Hypofunction of the spleen and stomach:

Main manifestations: Sallow complexion, vomiting after a big meal, loss of appetite, lassitude, weakness, slightly loose stool, pale tongue, thin, white tongue coating, thready and forceless pulse.

Analysis: Weakness of the spleen and stomach leads to hypoactivity of the yang in the middle jiao, which fails to receive food and water, so vomiting appears after a big meal. If the spleen fails in transportation and transformation, the essentials of water and food no longer supply the body for nourishment, there may appear lassitude, weakness, loss of appetite and slightly loose stool. Pale tongue, thin white tongue coating, and thready and forceless pulse are the signs of weakness of the spleen and stomach.

Treatment

Method: The points of Yangming and Taiyin Meridians of Foot are selected as the principal points to activate the descent of qi and to pacify the stomach. For retention of food, reducing is indicated, for attack of the stomach by the liver qi, even movement is usually used to soothe the liver and regulate the flow of qi, and for weakness of the spleen and stomach, reinforcing combined with moxibustion is used to strengthen the function of the spleen and warm up the middle jiao.

Prescription: Zhongwan (Ren 12), Zusanli (S 36), Neiguan (P 6), Gongsun (Sp 4).

Supplementary points:

Retention of food: Xiawan (Ren 10).

Attack of the stomach by the liver qi: Taichong (Liv 3).

Weakness of the spleen and stomach: Pishu (B 20).

Persistent vomiting: Jinjing, Yuye (Extra).

Explanation: Zusanli (S 36) is the He-(Sea) point of the Stomach Meridian and Zhongwan (Ren 12), the Front-Mu point of the stomach. The two points used together are effective in pacifying the stomach and activating the descent of qi. Neiguan (P 6) and Gongsun (Sp 4), one of the pair-points of the Eight Confluent points, relieve the fullness of the chest and stomach. Xiawan (Ren 10), a point located in the epigastrium, is able to regulate the stomach qi and remove stagnation by applying reducing method Needling at Taichong (Liv 3), the Yuan (Primary) point of the Liver Meridian regulates the function of the liver. Pishu (B 20), a point where the spleen qi is infused, used in combination with Zusanli (S 36) and Gongsun (Sp 4), may reinforce the spleen qi and invigorate the qi in the middle jiao to perform the function of transportation and transformation and to restore the normal activities of qi. Pricking Jinjing(Extra) and Yuye(Extra) to cause bleeding is an experienced method for checking vomiting.

Remarks

Vomiting as described here may be found in acute and chronic gastritis, cardiospasm, pylorospasm and neurotic vomiting.

5. Hiccup

Hiccup is an involuntary spasm of the glottis and diaphragm, causing the characteristic sound. Occasional attack of hiccup suggests a mild case and can be removed without medication, but if it persists, treatment is required. Hiccup is mostly caused by irregular diet, stagnation of the liver qi and presence of cold in the stomach, leading to upward perversion of the stomach qi instead of descending.

Etiology and Pathogenesis
Irregular food intake causes failure of the stomach qi to descend, or emotional frustration stagnates the liver qi, leading to upward perversion of the stomach qi.

The attack of the stomach by cold, over-eating of raw and cold food, or taking drugs of cold nature gives rise to retaining of the stomach yang and upward perversion of qi.

Differentiation
a) Retention of food:

Main manifestations: Loud hiccups, epigastric and abdominal distension, anorexia, thick, sticky tongue coating, rolling and forceful pulse.

Analysis: Retention of food in the stomach disturbs the function of the spleen and stomach in transportation and transformation and impedes the qi activities in the middle jiao. "The stomach is in normal function when its qi descends." Failure of its qi to descend may lead to loud hiccups, epigastric and abdominal distension, and anorexia. Thick, sticky tongue coating, and rolling, forceful pulse are the signs of retention of food.

b) Stagnation of qi:

Main manifestations: Continual hiccups, distending pain and feeling of oppression in the chest and hypochondrium, thin tongue coating, string-taut and forceful pulse.

Analysis: The liver qi, if stagnated, will attack the stomach, causing upward perversion of stomach qi, therefore, hiccup, distending pain in the chest and hypochondrium, and feeling of oppression appear. String-taut and forceful pulse is a sign of stagnation of qi due to depression of the liver.

c) Cold in the stomach:

Main manifestations: Slow and forceful hiccups which may be relieved by heat and aggravated by cold, discomfort in the epigastrium, white, moist tongue coating, slow pulse.

Analysis: The stomach qi fails to descend because of stagnated cold, so hiccup is forceful. In case of disturbance of the stomach qi, discomfort in the epigastrium occurs. If cold gets heat, smooth circulation of qi results, and then hiccup is relieved; but if cold gets worse, hiccup is aggravated. White, moist tongue coating and slow pulse indicate the presence of cold in the stomach.

Treatment
Method: The points of the Stomach Meridian and some other points related are selected as the principal points. Reducing is applied for retention of food and stagnation of qi, while both acupuncture and moxibustion are used for cold in the stomach. The treatment is aimed at pacifying the stomach, facilitating the descent of qi and checking hiccup.

Prescription: Geshu (B 17), Zhongwan (Ren 12), Neiguan (P 6), Zusanli (S 36).

Supplementary points:

Retention of food: Juque (Ren 14), Inner-Neiting (Extra).

Stagnation of qi: Tanzhong (Ren 17), Taichong (Liv 3).

Cold in the stomach: Shangwan (Ren 13).

Explanation: Zhongwan (Ren 12), Neiguan (P 6) and Zusanli (S 36) may pacify the stomach, subdue the ascending qi and relieve the oppression feeling in the chest. Geshu (B 17) is able to check the perversive ascending of qi and stop hiccup. Juque (Ren 14) and Inner-Neiting (Extra) pacify the stomach and remove stagnation. Tanzhong (Ren 17) relieves the depressed feeling in the chest and diaphragm and checks hiccup. Taichong (Liv 3) may pacify the liver qi. Moxibustion to Shangwan (Ren 13) may warm the middle jiao to dispel cold, promote the smooth distribution of yang and check hiccup.

Remarks
Cupping:

Commonly used points: Geshu (B 17), Geguan (B 46), Ganshu (B 18), Zhongwan (Ren 12), Rugen (S 18).

6. Abdominal Pain

Abdominal pain is a frequently encountered symptom in clinic, often accompanied with many zang-fu disorders, of which dysentery, epigastric pain, appendicitis, and gynecologic diseases will be discussed in other sections. In this section only accumulation of cold, hypoactivity of the spleen yang and retention of food are related.

Etiology and Pathogenesis
a) Since cold is characterized by causing contraction and stagnation, accumulation of cold due to invasion of the abdomen by the pathogenic cold or injury of the stomach and spleen yang due to overeating of raw and cold food impairs the transportation and transformation function, resulting in abdominal pain.

b) Hypoactivity of the spleen yang or general deficiency of yang qi leads to impairment of transportation and transformation, and stagnation of cold dampness, resulting in abdominal pain.

c) Retention of food due to voracious eating or intake of too much fatty and hot food impedes the function of the stomach and intestines in transmission and digestion, nutrients and wastes mixing together to obstruct qi, resulting in pain.

Differentiation
a) Accumulation of cold:
Main manifestations: Sudden onset of violent abdominal pain which responds to warmth and gets worse by cold, loose stool, absence of thirst, clear and profuse urine, cold limbs, thin white tongue coating, deep, tense or deep, slow pulse.

Analysis: Cold is of yin nature and characterized by causing contraction and stagnation. If cold enters the body, yang qi will get obstructed, then sudden violent pain and cold limbs appear. Since cold stays inside, thirst is absent. Clear and profuse urine and loose stool are due to weakness of the stomach and spleen yang and failure in transportation and transformation. The flow of yang qi is usually obstructed by cold and facilitated by warmth, so pain responds to warmth but gets worse by cold. Deep, tense or deep, slow pulse, and thin white tongue coating are the signs of accumulation of cold.

b) Hypoactivity of the spleen yang:
Main manifestations: Intermittent dull pain which may be relieved by warmth or by pressure and aggravated by cold or by hunger and fatigue, lassitude, aversion to

cold, thin, white tongue coating, deep, thready pulse.

Analysis: Intermittent dull pain which may be relieved by warmth or by pressure and aggravated by cold or by hunger and fatigue indicates cold of deficiency type. Hypoactivity of the spleen yang causes loose stool and aversion to cold. If the spleen qi is weak, lassitude occurs. Thin white tongue coating and deep, thready pulse also indicate cold of deficiency type.

c) Retention of food:

Main manifestations: Epigastric and abdominal distending pain which is aggravated by pressure, anorexia, foul belching and sour regurgitation, or abdominal pain accompanied by diarrhea and relieved after defecation, sticky tongue coating, rolling pulse.

Analysis: In case of retention of food in the intestines and stomach, epigastric and abdominal distending pain occurs. Pain is aggravated by pressure because of excess condition. Anorexia is due to retention of food, foul belching and sour regurgitation due to indigestion of food. Pain is relieved after diarrhoea because the circulation of qi in the fu organs becomes smooth. Sticky tongue coating is due to retention of food and collection of dampness, while rolling pulse is the sign of indigestion.

Treatment

a) Accumulation of cold:

Method: Points of the Ren Meridian, Taiyin and Yangming Meridians of Foot are selected as the principal points with reducing method applied in combination with moxibustion to warm the stomach and dispel cold.

Prescription: Zhongwan (Ren 12), Shenque (Ren 8), Zusanli (S 36), Gongsun (Sp 4).

Explanation: Zhongwan (Ren 12), Zusanli (S 36) and Gongsun (Sp 4) are used to strengthen the function of the spleen and stomach, and to warm and promote the flow of qi in the fu organs. Indirect moxibustion with salt is applied to warm the stomach and dispel cold.

b) Hypoactivity of the spleen yang:

Method: The Back-Shu points and the points of the Ren Meridian are selected as the principal points with reinforcing method applied in combination with moxibustion to warm and activate the spleen and stomach yang.

Prescription: Pishu (B 20), Weishu (B 21), Zhongwan (Ren 12), Zhangmen (Liv 13), Qihai (Ren 6), Zusanli (S 36).

Explanation: Pishu (B 20) and Zhangmen (Liv 13), Weishu (B 21) and Zhongwan (Ren 12) are selected, known as combinations of the Back-Shu and Front-Mu points. Both acupuncture and moxibustion are used to invigorate the spleen and stomach yang. Qihai (Ren 6) and Zusanli (S 36) are needled to strengthen the function of the spleen and stomach.

c) Retention of food:

Method: The points of the Ren Meridian and Yangming Meridian of Foot are selected as the principal points with reducing method applied to remove retention of food.

Prescription: Zhongwan (Ren 12), Tianshu (S 25), Qihai (Ren 6), Zusanli (S 36), Inner-Neiting (Extra).

Explanation: Zhongwan (Ren 12), Zusanli (S 36), Tianshu (S 25) and Qihai (Ren 6) are applied to regulate the flow of the stomach qi. Inner-Neiting (Extra) is an empirical point to treat indigestion. The above points are used together to remove retention of food and relieve pain by promoting the flow of qi.

7. Diarrhoea

Diarrhoea refers to abnormal frequency and liquidity of fecal discharges. It is usually due to disorders of the spleen, stomach, large and small intestines. In light of the manifestations of the disease and the course, it is clinically divided into acute and chronic. The former is mostly caused by indigestion due to excessive eating or improper diet and attack of external cold dampness, leading to dysfunction in transmission of intestinal contents, or caused by invasion of damp heat in summer or autumn; the latter is caused by deficiency of the spleen and stomach, leading to failure in transportation and transformation.

It is essential to distinguish diarrhoea and dysentery.

Etiology and Pathogenesis

The causative factors are complicated, but functional disturbance of the spleen and stomach is inevitably involved pathogenetically. The stomach dominates receiving food while the spleen dominates transportation and transformation. In case the spleen and stomach are diseased, the normal digestion and absorption of food is impaired, leading to mixing of food essence and wastes. When they descend through the large intestine, diarrhoea occurs.

As to the factors of diarrhoea due to functional disturbance of the spleen and stomach, there are many as follows.

Diarrhoea may be caused by the six exogenous pathogenic factors, among which mostly by cold, dampness and summer heat. The spleen is in preference to dryness but dislikes dampness, which usually causes diarrhoea. Besides the superficial portion of the body and the lung, the stomach and intestines may be affected by the pathogenic cold or summer heat, resulting in diarrhoea.

In the latter case, however, the diarrhoea is also often related to dampness.

Excessive intake of food, particularly greasy food, leading to impairment of the stomach and spleen in transportation and transformation, or eating of raw, cold, dirty food, injuring the spleen and stomach, all bring about diarrhoea.

Diarrhoea may also be caused by weakened function of the spleen and stomach due to irregular daily life or other factors. Since the spleen has the function in transformation and transportation, diarrhoea may occur if this function is affected.

The spleen yang is closely related to the kidney yang. The fire of Mingmen (Vital gate) (kidney yang) may help the spleen and stomach to "digest and transform food into chyme." In case the kidney yang is weak, the spleen yang is weak as well and fails to digest and transform food into chyme, thus diarrhoea occurs. Zhang Jingyue said: "The kidney is the passgate of the stomach and makes the urino-genital orifice and the anus as its openings. The passing of both urine and stool is dominated by the kidney. Now the kidney yang is weak, leading to decline of Mingmen (Vital gate) fire, and excess of cold; therefore, diarrhoea occurs."

Differentiation

a) Acute diarrhoea

i) Cold-dampness:

Main manifestations: Watery diarrhoea, abdominal pain and borborygmi, chilliness which responds to warmth, absence of thirst, pale tongue, white tongue coating, deep, slow pulse.

Analysis: When the cold-dampness attacks the stomach and the intestines, disturbing the function of the spleen in sending food essence and water upward and that of the stomach in sending the contents downward, the food essence and the waste can not be separated, moving downward together through the large intestine, so watery diarrhoea with borborygmi occurs. If the qi of the stomach and intestines is stagnated, abdominal pain appears. Cold-dampness is a combination of yin pathogenic factors and easy to damage yang qi. When yang qi is blocked, chilliness which responds to warmth and absence of thirst occur. Pale tongue, white tongue coating, and deep, slow pulse are the signs of excess of internal cold.

ii) Damp heat:

Main manifestations: Diarrhoea with abdominal pain, yellow, hot and fetid stools, burning sensation in the anus, scanty urine, or accompanied by general feverish feeling, thirst, yellow, sticky tongue coating, rolling and rapid pulse.

Analysis: When the intestines and stomach are attacked by the damp heat in summer or autumn, the transmitting and transformation function is disturbed, and diarrhoea appears. If the damp heat pours down, diarrhoea happens as soon as the abdominal pain is brought about. If the heat stays in the intestines, there appear diarrhoea with yellow, hot and fetid stools and burning sensation in the anus. When excessive heat evaporates the dampness, there are scanty urine, general feverish feeling and thirst. Yellow, sticky tongue coating, and rolling, rapid pulse are the signs of excess of damp heat.

iii) Retention of food:

Main manifestations: Abdominal pain relieved after bowel movements, borborygmi, diarrhoea with fetid stools, epigastric and abdominal fullness and distension, belching, anorexia, thick filthy tongue coating, rolling, rapid or deep, string-taut pulse.

Analysis: Retention of food impairs the stomach function in sending its contents downwards and the transmitting function of the intestines, so there are epigastric and abdominal fullness and distension, abdominal pain and borborygmi. After the undigested food turns putrid, diarrhoea with offensive fetid stools, belching and anorexia occur. After the wastes are discharged, abdominal pain relieves. Thick filthy tongue coating, and rolling, rapid or deep, string-taut pulse are the signs of retention of food.

b) Chronic diarrhoea:

i) Deficiency of the spleen:

Main manifestations: Loose stool with undigested food, anorexia, epigastric distress after eating, sallow complexion, lassitude, pale tongue, white tongue coating, thready, forceless pulse.

Analysis: In case of weakness of the spleen and stomach, the spleen qi fails to ascend and digestion is impaired; therefore, loose stool with undigested food appears. As the weakened spleen fails to digest and transport the food, anorexia and epigastric distress after eating occur. Persistent diarrhoea further weakens the spleen and stomach, affecting the production of food essence and formation of qi and blood, and thus resulting in the sallow complexion and lassitude. Pale tongue, white tongue coating, and thready, forceless pulse are the signs of weakness of the spleen and stomach.

ii) Deficiency of the kidney:

Main manifestations: Pain below the umbilicus, borborygmi and diarrhoea usually occurring at dawn, relieved after bowel movements, and aggravated by cold, abdominal distension sometimes, cold lower extremities, pale tongue, white tongue coating, deep, forceless pulse.

Analysis: Pain below the umbilicus and diarrhoea with borborygmi at dawn are due to hypoactivity of the kidney yang and the declined Mingmen fire. Zhang Jingyue stated: "Yin should be at maximum in case yang qi is not restored. The stomach fails to hold its contents because of the declined Mingmen fire, thus diarrhoea results." Abdominal aversion to cold, and sometimes distension, cold lower extremities, pale tongue, white tongue coating, deep, forceless pulse are the signs of deficiency of the yang qi in the spleen and stomach.

Treatment

a) Acute diarrhoea:

Method: The points of the Yangming Meridian of Foot are selected as the principal points.

Cold-dampness: Reducing method in combination with moxibustion (with ginger) is applied to warm the stomach and resolve dampness.

Damp heat: Reducing is used to eliminate heat and dampness.

Retention of food: Reducing is used to regulate the function of the spleen and stomach and remove stagnation.

Prescription: Tianshu (S 25), Zusanli (S 36).

Supplementary points:

Cold dampness: Zhongwan (Ren 12), Qihai (Ren 6).

Damp heat: Neiting (S 44), Yinlingquan (Sp 9).

Retention of food: Inner-Neiting (Extra)

Explanation: Tianshu (S 25), the Front-(Mu) point of the large intestine is applied to regulate the transmitting function of the intestines. Zusanli (S 36), the He-(Sea) point of Yangming Meridian of Foot, is used to adjust the flow of the stomach qi. Moxibustion to Zhongwan (Ren 12) and Qihai (Ren 6) is applied to warm the spleen

and stomach, dispel cold, regulate the flow of qi and resolve dampness. Neiting (S 44) and Yinlingquan (Sp 9) are needled to eliminate damp-heat from the large intestine. For retention of food, Inner-Neiting (Extra) is used to regulate the function of the spleen and stomach and remove retention.

b) Chronic diarrhoea:

i) Deficiency of the spleen:

Method: The points of the Spleen Meridian and some other points concerned are selected as the principal points with the reinforcing method and moxibustion to strengthen the function of the spleen and stop diarrhoea.

Prescription: Pishu (B 20), Zhangmen (Liv 13), Taibai (Sp 3), Zhongwan (Ren 12), Zusanli (S 36).

Explanation: Pishu (B 20), a Back-(Shu) point of the spleen, Zhangmen (Liv 13), the Front-(Mu) point of the spleen, Taibai (Sp 3), the Yuan-(Primary) point of the Spleen Meridian, in combination with Zhongwan (Ren 12) the Front-(Mu) point of the stomach, and Zusanli (S 36), the He-(Sea) point of the Stomach Meridian, are needled with moxibustion to invigorate the spleen yang, strengthen the function of transportation and transformation and stop diarrhoea.

ii) Deficiency of the kidney:

Method: The points of the Kidney Meridian, Ren and Du Meridians are selected as the principal points with the reinforcing method and moxibustion to warm and reinforce the kidney yang.

Prescription: Shenshu (B 23), Pishu (B 20), Mingmen (Du 4), Guanyuan (Ren 4), Taixi (K 3), Zusanli (S 36).

Explanation: Shenshu (B 23) is the Back-(Shu) point of the kidney and Taixi (K 3) is the Yuan-(Primary) point of the Kidney

Meridian. Needling to these two points with the reinforcing method can warm the kidney yang and invigorate the kidney qi. Moxibustion to Mingmen (Du 4) and Guanyuan (Ren 4) is able to reinforce the Mingmen fire and strengthen the kidney yang so as to warm the spleen and kidney and promote digestion. This is known as a treatment of the root cause. Pishu (B 20) and Zusanli (S 36) are used to strengthen the spleen function and stop diarrhoea.

Remarks

This condition may be involved in acute and chronic enteritis, indigestion, intestinal parasitic diseases, diseases of the pancreas, liver and biliary tract, endocrine and metabolic disorders, and neurotic troubles.

8. Dysentery

Dysentery is characterized by abdominal pain, tenesmus and frequent stools containing blood and mucus. It is a common epidemic disease in summer and autumn. It is called "red-white dysentery," "bloody dysentery," "purulent and bloody dysentery" or "heat dysentery," and known as "persistent dysentery" if it lasts for a long time, and "intermittent dysentery" if it comes on and off.

The common patterns are damp-heat dysentery, cold-damp dysentery, food-resistant dysentery and intermittent dysentery.

This disease is often due to the invasion by the epidemic damp heat and internal injury by intake of raw, cold and unclean food, which hinders and damages the stomach and intestines.

Etiology and Pathogenesis

The summer epidemic heat dampness invades the stomach and intestines, impeding the flow of their qi and blood. Pus and blood are formed from the stagnated qi and blood in struggling against heat dampness, and hence occurs dysentery. In case dampness is preponderant to heat, white dysentery results, in case heat preponderant to dampness, red dysentery appears, and in case both dampness and heat are excessive, red-white dysentery occurs.

Preference for fatty and sweet food, internal accumulation of damp heat plus irregular diet, or intake of unclean food leads to stagnation of qi and blood in the fu organs, which turns into pus and blood in the stool and results in dysentery.

Excessive intake of raw, cold, or dirty food leads to internal accumulation of cold dampness, impeding the stomach and intestines. The stagnated qi in the large intestine also injures the blood, leading to discharge of pus and blood and resulting in cold-damp dysentery.

Although the above-mentioned etiological factors can be classified into the exogeneous pathogenic factors and food intake, the two are usually mutually affected.

The disease is in the intestine, but closely related to the stomach. If the epidemic toxic and damp heat attack the stomach, which fails to receive food, food-resistant dysentery occurs. If dysentery lasts longer, the body resistance is weaker and the spleen qi becomes more insufficient, persistent or intermittent dysentery therefore appears.

Differentiation

a) Damp-heat dysentery:

Main manifestations: Abdominal pain, tenesmus, mixing of pus and blood in stool, burning sensation of the anus, scanty and yellow urine, or chills, fever, restlessness, thirst, yellow, sticky tongue coating, rolling, rapid or soft, rapid pulse.

Analysis: In case the damp heat stagnates in the intestines, the qi and blood are blocked, leading to disturbance of transmission, so abdominal pain and tenesmus occur. When the blood vessels of the intestine are injured by damp heat, blood, pus and mucus appear in stools. Burning sensation of the anus, and scanty yellow urine are also manifestations of down-pouring of damp heat. When the summer heat and dampness attack the body, the body resistance will fight against it, so there are chills and fever. In case of excess of pathogenic heat, restlessness and thirst result. Sticky tongue coating and rolling or soft pulse indicate dampness, while yellow tongue coating and rapid pulse suggest heat.

b) Cold damp dysentery:

Main manifestations: Difficult defecation, white mucus in stools, preference for warmth and aversion to cold, mostly accompanied with fullness in the chest and epigastrium, lingering abdominal pain, tastelessness in the mouth, absence of thirst, white, sticky tongue coating, deep, slow pulse.

Analysis: Accumulation of internal cold dampness damages the spleen and stomach and blocks the qi flow of the large intestine. Cold is characterized by causing contraction and stagnation, while dampness is characterized by turbidity, so there are fullness in the chest and epigastrium, difficult defecation, white mucus in stools. Cold dampness is a yin pathogenic factor and apt to damage yang qi. When the yang qi is blocked and fails to disperse, preference for warmth, aversion to cold and lingering abdominal pain result. Tastelessness in the mouth, absence of thirst, sticky tongue coating are the signs of accumulation of dampness. Deep, slow pulse is the sign of excessive cold.

c) Food-resistant dysentery:

Main manifestations: Frequent stools with blood and pus, total loss of appetite, nausea, vomiting, yellow, sticky tongue coating, soft, rapid pulse.

Analysis: This condition is developed from the damp-heat dysentery. The epidemic summer heat dampness, when accumulated in the intestines, may attack the stomach and impair its function in sending its contents downwards. Thus the stomach fails to receive food, and the appetite is totally lost. The stomach qi ascends instead of descends, so nausea and vomiting occur. Yellow, sticky tongue coating, and soft, rapid pulse are the signs of damp heat.

d) Intermittent dysentery:

Main manifestations: Dysentery occurring on and off, difficult to cure, lassitude, aversion to cold, somnolence, anorexia, pale tongue, sticky coating, soft pulse.

Analysis: In case of the weakened body resistance with existence of the pathogenic factors impairing the transmitting function of the stomach and intestine, the condition is complicated with mixed deficiency and excess, and so the disease is lingering and recurrent. When the spleen yang is weak, and the qi is short, there may be lassitude, aversion to cold and somnolence. Soft pulse and persistent sticky coating are the signs of continuing presence of dampness.

Treatment

Method: The points of Yangming Meridians of Hand and Foot as well as the Front-(Mu) point and Lower He-(Sea) point of the large intestine are selected as the principal points to remove stagnation from the intestines. Reducing is used for the damp-heat dysentery, both acupuncture and moxibustion are used for the cold-damp dysentery, and acupuncture and moxibustion, with both reinforcing and reducing methods, are used for the persistent dysentery.

Prescription: Tianshu (S 25), Shangjuxu (S 37).

Damp-heat dysentery: Quchi (L I 11), Hegu (L I 4) are added.

Cold-damp dysentery: Zhongwan (Ren 12) is added with moxibustion to Qihai (Ren 6) and Yinlingquan (Sp 9).

Food-resistant dysentery: Zhongwan (Ren 12) and Neiguan (P 6) are added.

Intermittent dysentery: Pishu (B 20), Weishu (B 21), Guanyuan (Ren 4) and Zusanli (S 36) are added.

Supplementary points:

Fever: Dazhui (Du 14).

Tenesmus: Zhonglushu (B 29).

Prolapse of rectum: Baihui (Du 20) with moxibustion, Changqiang (Du 1).

Explanation: It is recorded in *Internal Classic* that the He-(Sea) points are applied for the diseases of the fu organs. Therefore, Tianshu (S 25), the Front-(Mu) point of the large intestine, and Shangjuxu (S 37), the He-(Sea) point of the large intestine, are selected as the principal points to remove stagnation of qi in the large intestine. Dampness will be resolved in case qi is regulated. Quchi (L I 11) and Hegu (L I 4) may dispel the damp heat from the stomach and intestines. Moxibustion to Zhongwan (Ren 12) and Qihai (Ren 6) is applied to warm the spleen and stomach, remove cold and regulate the flow of qi. Yinlingquan (Sp 9) is needled to strengthen the spleen function to resolve dampness. For food-resistant dysentery, Zhongwan (Ren 12) and Neiguan (P 6) are used to pacify the stomach and resolve dampness. Acupuncture with both reinforcing and reducing methods and

moxibustion may warm the spleen and stomach and eliminate the intestinal stagnation. Guanyuan (Ren 4), the Front-(Mu) point of the small intestine, is applied to separate the food essence from the waste, reinforce qi and activate yang.

Remarks

This condition includes acute and chronic bacillary and amebic dysentery.

9. Abdominal Distention

Abdominal distention is common in clinic. Distention and fullness are likely to occur in both the upper and lower abdomen. The stomach is located in the upper abdomen, while the small and large intestines are in the lower; they jointly complete the storage, digestion, and assimilation of food and excretion of the wastes. Once the stomach and intestines lose their functions, abdominal distention and pain, belching, vomiting, etc. will occur. This section deals with the syndromes mainly manifested by abdominal distention due to disorders of the stomach and intestines.

Etiology and Pathogenesis

a) Irregular or excessive food intake impairs the stomach and intestines, causing dysfunction of transportation and transformation, thus the retained food is stagnated and blocks the flow of qi, or the stagnated food turns into heat, which enters the stomach and intestines, causing abdominal distention.

b) Because of the weakened function of the spleen and stomach or general debility due to long illness, the spleen and stomach fail in their transporting functions, so the circulation of qi in the stomach and intestines is impaired, resulting in abdominal distention.

In addition, abdominal distention may also follow an abdominal operation.

Differentiation

a) Excess condition

Main manifestations: Persistence of distention and fullness in the abdomen, which is aggravated by pressure, abdominal pain, belching, foul breath, dark yellow urine, constipation, sometimes associated with fever, vomiting, yellow thick tongue coating, rolling, rapid and forceful pulse.

Analysis: Indigested food retained in the stomach gives rise to distention and fullness in the epigastrium, foul breath, belching, and even vomiting, and when it is retained in the intestines, there will be fullness and pain in the abdomen and constipation. Retention of food is an excess condition. This is why the pain is aggravated by pressure. Fever, dark yellow urine, yellow thick tongue coating, rolling, rapid and forceful pulse are the signs of excessive heat in the stomach.

b) Deficiency condition

Main manifestations: Abdominal distention relieved by pressure, borborygmi, loose stools, loss of appetite, lassitude, listlessness, clear urine, pale tongue with white coating and forceless pulse.

Analysis: Qi deficiency of the spleen and stomach results in dysfunction of transportation and transformation. Consequently there are loss of appetite, borborygmi and loose stools. Pain relieved by pressure is due to deficiency. Failure in creating qi and blood due to impaired transportation and transformation is the cause of lassitude and listlessness. Pale tongue with white coating,

and forceless pulse are signs of qi deficiency in the spleen and stomach.

Treatment

Method: The points of Yangming Meridian of Foot are selected as the principal points. The excess condition is treated by the reducing method to regulate the qi flow in the fu organs while the deficiency condition is treated by the reinforcing method or combined with moxibustion to invigorate the function of the stomach and spleen and to adjust the circulation of qi to relieve the distention.

Prescription: Zhongwan (Ren 12), Tianshu (S 25), Zusanli (S 36), Shangjuxu (S 37).

Supplementary points:

Excess condition: Hegu (L I 4), Qihai (Ren 6), Yinlingquan (Sp 9).

Deficiency condition: Guanyuan (Ren 4), Taibai (Sp 3).

Explanation: Application of Zhongwan (Ren 12), the Front-(Mu) point of the stomach, Zusanli (S 36), the Lower He-(Sea) point of the stomach, Tianshu (S 25), the Front-(Mu) point of the large intestine and Shangjuxu (S 37), the Lower He-(Sea) point of the large intestine, are used as a combination of Front-(Mu) and Lower He-(Sea) points to regulate the function of the stomach and intestines in order to maintain normal flow of qi and relieve the distention. Hegu (L I 4) and Qihai (Ren 6) are combined to adjust the circulation of qi, while Yinlingquan (Sp 9) can eliminate damp heat. Taibai (Sp 3) and Guanyuan (Ren 4) are beneficial to strengthen the spleen and stomach and to help transportation and transformation.

Remarks

This condition is involved in gastroptosis, acute gastrectasia, enteroparalysis, intestinal obstruction, gastrointestinal neurosis, etc.

10. Jaundice

Jaundice is mainly manifested by yellow discoloration of the sclera, skin and urine, resulted from the dampness in the spleen and heat in the stomach, leading to abnormal circulation of the bile which spreads to the skin surface. It is divided into yang jaundice and yin jaundice according to its nature.

Etiology and Pathogenesis

The seasonal and epidemic pathogenic factors accumulate in the spleen and stomach, leading to internal formation and collection of damp heat. Dampness after mixed with heat is apt to penetrate deeper, while heat mixed with dampness is apt to get more exuberant. The liver and gallbladder are steamed by the heat in the spleen and stomach, leading to overflow of the bile to the skin surface, thus jaundice appears.

Irregular diet injures the spleen and stomach, causing disturbance in transportation and transformation and internal formation of dampness, which transforms into heat. Damp heat stains the skin yellow.

Overstrain or general weakness of the spleen qi may give rise to hypoactivity of the yang in the middle jiao, leading to failure in transportation and transformation and stagnation of cold dampness, thus yin jaundice results. As said in *A Guide to the Clinic Treatment*, "The cause of yin jaundice is the dampness produced from cold water. If the spleen yang fails to resolve the dampness, the normal distribution of bile is impaired, affecting the spleen, soaking into the muscles, and spreading to the skin which turns yellow as if it were smoked."

Yin jaundice can also result from an improperly treated yang jaundice which leads to injury of the yang qi, hypoactivity of the spleen yang, and internal collection of cold dampness.

Differentiation

a) Yang jaundice:

Main manifestations: Lustrous yellow skin and sclera, fever, thirst, scanty dark yellow urine, heaviness of the body, fullness in the abdomen, stuffiness of the chest, nausea, yellow, sticky tongue coating, string-taut, rapid pulse.

Analysis: Steaming of the damp heat makes the bile spread to the skin surface. Heat being a yang pathogenic factor, makes the yellow discoloration of the skin lustrous. Fever, thirst, scanty dark yellow urine are due to excessive damp heat, which damages the body fluid, and disturbs the activity of the bladder. When the dampness is collected, the pure yang fails to be distributed and heaviness of the body results. In case of obstruction of the qi in the fu organs, fullness in the abdomen occurs. Stuffiness of the chest and nausea are due to the steaming of damp heat, leading to upward perversion of the turbid contents of the stomach. Yellow sticky tongue coating is due to accumulation of damp heat, and string-taut, rapid pulse due to excessive heat in the liver and gallbladder.

b) Yin jaundice:

Main manifestations: Sallow skin, heaviness of the body, weakness, loss of appetite, epigastric stuffiness, lassitude, aversion to cold, absence of thirst, pale tongue, thick, white tongue coating, deep slow pulse.

Analysis: The stagnation of cold

dampness in the spleen and stomach impedes the distribution of yang qi, leading to overflow of the bile, thus the skin is sallow. In case the dampness stays in the spleen, the spleen yang is hypoactive and the transporting and transforming function is impaired, therefore, heaviness of the body, weakness, loss of appetite and epigastric stuffiness occur. Aversion to cold and lassitude are due to weakness of the yang qi. Since this case is of cold-damp nature, thirst is absent. Pale tongue, thick white tongue coating are due to deficiency of yang failing to resolve dampness. Deep, slow pulse is a sign of cold dampness staying in the yin system.

Treatment

Method: The points of Taiyin, Yangming and Shaoyang Meridians are selected as the principal points. Reducing is applied to remove heat and dampness in yang jaundice, while even movement with moxibustion is used to warm the middle jiao and resolve dampness in yin jaundice.

Prescription: Yinlingquan (Sp 9), Zusanli (S 36), Ganshu (B 18), Danshu (B 19), Zhiyang (Du 9).

Supplementary points:

Yang jaundice: Taichong (Liv 3), Yanglingquan (G 34).

Yin jaundice: Moxibustion to Pishu (B 20), Yanggang (B 48).

Explanation: Yinlingquan (Sp 9) and Zusanli (S 36) are used to strengthen the spleen and resolve dampness. Ganshu (B 18), Danshu (B 19) and Zhiyang (Du 9) are important points to treat jaundice. Since the damp heat resides in the gallbladder, Yanglingquan (G 34) is selected to reduce heat, and used in combination with Taichong (Liv 3) to regulate the flow of qi in the liver and gallbladder. Moxibustion to Pishu (B 20) and Yanggang (B 48) may resolve cold dampness by warmth and treat jaundice.

Remarks

This condition is seen in acute icteric hepatitis, obstructive jaundice and hemolytic jaundice. Acupuncture and moxibustion are more effective to treat hepatogenic jaundice.

11.   Constipation

Constipation is mainly caused by the disturbed transmitting function of the large intestine and also related to the function of the spleen, stomach and kidney. In view of the difference in etiology and pathogenesis, this illness can be divided into two types: deficiency and excess.

Etiology and Pathogenesis

After food is digested by the spleen and stomach, its refined nutrients are assimilated, and the wastes are egested through the transmission of the large intestine. If the stomach and intestines are diseased, various kinds of constipation occur in the following conditions: internal accumulation of dryness and heat, stagnation of qi, deficiency of qi with inability of transmission, blood deficiency with dryness of the intestines, and agglomeration of cold.

Constitutional yang preponderance, or indulgence in alcohol and spicy greasy food may lead to accumulation of heat in the stomach and intestines. Or after some febrile diseases, the remnant heat and insufficiency of body fluids give rise to dryness and heat in the intestines, and in addition, there may be disturbance of fluid distribution to the lower jiao. Constipation is present in any of the above cases.

Emotional factors, such as anxiety and depression, or lack of movement can cause stagnation of qi, impairing the transmitting function of the large intestine. As a result, the wastes are retained inside and unable to move downward, and hence constipation.

The coexistent deficiency of qi and blood can result from internal injury by overstrain or improper food intake, or happen after an illness or delivery or in the aged people. Qi deficiency results in weakness of the large intestine in transmission, while blood definciency gives rise to shortage of body fluid, then the large intestine can no longer be moistened. Apparently both qi and blood deficiency can cause difficult evacuation of the feces, and hence constipation.

Constitutional debility or senile decay results in retention of the endogenous cold in the stomach and intestines. Consequently the yang qi is obstructed and the body fluid fail in distribution. Difficulty of the large intestine in transmission leads to constipation.

Differentiation

a) Excess condition

Main manifestations: Infrequent and difficult defecation from every three to five days, or even longer. In case of accumulation of heat, there are fever, dire thirst, foul breath, rolling and forceful pulse, yellow, dry tongue coating; in case of stagnation of qi, there are fullness and distending pain in the abdomen and hypochondriac regions, frequent belching, loss of appetite, thin sticky tongue coating and string-taut pulse.

Analysis: The large intestine is concerned with transmission. When there is accumulation of heat in the stomach and intestines,

which consumes the body fluid or stagnation of qi, disturbing the normal function of the large intestine, constipation may result. Fever and dire thirst indicate internal preponderance of pathogenic heat. When the heat in the stomach and intestines causes evaporation, there is foul breath. The yellow and dry tongue coating reveals the damage of the body fluid by the heat, while the rolling and forceful pulse is a sign of excess in the interior. Emotional disturbance leads to stagnation of qi in the liver and spleen, thus resulting in frequent belching, and fullness and distending pain in the abdomen or hypochondrium. Since the spleen fails in transportation and transformation, there is loss of appetite. Thin, sticky tongue coating and string-taut pulse are the signs of disharmony between the liver and spleen.

b) Deficiency condition:

Main manifestations: In cases of deficiency of qi and blood, pale and lustreless complexion, lips and nails, dizziness and palpitation, lassitude, shortness of breath, pale tongue with thin coating, thready and weak pulse; in cases of agglomeration of cold, pain and cold sensation in the abdomen, preference for warmth and aversion to cold, pale tongue with white and moist coating, deep slow pulse.

Analysis: Constipation can be caused either by qi deficiency, resulting in failure of the large intestine in transmission, or by blood deficiency with shortage of body fluid unable to moisten the large intestine. Endogenous cold stays in the stomach and intestines, leading to agglomeration of yin qi, failure of yang qi in transportation, and weakened transmission of the large intestine, and hence difficulty of defecation. Deficiency of qi and blood fails to ascend to nourish the upper portion, so there are pale and lustreless complexion and lips, lassitude and shortness of breath. In case of blood deficiency, the heart is poorly nourished, hence palpitation. When the head and eyes fail to be nourished, dizziness results. Since the nail is the external manifestation of the liver, there will be lustreless nails when the liver blood is insufficient. When cold is agglomerated, the circulation of qi is impeded, this accounts for the cold pain in the abdomen. Cold is of yin nature, and disorders caused by cold can be relieved by warmth, so there is preference for warmth and aversion to cold. Pale tongue with thin coating, thready weak pulse are the signs of insufficiency of qi and blood, while pale tongue with white, moist coating shows the internal cold due to yang deficiency.

Treatment

Method: The Back-(Shu) and Front-(Mu) points of the Large Intestine Meridian are mainly selected. For the excess condition the reducing method is applied to eliminate the heat, moisten the intestine, and remove the stagnation of qi, while for deficiency condition, the reinforcing method is used to reinforce qi and nourish blood, and moisten the intestines for defecation. Constipation due to cold can be relieved by moxibustion to warm the fu organ for defecation.

Prescription: Dachangshu (B 25), Tianshu (S 25), Zhigou (S J 6), Zhaohai (K 6).

Accumulation of heat: Quchi (L I 11), Hegu (L I 4).

Stagnation of qi: Zhongwan (Ren 12), Taichong (Liv 3).

Deficiency of qi and blood: Pishu (B 20), Weishu (B 21), Zusanli (S 36).

Agglomeration of cold: Moxibustion to Shenque (Ren 8) and Qihai (Ren 6).

Explanation: The causes of constipation are different, but they are common in impairing the transmitting function of the large intestine. Therefore, Dachangshu (B 25) and the Front-(Mu) point of the large intestine are applied to promote the flow of qi in the large intestine, the transmission can be regained when the qi of the fu organ flows smoothly. Zhigou (S J 6) can promote the flow of qi in the three jiao. When the qi in the three jiao is in normal circulation, the qi of the fu organ will circulate freely. Zhigou (S J 6) combined with Zhaohai (K 6) is a principal point in treating constipation. Quchi (L I 11) and Hegu (L I 4) can reduce the heat from the large intestine. Zhongwan (Ren 12), the Influential Point of the fu organs, is selected to lower the qi of the fu organ. The reducing method applied to Taichong (Liv 3) is to soothe the liver qi. Reinforcing to Pishu (B 20), Weishu (B 21) and Zusanli (S 36) is able to reinforce qi in the spleen and stomach. Once the spleen and stomach qi is vigorous, qi and blood can be produced as a natural consequence, so this is the approach of treating the root cause of constipation in deficiency conditions. Moxibustion to Shenque (Ren 8) and Qihai (Ren 6) is offered to reduce cold and loosen the bowels.

12. Prolapse of Rectum

Prolapse of rectum likely happens to infants, the old aged, and those with general debility after a long illness.

Etiology and Pathogenesis

This disease is mostly caused by deficiency of the primary qi, sinking of the spleen and stomach qi and disability of restraining due to long-standing diarrhoea or dysentery, or due to constitutional weakness after severe diseases.

Differentiation

Main manifestations: The onset is slow, to start with distending and draggling sensation of rectum during defecation, and returning to normal after the bowel movement. If it is sustained without proper treatment, recurrence may happen by overstrain and the prolapsed rectum fails to return spontaneously without the aid of the hand.

Sometimes there are lassitude, weakness of limbs, sallow complexion, dizziness and palpitation. The tongue is pale with white coating, and the pulse thready and feeble.

Analysis: Deficiency of the primary qi leads to the sinking of the spleen qi, and failure of the large intestine in holding itself in its normal position, so the rectum prolapses. Insufficiency of the spleen and stomach qi brings about dysfunction of transportation and transformation, causing deficiency of qi and blood, thus lassitude and weakness of the limbs appear. Qi deficiency fails to nourish the upper portion of the body. Dizziness results from the failure of nourishing the head and eyes, and palpitation from the failure of nourishing the heart. Pale tongue with white coating, thready and feeble pulse are the signs of qi deficiency.

Treatment

Method: Points of the Du Meridian are mainly applicable with the reinforcing method and moxibustion.

Prescription: Baihui (Du 20), Dachangshu (B 25), Changqiang (Du 1), Zusanli (S 36).

Explanation: Rectum is the distal part of the large intestine. Reinforcing Dachangshu (B 25) can replenish the qi of the large intestine. Baihui (Du 20) is the meeting point of the Du Meridian and the three yang meridians, and qi pertains to yang, subjected to the Du Meridian, therefore moxibustion to Baihui (Du 20) can invigorate yang qi, and improve the elevating and contracting function. Changqiang (Du 1), a point of the collateral of the Du Meridian, located near the anus, is selected as a local point. Zusanli (S 36) can reinforce qi for elevation. The combination of Baihui (Du 20), Changqiang (Du 1) and Zusanli (S 36) follows a principle — to elevate when there is subsidence.

Remarks

Picking therapy: Pick any spot on the paraspinal muscle bilaterally in between the third lumbar vertebra and the second sacral vertebra.

13. Edema

Subcutaneous retention of fluid which leads to puffiness of the head, face, eyelids, limbs, abdomen and even the whole body is called edema. The causative factors are invasion of the body by the exogeneous pathogenic wind and water dampness, and internal injury by food or overstrain, which results in disturbance of water circulation and overflow of water. Since the water circulation in the body is related to the regulatory function of the lung qi, transporting function of the spleen qi, activity of the kidney qi and water communication of the three jiao, the functional derangement of the lung, spleen, kidney and three jiao may lead to edema. Clinically edema is divided into two patterns: yin edema and yang edema, according to their etiology and pathogenesis.

Etiology and Pathogenesis

a) Invasion of the wind upon the lung causes dysfunction of the lung in dispersion. The lung dominates the surface of the body and is associated with the skin and hair. If the lung is attacked by wind, the lung qi fails to regulate the water passages and send the water down to the bladder, leading to the confrontation between wind and water and the overflow of water to the superficial part of the body, and thus edema appears.

b) Living in a damp place, wading through water or drenching by rain makes water dampness attack the body. Irregular food intake causes failure of the spleen in normal transportation and transformation and impairment of downward flow of water dampness. In either case there may be overflow of water dampness to the superficial part of the body, resulting in edema.

c) Overstrain injures the spleen, leading to gradual weakness of the spleen qi, which fails to distribute the essence to the lung and to the whole body. Water is also retained if the spleen function in transporting and transforming fluid is impaired. Once the spleen fails to control water and lets it flow over, edema results.

d) Indulgent sexual activities damage the kidney qi, and also the function of the bladder. Retention of water follows and edema results.

According to the above-mentioned, edema resulting from invasion by wind, drenching by rain and irregular food intake is of yang nature, while that resulting from overstrain, internal injury and indulgent sexual activity, leading to weakness of the spleen and kidney, is of yin nature.

However, the prolonged yang edema may lead to gradual weakness of the body resistance and increased water retention, and turn into yin edema. Pathogenetically, edema is closely related to the dysfunction of the lung, spleen and kidney.

Differentiation

a) Yang edema:

Main manifestations: Abrupt onset of edema with puffy face and eyelids and then anasarca, lustrous skin, accompanied by chills, fever, thirst, cough, asthma and reduced urine output, thin white tongue coating, superficial or rolling, rapid pulse.

Analysis: In case of internal accumulation of water and external invasion by wind, confrontation between them causes an abrupt onset of edema starting from the upper portion of the body, as the wind is a pathogenic factor of yang nature and charaterized by upward going. If the function of the bladder is impaired, the urine output is reduced. When the wind water attacks the lung, cough, asthma, aversion to wind and chills result. If heat is dominant, there are thirst, fever and rolling rapid pulse. Thin white tongue coating and superficial pulse indicate wind water of cold nature.

b) Yin edema:

Main manifestations: Insidious onset of edema, at first on the pedis dorsum or eyelids, and then over the whole body, especially remarkable below the lumbar region, accompanied by sallow complexion, aversion to cold, cold limbs, soreness of the back and loins, general weakness, epigastric fullness, abdominal distension, loss of appetite, loose stools, pale tongue, white coating, deep, thready pulse.

Analysis: Because of weakness of yang in the spleen and the kidney, yin is in excess and qi fails to transport water, causing overflow of water dampness in the lower portion of the body, and hence appears pitting edema which is especially remarkable below the lumbar region. In case of lowered function of the spleen and kidney, qi is unable to nourish the face, so the complexion is sallow. Weakened kidney yang with declined Mingmen fire is insufficient to warm the body, so there is aversion to cold with cold limbs. The lumbus is the house of the kidney. If the kidney qi is weakened and water dampness excessive, soreness is felt in the back and loins. In case of hypoactivity of the spleen yang, the function of transportation and transformation is weak, so epigastric fullness, loss of appetite, abdominal distension and loose stools result. Pale tongue, white coating, deep, thready pulse are also signs of deficiency of the spleen and kidney yang with excess of water dampness.

Treatment

a) Yang edema:

Method: The points of the Lung and Spleen Meridians are selected as the principal points. Even movement is applied to clear the lung, relieve the exterior symptoms and remove the retained fluid. After the exterior symptoms are relieved, refer to method for yin edema.

Prescription: Lieque (L 7), Hegu (L I 4), Pianli (L I 6), Yinlingquan (Sp 9), Weiyang (B 39).

Explanation: Edema above the lumbus should be treated by diaphoresis, therefore, Lieque (L 7) and Hegu (L I 4) are used to clear the lung and relieve the exterior symptoms by diaphoresis, while edema below the lumbus should be treated by diuresis, then Pianli (L I 6) and Yinlingquan (Sp 9) are applied to remove dampness and promote diuresis. Weiyang (B 39) is able to

regulate the qi activity of the sanjiao and water passages.

b) Yin edema:

Method: The points of the Spleen and Kidney Meridians are selected as the principal points. Reinforcing in combination with moxibustion is applied to warm the spleen and kidney.

Prescription: Pishu (B 20), Shenshu (B 23), Shuifen (Ren 9), Guanyuan (Ren 4), Fuliu (K 7), Zusanli (S 36).

Supplementary points:

Facial puffiness: Shuigou (Du 26).

Edema on the pedis dorsum: Zulinqi (G 41), Shangqiu (Sp 5).

Explanation: Yin edema is caused by decline of the kidney yang that fails to control water and by weakness of the spleen qi that leads to impairment of transportation in the middle jiao. Acupuncture and moxibustion to Pishu (B 20), Shenshu (B 23) and Fuliu (K 7) may warm the primary yang of the spleen and kidney and remove cold water. Moxibustion to Shuifen (Ren 9) and Guanyuan (Ren 4) may promote the water circulation and reinforce the primary qi respectively. Reinforcing on Zusanli (S 36) promotes the transporting and tranforming function of the spleen and stomach, restoring normal distribution of the fluid.

Remarks

In the context of edema, acute and chronic nephritis and malnutrition are included.

14.   Nocturnal Enuresis

Nocturnal enuresis is referred to involuntary discharge of the urine occurring at night and during sleep. As a morbid condition, it is mostly seen in children over the age of three years and occasionally in adults. It is mainly caused by deficiency of kidney qi with disability of the bladder to restrain the urine discharge.

Etiology and Pathogenesis

The normal excretion of urine is mainly concerned with the activities of the kidney qi and the restraining function of the bladder. The kidney is in charge of micturition and defecation, and responsible for the formation of urine, while the bladder stores and excretes urine. If the kidney qi is insufficient, it will be unable to maintain the function of the bladder in restraining the urine discharge, and thus occurs enuresis. Ancient doctors therefore believed that enuresis is due to deficiency. As stated in *General Treatise on the Etiology and Symptomology of Diseases:* "Enuresis is caused by cold in the bladder of deficiency type, which renders the bladder unable to restrain the urine discharge." Dai Sigong once said, "Involuntary urination during sleep is due to cold in the kidney causing incontinence of urine."

Differentiation

Main manifestations: Involuntary micturition during sleep with dreams, once in several nights in mild cases, or several times a night in severe cases; sallow complexion, loss of appetite, and weakness in the prolonged cases, pale tongue, white coating, thready pulse weak at the *chi* region.

Analysis: Deficiency of the kidney qi with failure of the bladder in restraining the urine discharge causes nocturnal enuresis. Long duration of the disease undermines the kidney qi, and consequently the spleen falls into loss of warming, its function of transportation and transformation being disturbed. Therefore, the appetite is lost. Deficiency of the spleen qi fails to distribute

the essence of food to nourish the whole body. This is why the complexion is sallow and the patient is lacking in strength. Pale tongue with white coating, and thready pulse weak at *chi* region are signs of deficiency.

Treatment

Method: The Back-(Shu) and Front-(Mu) points of the kidney and bladder are selected as the principal points, with reinforcing or moxibustion to strengthen the kidney and reinforce qi.

Prescription: Shenshu (B 23), Pangguangshu (B 28), Zhongji (Ren 3), Sanyinjiao (Sp 6), Dadun (Liv 1).

Supplementary points:

Enuresis with dreams: Shenmen (H 7).

Loss of appetite: Pishu (B 20), Zusanli (S 36).

Explanation: The kidney is exteriorly-interiorly related to the bladder, so the Back-(Shu) points of the kidney and bladder are applied. Zhongji (Ren 3) is the Front-(Mu) point of the bladder. Combined use of the above three points contributes to reinforce the kidney qi and the restraining function. Sanyinjiao (Sp 6) is added to adjust the qi of the three yin meridians. Moxibustion to Dadun (Liv 1), the Jing-(Well) point of the Liver Meridian which curves round the genitals, can promote the circulation of qi of the meridian and strenghthen the therapeutic effect.

Remarks

The chief causative factor of this disease is the underdevelopment of cerebral micturition centre and treatment of acupuncture and moxibustion provides satisfactory effect. As for enuresis caused by organic diseases, such as deformity of urinary tract, cryptorachischisis, organic cerebral diseases and oxyuriasis, the treatment should be given to the primary disease.

15. Urination Disturbance

Urination disturbance is manifested by frenquency of urination, painful urination and incontinence of urination, resulting mainly from accumulation of heat in the bladder, and sometimes also from emotional factors and deficiency of the kidney.

According to the clinic manifestations, urination disturbance is divided into five kinds, i.e. dysuria caused by calculi, dysuria caused by qi dysfunction, dysuria with milky urine, dysuria caused by overstrain and painful urination with blood.

Etiology and Pathogenesis

Eating too much fatty or sweet food or drinking too much alcohol leads to accumulation of damp heat in the lower jiao, where the urine is condensed into calculi, which may be either small as gravel or large as stones, staying in various portions of the urinary tract from the kidney to the bladder or the urethra, causing dysuria.

In case the damp heat accumulates in the bladder, or the heart fire shifts to the bladder, the heat injures the blood vessels and forces the blood to extravasate, then painful urination with blood results. If the damp heat accumulates in the lower jiao, impairing the control of the flow of the chylous fluid, viscous urine like milk appears, known as dysuria with milky urine.

Damage of the liver by anger, production of fire from stagnated qi or obstruction of qi due to stagnation, leading to accumulation of qi and fire in the lower jiao, impedes the activity of the bladder. Therefore, urination is difficult, painful and incontinent, known as dysuria caused by dysfunction of qi.

Indulgent sexual activities or mental stress leading to deficiency of the kidney qi, or sinking of the spleen qi due to deficiency, causes painful urination which often recurs on overstrain, known as dysuria caused by overstrain.

Differentiation

a) Dysuria caused by calculi:

Main manifestations: Occasional presence of calculi in the urine, dysuria, dark yellow turbid urine, or sudden interruption of urination, unbearable pricking pain during urination, pain of the lumbus and abdomen, or presence of blood in the urine, normal tongue coating.

Analysis: When the gravel and stones formed by damp heat fail to be discharged in the urine, dark yellow turbid urine and painful urination occur. If a large stone obstructs the outer orifice of the bladder, urination may suddenly be interrupted, accompanied by unbearable pain. In case the calculi cause internal injury, bloody urine appears. When the calculi have been formed, the signs of internal heat may sometimes become obscure and the tongue coating turns to normal.

b) Dysuria caused by qi dysfunction:

Main manifestations: Difficult and hesitant urination, fullness and pain of the lower abdomen, thin, white tongue coating, deep, string-taut pulse.

Analysis: Emotional depression leads to qi dysfunction, failure of the liver in qi spreading and stagnation of qi in the bladder. So there are fullness and pain of the lower abdomen, and difficult and hesitant urination. In case of depression of the qi in the liver, deep, string-taut pulse occurs.

c) Painful urination with blood:

Main manifestations: Hematuria with pain and urgency of micturition, burning sensation and pricking pain in urination, thin, yellow tongue coating, rapid, forceful pulse.

d) Dysuria with milky urine:

Main manifestations: Cloudy urine with milky or creamy appearance, urethral burning pain in urination, red tongue proper, sticky coating, thready, rapid pulse.

Analysis: This condition is due to downward shift of damp heat, which accumulates in the bladder and affects the qi function. The bladder fails to check the downward flow of fatty liquid, so there are cloudy urine with milky or even creamy appearance and urethral burning pain in urination. Red tongue proper, sticky coating, thready rapid pulse are the signs of deficiency of kidney yin and stagnation of damp heat.

e) Dysuria caused by overstrain:

Main manifestations: Difficulty in urination with dribbling of urine, occurring off and on, exacerbated after overwork, and usually refractory to treatment, weak pulse.

Analysis: Overstrain, indulgence in sex and drinking, or taking too much drugs cold in nature for treating other kinds of dysuria lead to deficiency of the spleen and kidney, and failure of the yang qi to ascend. That is why urination is exacerbated after overwork and refractory to treatment. Weak pulse is the sign of qi deficiency.

Treatment

Method: The Back-(Shu) and Front-(Mu) points of the bladder are selected as the principal points. Reducing alone or combination of reinforcing and reducing methods is applied to promote the activity of the bladder.

Prescription: Pangguangshu (B 28),
Zhongji (Ren 3), Yinlingquan (Sp 9).

Supplementary points:

Dysuria caused by calculi: Weiyang (B 39).

Dysuria caused by qi dysfunction: Xingjian (Liv 2).

Painful urination with blood: Xuehai (Sp 10), Sanyinjiao (Sp 6).

Dysuria with milky urine: Shenshu (B 23), Zhaohai (K 6).

Dysuria caused by overstrain: Baihui (Du 20), Qihai (Ren 6), Zusanli (S 36).

Explanation: Urination trouble is chiefly due to affections of the bladder, so Pangguangshu (B 28) and Zhongji (Ren 3), the Front-(Mu) point of the bladder, are needled to promote the activity of the bladder. Yinlingquan (Sp 9), the He-(Sea) point of the Spleen Meridian, is combined to promote diuresis, restoring the qi function and free urination. Dysuria caused by calculi is due to the accumulation of damp heat in the lower jiao and condensation of urine. Therefore, Weiyang (B 39), a point of the Bladder Meridian of Foot-Taiyang and also the Lower He-(Sea) point of sanjiao, is applied to reduce damp heat from the lower jiao and strengthen the function of the bladder. Xingjian (Liv 2), the Ying-(Spring) point of the Liver Meridian, is used to dispel the fire from the Liver Meridian and relieve pain for dysuria caused by qi dysfunction. Xuehai (Sp 10) and Sanyinjiao (Sp 6) are applied to remove the heat from the lower jiao and stop bleeding. If dysuria with milky urine lasts longer, deficiency of the kidney fails to check the downward flow of fatty liquid, so Shenshu (B 23) and Zhaohai (K 6) are needled to reinforce the kidney qi. Dysuria caused by overstrain is due to weakness of both spleen and kidney. Baihui (Du 20), the meeting point of all the yang meridians, in combination with Qihai (Ren

6) and Zusanli (S 36) may reinforce the qi of the spleen and kidney.

Remarks

This morbid condition includes urinary infection and urolithiasis.

16. Retention of Urine

Retention of urine is a disease manifested by difficult urination, distending pain in the lower abdomen and even blockage of urine. The mild case refers to difficulty in urination and dripping of urine, while the severe case to failure in urination with distension and feeling of urgency.

This disease results from dysfunction of qi in the bladder. As said in *Internal Classics*: "The bladder is in charge of storing liquid. Normal urination suggests the qi is in function. Its dysfunction causes retention of urine."

Etiology and Pathogenesis

Heat accumulates in the bladder, or heat of the kidney shifts to the bladder. Accumulation of heat in the bladder impedes the qi function and leads to retention of urine.

The kidney and the bladder are exteriorly-interiorly related. The function of the bladder depends upon the warming function of the kidney yang. In case of weakness of the kidney yang and decline of Mingmen fire, the bladder may be too weak to discharge the urine.

Traumatic injury or surgical operation hindering the qi of the meridians or damaging the zang organs, causes retention of urine too.

Differentiation

a) Accumulation of heat in the bladder:

Main manifestations: Scanty hot urine or retention of urine, distension and fullness of the lower abdomen, thirst but without desire to drink, constipation, red tongue with yellow coating, rapid pulse.

Analysis: In case of accumulation of heat in the bladder, scanty hot urine or retention of urine appears. When water and heat combined together, impair the function of the bladder, distension and fullness of the lower abdomen occur. Since the body fluid fails to be normally distributed, thirst results but there is no desire to drink. Red tongue with yellow coating, rapid pulse, or constipation are due to accumulation of heat in the lower jiao.

b) Decline of Mingmen fire:

Main manifestations: Dribbling urination, attenuating in force of the urine discharge, pallor, listlessness, chilliness below the lumbus, weakness of the loins and knees, pale tongue, deep, thready pulse weak at the *chi* region.

Analysis: Dribbling urination, attenuating in force of the urine discharge is due to deficiency of the kidney yang which affects the transmitting function. Pallor, listlessness and pale tongue are due to decline of the Mingmen fire and failure of qi in reaching the bladder.

c) Damage of the qi of the meridian:

Main manifestations: Dribbling urination or retention of urine, distension and dull pain in the lower abdomen, purplish spots on the tongue, hesitant, rapid pulse.

Analysis: After a traumatic injury or surgical operation on the lower abdomen, the qi of the Bladder Meridian is damaged and blood stasis occurs, so there appear dribbling urination, retention of urine, distension and pain in the lower abdomen. Purplish spots on the tongue, hesitant, rapid pulse are the signs of blood stasis.

Treatment

a) Accumulation of heat in the bladder:

Method: The Back-(Shu) points and Front-(Mu) points are selected as the principal points. Reducing method is applied to remove heat and promote diuresis.

Prescription: Pangguangshu (B 28), Zhongji (Ren 3), Sanyinjiao (Sp 6), Weiyang (B 39).

Explanation: Pangguangshu (B 28), the Back-(Shu) point of the bladder, and Zhongji (Ren 3), the Front-(Mu) point of the bladder, are needled to reduce heat from the bladder and adjust its function. Sanyinjiao (Sp 6) may dispel heat from the lower jiao. Weiyang (B 39), the Lower He-(Sea) point of sanjiao, promotes the circulation of water. These points, used together, reduce heat and promote diuresis.

b) Decline of the Mingmen Fire:

Method: The points relating to the Kidney Meridian are selected as the principal points. Reinforcing or moxibustion is applied to warm the kidney yang.

Prescription: Mingmen (Du 4), Shenshu (B 23), Baihui (Du 20), Guanyuan (Ren 4), Yangchi (S J 4).

Explanation: In case of deficiency of the kidney qi and decline of the Mingmen fire, the kidney qi should be reinforced, so Mingmen (Du 4) and Shenshu (B 23) are needled to reinforce the kidney yang. Moxibustion to Baihui (Du 20) and

Guanyuan (Ren 4) is to invigorate the kidney qi. Urination will be free in smooth qi circulation. Since deficiency of the kidney qi makes sanjiao fail to promote the circulation of water, Yangchi (S J 4), the Yuan-(Primary) point of sanjiao, is needled to strengthen the function of sanjiao and promote circulation of water.

c) Damage of the qi in the meridian:

Method: The Front-(Mu) point of the bladder is selected as the principal point. Even movement is applied to promote circulation of the qi in the meridian and restore the function of the bladder.

Prescription: Zhongji (Ren 3), Sanyinjiao (Sp 6), Shuidao (S 28), Shuiquan (K 5).

Explanation: A traumatic injury or surgical operation can injure the blood vessels and impede the activity of the bladder, thus urodialysis appears. Zhongji (Ren 3), the Front-(Mu) point of the bladder, is needled to adjust the function of the bladder and promote urination. Sanyinjiao (Sp 6) may promote the circulation of blood and qi in the meridian. Shuiquan (K 5), the Xi-(Cleft) point of the Kidney Meridian of Foot-Shaoyin, combined with Shuidao (S 28), may promote urination, and relieve distension and pain.

17.   Impotence
(*Appendix:* Seminal Emission)

Impotence is referred to lack of copulative power in males.

Etiology and Pathogenesis

Impotence is generally due to indulgence in sex or excessive masturbation, which makes Mingmen fire decline and exhausts the kidney essence. It may also be due to fear, fright or worry, which damages the qi of the heart, spleen and kidney. Just as said in *Treatment of Internal Disorders:* "The inability of penis to erect is due to the injury of the internal organs, which is mainly caused by the exhaustion of kidney essence from indulgent sexual activity, or by worry damaging the mind, or by fright leading to dysfunction of the kidney."

Greasy food and wine may damage the function of the spleen and stomach in transportation and transformation, causing dampness to turn into heat. The damp heat drives downward to make the penis unable to erect, resulting in impotence. However, impotence of the damp heat type is not very common. Zhang Jingyue said, "Seven to eight out of ten impotent patients are caused by the decline of fire. Only a few of them are due to excess of fire."

Differentiation

a) Decline of Mingmen Fire:

Main manifestations: Failure of the penis in erection, or weak erection, pallor, cold extremities, dizziness, listlessness, soreness and weakness of the loins and knees, frequent urination, pale tongue with white coating, deep thready pulse. If the heart and spleen qi is damaged, palpitations and insomnia may be present.

Analysis: The kidney dominates reproduction and opens into the urethra, spermatic duct and the anus. Insufficiency of the kidney yang and the decline of Mingmen fire wither up the reproductive ability, leading to impotence. Owing to yang deficiency, the body cannot be warmed, resulting in pallor, cold extremities, dizziness, and listlessness. As the lumbar region is the house of the kidney, kidney deficiency gives rise to soreness and weakness of the loins and knees. Only with the help of the activity of the kidney, can normal urination be performed. If the kidney yang fails in controlling urination, there appears frequent urination. Pale tongue with white coating, and deep, thready pulse are the signs of yang insufficiency. If the heart and spleen qi is damaged, there is poor production of qi and blood. If blood is inadequate for nourishing the heart, palpitations and insomnia occur.

b) Downward flowing of damp heat:

Main manifestations: Inability of the penis to erect, complicated with bitter taste in the mouth, thirst, hot and dark red urine, soreness and weakness of the lower extremities, yellow, sticky tongue coating, soft, rapid pulse.

Analysis: The penis consists of two cylindrical bodies. As said in *Internal Classic:* "If the damp heat stagnates in the penis, the major body becomes soft and short, and the small body gets loose and long. The former is known as contracture, while the latter known as atrophy and weak." The downward flowing of the damp heat makes the cylindrical bodies loose and weak, resulting in inability of the penis to erect. If the damp heat ascends, there will be bitter taste in the mouth or thirst. If the damp heat is transmitted to the small intestine, and then to the bladder, hot and dark red urine occurs. Soreness and weakness of the lower extremities, yellow, sticky tongue coating, and soft, rapid pulse indicate the presence of damp heat.

Treatment

a) Decline of Mingmen Fire:

Method: Points of the Ren and Kidney Meridians are selected as the principal points. Reinforcing method with moxibustion is applied to invigorate the kidney yang.

Prescription: Guanyuan (Ren 4), Mingmen (Du 4), Shenshu (B 23), Taixi (K 3).

Supplementary points: For damage of the qi of the heart and spleen: Xinshu (B 15), Shenmen (H 7), Sanyinjiao (Sp 6).

Explanation: Guanyuan (Ren 4) is the meeting point of the Ren Meridian and the three foot yin meridians. Reinforcing is used to promote the primary qi and invigorate the kidney function. Mingmen (Du 4), Shenshu (B 23) and Taixi (K 3) are used to strengthen the kidney yang. Xinshu (B 15), Shenmen (H 7) and Sanyinjiao (Sp 6) are good for activating the qi of the heart and spleen.

b) Downward flowing of damp heat:

Method: Points of the Ren and Spleen Meridians are selected as the principal points. Reducing method is applied to eliminate the damp heat.

Prescription: Zhongji (Ren 3), Sanyinjiao (Sp 6), Yinlingquan (Sp 9), Zusanli (S 36).

Explanation: This condition is caused by the downward flowing of damp heat from the Spleen Meridian, Zhongji (Ren 3), Sanyinjiao (Sp 6) and Yinlingquan (Sp 9) are therefore selected to soothe and regulate the qi of Spleen Meridian to eliminate the damp heat. Zusanli (S 36) is the He-(Sea) point of the Stomach Meridian of Foot Yangming. Because of the interior-exterior relationship between the Spleen and Stomach Meridians, Zusanli (S 36) is chosen to dispel dampness by improving the function of the spleen in transportation and transformation. Heat will disappear when dampness is dispelled. The above points combined together are suitable for the treatment of impotence caused by damp heat.

Remarks

Impotence in most cases is a functional disorder, for instance, sexual neurasthenia.

Appendix: Seminal Emission

Seminal emission may be divided into two types: nocturnal emission and spermatorrhea. Generally, in adult males, unmarried or married, occasional emission is not pathological.

a) Nocturnal emission:

Nocturnal emission is mainly due to overcontemplation or excessive sexual activities which lead to disharmony between the heart and kidney. If the heart fire fails to descend and control the kidney water, the kidney water cannot ascend and cool the heart fire. When water deficiency and fire excess disturb the essence, nocturnal emission happens in dreams. Moreover, there are dizziness, palpitation, listlessness, lassitude and scanty yellow urine, red tongue, and thready, rapid pulse. Treatment is given by applying acupuncture with reducing method to the points of the Heart Meridian of Hand Shaoyin and with reinforcing method to the points of the Kidney Meridian of Foot Shaoyin.

Prescription: Shenmen (H 7), Xinshu (B 15), Taixi (K 3), Zhishi (B 52).

Explanation: Shenmen (H 7) and Xinshu (B 15) are needled to lower the heart fire and harmonize the heart and kidney. Taixi (K 3) is used to activate the kidney qi, and Zhishi (B 52) to control the essence.

b) Spermatorrhea:

Spermatorrhea is usually due to damage of the kidney after a prolonged illness, indulgent sexual activity, or stubborn nocturnal emission. In exhaustion of the kidney essence, the loss of yin affects yang. The primary qi of the kidney becomes insufficient, the storage of essence fails and seminal fluid is discharged involuntarily. Clinical manifestations are frequent spermatorrhea at day or night, particularly if there is a desire for sex, pallor, lassitude, listlessness, pale tongue, and deep, thready, weak pulse. Treatment is given by applying acupuncture with reinforcing method and moxibustion to the points mainly selected from the Foot-Shaoyin (Kidney) and Ren Meridians to strengthen the kidney and control the essence and seminal fluid.

Prescription: Shenshu (B 23), Dahe (K 12), Sanyinjiao (Sp 6), Guanyuan (Ren 4), Qihai (Ren 6).

Explanation: Shenshu (B 23) and Sanyinjiao (Sp 6) are needled to reinforce the kidney qi. Guanyuan (Ren 4), the meeting point of the Ren and three foot yin meridians, and Qihai (Ren 6) are two important points for invigoration. Moxibustion applied to these two points can warm and strengthen the primary yang. Dahe (K 12) is combined to assist the control of the kidney essence.

18. Insomnia
(*Appendix:* Poor Memory)

Insomnia has different patterns: difficulty in falling asleep after retiring, early awakening, intermittent waking through the period of attempted sleep, and even inability to sleep all the night.

Insomnia is often accompanied by dizziness, headache, palpitation, poor memory and mental disorders.

Etiology and Pathogenesis

a) Anxiety and overwork damage the heart and spleen. Blood is exhausted and the mind is disturbed in case of damage of the heart, while qi and blood production becomes poor in case of deficiency of the spleen qi. Blood deficiency is unable to nourish the heart, leading to insomnia. Just as Zhang Jingyue described, "Overwork and

anxiety cause exhaustion of blood and disturb the mind. As a result, insomnia follows."

b) Congenital deficiency, indulgent sexual activity, or a prolonged illness damages the kidney yin. The kidney water fails to ascend smoothly to the heart to check the heart fire, and the heart yang is therefore hyperactive alternatively. A violent emotional fit can induce flaring of the heart fire which fails to descend to the kidney to control the kidney water. The kidney yin is therefore deficient. Deficiency of kidney yin injures the will and excess of the heart fire disturbs the mind. In either case there is a disharmony between the heart and the kidney, and hence insomnia.

c) Emotional depression causes the stagnation of qi in the liver. The stagnant qi of long duration is transformed into fire, which flares up to disturb the mind, and then insomnia occurs.

d) Irregular food intake damages the spleen and stomach. The accumulated undigested food produces phlegm heat in the middle jiao, which in turn causes dysfunction of the stomach and insomnia, as stated in *Internal Classic* that sleep is disturbed if the function of the stomach is in disharmony.

In summary, insomnia is related to dysfunction of the heart, spleen, liver and kidney, although there are many other causative factors. Blood is made from food essence and supplies the heart with nourishment. Blood is stored in the liver and the liver is soothed by the blood. Blood is controlled by the spleen, where production of essence from blood continues. The essence is stored in the kidney. When the kidney essence ascends to the heart and the heart qi descends to the kidney. With harmonious condition between the heart and kidney, the mind is at ease. Whenever there is anxiety, depression, or overwork to damage the heart, spleen, liver or kidney, essence and blood are consumed and mutually affected, resulting in insomnia.

Differentiation

a) Deficiency of both the heart and spleen qi:

Main manifestations: Difficulty in falling asleep, dream-disturbed sleep, palpitation, poor memory, lassitude, listlessness, anorexia, sallow complexion, pale tongue with a thin coating, thready, weak pulse.

Analysis: When there is impairment of the heart and spleen, blood is insufficient to house the mind, so dream-disturbed sleep, poor memory and palpitation occur. Sallow complexion and pale tongue are manifestations of a poor blood supply which is unable to nourish the upper part of the body. Dysfunction of the spleen and stomach in transportation and transformation causes anorexia. Deficiency of qi and blood leads to qi declining and blood shortage, resulting in lassitude, listlessness, thready and weak pulse.

b) Disharmony between the heart and kidney:

Main manifestations: Restlessness, insomnia, dizziness, tinnitus, dry mouth with little saliva, burning sensation of the chest, palms and soles, red tongue, thready rapid pulse, or nocturnal emission, poor memory, palpitation, low back pain.

Analysis: Restlessness, poor memory, palpitation, nocturnal emission and low back pain are due to deficiency of the kidney and hyperactivity of the heart fire. Dry mouth with little saliva, burning sensation of the chest, palms and soles, red tongue and thready rapid pulse are the signs of yin deficiency in the lower jiao with fire flaring up. Dizziness and tinnitus result from the flaring up of the ministerial fire due to deficiency of the kidney yin.

c) Upward disturbance of the liver fire:

Main manifestations: Irritability, dream-disturbed sleep, fright and fear accompanied with headache, distending pain in the costal region, bitter taste in the mouth and string-taut pulse.

Analysis: The liver fire flares up to disturb the mind, causing dream-disturbed sleep, fright and fear. When the flaring fire of the liver attacks the head, headache occurs. The liver qi in long stagnation is transformed into fire, leading to irritability. The liver fire flares up with upward flow of the bile, producing bitter taste in the mouth. When the fire stagnates in the Liver Meridian, there is distending pain in the costal region. The string-taut pulse is a sign of hyperactivity of the liver.

d) Dysfunction of the stomach:

Main manifestations: Insomnia, suffocating feeling and distending pain in the epigastric region, belching, or difficult defecation, sticky tongue coating, and rolling pulse.

Analysis: With the dysfunction of the spleen and stomach in transportation and transformation, the food accumulates in the middle jiao, obstructing the passage, and thus giving rise to suffocating feeling and distending pain in the epigastric region and difficulty in defecation. Therefore, sleep is disturbed. The undigested food staying in the middle jiao forms dampness and produces phlegm, so the tongue coating is sticky and the pulse rolling.

Treatment

Method: Points of the Heart Meridian are selected as the main points to calm the heart and soothe the mind.

Deficiency of the heart and spleen:

Reinforcing method with moxibustion in combination is applied to strengthen the heart and spleen.

Disharmony between the heart and kidney: Even movement is applied to harmonize the heart and kidney.

Upward disturbance of the liver fire: Reducing is applied to subdue the liver fire.

Dysfunction of the stomach: Reducing is applied to regulate the stomach qi.

Prescription: Shenmen (H 7), Sanyinjiao (Sp 6), Anmian (Extra).

Supplementary points:

Deficiency of the heart and spleen: Pishu (B 20), Xinshu (B 15), Yinbai (Sp 1, moxibustion with small moxa cones).

Disharmony between the heart and kidney: Xinshu (B 15), Shenshu (B 23), Taixi (K 3).

Upward disturbance of the liver fire: Ganshu (B 18), Danshu (B 19), Wangu (G 12).

Dysfunction of the stomach: Weishu (B 21), Zusanli (S 36).

Explanation: Shenmen (H 7), the Yuan-(Primary) point of the Heart Meridian, calms the heart and soothes the mind. Sanyinjiao (Sp 6), the crossing point of the Liver, Spleen and Kidney Meridians, regulates the three meridians. Anmian (Extra) is an extra point for insomnia. Xinshu (B 15), the Back-(Shu) point of the heart, and Pishu (B 20), the Back-(Shu) point of the spleen, are combined to reinforce the spleen and nourish the heart. Yinbai (Sp 1), the Jing-(Well) point of the Spleen Meridian, is effective for dream-disturbed sleep. Xinshu (B 15) reduces heart fire. Shenshu (B 23) and Taixi (K 3) reinforce kidney water. The combination of these points is to harmonize the heart and kidney. The combination of Ganshu (B 18), Danshu (B 19) and Wangu (G 12) is to subdue the fire

of the liver and gallbladder. The combination of Weishu (B 21) and Zusanli (S 36) is to regulate the stomach and soothe the mind.

Remarks

Tapping-needling: Tap Sishenchong (Extra), Back-(Shu) points or Huatuojiaji (Extra) slightly from above downward two to three times. Treat once daily or every other day. Ten treatments constitute a course. Next course of treatment begins after an interval of two to three days.

Appendix: Poor Memory

Poor memory is a trouble characterized by the functional decline of the brain, hypomnesia and forgetfulness. It differs from lack of intelligence and natural endowments. The condition in most cases is caused by insufficiency of the heart and spleen and deficiency of the kidney essence. As Wang Yang said, "Essence and will are both stored in the kidney. If the kidney essence is deficient, the will is weakened. Poor memory appears when the will fails to cooperate with the heart." In *Prescriptions Based on Three Pathogenic Factors,* it says: "The spleen dominates the recollection and thinking. Recollection refers to the power of calling back the past facts to the mind, and thinking depends also on the action of the heart.... Since the spleen is troubled, collection is impaired, and the mind is uneasy, so memory is poor." The heart and spleen dominate the blood. Overthinking injuring the heart and spleen consumes blood and leads to poor memory. The kidney dominates essence and marrow, which can be consumed or exhausted by indulgent sexual activity. The brain is therefore poorly nourished, causing forget-fulness. The old aged also tend to have poor memory due to the kidney decline.

The treatment is mainly to replenish the blood of the heart and reinforce the spleen and kidney. Reinforcing method is applied to Sishencong (Extra), Xinshu (B 15), Pishu (B 20), Zusanli (S 36), Shenshu (B 23), and Zhaohai (K 6).

Explanation: Sishencong (Extra) is an empirical point for treatment of poor memory. Xinshu (B 15) and Pishu (B 20) are applied to strengthen the heart and spleen. Shenshu (B 23) and Zhaohai (K 6) promote the kidney essence, produce marrow and replenish the brain. Zusanli (S 36) reinforces the spleen and stomach in transportation and transformation, and replenishes qi and blood.

19. Palpitation

Palpitation refers to unduly rapid action of the heart which is felt by the patient and accompanied by nervousness and rest-lessness.

Mild palpitation is mostly due to a sudden fright and overstrain. The general condition is comparatively good and the symptoms are of short duration. A serious case is often due to prolonged internal injury. The general condition is comparatively poor and the symptoms are severe.

Etiology and Pathogenesis
a) Disturbance of the mind:
A timid person is likely to have palpitation when he or she is frightened by strange noises, surprising objects, or dangerous environments. In Chapter 19 of *Plain Questions,* it says: "Fright makes qi disturbed because the heart has nothing to rely on, the mind has no place to house and the thinking has nothing to focus on." There are other pathogenic factors causing palpitation, such as internal accumulation of phlegm heat, mental depression and anger, dysfunction of the stomach and upward perversion of phlegm fire.

b) Insufficiency of qi and blood:
Persistent disease, weak constitution, loss of blood, or overthinking damages the heart and spleen, and impedes the production of qi and blood. Deficiency of qi and blood fails to nourish the heart, which affects the housing of the mind, causing palpitation.

c) Hyperactivity of the fire due to yin deficiency:
Injury of kidney yin by indulgent sexual activity, or debility after a prolonged disease renders the kidney water unable to check the heart fire. Disharmony between the heart and kidney with flaring fire disturbing the mind causes palpitation.

d) Retention of harmful fluid:
Retention of harmful fluid due to depression of the heart yang or due to deficiency of the spleen and kidney yang disturbs the heart, resulting in palpitation.

Differentiation:
a) Disturbance of the mind:
Main manifestations: Palpitation, fear and fright, irritability, restlessness, dream-disturbed sleep, anorexia, white, thin tongue coating, a little bit rapid pulse. In cases of phlegm heat, yellow, sticky tongue coating, rolling, rapid pulse.

Analysis: Fear makes the qi flow disordered, and fright makes qi descend. A disturbed mind is out of self-control, so there are palpitation, fear and fright, dream-disturbed sleep, irritability and restlessness. White thin tongue coating and a little bit rapid pulse are the signs of disturbance of the mind. Yellow sticky coating, and rolling, rapid pulse indicate the presence of phlegm heat.

b) Insufficiency of qi and blood:

Main manifestations: Palpitation, lustre-less complexion, dizziness, blurring of vision, shortness of breath, lassitude, pale tongue with tooth prints, thready, weak or intermittent pulse.

Analysis: Palpitation is due to insuffi-ciency of qi and blood, which fails to nourish the heart. Lustreless complexion is due to the insufficient qi and blood unable to lustre the complexion. Dizziness is due to the poor nourishment of the brain by the insufficient qi and blood. The heart dominates the blood and vessels and is manifested in the tongue. Therefore insufficient qi and blood makes the tongue pale with tooth prints, and the pulse thready, weak or intermittent.

d) Fire hyperactivity due to yin deficiency:

Main manifestations: Palpitation, rest-lessness, irritability, insomnia, dizziness, blurring of vision, tinnitus, red tongue with little coating, thready, rapid pulse.

Analysis: Kidney yin in deficiency state fails to check the heart fire, leading to disturbance of the mind, and resulting in palpitation, irritability and insomnia. When yin deficiency is present in the lower part of the body, and yang hyperactivity in the upper, there may be dizziness and tinnitus. Red tongue with little coating, and thready rapid pulse are the signs of yang hyperactivity due to yin deficiency.

e) Rentention of harmful fluid:

Main manifestations: Palpitation, ex-pectoration of mucoid sputum, fullness in the chest and epigastric region, lassitude, weakness, cold extremities, white tongue coating, string-taut, rolling pulse. In case of deficiency of yang in the spleen and kidney, scanty urine, thirst without desire to drink, white, slippery tongue coating, deep, string-taut or rapid pulse.

Analysis: Accumulation of dampness forms the harmful fluid, which depresses the heart yang. When the yang qi is unable to reach the extremities, they are cold and weak. White tongue coating, string-taut, rolling pulse suggest the presence of harmful fluid. Unsmooth circulation of qi resulting from yang deficiency of the spleen and kidney gives rise to scantiness of urine and thirst without desire to drink. White, slippery tougue coating and deep, string-taut pulse are due to yang deficiency of the spleen and kidney and retention of fluid. Rapid pulse indicates the decline of the heart yang.

Treatment

Method: The Back-(Shu) and Front-(Mu) points of the heart, and points of the Heart and Pericardium Meridians are selected as the main points. Even movement is applied for disturbance of the mind to clam the heart. Reinforcing is used for insufficiency of qi and blood to nourish the heart and ease the mind. Reinforcing combined with reducing is applied for fire hyperactivity due to yin deficiency to nourish yin and subdue the fire. For retention of harmful fluid, reducing method is applied first and then reinforcing in combination with moxibus-tion to warm yang and dissolve the harmful fluid.

Prescription: Xinshu (B 15), Juque (Ren 14), Shenmen (H 7), Neiguan (P 6).

Supplementary points:

Disturbance of the mind: Tongli (P 5),

Qiuxu (G 40); if accompanied with phlegm heat: Fenglong (S 40), Danshu (B 19).

Insufficiency of qi and blood: Pishu (B 20), Weishu (B 21), Zusanli (S 36).

Fire hyperactivity due to yin deficiency: Jueyinshu (B 14), Shenshu (B 23), Taixi (K 3).

Retention of harmful fluid: Shuifen (Ren 9), Guanyuan (Ren 4), Shenque (Ren 8), Yinlingquan (Sp 9).

Explanation: The combination of Shenmen (H 7), the Yuan-(Primary) point of the Heart Meridian, and Xinshu (B 12) with Juque (Ren 14), the Front-(Mu) point of the heart, and Neiguan (P 6), the Luo-(Connecting) point of the Pericardum Meridian can regulate qi and blood of the heart to ease the mind. The combination of Tongli (H 5), the Luo-(Connecting) point of the Heart Meridian, and Qiuxu (G 40), the Yuan-(Primary) point of the Gallbladder Meridian, can calm the mind and regulate the gallbladder. Fenglong (S 40), the Luo-(Connecting) point of the Stomach Meridian, and Danshu (B 19), the Back-(Shu) point of the gallbladder, can dissolve phlegm and dispel heat. Pishu (B 20) and Weishu (B 21) can regulate the spleen and stomach to promote qi and blood production. Zusanli (S 36) is an important point to reinforce qi and blood. Shenshu (B 23) and Taixi (K 3) can replenish kidney yin. Jueyinshu (B 14) can clear heart fire. Guanyuan (Ren 14), Shuifen (Ren 9) and Yinlingquan (Sp 9) can invigorate the heart yang, strengthen the spleen and remove the harmful fluid.

Remarks

Palpitation described here may be involved in neurosis, functional disorders of the vegetative nervous system and cardiac arrhythmia of various origins.

20.   Manic-Depressive Disorder

Depressive disorder is manifested by mental dejection, reticence or incoherant speech, while manic disorder by shouting, restlessness and violent behaviours. As described in *Classic on Medical Problems*, depressive disorder is caused by excessive yin, while manic disorder by abundant yang.

The most important etiological factor of manic-depressive disorder is emotional injury. Pathogenetically, phlegm plays the primary role. Depressive disorder is due to stagnation of phlegm combined with qi, while manic disorder is due to phlegm fire. Although they are different in symptomatology, they are related to each other. A prolonged depressive disorder, in which fire is produced by phlegm stagnation, may change into manic disorder, while a protracted manic disorder, in which the stagnated fire is gradually dispersed, but the phlegm is still existing, can change into depressive disorder. Therefore, they are termed together as manic-depressive.

Etiology and Pathogenesis:

a) Depressive disorder:

In most cases it is caused by over-contemplation and emotional depression, which lead to dysfunction of the liver and spleen. There are stagnant liver qi and accumulated fluid due to impaired transportation, which turns into phlegm. Then the phlegm pervertedly goes upward to invade the mind.

b) Manic disorder:

In most cases it is caused by anger that injures the liver, leading to its failure in dispersing. The stagnated qi transforms into fire, which evaporates the body fluid to produce phlegm fire. The phlegm fire pervertedly rushes upward and disturbs the mind.

In addition, this disease has a hereditary trend and often a positive family history.

Differentiation:

a) Depressive disorder:

Main manifestations: Gradual onset, emotional dejection and mental dullness at the initial stage, followed by incoherent speech, changing moods, or muteness, somnolence, anorexia, thin, sticky tongue coating, string-taut, thready or string-taut rolling pulse.

Analysis: Overcontemplation and emotional dejection make the liver qi stagnated and the spleen qi fail to ascend. The stagnated qi combined with the phlegm disturbs the mind, leading to mental disorders. The stagnated phlegm in the middle jiao gives rise to anorexia and thin, sticky tongue coating. String-taut thready or string-taut rolling pulse is due to the accumulation of phlegm and qi.

b) Manic disorder:

Main manifestations: Sudden onset, irritability, being easy to anger, insomnia, loss of appetite, followed by excessive motor activity with increased energy and violent behaviours, yellow, sticky tongue coating. String-taut, rolling and rapid pulse.

Analysis: Anger damages the liver. The liver fire flares up and agitates the phlegm heat of Yangming to disturb the mind. Therefore, the patient is irritable, unable to fall asleep and easy to anger. Because of the disturbance of the mind by the phlegm heat, violent behaviours take place. The limbs are the foundation of all the yang actions. Preponderant yang makes the limbs more energetic, thus, the physical strength and motor activity are increased. The combination of phlegm and heat, leads to yellow,

sticky tongue coating, string-taut, rolling and rapid pulse.

Treatment

a) Depressive disorder:

Method: Even movement is applied to the points of the Heart and Liver Meridians to soothe the liver, calm the heart and dissolve the phlegm.

Prescription: Xinshu (B 15), Ganshu (B 18), Pishu (B 20), Shenmen (H 7), Fenglong (S 40).

Explanation: This condition is caused by the stagnation of phlegm and qi, which injures the heart, liver and spleen. Xinshu (B 15) is used to clear the heart, Ganshu (B 18) to remove the liver stagnation, Pishu (B 20) to promote the spleen qi circulation, Shenmen (H 7) and Fenglong (S 40) to dissolve the phlegm for calming the mind.

b) Manic disorder:

Method: Reducing is applied to the main points of the Du Meridian and Pericardium Meridian of Hand Jueyin to calm the heart, ease the mind, reduce the heat and dissolve the phlegm.

Prescription: Dazhui (Du 14), Fengfu (Du 16), Shuigou (Du 26), Neiguan (P 6), Fenglong (S 40).

Supplementary points:

Mania with extreme heat: Prick the twelve Jing-(Well) points on hand (L 11, H 9, P 9, L I 1, S J 1, S I 1) to bleeding for reducing heat.

Explanation: Dazhui (Du 14) and Shuigou (Du 26) are used to reduce heat for clearing the mind. Fengfu (Du 16) is selected for mental disorders as *Miraculous Pivot* states: "The brain is the sea of marrow, its upper part reaches the vertex of the cranium, and its lower part reaches point Fengfu (Du 16)." Neiguan (P 6) is combined with Fenglong (S 40) to clear the heart and dissolve the phlegm.

Remarks

a) The condition described here includes the depressive and manic types of schizophrenia in modern medicine.

b) Thirteen points for manic-depressive disorder: Prick to bleed according to the order of Shuigou (Du 26), Shaoshang (L 11), Yinbai (Sp 1), Daling (P 7), Shenmai (B 62), Fengfu (Du 16), Jiache (S 6), Chengjiang (Ren 24), Laogong (P 8), Shangxing (Du 23), Huiyin (Ren 1), Quchi (L I 11), and Shexiazhongfeng (an extra point located at the midline of the under side of the tongue).

21.   Epilepsy

Epilepsy occurs in seizures, manifested by falling down in a fit, loss of consciousness, foam on the lips, or screams with eyes staring upward, and convulsions. After some minutes, consciousness returns, and the patient's condition becomes normal.

Besides the typical seizures, there may be variations. It can be a momentary loss of attention or consciousness with eyes staring directly forward, or prolonged loss of consciousness associated with convulsions and foam on the lips. Epileptic fits may occur at any time, in various frequency and with different severity. It is often preceded by an "aura" of dizziness, depression sensation of the chest, and listlessness. Generally speaking, epilepsy is an excess condition, but frequent recurrence can lower the body resistance.

Etiology and Pathogenesis

a) Fear and fright: Fear makes qi disordered and fright makes qi descend, affecting the liver and kidney and leading to stirring of the deficiency wind.

b) Dysfunction of the liver in smoothing flow of qi, or irregular food intake damaging the spleen and stomach, makes the dampness of food and drinks accumulate as phlegm, which combined with the stagnated liver qi, disturbs the mind and causes epilepsy.

c) Epilepsy may result from hereditary factors, but in most of the hereditary cases it comes on in early childhood.

Differentiation

a) During seizure

Main manifestations: A typical seizure is preceded by dizziness, headache and suffocating sensation in the chest, and immediately followed by falling down with loss of consciousness, pallor, clenched jaws, upward staring of the eyes, convulsion, foam on the lips, screaming as pigs or sheep, and even incontinence of urine and feces. Gradually, the patient regains consciouseness, and the symptoms disappear. Apart from fatigue and weakness, the patient can live a normal life. White sticky tongue coating, and string-taut, rolling pulse.

Analysis: Dizziness, headache and suffocated sensation in the chest are the prodromal symptoms which show the upward perversion of the wind phlegm. The liver wind stirs up with the phlegm to disturb the mind. Therefore, there are loss of consciousness, convulsions and upward staring of the eyes. The foam on the lips is owing to the ascending wind phlegm. White, sticky tongue coating and rolling pulse are the signs of retaining of the phlegm. Since the wind phlegm is irregularly accumulated and dispersed, the seizures are paroxysmal, and the patient behaves as normal after the seizure.

b) After seizure:

Main manifestations: Listlessness, lustreless complexion, dizziness, palpitation, anorexia, profuse sputum, weakness and soreness of the loins and limbs, pale tongue with white coating and thready, rolling pulse.

Analysis: Listlessness is due to damage of the vital qi by frequent epileptic fits. With insufficiency of blood, the complexion is lustreless. There is dizziness if the brain lacks blood supply, and palpitation if the heart is poorly supplied with blood. Due to the depression of the spleen yang, the food cannot be transformed into essence, and dampness and phlegm are produced, so there are anorexia and profuse sputum. Deficiency of the kidney essence causes soreness and weakness of the loins and limbs. Pale tongue with white coating and thready, rolling pulse suggest consumption of qi and blood and accumulation of phlegm dampness.

Treatment

a) During seizure:

Method: Points of the Du, Ren and Liver Meridians are selected as the main points with reducing method to dissolve the phlegm, induce resuscitation, soothe the liver and dispel the wind.

Prescription: Shuigou (Du 26), Jiuwei (Ren 15), Jianshi (P 5), Taichong (Liv 3), Fenglong (S. 40).

Explanation: Shuigou (Du 26) and Jiuwei (Ren 15) are used for resuscitation. Jianshi (P 5), Fenglong (S 40) and Taichong (Liv 3) are used to calm the heart, ease the mind, dissolve the phlegm and dispel the wind.

b) After seizure:

Method: Points of the Heart, Spleen and Kidney Meridians are selected as the main points with even movement to nourish the heart, ease the mind, strengthen the spleen and reinforce the kidney.

Prescription: Xinshu (B 15), Yintang (Extra), Shenmen (H 7), Sanyinjiao (Sp 6), Taixi (K 3), Yaoqi (Extra).

Supplementary points:

Daytime seizure: Shenmai (B 62).

Night seizure: Zhaohai (K 6).

Phlegm stagnation: Zhongwan (Ren 12), Fenglong (S 40).

Severe deficiency of qi and blood: Guanyuan (Ren 4), Zusanli (S 36).

Explanation: Xinshu (B 15), Yintang (Extra) and Shenmen (H 7) are used for nourishing the heart and easing the mind, and Sanyinjiao (Sp 6) and Taixi (K 3), for strengthening the spleen and reinforcing the kidney. Yaoqi (Extra) is an empirical point for epilepsy. Shenmai (B 62), a point of Yangqiao Meridian, is needled for the daytime seizure, while Zhaohai (K 6), a point of Yinqiao Meridian, is needled for night seizure. Zhongwan (Ren 12) and Fenglong (S 40) are applied to regulate the stomach and dissolve the phlegm. Guanyuan (Ren 4) and Zusanli (S 36) are used to regulate and replenish qi and blood.

Remarks

The above description refers to many types of epileptic seizures including grand mal, petit mal, psychomotor and focal seizures. For secondary epilepsy, the primary disease should be treated actively.

22. Dizziness

The mild case can be relieved by closing one's eyes, while the serious case has an illusion of bodily movement with rotatary sensation like sitting in a sailing boat or moving car, and even accompanied by nausea, vomiting and sweating.

Etiology and Pathogenesis

a) Hyperactivity of the liver yang:

The liver is analogized as wind and wood, characterized by movement and ascending. Overcontemplation, anxiety, depression or anger can damage the liver yin, resulting in hyperactivity of liver yang. Dizziness occurs in case the liver yang moves as the wind and ascends to attack the brain. Or the kidney water, generally in deficiency, fails to nourish the liver. Dizziness occurs in case the liver is lack of nourishment, which leads to hyperactivity of liver yang. In both situations there is deficiency in the lower but excess in the upper part of the body.

b) Deficiency of qi and blood:

The heart and spleen are damaged by overwork and over contemplation in case of a weak constitution after a disease. The damaged spleen fails to produce qi and blood, leading to deficiency. In case the brain is poorly nourished by qi and blood, dizziness occurs.

c) Interior retention of phlegm dampness:

In a person with generally abundant phlegm dampness, irregular food intake and overwork damage the stomach and the spleen, impairing their function in transportation and transformation and leading to production of dampness and phlegm. Then the stagnant phlegm and qi may impede the ascending of clear yang and the descending of the turbid yin, and thus dizziness occurs.

Differentiation

a) Hyperactivity of liver yang:

Main manifestations: Dizziness aggravated by anger, irritability, flushed face, red eyes, tinnitus, bitter taste in the mouth, dream-disturbed sleep, red tongue proper with yellow coating, string-taut, rapid pulse.

Analysis: Anger damages the liver yin, causing hyperactivity of the liver yang, which transforms into fire. When the fire flares up, flushed face, red eyes and irritability appear. The spirit stored in the liver is upset by disorders of the liver, then dream-disturbed sleep occurs. The red tongue proper with yellow coating, bitter taste in the mouth, string-taut, rapid pulse are the signs of yin deficiency resulting in fire hyperactivity.

b) Deficiency of qi and blood:

Main manifestations: Dizziness accompanied by pallor and lustreless complexion, weakness, palpitation, insomnia, pale lips and nails, lassitude, pale tongue proper, thready and weak pulse. Dizziness occurs mostly after a serious disease or loss of blood and is aggravated by overwork. Loss of consciousness happens in severe cases.

Analysis: Dizziness is inevitable because deficiency of qi and blood fails to nourish the brain. The heart dominates the blood and is manifested in the complexion. The spleen dominates the transportation and transformation to manufacture qi and blood. If the heart and spleen are injured, qi and blood will be insufficient, thereby, the complexion is lustreless, and the lips and the nails are pale. Deficiency of blood leads to palpitation and insomnia. Deficiency of qi gives rise to weakness, lassitude, anorexia, and is aggravated by overwork. Pale tongue and thready, weak pulse are the signs of deficiency of qi and blood.

c) Interior retention of phlegm dampness:

Main manifestations: Dizziness with a heavy feeling of the head and suffocating sensation in the chest, nausea, profuse sputum, anorexia, somnolence, white, sticky tongue coating, soft, rolling pulse.

Analysis: Dizziness with a heavy feeling of the head is the sign of the pure yang disturbed by phlegm dampness. Suffocating sensation in the chest and nausea are caused by qi obstructed in the middle jiao. Anorexia and somnolence are due to the spleen yang deficiency. White, sticky tongue coating, soft and rolling pulse are the signs of phlegm dampness.

Treatment

a) Hyperactivity of liver yang:

Method: Points of the Liver Meridian and Kidney Meridian are selected as the main points to nourish yin and pacify yang. Reinforcing and reducing methods are applied with either one first according to the condition of the disease.

Prescription: Fengchi (G 20), Ganshu (B 18), Shenshu (B 23), Taixi (K 3), Xingjian (Liv 2).

Explanation: The reinforcing method applied to Shenshu (B 23) and Taixi (K 3) is to replenish the kidney water, while the reducing to Ganshu (B 18), Xingjian (Liv 2) and Fengchi (G 20) is to pacify the liver yang.

b) Deficiency of qi and blood:

Method: Points of the Ren Meridian and the Bladder and Stomach Meridians are selected as the main points with reinforcing in combination with moxibustion to replenish qi and blood.

Prescription: Baihui (Du 20), Pishu (B 20), Guanyuan (Ren 4), Zusanli (S 36), Sanyinjiao (Sp 6).

Explanation: Moxibustion to Baihui (Du 20), which is located at the vertex, is to make qi and blood ascend to the head to nourish the brain and check dizziness. Guanyuan (Ren 4) is used to strengthen the primary qi. Pishu (B 20) and Sanyinjiao (Sp 6) are for invigorating the spleen and stomach to produce qi and blood.

c) Interior retention of phlegm dampness:

Method: The Back-(Shu) and Front-(Mu) points of the spleen and stomach are selected as the main points with even movement to resolve phlegm and eliminate dampness.

Prescription: Touwei (S 8), Pishu (B 20), Zhongwan (Ren 12), Neiguan (P 6), Fenglong (S 40).

Explanation: Pishu (B 20) and Zhongwan (Ren 12) are needled to strengthen the spleen and stomach for eliminating dampness. Fenglong (S 40), the Luo-(Connecting) point of the stomach, is to make qi descend and resolve phlegm. Touwei (S 8) is for dizziness. Neiguan (P 6) is for relaxing the chest, regulating qi and harmonizing the stomach to check vomiting.

Remarks

a) Dizziness may be explained as derangement of the equilibrium of the senses in modern medicine. Clinically, the symptom is mostly seen in hypertention, arteriosclerosis, neurosis, and otogenic diseases.

b) Tapping needling:

Main points: Baihui (Du 20), Taiyang (Extra), Yintang (Extra), and Huatuojiaji (Extra).

Method: Tap once or twice daily with moderate stimulation. Five to ten treatments constitute one course.

23. Melancholia

Melancholia is a general term for disorders resulted from emotional depression and stagnation of qi. The symptoms due to emotional frustration, and depression of qi which lead to stagnation of blood, accumulation of phlegm, retention of food, collection of fire, and disharmony of the zang-fu organs fall into this category. Zhu Danxi said, "There is no disease when qi and blood are in harmony. Once depression occurs, disease results."

Etiology and Pathogenesis:

Generally speaking, melancholia is caused by emotional injuries resulting in disharmony of the activity of the zang organs. As said in Chapter 28 of *Miraculous Pivot:* "Grief, sorrow, worry and anxiety disturb the mind and disturbance of the mind will affect all the five zang and six fu organs."

a) Depressed anger may give rise to many disorders of the liver with impairment of the free flow of qi. Then the liver qi may go upward to attack the mind, or conquer the spleen and stomach, or counteract the lung, or go downward to the intestines, leading to various illnesses.

b) Too much worry may depress the liver and suppress the spleen, causing the failure of the spleen in transportation and transformation, which brings about accumulation of dampness and phlegm and retention of undigested food. Agglomeration of the dampness, phlegm and undigested food in a long duration is apt to produce fire. Overanxiety may also lead to dysfunction of the qi and consumes yin (nutrients and blood,) generating many symptoms.

Differentiation

a) Depression of the qi in the liver:

Main manifestations: Mental depression, distress of the chest, hypochondriac pain, abdominal distension, belching, anorexia, or abdominal pain, vomiting, abnormal bowel movement, thin, sticky tongue coating, string-taut pulse.

Analysis: In case of emotional injury, the liver fails to be harmonious and flourishing, so mental depression appears. The Liver Meridian of Foot-Jueyin runs up to the lower abdomen and curves around the stomach and then branches out in the costal and hypochondriac regions. In case of stagnation of the qi of the liver, there may appear distress in the chest, hypochondriac pain and abdominal distension. If the stomach qi fails to descend, belching and anorexia occur. When the liver qi encroaches the spleen, abdominal pain, vomiting and abnormal bowel movement result. Thin, sticky tongue coating and string-taut pulse are the signs of disharmony between the liver and stomach.

b) Transformation of depressed qi into fire:

Main manifestations: Headache, dryness and bitter taste in the mouth, irritability, distress of the chest, hypochondriac distension, acid regurgitation, constipation, red eyes, tinnitus, red tongue with yellow coating, string-taut, rapid pulse.

Analysis: When the depressed qi is transformed into fire, it flares up along the Liver Meridian, resulting in headache, red eyes and tinnitus. When the liver fire evaporates the fluid and heat accumulates in the stomach and intestines, dryness and bitter taste in the mouth and constipation occur. If the liver is hyperactive, it will encroach the stomach, leading to failure of the stomach in descending function, then distress of the chest, hypochondriac distension, and acid regurgitation occur. Irritability, yellow tongue coating, string-taut, rapid pulse are the signs of the fire in the liver.

c) Stagnation of phlegm (also known as globus hystericus):

Main manifestations: Feeling of a lump choking in the throat, hard to spit it out or to swallow it, thin, sticky tongue coating, string-taut, rolling pulse.

Analysis: The depressed liver qi acts over the spleen and stomach, leading to disturbance of transportation and transformation. Dampness derived from the water and food taken is gathered and turned into phlegm, which combined with qi, stays in the throat, giving rise to choking feeling. Thin, sticky tongue coating and string-taut, rolling pulse are the signs of the stagnation of phlegm with qi.

d) Insufficiency of blood (also known as hysteria):

Main manifestations: ˙Grief without reasons, capricious joy or anger, suspicions, liability to get frightened, palpitation, irritability, insomnia, or sudden distress of the chest, hiccup, sudden aphonia, convulsion, or loss of consciousness in severe cases, thin, white tongue coating, string-taut, thready pulse.

Analysis: Because of overcontemplation and emotional frustration, the qi function is impaired and the blood is gradually consumed, leading to poor nourishment of the mind, thus the above-mentioned symptoms occur. In case the qi is blocked, there may be sudden distress of the chest, hiccup, sudden aphonia and convulsion. Thin white tongue coating, and string-taut thready pulse are the signs of a long-standing stagnation of qi that damages blood.

Treatment

a) Depression of qi in the liver:

Method: The Influential point of qi and the points of the Liver Meridian are selected as the principal points. Even movement is applied to soothe the liver, strengthen the spleen and harmonize the stomach.

Prescription: Ganshu (B 18), Tanzhong (Ren 17), Zhongwan (Ren 12), Zusanli (S 36), Gongsun (Sp 4), Taichong (Liv 3).

Explanation: Tanzhong (Ren 17), the Influential point of qi, is able to regulate the flow of qi. Ganshu (B 18) and Taichong (Liv 3) are the Back-(Shu) point and Yuan-(Primary) point of the liver respectively. When used in combination, they may soothe the liver and remove depression. Zhongwan (Ren 12) and Zusanli (S 36) may harmonize the stomach and make the stomach qi descend. Gongsun (Sp 4), the Luo-(Connecting) point of the Spleen Meridian, may strengthen the spleen and harmonize the stomach.

b) Transformation of depressed qi into fire:

Method: Points of the Liver, Gallbladder and Stomach Meridians are selected as the principal points. Reducing method is used to dispel the fire from the liver and strengthen the stomach function.

Prescription: Shangwan (Ren 13), Zhigou (S J 6), Yanglingquan (G 34), Xingjian (Liv 2), Xiaxi (G 43).

Explanation: Xingjian (Liv 2) and Xiaxi (G 43), the Ying-(Spring) points of the Liver and Gallbladder Meridians, may dispel fire from the liver and gallbladder. Zhigou (S J 6) in combination with Yanglingquan (G 34) may treat distress of the chest, hypochondriac distension, bitter taste in the mouth and constipation. Shangwan (Ren 13) may harmonize the stomach and regulate the flow of qi to treat acid regurgitation.

c) Stagnation of phlegm:

Method: Points of the Liver Meridian and Ren Meridian are selected as the principal points. Even movement is applied to soothe the liver, remove the depression, regulate the flow of qi and resolve phlegm.

Prescription: Tiantu (Ren 22), Tanzhong (Ren 17), Neiguan (P 6), Fenglong (S 40), Taichong (Liv 3).

Explanation: Taichong (Liv 3) is applied to soothe the liver and remove the depression. Tiantu (Ren 22) is needled to descend the qi and treat the throat trouble. Neiguan (P 6) is used to remove depression from the chest and regulate the flow of qi. Tanzhong (Ren 17), the Influential point of qi, Fenglong (S 40), the Luo-(Connecting) point of the stomach, used together, may promote the circulation of qi and resolve phlegm.

d) Insufficiency of blood:

Method: Points of the Heart and Liver Meridians are selected as the principal points. Even movement is applied to nourish blood, soothe the liver and refresh and tranquilize the mind.

Prescription: Juque (Ren 14), Shenmen (H 7), Sanyinjiao (Sp 6), Taichong (Liv 3).

Supplementary points:

Distress of the chest: Neiguan (P 6), Tanzhong (Ren 17).

Hiccup: Gongsun (Sp 4), Tiantu (Ren 22).

Sudden aphonia: Tongli (H 5), Lianquan (Ren 23).

Convulsion: Hegu (L I 4), Yanglingquan (G 34).

Loss of consciousness: Shuigou (Du 26), Yongquan (K 1).

Explanation: Taichong (Liv 3) is selected to soothe the liver and remove depression. Juque (Ren 14), the Front-(Mu) point of the Heart Meridian, Shenmen (H 7), the Yuan-(Primary) point, combined with Sanyinjiao (Sp 6) of the Spleen Meridian, may nourish blood, refresh and tranquilize the mind. Neiguan (P 6) and Tanzhong (Ren 17) may remove the depression of the chest. Gongsun (Sp 4) and Tiantu (Ren 22) causes the qi to descend and checks hiccup. Tongli (H 5) and Lianquan (Ren 23) are effective in the treatment of aphonia. Hegu (L I 4) is taken to regulate the flow of qi. Yanglingquan (G 34), the Influential point of the tendons, is used to check convulsion and relieve pain. Shuigou (Du 26) and Yongquan (K 1) are

used for resuscitation.

Remarks

This condition is seen in hysteria and neurosis in Western medicine.

III.   DISEASES OF HEAD, TRUNK AND LUMBAR REGIONS

1.   Headache

Headache is a subjective symptom. It can be induced by various acute and chronic diseases. As it covers a wide sphere, this section only deals in detail with headache as the predominant symptom. If headache is an accompanying symptom in the development of a certain disease, it will disappear automatically as soon as the disease is cured. This type of headache is not to be discussed here.

The head is the place where all the yang meridians of hand and foot meet, and qi and blood of the five zang organs and six fu organs all flow upward to the head. Attacks of endogenous or exogenous factors may cause headache due to derangement of qi and blood in the head and retardation of circulation of qi in the meridians that traverse the head. Headache caused by exogenous pathogenic factors is mostly due to invasion of pathogenic wind into the meridians and collaterals. It is said: "When the pathogenic wind invades the human body, it first attacks the upper portion of the body." Headache caused by endogenous factors often originates from hyperfunction of the liver yang, or deficiency of both qi and blood.

Etiology and Pathogenesis

a) Invasion of pathogenic wind into the upper meridians and collaterals causes derangement and obstruction of qi and blood. With stagnation in the collaterals, sudden weather change or exposure to wind usually precipitates an attack of headache.

b) In patients with excessive yang of body constitution, headache may be caused by upsurge of liver yang due to stagnation of qi or injury of the liver after a fit of anger, which damages the yin.

c) Headache may also be caused by deficiency of both qi and blood because of irregular food intake, overstrain and stress, poor health with a chronic disease, or congenital deficiency. Deficiency of qi prevents the clear yang from ascending, and deficiency of blood does not nourish the mind, so there is headache.

Differentiation

a) *Headache due to invasion of pathogenic wind into the meridians and collaterals:*

Main manifestations: Headache occurs on exposure to wind. The pain may extend to the nape of the neck and back regions. It is a violent, boring and fixed pain, accompanied by string-taut pulse and thin white tongue coating. Such a syndrome is also termed "head wind."

Analysis: Pain comes from obstruction of qi in the meridians and collaterals on the head caused by invasion of the exogenous pathogenic wind. Owing to the excess of the pathogenic factor, the pain is violent and boring. Wind is a yang pathogenic factor and apt to attack the upper portion of the body. So the pain caused by wind may extend to the nape of the neck and back region. The fixed pain is due to blood stagnation derived from qi stagnation. String-taut pulse and thin white tongue

coating are the signs of meridians and collaterals being invaded by pathogenic wind.

b) *Headache due to upsurge of liver-yang:*

Main manifestations: Headache, blurred vision, severe pain on the bilateral sides of the head, irritability, hot temper, flushed face, bitter taste in the mouth, string-taut and rapid pulse, reddened tongue with yellow coating.

Analysis: Headache and blurred vision are due to rising of excessive liver-yang which attacks the head. Bitter taste in the mouth suggests accumulation of heat in the Gallbladder Meridian derived from the upsurge of liver-yang which affects the gallbladder, as the liver and gallbladder are externally and internally related. Severe pain on the bilateral sides of the head is because the Gallbladder Meridian travels bilaterally on the side of the head. String-taut and rapid pulse, reddened tongue with yellow coating are signs of heat in the gallbladder and liver.

c) *Headache due to deficiency of both qi and blood:*

Main manifestations: Lingering headache, dizziness, blurred vision, lassitude, lustreless face, pain relieved by warmth and aggravated by cold, overstrain or mental stress, weak and thready pulse, pale tongue with thin and white coating.

Analysis: Lingering headache is due to the head being affected by the deficiency of qi that fails to make the clear yang ascend and the turbid yin descend. Pain aggravated by overstrain and stress is due to further consumption of qi. Lassitude, pain which is relieved by warmth and aggravated by cold suggest failure in distribution of yang qi. Lustreless face, dizziness and blurred vision indicate poor nourishment of the face and head due to deficiency of blood. Pale tongue with thin white coating and weak, thready pulse are signs of deficiency of both qi and blood.

Clinically, varieties of headache should be also differentiated according to the locality and the related meridians and collaterals. Pain in the occipital region and nape of the neck is related to the Bladder Meridian of Foot-Taiyang, pain at the forehead and supraorbital region is related to the Stomach Meridian of Foot-Yangming, pain in bilateral or unilateral temporal region is related to the Gallbladder Meridian of Foot-Shaoyang, and that in the parietal region is related to the Liver Meridian of Foot-Jueyin.

Treatment

a) Headache due to invasion of pathogenic wind into meridians and collaterals:

Method: To dispel the wind, remove obstruction in the meridians and collaterals, regulate the qi and blood and check the pain by puncturing the local points combined with distal points along the related meridians. The reducing method with needle retention is used.

Prescription: Occiptal headache: Fengchi (G 20), Kunlun (B 60), Houxi (S I 3).

Frontal headache: Touwei (S 8), Yintang (Extra), Shangxing (Du 23), Hegu (L I 4), Neiting (S 44).

Temporal headache: Taiyang (Extra), Shuaigu (G 8), Waiguan (S J 5), Zulinqi (G 41).

Parietal headache: Baihui (Du 20), Houxi (S I 3), Zhiyin (B 67), Taichong (Liv 3).

Explanation: The above prescriptions are formulated by combining local points with distal points according to the location of headache and the affected meridian.

Occipital headache — points of the Tai-yang Meridians of Hand and Foot.

Frontal headache — points of the Yang-ming Meridians of Hand and Foot.

Temporal headache — points of the Shao-yang Meridians of Hand and Foot.

Parietal headache — points of the Tai-yang Meridians of Hand and Foot plus those of the Jueyin Meridian of Foot.

b) Headache due to upsurge of liver yang:

Method: Select points of Jueyin and Shaoyang Meridians of Hand and Foot as the principal points to pacify the liver yang. Puncture with the reducing method.

Prescription: Fengchi (G 20), Baihui (Du 20), Xuanlu (G 5), Xiaxi (G 43), Xingjian (Liv 2).

Explanation: The Jueyin Meridian of Foot reaches the parietal region and the Shaoyang Meridians run up to the bilateral sides of the head. Combining the local points with distal points can reduce heat in the meridians and pacify the liver yang.

c) Headache due to deficiency of both qi and blood:

Method: To tonify and regulate circulation of qi and blood, promoting the clean qi to ascend and the turbid qi to descend by needling points of the Du and Ren Meridians and the corresponding Back-(Shu) points. Puncture with the reinforcing method.

Prescription: Baihui (Du 20), Qihai (Ren 6), Ganshu (B 18), Pishu (B 20), Shenshu (B 23), Zusanli (S 36).

Explanation: Qihai (Ren 6) is chosen to tonify the primary qi, and Baihui (Du 20) is for lifting up the clean yang. Ganshu (B 18), Pishu (B 20), and Shenshu (B 23) are the points associated with the liver, spleen and kidney. Since the liver stores blood, the spleen controls blood, and the kidney stores and produces essence and blood, these three points can be used to strengthen essence in the kidney and to tonify qi and blood.

Zusanli (S 36), punctured with the reinforcing method, can benefit the stomach which is the productive source of qi and blood.

Remarks

a) Headache occurs in various diseases of modern internal medicine, surgery, neurology, psychosis, ear, nose, throat, etc. Acupuncture gives gratifying results in migraine, and in vascular and neurotic headache.

b) Tapping with cutaneous needles and cupping method:

Main points: Area along L1 to S 4

Secondary points: Fengchi (G 20), Taiyang (Extra), Yangbai (G 14).

Method: Tap on the area from L1 to S 4. Then tap on the local area and along the afflicted meridians. For acute pain, Taiyang (Extra) and Yangbai (G 14) may be tapped to slight bleeding, then apply cupping.

2. Facial Pain

Facial pain is a kind of severe pain occurring in transient paroxysms in a certain facial region. It mostly occurs in one side of the forehead, maxillary region or mandibular region. The onset is abrupt like an electric shock, and the pain is cutting, burning and intolerable. Frequent recurrence denotes a chronic disease. In most cases it starts after middle age in women.

Etiology and Pathogenesis

A sudden attack of this disease is due to invasion of the meridians and collaterals on the face by pathogenic wind cold which contracts the meridians and collaterals and retards the circulation of qi and blood. In Chapter 38 of *Plain Questions,* it says:

"When pathogenic cold comes and stays in the meridians it impedes and slows down the circulation. If it lodges outside the vessels, the blood supply is decreased, and if it remains in the vessels, the passage of qi is obstructed, resulting in a sudden attack of pain."

Facial pain may also arise from excessive fire of the liver and stomach which flares up and attacks the face. The fire in the stomach is produced by retention of food caused by irregular food intake. The fire of the liver is due to the stagnation of qi in the liver. Furthermore, facial pain may be due to deficiency of yin producing excess of fire in the patients with a body constitution of yin deficiency and excessive sexual activity which consumes essence. In addition, diseases of the teeth, mouth, ear, nose, or mental disorders may also induce facial pain.

Differentiation

a) Facial pain due to invasion by pathogenic wind and cold:

Main manifestations: Abrupt onset of pain occurs like an electric shock. The pain is cutting, boring and intolerable, but transient and paroxysmal. Each attack lasts a few seconds or one to two minutes. It may recur several times a day. Tender points can be found on the supraobital foramen, infraorbital foramen, cheek foramen, lateral side of ala nasi, angle of the mouth, and nasolabial groove, where pressure induces the attack of pain. The pain is often accompanied by local spasm, running nose and lacrimation, salivation, or by exterior symptoms with string-taut and tense pulse.

Analysis: Pain is caused by the obstruction of circulation of qi and blood in the meridians and collaterals on the face due to invasion of pathogenic wind and cold.

Pain aggravated by pressure suggests that the pathogenic factors are in excess. Burning pain comes from the fierce fight between the antipathogenic qi and pathogenic factors. String-taut and tense pulse is the sign of invasion by pathogenic wind cold. Endogenous wind heat comes from prolonged accumulation of exogenous pathogenic cold wind, giving rise to spasm, running nose, lacrimation and salivation.

b) Facial pain due to excessive fire in the liver and stomach:

Main manifestations: The attack of pain as described above is accompanied by irritability, hot temper, thirst, constipation, yellow and dry tongue coating, and string-taut, rapid pulse.

Analysis: Irritability and hot temper are due to fire caused by prolonged depression of the liver qi. Burning pain is caused by endogenous heat coming from prolonged retention of food in the stomach, which rises to the face through the Stomach Meridian. Thirst and constipation are due to heat in the stomach. Yellow dry tongue coating, string-taut and rapid pulse are signs of accumulation of fire in the liver and stomach.

c) Facial pain due to deficiency of yin and excessive fire:

Main manifestations: Insidious pain, emaciation, malar flush, soreness in the lumbar region, lassitude, pain aggravated by fatigue, thready and rapid pulse, reddened tongue with little coating.

Analysis: The kidney stores essence and dominates water. When the kidney essence is insufficient, lassitude, soreness in the lumbar region and emaciation occur. Insufficiency of kidney water fails in controlling fire, which flares up along the meridians and reaches the face, causing malar flush and facial pain. Thready, rapid pulse, reddened

tongue with little coating are signs of deficiency of yin with flaming fire.

Treatment

Method: Select the local points in combination with distal points according to the location of pain and the meridians affected. For facial pain due to invasion of pathogenic wind and cold, reducing method is used to promote the circulation of qi and blood in the diseased area. For facial pain due to excessive fire in the liver and stomach, the points along the Foot-Jueyin and Yangming Meridians are punctured with the reducing method to bring down the fire. For facial pain due to deficiency of yin and excessive fire, the points along the Foot-Shaoyin Meridian should be added and punctured with the reinforcing method to nourish the yin and to dissipate the fire.

Prescription: Pain at supraorbital region: Yangbai (G 14), Taiyang (Extra), Zanzhu (B 2), Waiguan (S J 5).

Pain at maxillary region: Sibai (S 2), Quanliao (S I 18), Yingxiang (L I 20), Hegu (L I 4).

Pain at mandibular region: Xiaguan (S 7), Jiache (S 6), Daying (S 5), Jiachengjiang (Extra), Hegu (L I 4).

Supplementary points:

Invasion by pathogenic wind and cold: Fengchi (G 20).

Excessive fire in the liver and stomach: Taichong (Liv 3), Neiting (S 44).

Deficiency of yin and excessive fire: Zhaohai (K 6), Sanyinjiao (Sp 6).

Explanation: The above prescriptions are formulated by combining the local points with the distal points according to the location of pain and the meridians affected. For instance, Xiaguan (S 7), Jiache (S 6) and Jiachengjiang (Extra) are the points located at the mandibular region. Hegu (L I 4) and

Waiguan (S J 5) are the points along the Hand-Yangming and Hand-Shaoyang Meridians which go upward to the facial region. The above prescription has the effect of promoting circulation of qi of the meridians and collaterals in the affected area, and the function of reducing excess and relieving pain. Fengchi (G 20), the meeting point of the Foot-Shaoyang and Yangwei Meridians, can be used to dispel wind and to check pain. Taichong (Liv 3) and Neiting (S 44) can be chosen for the purpose of eliminating excessive fire in the liver and stomach. Zhaohai (K 6) and Sanyinjiao (Sp 6) nourish the yin and reduce the fire. For a chronic disease, local points on the affected side can be punctured with the reinforcing method, shallow insertion and needle retention. Or the reducing method with long retaining of needles can be applied to the corresponding local points of the healthy side.

Remarks

a) Facial pain is referred to trigeminal neuralgia in modern medicine.

b) Acupuncture is effective in pain of primary trigeminal neuralgia. For secondary trigeminal neuralgia accompanying intracranial diseases or lesions of the nervous system, in which the pain is usually continuous with paroxysms of aggravation, treatment should be aimed at its primary cause.

3. Deviation of Eye and Mouth

Deviation of the eye and the mouth is derived from invasion of the meridians and collaterals and muscle meridians in the facial region by exogeneous pathogenic wind and cold. It can occur in patients of any age, but mostly at the age of twenty to forty, and more frequently in males.

Etiology and Pathogenesis

Deviation of the eye and the mouth is due to paralysis of the facial muscles caused by the attack of pathogenic wind and cold on Yangming and Shaoyang Meridians, which leads to malnutrition of the muscle regions of the meridians.

Differentiation

Main manifestations: Sudden onset, usually right after waking up, incomplete closure of the eye in the affected side, drooping of the angle of the mouth, salivation and inability to frown, raise the eyebrow, close the eye, blow out the cheek, show the teeth or whistle, and in some cases pain in the mastoid region or headache, thin white tongue coating, superficial tense or superficial slow pulse.

Analysis: It is known that the Foot and Hand Yangming and Shaoyang Meridians supply the facial region, and the Muscle Meridians of Hand and Foot Yangming and Shaoyang also reach the forehead, cheek, and the front of the ear. The above manifestations of deviation of the eye and the mouth are due to the flaccidity of affected muscles leading to the imbalance of facial muscles between the two sides. The paralytic muscles are caused by stagnation of qi in the meridians and malnutrition of the regions of the muscle meridians after the invasion of pathogenic wind and cold.

Treatment

Method: To eliminate wind and remove the obstruction of meridians by applying even-movement mainly to the points of Hand and Foot Yangming Meridians, and also to the points of Shaoyang Meridians.

Prescription: Yifeng (S J 17), Yangbai (G 14), Taiyang (Extra), Quanliao (S I 18),

Xiaguan (S 7), Dicang (S 4), Jiache (S 6), Hegu (L I 4).

Supplementary points:

Headache: Fengchi (G 20).

Difficulty in frowning and raising the eyebrow: Zhanzhu (B 2), Sizhukong (S J 23).

Incomplete closing of the eye: Zanzhu (B 2), Jingming (B 1), Tongziliao (G 1), Yuyao (Extra), Sizhukong (S J 23).

Difficulty in sniffing: Yingxiang (L I 20).

Deviation of the philtrum: Renzhong (Du 26).

Inability to show the teeth: Juliao (S 3).

Tinnitus and deafness: Tinghui (G 2).

Tenderness at the mastoid region: Wangu (G 12), Waiguan (S J 5).

Explanation: Hegu (L I 4), the Yuan-(Primary) point of the Large Intestine Meridian of Hand-Yangming, can eliminate pathogenic wind from the head and facial region. Wangu (G 12) and Tinghui (G 2) can eliminate wind and relieve headache. Yangbai (G 14), Taiyang (Extra), Zanzhu (B 2), Sizhukong (S J 23), Tongziliao (G 1), Yuyao (Extra), Juliao (S 3), Renzhong (Du 26), Dicang (S 4), Jiache (S 6), Yingxiang (L I 20) and Quanliao (S J 17) are all local points of the involved meridians and have the effect of elininating wind and invigorating circulation of meridians.

Remarks

a) This condition is seen in peripheral facial paralysis or Bell's palsy in modern medicine.

b) In long-standing cases, the warming needle or moxibustion may be used to the points Taiyang (Extra), Jiache (S 6), Dicang (S 4), Juliao (S 3), and Xiaguan (S 7).

c) Cupping: Cupping may be used as an adjuvant method to acupuncture. The affected side may be treated with small cups once every three to five days.

d) If the healthy side of the face is stiff, shallow puncture and needle retaining at the local points of the healthy side can be applied in combination with needling of the affected side.

4.   Pain in Hypochondriac Region

Hypochondriac pain is a subjective symptom commonly seen in the clinic. It may be unilateral or bilateral. The classic book *Miraculous Pivot* points out: "Pathogenic factors in the liver give rise to hypochondriac pain." Chapter 22 of *Plain Questions* says: "When the liver is diseased, it causes pain below the ribs on both sides, and then refers to the lower abdomen." As the meridian of the liver supplies the hypochondriac regions, and the liver is externally and internally related with the gallbladder, the occurrence of hypochondriac pain is mostly concerned with disorders of the liver and gallbladder.

Etiology and Pathogenesis

a) The liver is situated in the hypochondriac region. Its meridians supply bilateral hypochondriac regions. If it is diseased, it will cause hypochordriac pain. The liver is the organ in the category of wind and wood of Five Elements, and prefers to be in a harmonious state with free flow of qi. Emotional depression may restrain the liver function, causing poor circulation of qi in the meridians, often resulting in hypochondriac pain.

b) The prolonged stagnation of the liver qi, or traumatic injuries such as sprain and contusion may cause stasis of blood in collaterals, resulting in hypochondriac pain.

c) Poor health associated with chonic disease, overstrain and stress, may cause deficiency of essence and blood, which in turn produces poor nourishment of the liver and its collaterals, resulting in hypochondriac pain.

Differentiation

a) Excess type:

i) Stagnation of qi:

Main manifestations: Distending pain in the costal and hypochondriac region, stifling sensation in the chest, sighing, poor appetite, bitter taste in the mouth, thin white tongue coating, string-taut pulse. Severity of the symptoms varies with the changes of emotional state.

Analysis: Distending pain in the costal and hypochondriac region suggests obstruction of the collaterals due to failure of the liver in maintaining the free flow of qi. Severity of the symptoms varies with the emotional state because of the close relationship between emotional changes and stagnation of qi. Stifling sensation in the chest and sighing indicate uneven qi activity. Poor appetite shows that the spleen is being attacked by the liver qi. Thin white tongue coating and string-taut pulse are the signs of depression of the liver.

ii) Stagnation of blood:

Main manifestations: Fixed stabbing pain in the hypochondriac region, intensified by pressure and at night, dark purplish tongue proper, deep and hesitant pulse.

Analysis: Fixed stabbing pain in the hypochondriac region is caused by stagnation of blood following stagnation of qi in the hypochondriac region. Pain intensified at night suggests that blood as a yin factor is apt to stagnate at night which is the yin time of a day. Pain due to stagnation of blood is a condition of excess, so it is aggravated by pressure. Dark purplish tongue proper, and deep, hesitant pulse are the signs of blood stagnation.

b) Deficiency type:

Main manifestations: Dull pain lingering in the costal and hypochondriac region, dryness of the mouth, irritability, dizziness, blurring of vision, red tongue with little coating, weak, or rapid and thready pulse.

Analysis: Dull pain in the costal and hypochondriac region indicates deficiency of essence and blood which causes poor nourishment of the collaterals of the liver. Dryness of the mouth and irritability suggest deficiency of yin with endogenous heat. Dizziness and blurring of vision are due to the shortage of essence and blood. Red tongue with little coating, and weak or rapid and thready pulse are signs of deficiency of essence and blood with endogenous heat.

Treatment

a) Excess type:

Method: Points are mainly selected from Jueyin and Shaoyang Meridians of Foot to remove the stagnation of liver qi and the obstruction in the collaterals. Needling with reducing method is to be applied.

Prescription: Qimen (Liv 14), Zhigou (S J 6), Yanglingquan (G 34).

Supplementary points:

Stagnation of qi: Taichong (Liv 3), Qiuxu (G 40).

Stagnation of blood: Geshu (B 17), Ganshu (B 18).

Explanation: The Shaoyang Meridian supplies the lateral aspect of the body, so Zhigou (S J 6) and Yanglingquan (G 34) are used to relieve pain by regulating the qi of the Shaoyang Meridian. Qimen (Liv 14), the Front-(Mu) point of the Liver Meridian, eases the liver and relieves pain in the hypochondrum. Taichong (Liv 3) and Qiuxu (G 40) regulate the qi of the liver and gallbladder. Geshu (B 17) and Ganshu (B

18) can activate blood circulation and remove stasis.

b) Deficiency type:

Method: Nourish essence and blood, invigorate circulation of qi, and relieve pain by applying reinforcing method to points of the Foot-Jueyin Meridian and Back-(Shu) points.

Prescription: Qimen (Liv 14), Ganshu (B 18), Shenshu (B 23), Zusanli (S 36), Sanyinjiao (Sp 6), Taichong (Liv 3).

Explanation: Ganshu (B 18), the Back-(Shu) point of the liver, Shenshu (B 23), the Back-(Shu) point of the kidney, Qimen (Liv 14), the Front-(Mu) point of the liver, Taichong (Liv 3), the Yuan-(Primary) point of the Liver Meridian, used in combination, can nourish essence and blood, readjust the liver and relieve pain. Zusanli (S 36) and Sanyinjiao (Sp 6) strengthen the function of the spleen and stomach which are the main source of producing qi and blood.

Remarks

a) Hypochondriac pain is seen in diseases of the liver and gallbladder, contusion of the hypochondriac region, intercostal neuralgia and costal chondritis.

b) Application of Huatuojiaji points of the corresponding segments gives gratifying effect to relieve pain in the treatment of intercostal neuralgia.

c) Cutaneous needling: Tap the skin over the affected hypochondriac area, and then apply cupping. This method is indicated in hypochondriac pain due to sprain or contusion. It has the action of removing stasis and relieving pain.

5. Low Back Pain

Low back pain (pain in the lumbar region) is closely associated with disorders of the kidney for the lumbus is the seat of the kidney.

Clinically, low back pain can be found in various diseases. This section only deals with the following etiological factors: 1. Invasion of exogenous pathogenic cold and damp; 2. Deficiency of qi of the kidney; and 3. Sprain or contusion.

Etiology and Pathogenesis

a) Invasion by pathogenic cold and damp:

In this case low back pain is due to obstruction of circulation of qi in meridians and collaterals. The precipitating factors may be living in cold and damp places, exposure to the rain or wading in water, or being drenched with sweat.

b) Deficiency of the kidney qi:

In this case low back pain is generally due to excessive sexual activity that consumes essence and qi, resulting in poor nourishment of the meridians in the lumbar region.

c) Trauma due to sprain or contusion:

Trauma may cause injury of qi and blood in the meridians and collaterals, leading to stagnation of qi and blood, thus producing low back pain.

Differentiation

a) Cold damp:

Main manifestations: Low back pain usually occuring after exposure to cold and damp and aggravated on rainy days, heavy sensation and stiffness of the muscles in the dorsolumbar region, limitation of extension and flexion of the back, pain radiating downwards to the buttocks and lower limbs, cold feeling of the affected area, white and sticky tongue coating, deep and weak, or deep and slow pulse.

Analysis: Pathogenic cold and damp characterized by viscosity and stagnation block the meridians and collaterals, causing retarded circulation of qi and blood. This produces heaviness, cold sensation and pain in the lumbar region and limitation of extension and flexion of the back. Stagnation of qi and blood becomes worse on cloudy and rainy days, and so does the pain. Accumulation of cold and damp gives rise to the white sticky tongue coating and the deep, weak or deep, slow pulse.

b) *Kidney deficiency:*

Main manifestations: Insidious onset of protracted pain and soreness, accompanied by lassitude and weakness of the loins and knees, aggravated by fatigue and alleviated by bed rest. In case of deficiency of kidney yang, cramp-like sensation in the lower abdomen, pallor, normal taste in the mouth, cold limbs, pale tongue, deep thready or deep slow pulse. In case of deficiency of kidney yin, irritability, insomnia, dry mouth and throat, flushed face, feverish sensation in the chest, palms and soles, reddened tongue proper with scanty coating, thready weak or thready rapid pulse.

Analysis: The lumbar region is said to be the "dwelling house of the kidney." The kidney dominates the bones, produces marrow and stores essence. When the kidney has insufficient essence, the bone is lacking of marrow, and the result is soreness and pain in the lumbar region accompanied by weakness of the knees. Over strain and stress consume essence and qi, and make the pain worse. Pain is lessened by bed rest, which makes qi quiescent. In case of deficiency of kidney yang, the kidney fails to warm the lower abdomen and the limbs. This gives rise to cramp-like sensation in the lower abdomen and cold limbs. Deficiency of yang causes pallor, pale tongue, deep thready or deep slow pulse. When yin is deficient, kidney water is unable to ascend to reduce the heart fire. This results in irritability and

insomnia. Deficiency of yin causes excessive internal heat, which gives rise to the following symptoms: flushed face, feverish sensation in the chest, palms and soles, dryness of the mouth and throat, reddened tongue with little coating, thready weak or thready rapid pulse.

c) *Trauma:*

Main manifestations: History of sprain of the lumbar region, rigidity and pain of the lower back which is generally fixed in a certain area, and is aggravated by pressure and by turning the body, pink or dark purplish tongue proper, string-taut hesitant pulse.

Analysis: Muscular strain in the lumbar region causes retardation of qi and blood and further leads to stagnation of blood in the meridians and collaterals. The result is the fixed severe pain which can be aggravated by pressure. String-taut pulse is associated with pain, dark purplish tongue proper and hesitant pulse are signs of blood stasis.

Treatment

Method: Points are mainly selected from the Du and the Foot-Taiyang Meridians to promote the circulation of qi and blood, to relieve pain, to relax the muscles and to activate the blood circulation in the collaterals. Acupuncture and moxibustion are applied together for cold-damp type. in case of deficiency of the kidney yang, apply needling with reinforcing method and moxibustion. For deficiency of the kidney yin, puncture with reinforcing method. For traumatic low back pain, apply reducing method or pricking to cause bleeding.

Prescription: Shenshu (B 23), Yaoyang-guan (Du 3), Weizhong (B 40).

Supplementary points:

Cold damp: Dachangshu (B 25), Guanyuanshu (B 26).

Deficiency of the kidney yang: Mingmen (Du 4), Yaoyan (Extra).

Deficiency of the kidney yin: Zhishi (B 52), Taixi (K 3).

Traumatic injury: Renzhong (Du 26), Yaotongxue (Extra), Ahshi point.

Explanation: The low back is the "dwelling house of the kidney." Shenshu (B 23) can be selected to tonify the qi of the kidney. Moxibustion may also be applied to this point to eliminate cold and damp. Yaoyangguan (Du 3) is a local point. Weizhong (B 40) is one of "Four Key Points," and an important distal point for the treatment of low back pain. Dachangshu (B 25) and Guanyuanshu (B 26) can dispel wind and cold, remove obstruction in meridians, and relieve pain. Combination of acupuncture and moxibustion applied to Mingmen (Du 4) and Yaoyan(Extra) can tonify the kidney yang and strengthen the kidney essence as well. Zhishi (B 52) and Taixi (K 3) are selected for the purpose of nourishing the kidney yin. As the Du Meridian travels along the spine, Renzhong (Du 26) is a distal point effective for treating rigidity and pain of the lumbar region. Yaotongxue (Extra) is an empirical point used in treating sprain of the lumbar region.

Remarks

a) Low back pain may be seen in renal diseases, rheumatism, rheumatoid arthritis, hyperplastic spondilitis, muscle strain or traumatic injury of the lumbar region.

b) When the lumbar vertebrae are diseased, the corresponding Huatuojiaji points may be punctured perpendicularly 1.0-1.5 inches. Needles are retained. Here, acupuncture therapy is only a supplementary method of treatment.

6. Bi Syndromes

Bi syndromes are the syndromes characterized by obstruction of qi and blood in meridians and collaterals due to invasion of pathogenic wind, cold and damp, and manifested by soreness, pain, numbness and heavy sensation of the limbs and joints, and limitation of movement.

Clinically, bi syndromes are common in the areas where the weather is cold, wet and windy, occurring in persons of either sex and any age. In mild cases there are only soreness and pain in limbs and joints, aggravated by the change of weather. In severe cases the soreness and pain are marked and recur repeatedly, accompanied by swelling of the joints and even deformity and limitation of movement.

Bi syndromes may be classified into four types according to etiology and manifestations: 1. Wandering bi is characterized by migrating pain and caused chiefly by pathogenic wind; 2. Painful bi is characterized by severe pain and caused chiefly by pathogenic cold; 3. Fixed bi is characterized by marked soreness, numbness and heaviness and caused chiefly by pathogenic damp; and 4. Heat bi is characterized by heat manifestations and sudden onset.

Etiology and Pathogenesis

a) Attack of pathogenic factors on individuals with weakened body resistance:

Bi syndromes are caused by obstruction of qi and blood due to 1. invasion of the meridians and collaterals by pathogenic wind, cold and damp; 2. general weakness of the body with deficiency of yang qi; and 3. dysfunction of the pores, and weakness of defensive yang. The book *Prescriptions for Succouring the Sickness* points out, "It is because of weakness of the body with poor function of the pores that invasion of wind, cold and damp to produce Bi syndromes is possible."

b) *Body constitution:*

The body constitution differs in the natures of heat and cold. In case of the body constitution with exuberant yang qi and accumulated heat, invasion of pathogenic wind, cold and damp will give rise to heat bi. Furthermore, long-standing wind, cold and damp Bi syndromes may turn into heat Bi as the pathogenic factors in the meridians and collaterals are transformed into heat.

Differentiation

a) *Wandering bi:*

Main manifestations: Wandering pain in the joints, especially the wrists, elbows, knees and ankles; limitation of movement, chills and fever, thin and sticky tongue coating, superficial and tight or superficial and slow pulse.

Analysis: Pain in the joints is a common manifestation of all the Bi syndromes caused by wind, cold and damp that obstruct qi and blood circulation in meridians and collaterals. As stated in Chinese medicine, "There is pain if there is obstruction." Wandering pain is due mainly to invasion by pathogenic wind which is characterized by constant movement and changes. Chills and fever result from the struggle between antipathogenic factors and pathogenic factors after the invasion. Superficial tense or superficial slow pulse indicates invasion of exogenous pathogenic wind on the exterior of body; and thin and sticky tongue coating shows the initial stage of invasion by pathogenic wind, cold and damp.

b) *Painful bi:*

Main manifestations: Severe stabbing pain in the joints, alleviated by warmth and aggravated by cold, with fixed localization

but no local redness and hotness, thin and white tongue coating, string-taut and tense pulse.

Analysis: Severe pain is due to retarded circulation of qi and blood in the meridians and collaterals caused by excessive cold. Cold is a yin pathogenic factor, characterized by causing contraction. The pain is localized because of the congealing effect of cold. Pain alleviated by warmth suggests that heat improves the circulation of blood. Cold causes further stagnation of blood, and hence aggravates the pain. The absence of local redness and hotness is characteristic of affection by pathogenic cold. String-taut and tense pulse is associated with cold and pain. White tongue coating is a sign of pathogenic cold.

c) *Fixed bi:*

Main manifestations: Numbness and heavy sensation of the limbs, soreness and fixed pain of the joints, aggravated on cloudy and rainy days, white and sticky tongue coating and soft pulse.

Analysis: Pathogenic damp is characterized by heaviness. When it is in an excessive state, it invades the limbs and joints, causing retarded circulation of qi and blood, and resulting in numbness and heaviness. Pathogenic damp is a yin factor, characterized by viscosity and stagnation. So the pain caused by damp is also fixed in location. The condition becomes worse on cloudy and rainy days for the weather change brings about more stagnation of qi and blood. Soft pulse and white sticky tongue coating indicate the presence of pathogenic damp.

d) *Heat bi:*

Main manifestations: Arthralgia involving one or several joints, local redness, swelling and excruciating pain with limitation of movement, accompanied by fever and thirst, yellow tongue coating, rolling and rapid pulse.

Analysis: Local redness, swelling and pain of the joints are the result of the transformation of pathogenic factors into heat. Movement is limited because of swelling and deformity of joints. Fever, thirst, yellow tongue coating, rolling and rapid pulse are the signs of excessive heat.

In addition, bi syndromes may also be classified according to the locality of the diseased area as follows:

Skin bi: Numbness of the skin with cold sensation.

Muscle bi: Soreness, numbness and pain of the muscles.

Tendon bi: Soreness, pain and stiffness of the tendons and muscles.

Vessel bi: Pain due to blockage of vessels.

Bone bi: Soreness, heaviness and pain of joints which fail to perform their functions of lifting, extension and flexion.

Treatment

Ahshi points together with the local and distal points along the yang meridians supplying the diseased areas are selected for the purpose of eliminating wind, cold and damp. Wandering bi, heat bi and tendon bi are mainly treated by the reducing method. Subcutaneous needles may also be applied. For painful bi and vessel bi, it is better to use moxibustion, and apply needling as an adjuvant treatment with deep insertion and prolonged retaining of the needles. For severe pain, intradermal needles or indrect moxibustion with ginger may be used. Fixed bi, skin bi, muscle bi and bone bi may also be treated by combined acupuncture and moxibustion, or together with warming needle, or tapping plus cupping.

Prescriptions:

Pain in the shoulder joint: Jianyu (LI 15), Jianliao (SJ 14), Jianzhen (SJ 19), Naoshu (SI 10).

Pain in the scapula: Tianzong (SI 11), Bingfeng (SI 12), Jianwaishu (SI 14), Gaohuang (B 43).

Pain in the elbow: Quchi (LI 11), Chize (L5), Tianjing (SJ 10), Waiguan (SJ 5), Hegu (LI 4).

Pain in the wrist: Yangchi (SJ 4), Yangxi (LI 5), Yanggu (SI 5), Waiguan (SJ 5).

Stiffness of the fingers: Yanggu (SI 5), Hegu (LI 4), Houxi (SI 3).

Numbness and pain in the fingers: Houxi (SI 3), Sanjian (LI 3), Baxie (Extra).

Pain in the lumbar region: Renzhong (Du 26), Shenzhu (Du 12), Yaoyangguan (Du 3).

Pain in the hip joint: Huantiao (G 30), Juliao (G 29), Xuanzhong (G 39).

Pain in the thigh region: Zhibian (B 54), Chengfu (B 36), Yanglingquan (G 34).

Pain in the knee joint: Heding (Extra), Dubi (S 35), Medial Xiyan (Extra), Yanglingquan (G 34), Yinlingquan (Sp 9).

Numbness and pain in the leg: Chengshan (B 57), Feiyang (B 58).

Pain in the ankle: Jiexi (S 41), Shangqiu (Sp 5), Qiuxu (G 40), Kunlun (B 60), Taixi (K 3).

Numbness and pain in the toes: Gongsun (Sp 4), Shugu (B 65), Bafeng (Extra).

Pain in the back: Shuigou (Du 26), Shenzhu (Du 12), Yaoyangguan (Du 3).

General pain: Houxi (SI 3), Shenmai (B 62), Dabao (Sp 21), Geshu (B 17), Jianyu (LI 15), Quchi (LI 11), Hegu (LI 4), Yangchi (SJ 4), Huantiao (G 30), Yanglingquan (G 34), Xuanzhong (G 39), Jiexi (S 41).

Supplementary points: 1. Wandering bi, vessel bi: Geshu (B 17), Xuehai (Sp 10); 2. Painful bi: Shenshu (B 23), Guanyuan (Ren 4); 3. Fixed bi: Zusanli (S 36), Shangqiu (Sp 5); 4. Heat bi: Dazhui (Du

14), Quchi (LI 11); 5. Tendon bi: Yanglingquan (G 34); and 6. Bone bi: Dazhu (B 11), Xuanzhong (G 39).

Explanation: The above prescriptions are formulated by selection of the local and distal points on the meridians supplying the diseased areas. The principle of the treatment is to remove obstruction from the meridians and collaterals and to regulate ying (nutrient qi) and wei (defensive qi) for elimination of wind, cold and damp. When the skin and muscles are diseased, shallow insertion should be used. When bones and tendons are affected, deep insertion with retaining of the needles is recommended. The methods of acupuncture and moxibustion depend on symptoms and signs. Houxi (SI 3) communicates with the Du Meridian, and Shenmai (B 6) with the Yangqiao Meridian. They are a set of the Eight Confluent points for the treatment of the diseases of the shoulder, back, lumbar region, legs, muscles, tendons and bones. Dabao (Sp 21) is the major Luo-(Connecting) point of the spleen which connects qi of the whole body, and Geshu (B 17) is the Influential Point of the blood. Combination of these two points can be used to treat general pain. Dazhui (Du 14) and Quchi (LI 11) are used to treat heat bi. Geshu (B 17) and Xuehai (Sp 10) have the function of activating and nourishing the blood. The selection is based on the principle: "Wind will be naturally eliminated if blood circulates smoothly." Fengchi (G 20), the most important point for dispelling wind, can be combined with Geshu (B 17) and Xuehai (Sp 10) to treat wandering bi and vessel bi. Shangqiu (Sp 5) and Zusanli (S 36) strengthen the function of spleen and stomach and eliminate damp to relieve the fixed bi. Guanyuan (Ren 4) and Shenshu (B 23) strengthen the kidney

fire and relieve the painful bi. Yanglingquan (G 40), the Influential Point of the tendon, is used to treat the tendon bi. Dazhu (B 11), the Influential Point of the bone, Xuanzhong (G 39), the Influential Point of the marrow, can be used together in treating the bone bi.

Remarks

a) Bi syndromes may include such diseases as rheumatic fever, rheumatic arthritis, rheumatoid arthritis, fibrositis, neuralgia and gout.

b) Cutaneous needle and cupping: Heavy tapping to induce slight bleeding along the two sides of the spine or the local area of the affected joint plus cupping is often used for the treatment of skin bi and muscle bi associated with numbness, and bone bi characterized by stiffness and limitation of movement or deformity of the joint.

c) Acupuncture is effective in treating mild bi syndromes. For severe cases, a long period of treatment is necessary. In chronic cases with exhaustion of ying (nutrient qi) and wei (defensive qi) and undernourishment of tendons and muscles, the bi syndrome may turn into a wei syndrome.

7. Wei Syndromes

The wei syndrome is characterized by flaccidity or atrophy of the limbs with motor impairment. It is also called "flaccid lame," for the leg is usually involved. The wei syndrome was first described in Chapter 44 of *Plain Questions* as a syndrome mainly caused by heat in the lung with the lobes scorched. The physicians of later generations further developed this theory. Zhang Jingyue (1156-1228 A.D.) pointed out, "It is not a few cases of wei syndromes that are due to the injury of primary qi leading to deficiency of essence which fails to irrigate, or deficiency of blood which fails to nourish."

On the treatment of wei syndromes, Chapter 44 of *Plain Questions* puts forward the theory: "Only points along the Yangming Meridians are selected in treating wei syndromes." The stomach is believed to be the sea of water and food, and the source of acquired essence. The Foot-Yangming Meridian is enriched with qi and blood. The twelve meridians, tendons, bones, and muscles need the acquired qi and blood for nourishment, while the production of blood in the liver and essence in the kidney depends upon the transformation of water and food. Therefore, regulating the function of the Stomach Meridian of Yangming is the main principle in treating the wei syndromes. In clinical practice, treatment is determined according to differentiation of the syndrome as well as locality, etiology and pathogenesis of the disease. In a chronic bi syndrome there may be prolonged motor impairment of the joint because of pain. In this case there develops muscular atrophy or flaccidity of the limb on account of disuse. It should be differentiated from the wei syndrome which is characterized by absence of pain.

Etiology and Pathogenesis

a) Burning heat in the lung:

The muscular flaccidity or atrophy of the limb results from malnourishment of the tendons due to exhaustion of body fluid. This condition may be caused by invasion of the lung by exogenous pathogenic heat, or excessive heat remaining in the lung after an illness.

b) Damp heat:

Exogenous pathogenic damp invades in the body, and the accumulation of damp is

eventually transformed into heat which damages the muscles and tendons. Hence, the muscles and tendons become flaccid. The wei syndromes may also be caused by excessive intake of greasy food which produces internal accumulation of damp-heat, resulting in stagnation of qi and blood in the meridians and collaterals.

c) Deficiency of yin in the liver and kidney:

Since the liver stores blood and controls the tendons, and the kidney stores essence and dominates the bones, prolonged illness or indulgent sexual activity causes loss of essence and blood, resulting in malnutrition of the tendons. Conditions affecting the proper function of the liver and kidney may therefore also give rise to the wei syndrome.

d) Trauma:

Contusion causes injury of the meridians and leads to retarded flow of qi and blood in the meridians. As a result, the muscles and tendons are poorly nourished, and become flaccid. Thus occurs the wei syndrome.

Differentiation

a) Heat in the lung:

Main manifestations: Muscular flaccidity of the lower limbs with motor impairment, accompanied by fever, cough, irritability, thirst, scanty and brownish urine, reddened tongue with yellow coating, thready and rapid or rolling and rapid pulse.

Analysis: Fever and cough are the results of the invasion of the lung by the pathogenic heat. Irritability, thirst and scanty, brownish urine indicate that the body fluid has been damaged by the internal heat. Muscular flaccidity and motor impairment result from malnutrition of the tendons and muscles and damage of essence and body fluid. The thready, rapid pulse and reddened tongue with yellow coating indicate that the body fluid has been injured by heat. The rolling, rapid pulse is associated with excessive heat.

b) Damp heat:

Main manifestations: Flaccid or slight swollen legs, a little hot sensation on touch, general heaviness, sensation of fullness in the chest and epigastric region, painful urination, hot and brownish urine, yellow sticky tongue coating, soft and rapid pulse.

Analysis: Flaccidity of the legs is due to the stagnation of qi and blood in the tendons and muscles caused by prolonged accumulation of internal damp-heat. General heaviness is also due to accumulation of damp-heat. When damp-heat is accumulated in the chest, fullness sensation in the chest and epigastrium results. Hot, brownish urine, and painful urination suggest the downward flow of damp heat. Yellow sticky tongue coating, and soft rapid pulse are signs of damp-heat.

c) Deficiency of yin of the liver and kidney:

Main manifestations: Muscular flaccidity of the lower limbs with motor impairment, combined with soreness and weakness of the lumbar region, seminal emission, prospermia, leukorrhoea, dizziness, blurring of vision, reddened tongue, thready and rapid pulse.

Analysis: In deficiency of yin of the liver and kidney the muscles, tendons and bones are poorly nourished by essence and blood, and hence occurs muscular flaccidity with motor impairment. Soreness and weakness of the lumbar region, seminal emission and leukorrhoea are the result of deficiency of essence in the kidney. Since the kidney is located in the lumbar region, it stores essence, and its meridians connect with the Chong Meridian and the Ren Meridian. Dizziness and blurring of vision are caused by preponderance of yang in the liver arising from deficiency of yin in the kidney.

Reddened tongue, thready and rapid pulse are signs of deficiency of yin of the liver and kidney.

d) Trauma:

Main manifestations: History of trauma, flaccid paralytic limbs, may be accompanied with incontinence of urine and feces, relaxed or hesitant pulse, pink or dark purplish tongue with thin white coating.

Analysis: Flaccid paralytic limbs arise from obstruction of the circulation of qi and blood at the injured site of trauma. Incontinence of urine and feces is mainly due to dysfunction of the kidney which fails to control urine and feces. In case of trauma, the Du Meridian which dominates the yang qi of the whole body is affected, and the qi activity of all zang-fu organs may be impaired, including the function of the kidney in controlling urine and feces. Damage of qi of the kidney causes incontinence of urine and feces. Hesitant pulse and dark purplish tongue indicate blood stasis.

Treatment

Method: Main points are selected from the Yangming Meridians to promote circulation of qi in the meridians, and to nourish the tendons and bones. If heat or damp heat in the lung is the main etiological factor, the reducing method should be used to dissipate heat. In case of deficiency of yin in the liver and kidney, the reinforcing method should be employed. For trauma, puncture the points on the affected side with even movement.

Prescription:

Upper limb: Jianyu (LI 15), Quchi (LI 11), Hegu (LI 4), Waiguan (SJ 5).

Lower limb: Biguan (S 31), Huantiao (G 30), Xuehai (Sp 10), Liangqiu (S 34), Zusanli (S 36), Yanglingquan (G 34), Jiexi (S 41),

Xuanzhong (G 39).

Supplementary points:

Heat in the lung: Chize (L 5), Feishu (B 13).

Damp heat: Pishu (B 20), Yinlingquan (Sp 9).

Deficiency of yin in the liver and kidney: Ganshu (B 18), Shenshu (B 23).

Trauma: Huatuojiaji points at the corresponding level of spinal injury.

Incontinence of urine: Zhongji (Ren 3), Sanyinjiao (Sp 6).

Incontinence of feces: Dachangshu (B 25), Ciliao (B 32).

Explanation: In the above prescription points the Yangming Meridians are predominating. This is based upon the statement in *Internal Classic:* "Only points along the Yangming Meridians are selected to treat paralysis of the limbs." Yanglingquan (G 34) and Xuanzhong (G 39), the Influential Points of tendon and marrow respectively, are added to enhance the effect of nourishing the tendons and bones. Feishu (B 13) and Chize (L 5) are used to dissipate heat from the lung. Pishu (B 20) and Yinlingquan (Sp 9) eliminate damp heat. Ganshu (B 18) and Shenshu (B 23) are chosen to tonify the yin in the liver and kidney. Huatuojiaji points are selected to regulate qi in the Du Meridian. Zhongji (Ren 3) and Sanyinjiao (Sp 6) are taken to adjust the qi in the kidney and bladder. Dachangshu (B 25) and Ciliao (B 32) improve the function of the large intestine.

Remarks

a) The wei syndrome is seen in acute myelitis, progressive myatrophy, myathenia gravis, multiple neuritis, sequellae of poliomyelitis, periodic paralysis, hysterical paralysis, traumatic paraplegia, etc.

b) Since the wei syndrome needs a long period of treatment, the patients should cooperate with the doctor during the treatment. Tapping with subcutaneous needles in the affected areas and along the affected meridians may also be added to the treatment.

Chapter 18

GYNECOLOGICAL AND OTHER DISEASES

I. GYNECOLOGICAL DISEASES

1. Irregular Menstruation

Irregular menstruation refers to any abnormal change in menstrual cycle, in quantity and color of flow, and other accompanying symptoms. Commonly seen cases are antedated and postdated menstruation, irregular menstrual cycle. Menstruation earlier than due time by seven to eight days, or even twice a month, is regarded as antedated menstruation, while menses later than due time by eight to nine days or even once every forty to fifty days is considered as postdated menstruation.

Menopathy is caused by many factors, such as the exogenous pathogenic cold, heat and damp, emotional disturbances — worries, depressed rage, indulgence in sexual life, grand multiparity, etc., leading to the disharmony between qi and blood and the injury of the Chong and Ren Meridians.

Etiology and Pathogenesis
a) Antedated menstruation:
i) Heat in the blood:
It is due to abundance of the internal heat, yin deficiency and yang excess, or overtake of pungent food, overdosage of the warm property drugs acting on uterus, or to fire transformed from stagnated liver qi, etc. All of these lead to the injury of the Chong and

Ren Meridians by excessive heat, bringing about antedated menstruation.
ii) Qi deficiency:
This is caused by overexertion, improper diet leading to weakness of the spleen qi and insufficient qi in the middle jiao, which fails to control the menstrual flow, resulting in antedated menses. Dr. Zhang Jingyue pointed out, "If the pulse does not reflect excessive heat internally it means antedated menstruation is caused by qi deficiency of the heart and spleen that fail to control the blood."
b) Postdated menstruation:
i) Blood deficiency:
The blood may be marred due to chronic hemorrhage, debility resulted from chronic diseases and multiparity. Irregular diet and overexertion may injure the spleen and stomach, causing insufficiency of blood in the Chong and Ren Meridians. Finally, postdated menstruation occurs.
ii) Cold in the blood:
It is due mostly to constant yang deficiency and internal growth of cold, or due to overtake of raw and cold food, exposure to rain and cold during the menstrual periods. Then the pathogenic cold invades the Chong and Ren Meridians, impeding the free flow of blood, hence the menstrual cycle delays.
iii) Qi stagnation:

It is due to emotional depression, disturbing the qi activity and resulting in qi stagnation. The stagnated qi impairs the smooth flow of blood which leads to abnormal function of the Chong and Ren Meridians. The sea of blood cannot be filled up at due time, and postdated menstruation occurs.

c) Irregular menstrual cycles:

i) Qi stagnation in the liver:

It is due usually to depressed rage that hurts the liver and disturbs the storage of blood, which leads to dysfunction of the blood in the Chong, Ren Meridians and uterus, hence irregular menstrual cycles.

ii) Kidney deficiency:

It is due to marriage at an immature age, indulgence of sexual life, grand multiparity, etc., which consume the essence and blood. The kidney qi fails to conduct its function in storing essence and adjusting the Chong and Ren Meridians, resulting in irregular menstrual cycles.

Differentiation

a) Antedated menstruation:

i) Heat in blood:

Main manifestations: Shortened cycle, dark red and thick blood flow in large quantities, restlessness, fullness in the chest, brown urine, reddened tongue with yellow coating, rapid and forceful pulse.

Analysis: Dark red, thick and profuse menses indicate internal excessive heat, which impairs the heart and liver, leading to restlessness and fullness in the chest. When the heat shifts from the heart down to the small intestine there appears scanty and dark yellow urine. The yellow tongue coating and the rapid pulse are signs of internal heat.

ii) Qi deficiency:

Main manifestations: Profuse, thin and light red menses in shortened cycle, lassitude, palpitation, shortness of breath, subjective empty and heavy sensation in the lower abdomen, pale tongue with thin coating, weak pulse.

Analysis: The spleen qi dominates the middle jiao and controls blood. Qi insufficiency fails to check the blood, there occurs disturbance of the Chong and Ren Meridians, leading to profuse, thin and light red menses in shortened cycle. Lassitude, shortness of breath and empty heavy sensation are manifestations of qi deficiency. Palpitation and pale tongue account for blood deficiency, and the weak pulse is a sign of qi deficiency.

b) Postdated menstruation:

i) Blood deficiency:

Main manifestations: Scanty and light red menses in delayed cycle, empty and painful feeling in the lower abdomen, emaciation, sallow complexion, lusterless skin, dizziness and blurred vision, palpitation and insomnia, pink tongue with little coating, weak and thready pulse.

Analysis: Owing to a chronic disease, weak body constitution or chronic hemorrhage, blood cannot form the timely tide in the sea of blood, bringing about scanty and light red menses in delayed cycle. When the blood fails to nourish the uterus, there is an emptiness and pain in the lower abdomen. When the meridians, vessels, muscles and skin are undernourished, there may appear emaciation, sallow complexion and lustreless skin. When the liver and heart fail to be nourished by blood, dizziness, blurred vision, palpitation and insomnia occour. If the tongue is malnourished and the vessels are not filled up, there present pink tongue and weak thready pulse.

ii) Cold in the blood:

Main manifestations: Scanty and dark-coloured menses in delayed cycle, colic pain in the lower abdomen, slightly alleviated by warmth, cold limbs, thin and white tongue, deep and slow pulse.

Analysis: The invasion of pathogenic cold during menstruation impedes blood flow, leading to scanty and dark-coloured menses in delayed cycle. Cold in the uterus hinders the smooth flow of qi and blood and then there appears colic pain. Cold, yin by nature, injures yang qi and brings about cold limbs. Thin and white tongue coating, deep and slow pulse are signs of cold syndromes.

iii) Qi stagnation:

Main manifestations: Scanty and dark red menses in delayed cycle, distending pain in the lower abdomen, mental depression, stuffy chest alleviated by belching, distension in the hypochondria and breast region, thin, white tongue coating and string-taut pulse.

Analysis: Stagnated qi of the liver brings about retarded blood flow and results in scanty and delayed menses with distending pain in the lower abdomen. When the qi fails to travel smoothly, mental depression and stuffy chest present. Since the Liver Meridian runs through the costal and hypochondriac regions, the stagnated liver qi gives rise to the distension in the hypochondrium and breast. String-taut pulse is a typical sign of liver disorder and qi stagnation.

c) *Irregular menstrual cycles:*

i) Qi stagnation in the liver:

Main manifestations: Alteration of menstrual cycles and quantity of blood flow, thick, sticky, and purple colored menses difficult to flow, distension in the hypochondriac region and breast, distending pain in the lower abdomen, mental depression, frequent sighing, thin white tongue coating and string-taut pulse.

Analysis: Depressed rage injuries the function of the liver, leading to unsmooth flow of qi and blood and disturbance in the sea of blood, and finally to the alteration of menstrual cycles and quantity of blood flow. The stagnation of liver qi causes impeded flow of blood, bringing about difficult menstruation, distension in the hypochondriac region and breast, and distending pain in the lower abdomen. Frequent sighing may help to relieve the stagnated qi. String-taut pulse is a typical sign of liver qi stagnation.

ii) Kidney deficiency:

Main manifestations: Scanty, light red blood flow in altering cycles, dizziness and tinnitus, weak and aching of the lower back and knees, frequent night urination, loose stools, pale tongue with thin coating, deep and weak pulse.

Analysis: When there is insufficiency of kidney qi, disharmonized Chong and Ren Meridians bring on the derangement of the flow and ebb of tide in the sea of blood, resulting in the alteration of menstrual cycles. Insufficient kidney qi decreases the essence and blood, leading to scanty, thin and light red menses. Since the kidney dominates bones, generates marrow, and has its opening in the ear, and the Kidney Meridian runs through the waist, deficiency condition of the kidney causes lack of marrow, impairs audibility and mal-nourishes the waist, bringing on dizziness, tinnitus, sore and weak in knees and the lower back. When the kidney fails to control urination and defecation there appear frequent urination and loose stools. Pale tongue with thin coating and deep weak pulse indicate kidney yang deficiency.

Treatment

a) *Antedated menstruation:*

i) Heat in the blood:

Method: Points of the Spleen and Kidney Meridians are selected as the principal points. Acupuncture with the reducing method is applied to regulate the Chong and Ren Meridians and, clear off heat from blood.

Prescription: Quchi (L I 11), Zhongji (Ren 3), Xuehai (Sp 10), Shuiquan (K 5).

Supplementary points:

Liver qi transforming into fire: Xingjian (Liv 2).

Yin deficiency with internal heat: Rangu (K 2).

Explanation: Quchi (L I 11) is the He-Sea Point of the Hand-Yangming Meridian while Xuehai (Sp 10) is the Jing-River Point of the Foot-Taiyin Meridian. When they are used together, heat is removed from blood. Zhongji (Ren 3), the intersecting point of the three yin meridians of foot, works to regulate the Chong and Ren Meridians and remove internal heat from the lower jiao. Shuiquan (K 5), Xi-Cleft Point of the Kidney Meridian, strengthens yin, reduces heat and regulates menses. All the points used together serve the purpose of clearing off heat and regulating menstruation. Xingjian (L 2) is added to clear away the heat from the liver in case of stagnated liver qi transforming into fire. Rangu (K 2) is used to nourish yin, reduce heat and to regulate menses.

ii) Qi deficiency:

Method: Select the main points from the Ren, Foot-Taiyin and Foot-Yangming Meridians to replenish qi so as to restore its function in controlling blood. Acupuncture is applied with the reinforcing method.

Prescription: Qihai (Ren 6), Sanyinjiao (Sp 6), Zhongwan (Ren 12), Zusanli (S 36).

Explanation: Qihai (Ren 6) can regulate qi of the whole body. Qi is the commander of blood and when it is abundant blood is totally controlled by it. Sanyinjiao (Sp 6), Zhongwan (Ren 12) and Zusanli (S 36) are chosen to build up the spleen qi, and strengthen spleen qi, controls blood. All the points applied together attain the purpose of replenishing qi and controlling blood.

b) Postdated menstruation:

i) Blood deficiency and cold in the blood:

Method: Points of the Ren and Foot-Taiyin Meridians are selected as the principal points. In case of blood deficiency, acupuncture is applied with the reinforcing method to replenish qi and nourish blood. Moxibustion is also advisable. In case of cold in the blood, acupuncture is given with the even movement. Strong stimulation of moxibustion is used to warm up the meridians and disperse cold.

Prescription: Guanyuan (Ren 4), Qihai (Ren 6), Sanyinjiao (Sp 6).

Supplementary points:

Dizziness and blurred vision: Baihui (Du 20),

Palpitation and insomnia: Shenmen (H 7).

Explanation: Guanyuan (Ren 4), an intersecting point of the three yin meridians of foot connects the uterus. When the reinforcing method is applied to Guanyuan (Ren 4) and Sanyinjiao (Sp 6), qi and blood are promoted, the Chong and Ren Meridians are regulated and then cold is dispelled from them. Qihai (Ren 6) assists to adjust qi and blood so that the Chong and Ren Meridians are well regulated and menses comes on time. Baihui (Du 20) helps ascend qi and blood, nourishing the head and eliminating dizziness and blurred vision. Shenmen (H 7) pacifies the mind in case of palpitation and insomnia.

ii) Qi stagnation:

Method: Points of the Foot-Jueyin and Foot-Yangming Meridians are selected as the principal points. Acupuncture is applied with the reducing method to activate qi and blood flow.

Prescription: Tianshu (S 25), Qixue (K 13), Diji (S 8), Taichong (Liv 3).

Supplementary points:

Fullness of the chest: Neiguan (P 4).

Distension in the hypochondriac region and breast: Qimen (Liv 74).

Analysis: Tianshu (S 25) and Qihai (Ren 6) are located on the Foot-Yangming Meridian. Qixue (K 13) can promote qi and blood flow and regulate the Chong and Ren Meridians. Diji (Sp 8), a qi point of the blood system can adjust blood and qi circulation. Taichong (Liv 3), the Yuan-(Primary) Point of the Liver Meridian can soothe the liver and regulate liver qi. The points are used together to achieve free flow of qi and blood. Neiguan (P 6) is chosen to remove fullness from the chest and adjust qi. Qimen (Liv 14) is added to regulate qi so as to weed out the distension in the hypochondriac region and breast.

c) Irregular menstrual cycles:

i) Qi stagnation in the liver:

Method: Points of the Ren and Jueyin Meridians are selected as the principal points to ease the liver and regulate the Chong and Ren Meridians. Acupuncture is given with the even movement.

Prescription: Qihai (Ren 6), Siman (K 14), Jianshi (P 5), Ligou (Liv 5).

Supplementary points:

Distension in the hypochondriac region and breast: Tanzhong (Ren 17), Qimen (Liv 14).

Mental depression: Shenmen (H 7), Taichong (Liv 3).

Explanation: Qihai (Ren 6) and Siman (K 14) can promote the flow of qi and blood, regulate Chong and Ren Meridians. Located on the Jueyin Meridians, Jianshi (P

5) and Ligou (Liv 5) remove stagnation of the liver qi and treat disordered menses. The irregular menstrual cycles will be removed once the liver restores its normal function and the Chong and Ren Meridians are harmonized. Tanzhong (Ren 17) and Qimen (Liv 14) are included in the prescription to soothe the liver and relieve the stagnated qi of the liver and distending pain in the hypochondriac region and breast. Shenmen (H 7) and Taichong (Liv 3) ease the mind and relieve depression.

ii) Kidney deficiency:

Method: Points on the Ren and Foot-Shaoyin Meridians are selected as the principal points. Acupuncture is given with the reinforcing method. Moxibustion is used to replenish the kidney qi and regulate the Chong and Ren Meridians.

Prescription: Guanyuan (Ren 4), Shenshu (B 23), Jiaoxin (K 8).

Supplementary points:

Sore and weak low back and knees: Yaoyan (Extra), Yingu (K 10).

Dizziness and tinnitus: Baihui (Du 20), Taixi (K 3).

Explanation: Shenshu (B 23) the Back-Shu point of the kidney, can strengthen congenital essence when used together with Guanyuan (Ren 4) and Jiaoxin (K 8). The irregular menstrual cycles get redressed naturally once the kidney can carry out well its function in storing essence. Yaoyan (Extra) aims at the sore and weak low back and knees, while Yingu (K 10) strengthens the bones through kidney activation. Taixi (K 3) and Baihui (Du 20) are added to promote marrow and nourish the brain by means of tonifying kidney to treat dizziness and tinnitus.

Remarks

Included in this disorder is the irregular

menorrhea resulted from dysfunction of antehypophysis or from ovarian dysfunction.

2. Dysmenorrhea

Dysmenorrhea refers to the pain appearing in the lower abdomen and lower back before, after or during menstruation. The pain, sometimes intolerable, occurring during the cycle of menses is known as painful menstruation.

Dysmenorrhea is principally ascribed to the impeded flow of qi and blood in the uterus. Deficiency or stagnation of qi and blood may cause unsmooth flow of menstruation. Dysmenorrhea is clinically classified into dificiency and excess type.

Etiology and Pathogenesis

a) Excess syndrome:

It is due to stagnation of the liver qi, which fails to carry the free flow of blood. The impaired flow of blood causes disharmony between the Chong and Ren Meridians and stagnation of blood in the uterus, resulting in pain. Another cause is the affection of external cold or intake of cold drinks during menstrual periods, which hurts the lower jiao, and makes the cold retain in the uterus. Finally there appears retarded menstruation with pain.

b) Deficiency syndrome:

In circumstances of qi and blood deficiency due to either weak body-build or chronic disease, menstruation drains up the sea of blood and deprives the uterus from nourishment, then pain occurs.

Differentiation

a) Excess syndrome:

Main manifestations: Pain in the lower abdomen, usually starting before menstruation, retarded and scanty and dark purple menses with clots, distending pain in the lower abdomen, alleviated by passing out the clots, distension in the hypochondriac region and breast, purplish tongue with purple spots on its edge, deep and string-taut pulse; pain and cold feeling in the lower abdomen referring to the waist and back, alleviated by warmth, scanty dark red menses with clots, sticky and white tongue coating, deep string-taut pulse.

Analysis: The depressed liver qi gives rise to the distending pain in the lower abdomen, hypochondriac region and breast, and scanty and impeded menses. Qi stagnation inevitably leads to blood stasis, so the menses appears dark purple with clots. The release of clots helps to weed out a little stagnation, alleviating the pain. Purplish tongue with purple spots on its edge, deep and string-taut pulse are signs of qi stagnation and blood stasis. When the cold and damp retain in the uterus and surround the blood, there present impeded scanty menses with clots and pain in the lower abdomen. Since the uterus connects with the kidney, severe pain refers to the waist and back. Warmth alleviates the pain for it accelerates the flow of blood. White tongue coating, deep and string-taut pulse are signs of collection of internal cold and damp.

b) Deficiency syndrome:

Main manifestations: Dull pain appearing by the end of or after menstruation, alleviated by warmth and pressure, pink, scanty and thin menses, thready and weak pulse accompanied by aversion to cold, cold extremities, pale complexion, palpitation and dizziness.

Analysis: When qi and blood is insufficient the sea of blood is not able to provide enough nutrients to the uterus. This is the cause of dull pain, which can be alleviated by pressure and warmth. Deficiency of both qi and blood also gives ground to scanty pink and thin menses. Severe deficiency of qi and blood causes the failure of the heart and head to be nourished, leading to palpitation, dizziness and pale compexion. The weakened yang qi after a chronic disease is the cause of aversion to cold and cold extremities. Thready and weak pulse indicates deficiency of both qi and blood.

Treatment

a) Excess syndrome:

Method: Acupuncture is given with the reducing method. Points of the Ren and Foot-Taiyin Meridians are selected as the principal points. Both acupuncture and moxibustion are used in case of cold syndromes to adjust qi activities, invigorate blood flow and restore the functions of meridians.

Prescription: Zhongji (Ren 3), Ciliao (B 32), Hegu (L I 4), Xuehai (Sp 10), Diji (Sp 8), Taichong (Liv 3).

Supplementary points:

Distending pain in the lower abdomen: Siman (K 14), Shuidao (S 28).

Pain with cold feeling in the lower abdomen: Guilai (S 29), Daju (S 27).

Explanation: Zhongji (Ren 3) serves to regulate the qi in the Chong and Ren Meridians. When it is applied together with Xuehai (Sp 10), Diji (Sp 8), the Xi-(Cleft) Point of the Spleen Meridian, may invigorate blood flow and menstruation. Taichong (Liv 3), the Yuan-(Primary) Point of the Liver Meridian can free the stagnated liver qi, paired with Hegu (L I 4) can regulate qi and blood flow and eliminate pain. Ciliao (B 32) is an empirical point for dysmenorrhea. For distending pain in the lower abdomen it is used together with

Siman (K 14), Shuidao (S 28) to regulate the Chong and Ren Meridians and remove blood stasis and pain. Moxibustion applied to Guilai (S 29) and Daju (S 27) warms up the related meridians and eliminates pain in the lower abdomen. The above points used together are to promote the flow of qi, remove blood stasis, warm up meridians and dissipate cold. Thus dysmenorrhea gets cured when the Chong and Ren Meridians are well adjusted.

b) Deficiency syndrome:

Method: Points of the Ren, Spleen and Kidney Meridians are selected as the principal points. Acupuncture is given with the reinforcing method and moxibustion to regulate qi and blood, warm up and nourish the Chong and Ren Meridians.

Prescription: Guanyuan (Ren 4), Pishu (B 20), Shenshu (B 23), Zusanli (S 36), Sanyinjiao (Sp 6).

Explanation: Guanyuan (Ren 4) is an intersecting point of the three foot-yin meridians. When moxibustion is applied to it and Shenshu (B 23), it may warm up the lower jiao, benefit essence, blood and finally the Chong and Ren Meridians. Pishu (B 20), Zusanli (S 36) and Sanyinjiao (Sp 6) grouped together can tonify the spleen and stomach, and benefit qi and blood. Dysmenorrhea is naturally removed when the uterus is nourished by abundant qi and blood, and the balanced equilibrium of the Chong and Ren Meridians.

Remarks

This disorder often involves in pathological changes of the genitalia, and relates to endocrinal and neuropsychiatrical factors. If dysmenorrhea is secondary, treatment should be given to the primary cause.

3. Amenorrhea

Menstrual flow begins at about fourteen in healthy girls. Menstruation that does not come until 18 or suppression of menstruation for over three months is called amenorrhea. Stop of menses during gestation period and lactation period is of normal physiological phenomena. The causative factors of amenorrhea fall into deficiency and excess types. The deficiency type is mostly seen due to deficiency of blood, and the excess type is caused by excessive pathogenic factors obstructing the passage of menses.

The clinical differentiation and treatment are usually conducted in the light of blood stagnation and blood depletion.

Etiology and Pathogenesis
a) Blood stagnation:
It is due to the seven emotional disturbances, stagnation of liver qi, resulting in retardation of both qi and blood in the uterus and obstruction in the passage of menses.

b) Blood depletion:
Improper intake of food or overstrain undermines the reproducing source of qi and blood, severe or chronic diseases that consume blood, or by grand multipara or indulgence in sexual life that exhaust essence and blood, all of which may drain the sea of blood, deprive the Chong and Ren Meridians of nourishment and result in amenorrhea.

Differentiation
a) Blood stagnation:
Main manifestations: Absence of menses for months, lower abdominal distending pain aggravated by pressure, hard mass in lower abdomen, distension and fullness in the chest and hypochondriac region, dark purple tongue coating with purplish spots on its borders, deep string-taut pulse.

Analysis: Worry and anger cause qi stagnation and failure of it to control blood, bringing on blockage of the Chong and Ren Meridians and amenorrhea. The abnormal function of qi gives rise to lower abdominal distending pain and fullness in the chest and epigastrium. Blood stasis retaining in the sea of blood hinders menstrual flow, manifested by the abdominal pain aggravated by pressure and hard mass in the lower abdomen. Purple tongue coating with purplish spots on its borders and deep string-taut pulse are signs of stagnation of qi and blood.

b) Blood depletion:
Main manifestations: Delayed menstrual cycle, gradual decrease of menses and amenorrhea, sallow complexion in prolonged cases, lassitude, vertigo and dizziness, poor appetite, loose stools, dry skin, pale tongue with white coating, slow weak pulse, all of which are signs of deficiency of qi and blood; dizziness and tinnitus, sore and weak low back and knees, dry mouth and throat, hot sensation in the palms, soles and epigastrium, afternoon fever and night sweating, pale tongue with little coating, string-taut and thready pulse, all of which are signs of deficiency of essence and blood.

Analysis: Blood is transferred from food through the function of transportation and transformation of the spleen, and dysfunction of the spleen leads to blood deficiency. Blood deficiency causes malnutrition of the Chong and Ren Meridians and the voidness in the sea of blood. Hemorrhage causes exhaustion of blood, and finally delayed menstrual cycle and the gradual decrease of menses till amenorrhea. Blood deficiency fails to nourish the muscles, skin and head, bringing on sallow complexion, dry skin, vertigo and dizziness and lassitude. Dysfunction of transportation and transformation of the spleen gives rise to poor appetite and loose stools. Pale tongue with white coating and slow, weak pulse are signs of blood depletion. Since the kidney dominates bone and marrow, while the brain is the sea of marrow, deficiency in the kidney may lead to dizziness, tinnitus, sore and weak low back and knees. Yin deficiency produces internal heat manifested by the dry mouth and throat, hot sensation in palms, soles and epigastrium, afternoon fever and the night sweating. Pale tongue and string-taut thready pulse are signs of deficiency of essence and blood.

Treatment

a) Blood stagnation:

Method: Points of the Ren, Foot-Taiyang and Foot-Jueyin Meridians are selected as the principal points. Acupuncture with the reducing method is used to remove the stagnation and regulate the circulation of qi and blood in the meridians.

Prescription: Zhongji (Ren 3), Guilai (S 29), Xuehai (Sp 10), Taichong (Liv 3), Hegu (L I 4), Sanyinjiao (Sp 6).

Supplementary points:

Pain in the lower abdomen with hard mass aggravated by pressure: Siman (K 14).

Explanation: Zhongji (Ren 4), an intersecting point of the three foot-yin meridians, may regulate the Chong and Ren Meridians and dredge the blockage from the lower jiao. Guilai (S 29) is chosen as a local point to remove blood stasis from the uterus. Xuehai (Sp 10) and Taichong (Liv 3) applied together can regulate the liver qi, and relieve stagnation and stasis. Hegu (L I 4)and Sanyinjiao (Sp 6) can get qi and blood down to restore the normal menstruation. Siman

(K 14) may be added when there is pain and hard mass in the lower abdomen aggravated on pressure.

b) Blood depletion:

Method: Select points of the Ren, Liver, Spleen and Kidney Meridians. Acupuncture is used with the reinforcing method. Moxibustion is applied sometimes to tonify blood and restore menses.

Prescription: Guanyuan (Ren 4), Ganshu (B 18), Pishu (B 20), Shenshu (B 23), Zusanli (S 36), Sanyinjiao (Sp 6).

Explanation: The spleen, the foundation of the acquired essence, abstracts nutrient particles from food and transforms them into qi and blood. When blood supply is abundant the menstrual cycle is normal. So Pishu (B 20), Zusanli (S 36) and Sanyinjiao (Sp 6) are selected to strengthen the function of the spleen and stomach. The kidney is the foundation of congenital essence, and ample kidney qi guarantees sufficient qi and blood. For this reason Shenshu (B 23) and Guanyuan (Ren 4) are chosen to replenish kidney qi. Ganshu (B 18) is selected to promote the blood in the liver, where blood is stored. When the spleen, liver and kidney carry out well their functions of controlling blood, storing blood and essence respectively, the Chong and Ren Meridians are well nourished and amenorrhea is cured.

Remarks

Included in this disease is amenorrhea resulted from endocrinal and neuropsychiatrical factors.

4. Uterine Bleeding

Vaginal hemorrhage beyond menstrual period, either copious or continuously dripping, is generally defined as metrorrhagia. The copious bleeding with a sudden onset is referred to as profuse metrorrhagia, and the scanty bleeding with a gradual onset as continuous scanty uterine bleeding. Although they are different in manifestations, the two are intertransmutable during the process of the disease course. Chronic profuse bleeding consumes qi and blood, leading to continuous scanty bleeding, whereas prolonged scanty bleeding becomes worse, it inevitably turns to profuse bleeding. In terms of severity, the profuse bleeding is severe and the scanty bleeding is comparatively mild. It says in *Recipes for Saving Lives,* "Vaginal bleedings are of the same scope of a disease, while the mild one is called continuous scanty bleeding and the severe one is named profuse metrorrhagia."

Etiology and Pathogenesis

a) Excessive heat:

The causative factors may be constant excess of yang, exposure to external pathogenic heat, indulgence in spicy food and disturbance of the seven emotions, etc., which transform into internal fire. The Chong and Ren Meridians are injured by heat and there appears bleeding. It may also be due to exasperation that hurts the liver. Abundant liver fire expels the blood out of its shedding house, causing metrorrhagia.

b) Qi deficiency:

Worries, irregular intake of food and overstrain may damage the spleen qi. A weakened spleen is unable to restrict blood, instablizes the activities of the Chong and Ren Meridians and finally metrorrhagia presents.

Differentiation

a) Excessive heat:

Main manifestations: Sudden onset of profuse or prolonged continuous vaginal bleeding in deep red colour, fidgets, insomnia, dizziness, red tongue with yellow coating, rapid pulse.

Analysis: The blood escape is due to excessive internal heat. When the heat disturbs the mind there present fidgets and insomnia. Dizziness is caused by the upward going of heat. Red tongue with yellow coating and rapid pulse are signs of heat in the blood.

b) Qi deficiency:

Main manifestations: Sudden profuse bleeding or continuous scanty bleeding marked by light red and thin blood, lassitude, shortness of breath, apathy, anorexia, pale tongue, thready weak pulse.

Analysis: It is caused by the failure of the qi in control of blood and the disordered Chong and Ren Meridians. Lassitude, shortness of breath and apathy are manifestations of qi deficiency in the middle jiao. Anorexia derives from the dysfunction of the spleen in transportation and transformation. The light-coloured and thin blood is due to failure of blood to be warmed up. The pale tongue and thready weak pulse are signs of deficiency of qi and blood.

Treatment

a) Excessive heat:

Method: Mainly select points of the Ren and Foot-Taiyin Meridians. Acupuncture with the reducing method is used to clear off heat and stop bleeding.

Prescription: Zhongji (Ren 3), Xuehai (Sp 10), Yinbai (Sp 1), Ququan (Liv 8).

Supplementary points:

Affection of external heat: Quchi (L I 11).

Excessive heart fire: Shaofu (H 8).

Excessive liver fire: Taichong (Liv 3).

Explanation: Zhongji (Ren 3), the meeting point of the three foot yin meridians and the Ren and Chong Meridians, is used to adjust the qi of the Chong and Ren Meridians so as to check the escape of blood.

Yinbai (Sp 1), the Jing-(Well) Point of the Spleen Meridian, is often helpful to metrorrhagia. Ququan (Liv 8) functions to sooth and regulate the liver qi. Xuehai used (Sp 10) with the reducing method may remove heat from blood to stop bleeding. All the points functioning together can clear heat, reduce fire, regulate meridians and cease bleeding. In case of varied symptoms, Quchi (L I 11) is added to dissipate the pathogenic heat, and Shaofu (H 8) is used to clear away the heart fire, and Taichong (Liv 3) to reduce the liver fire.

b) Qi deficiency:

Method: Select the points of the Ren and Foot-Taiyin Meridians as the principal points. Acupuncture with the reinforcing method and moxibustion are employed to promote the restricting function of qi.

Prescription: Baihui (Du 20), Guanyuan (Ren 4), Zusanli (S 36), Sanyinjiao (Sp 6), Yinbai (Sp 1), Yangchi (S J 4).

Supplementary points:

Spleen qi deficiency manifested by anorexia and loose stools: Pishu (B 20), Weishu (B 21).

Explanation: Guanyuan (Ren 4) can adjust the Chong and Ren Meridians, promote the restricting function of qi and stop uterine bleeding. Sanyinjiao (Sp 6), Yinbai (Sp 1) and Zusanli (S 36) are together used to tonify the spleen and foster the restriction of qi on blood. Moxibustion applied to Baihui (Du 22) helps the ascending of yang qi, an application of the principle of using upper points for lower disorders. Yangchi (S J 4) is the Yuan-(Primary) Point of the Sanjiao Meridian, which maintains the qi in general. Needling Yangchi (S J 4) with the reinforcing method may build up the functions of the Chong and Ren Meridians and foster the restriction of qi on blood.

Remarks

This disease includes functional uterine bleeding due to ovarian dysfunction, but organic disorders of the reproductive system must be excluded.

5. Morbid Leukorrhea

Morbid leukorrhea is a disease symptomized by persistent excessive mucous vaginal discharge.

The chief causative factors of leukorrhea are deficiency of the spleen qi and stagnation of the liver qi, downward infusion of damp heat or kidney qi deficiency, leading to dysfunctions of the Chong, Ren and Dai Meridians, and leukorrhea. The ancient doctors classified the condition by its colour into white, yellow, red, red-white and multicoloured leukorrhea, among which white and yellow leukorrhagia are commonly seen in clinic.

Etiology and Pathogenesis

a) Deficiency in the spleen:

Improper diet and overstrain hinder the spleen qi from transforming and transporting nutrient particles, which accumulate in the lower jiao and turn to damp and finally leukorrhea appears.

b) Deficiency in the kidney:

Constant deficiency of kidney qi, grand multipara, dysfunctions of the Dai and Ren Meridians lead to leukorrhea.

c) Damp heat:

The presence of excessive damp due to deficiency in the spleen, changes into heat. Prolonged stagnated liver qi may transform into heat and amalgamate with the damp. The downward infusion of damp heat turns out to be leukorrhea.

Differentiation

a) Deficiency in the spleen:

Main manifestations: Profuse thick, white

or light yellow vaginal discharge without smell, pale or sallow complexion, lassitude, poor appetite and loose stools, edema in the lower limbs, pale tongue with white sticky coating, slow weak pulse.

Analysis: On account of deficiency in the spleen, the downward infusion of water and damp form leukorrhea. With deficiency in the spleen, the sapped yang qi in the middle jiao gives rise to poor appetite, loose stools and edema in the lower limbs, lustreless and pale or sallow complexion, cold extremities and lassitude. Pale tongue with white sticky coating and slow pulse are signs of deficiency in the spleen.

b) Deficiency in the kidney:

Main manifestations: Profuse and continuous discharge of thin and transparent whites, severe soreness of the low back, cold sensation in the lower abdomen, frequent and excessive urine, loose stools, pale tongue with thin coating, and deep pulse.

Analysis: Deficient kidney yang causes Dai and Ren Meridians to slacken its restriction of essence, resulting in the continuous vaginal discharge. The dimmed fire in the Mingmen is too weak to warm up the bladder and spleen and brings on frequent urine in large volume and loose stools. Sore low back is due to a weakened kidney that is situated here. When the weak kidney yang fails to keep the uterus warm, there appears a cold sensation in the lower abdomen. Pale tongue with thin white coating and deep pulse are signs of deficiency of the kidney yang.

c) Damp heat:

Main manifestations: Sticky, viscous and stinking yellow leukorrhea in large quantity, itching in the vulva, dry stool, scanty and yellow urine, soft and rapid pulse, sticky yellow coating, or leukorrhea in reddish yellow colour, bitter taste in the mouth, dry throat, irritability with a feverish sensation, palpitation, insomnia, yellow coating, string-taut and rapid pulse.

Analysis: The downgoing damp and heat hurt the Ren and Dai Meridians. This is the cause of leukorrhagia. The pathogenic heat amalgamated with damp gives rise to the yellow colour, visicosity and stench of the whites and the itching in the vulva. The internal accumulation of the pathogenic damp is the cause of dry stools and scanty yellow urine. Soft rapid pulse and yellow sticky tongue coating are signs of damp and heat. There appear irritability, bitter taste in the mouth and dry throat, when the pathogenic heat is transformed from the stagnated liver qi. Heat in the blood causes reddish leukorrhea. When heat disturbs the mind there present irritability, feverish sensation, palpitation and insomnia. The string-taut rapid pulse and yellow coating imply accumulated heat in the Liver Meridian.

Treatment

a) Deficiency in the spleen:

Method: Main points are selected from the Ren, Foot-Taiyin and Yangming Meridians. Acupuncture with the reinforcing method and moxibustion is used to build up the spleen and remove damp, regulate Ren Meridian and stabilize Dai Meridian.

Prescription: Daimai (B 26), Qihai (Ren 6), Baihuanshu (B 30), Yinlingquan (Sp 9), Zusanli (S 36).

Explanation: Daimai (B 26), an intersecting point of the Dai and Foot-Shaoyang Meridians, stabilizes the Dai Meridian and is a cure for leukorrhagia. Qihai (Ren 6) regulates qi, resolves damp, adjusts the Ren Meridian and stabilizes the Dai Meridian. Baihuanshu (B 30) is selected as an adjacent point to check leukorrhagia. Yinlingquan (Sp 9) and Zusanli (S 36), major points in this prescription, are paired to build up the spleen and remove damp.

b) Deficiency in the kidney:

Method: Select points mainly from the Ren and Foot-Shaoyin Meridians. Acupuncture with the reinforcing method and moxibustion are used to promote yang qi, tonify the kidney and stablize the Ren and Dai Meridians.

Prescription: Shenshu (B 23), Guanyuan (Ren 4), Dahe (K 12), Daimai (B 26), Fuliu (K 7).

Explanation: Shenshu (B 23), Guanyuan (Ren 4), Dahe (K 12) and Daimai (B 26), a combination of adjacent and distal points, are applied together to promote yang qi and tonify the kidney so as to restore its storing function, and stabilize the Ren and Dai Meridians, and finally check leukorrhagia. Daimai (B 26) is selected aiming at leukorrhagia.

c) Damp heat:

Method: Mainly select points from the Ren and Foot-Taiyin Meridians. Acupuncture with the reducing method is employed to clear heat, remove damp, adjust the Ren Meridian and stabilize the Dai Meridian.

Prescription: Zhongji (Ren 3), Ciliao (B 32), Sanyinjiao (Sp 6), Taichong (Liv 3).

Supplementary points:

Itching in the vulva: Ligou (Liv 5).

Reddish leukorrhea: Xuehai (Sp 10).

Excessive heat: Quchi (L I 11).

Explanation: Zhongji (Ren 3) is the Front-(Mu) Point of the bladder. It works to clear damp heat of the lower jiao when it is applied with the reducing method. Ciliao (B 32) clears heat and resolves damp to check leukorrhagia. Sanyinjiao (Sp 6), an intersecting point of the three yin meridians of foot tonifies the spleen, removes damp

and reduces the liver fire. The above points grouped together serve the purpose of clearing heat, resolving damp, adjusting the Ren Meridian and stabilizing the Dai Meridian. Ligou (Liv 5) cures the itching in the vulva by removing damp and heat away from the Liver Meridian. Xuehai (Sp 10) eliminates reddish leukorrhea by clearing heat from blood. In case of excessive heat, Quchi (L I 11) is used to clear the heat. The right usage of the auxilliary point can enhance the therapeutic results.

Remark

This disease covers infections in the reproductive organs such as vaginitis, cervicitis, endometritis and anexitis, etc.

6. Morning Sickness

Morning sickness is marked by a group of symptoms including nausea, vomiting, dizziness, anorexia within the first trimester of gestation. It is a commonly seen disorder appearing in early stage of pregnancy. Severe condition may emaciate the pregnanted woman very quickly and trigger off other diseases.

The factors are due mostly to deficiency of stomach qi, upward flux of the fetal qi invading the stomach, and perversive flow of stomach qi.

Etiology and Pathogenesis

It is caused by constant deficiency of the stomach qi, ceasation of menstruation after pregnancy and hyperfunction of the Chong Meridian, which further affect the Yangming Meridian, leading to perversive flowing of the feeble stomach qi together with the qi in the Chong Meridian, hence nausea and vomiting. In some cases, when the blood flows to nurture the fetus there results in insufficient liver blood and hyperactivity of liver yang accompanied by weakened spleen and stomach, leading to nausea and vomiting.

Differentiation

a) Deficiency in the spleen and stomach:

Main manifestations: Nausea and vomiting of liquid or indigested food immediately after meals, fullness and distending feeling in the chest, lassitude and sleepiness, pale tongue with white coating, slippery and weak pulse during the first trimester of pregnancy.

Analysis: Blood centred in the lower abdomen after pregnancy, the qi of the Chong Meridian gushes upward and the stomach qi is unable to descend due to the weakened spleen and stomach. The stomach qi does not go downward, instead, upward with the qi of the Chong Meridian, causing nausea, anorexia and vomiting right after intake of food. Weakened spleen and stomach leads to the insufficiency of yang qi in the middle jiao, manifested by fullness and distension in the epigastrium, lassitude and sleepiness, and vomiting of liquid. Pale tongue with white coating and weak slippery pulse are signs of deficiency in the spleen and stomach after pregnancy.

b) Disharmony between the liver and stomach:

Main manifestations: Vomiting of bitter or sour liquid, epigastric fullness and hyperchondriac pain, frequent belching and sighing, mental depression, dizziness and eye distension, yellowish tongue coating and string-taut slippery pulse in the early stage of gestation.

Analysis: The stagnated liver qi travels adversely along the Liver Meridian via the stomach to diaphram, hypochondrium and chest, which causes nausea, vomiting, epigastric fullness, distending·pain in the chest and hypochondrium, frequent belching and mental depression. Dizziness and eye distension are consequence of the upward influx of the liver qi. The liver and gallbladder are interiorly-exteriorly related. When there is internal liver heat fire of the gallbladder discharges, resulting in vomiting of bitter or sour liquid. Yellowish coating and string-taut slippery pulse are signs of disharmony between the liver and stomach.

Treatment

a) Deficiency in the spleen and stomach:

Method: Select points mainly from the Foot-Yangming and Foot-Taiyin Meridians. Acupuncture with the even movement is applied to build up the spleen, harmonize the stomach and quell the perversive flowing of qi so as to check vomiting.

Prescription: Zhongwan (Ren 12), Shangwan (Ren 13), Neiguan (P 6), Zusanli (S 36), Gongsun (Sp 4).

Explanation: Zhongwan (Ren 12), the Confluential Point of the fu organs and Front-(Mu) Point of the stomach, functions to harmonize the stomach when adopted together with Shangwan (Ren 13). Zusanli (S 36), the He-(Sea) Point of the Stomach Meridian, can tonify the spleen, harmonize the stomach and quell the adversive flow of the stomach qi. Gongsun (S 4) is the Luo-(Connecting) Point of the Spleen Meridian as well as the Confluential Point linking the Chong Meridian. When it is paired with Neiguan (P 6), it amplifies its function of quelling the upward going of stomach qi and checking vomiting. All the points grouped together achieve the aim of tonifying the spleen, harmonizing the stomach, descending the stomach qi and stopping vomiting.

b) Disharmony between the liver and stomach:

Method: Select points chiefly from the Foot-Yangming and Jueyin Meridians. Acupuncture with the even movement is used to relieve liver stagnation and harmonize the stomach so as to check vomiting.

Prescription: Tanzhong (Ren 17), Zhongwan (Ren 12), Neiguan (P 6), Zusanli (S 36), Taichong (Liv 3).

Explanation: Since deficiency in the spleen and stomach and upward flow of liver qi are significant to the disease, Zhongwan (Ren 12) and Zusanli (S 36) are used to tonify the spleen and harmonize the stomach, Tanzhong (Ren 17) the Influential Point of qi, is to bring qi down. Neiguan (P 6), Taichong (Liv 3) from the Jueyin Meridians are to sooth the liver, regulate the qi, counteract the abnormal upflow of qi and check vomiting.

Remarks

a) Acupuncture should not be applied to many points, nor with strong stimulation when the fetus is still young in the early stage of gestation, lest the fetal qi should be affected.

b) It is appropriate to keep the patient in bed and away from raw, cold or greasy food. In the hope of adjusting and replenishing the stomach qi, multiple meals with a little intake of food is advisable.

7. Prolonged Labour
(*Appendix:* Malposition of Fetus)

Parturition lasting over twenty-four hours is defined as prolonged labour. It is often due to weak contraction and forceless contraction of the womb, or narrow pelvic fetal and malposition of fetus.

Etiology and Pathogenesis
a) Deficiency of qi and blood:

Weak constitution with insufficient qi, exhaustion through premature contraction, premature amniorrhea, and depletion of blood due to hemorrhage, all lead to prolonged labour. In *Understanding of Childbirth,* it says, "Physical weakness and early exertion of force have exhausted the mother before the baby is delivered and thus the baby gets stuck. Dryness in the vagina also brings about difficult delivery."

b) Qi stagnation and blood stasis:

Fear or too much worry over the forthcoming delivery retards qi and stagnates blood. Extreme leisure during gestation leads to impaired flow of qi and blood. Affection of external cold during delivery hinders the circulation of qi and blood. All of them are causative factors of prolonged labour. Just as *Golden Mirror of Medicine* says, "Prolonged labour derives from various factors such as seeking comfort and ease and too much sleep, both of which lead to retarded flow of qi; or from fright and worry over the oncoming labour... and obstruction of vagina by blood stasis from an injured uterus."

Differentiation
a) Deficiency of qi and blood:

Main manifestations: Dull and paroxzysmal labour pains with mild weighing and distending sensation, or profuse hemorrhage in light colour, pale complexion, lassitude, palpitation, shortness of breath, pale tongue, weak pulse.

Analysis: Since both qi and blood are deficient and the puerperant is too weak to have uterus contraction, there are mild abdominal pain, mild heavy and distending sensation, and the delivery duration is prolonged. Qi deficiency leads to profuse hemorrhage in light colour, pale complexion, lassitude, palpitation, and shortness of breath. Pale tongue and weak pulse are signs of deficiency of qi and blood.

b) Qi stagnation and blood stasis:

Main manifestations: Sharp pains in the waist and abdomen, scanty hemorrhage in dark red colour, prolonged delivery course, dark bluish complexion, depressive mood, fullness in the chest and epigastruim, frequent nausea, dark tongue, deep forceful pulse.

Analysis: The retarded circulation of qi and blood gives rise to the sharp pain in the waist and abdomen and prolonged course of delivery. The stagnated qi does not ascend as usual, bringing about the dark bluish complexion, fullness and distension in the chest and epigastrium, and frequent nausea. The dark tongue, deep and forceful pulse indicate qi stagnation and blood stasis.

Treatment

a) Deficiency of qi and blood:

Method: Points are chiefly chosen from the Foot-Yangming and Foot-Taiyang Meridians. Acupuncture is given with the reinforcing method with moxibustion to tonify qi and blood, and quicken the delivery.

Prescription: Zusanli (S 36), Sanyinjiao (Sp 6), Zhiyin (B 67).

Explanation: Zusanli (S 36) and Sanyinjiao (Sp 6) may generate qi and blood and tonify the spleen and stomach, while Zhiyin (B 67) is an effective and empirical oxytocic point. The three points thus used together fulfil the set purpose of tonifying qi and blood and quickening the delivery.

b) Stagnation of qi and blood:

Method: Points are chiefly chosen from the Hand-Yangming and Foot-Taiying Meridians. Acupuncture is given with the reducing method to regulate qi and blood, activate qi so as to quicken the delivery.

Prescription: Hegu (L I 4), Sanyinjiao (Sp 6), Zhiyin (B 67).

Explanation: Hegu (L I 4) is the Yuan-(Primary) Point of the Hand-Yangming Meridian and Sanyinjiao (Sp 6) is an intersecting point of the three foot yin meridians. The two paired together may regulate qi and blood, clear off stasis and speed up the delivery. Zhiyin (B 67) is an effective and empirical oxytocic point.

Remarks

Acupuncture and moxibustion carry an oxytocic effect to the prolonged labour due to weak uterine contraction. Measures other than acupuncture and moxibustion should be taken in case of prolonged labour caused by uterine deformity or contracted pelvis.

Appendix: Malposition of Fetus

Malposition of fetus refers to the lying of the fetus in uterus for thirty weeks after conception. It is usually seen in multipara or those with lax abdominal wall. No symptoms are found in most cases. It is only made known by prenatal examination. The commonly seen are breech, transverse position, etc.

Treatment

Zhiyin (B 67) is selected.

Method: Moxibustion is applied to Zhiyin (B 67) bilaterally for fifteen to twenty minutes while the pregnant woman sits in chair or lies supinely in bed with the belt unclasped. Give the treatment once or twice every day till the fetal position is corrected. Zhiyin (B 67) is the Jing-(Well) Point of the Foot-Taiyang Meridian, and an empirical point for fetal malposition. The reported success rate is over 80%. It works more effectively in multiparae than primiparae. Moxibustion is much more widely adopted than acupuncture, the latter is sometimes served for the same purpose though.

There are many causative factors of the fetal malposition, they should be examined carefully. Other measures should be taken if the malposition is resulted from such factors as contracted pelvis, uterine deformity, etc.

8. Insufficient Lactation (*Appendix:* Lactifuge Delactation)

Insufficient lactation refers to the common clinical symptom that milk secretion of a nursing mother is insufficient to feed the baby. In some cases there may even be no secretion of milk at all. Ancient people named it as lack of milk and halted milk flow due to deficiency of qi and blood or to stagnation of the liver qi. It is clinically devided into deficiency and excess types.

Etiology and Pathogenesis
a) Deficiency of qi and blood:
Milk is transformed from qi and blood, the origin of which are nutrient substances of food or the acquired essence. Either the weakness of the spleen and stomach or profuse loss of qi and blood during delivery may effect the formation of milk. Zhang Jingyue in his book *Observations of Women* points out, "The qi and blood in women's Chong and Ren Meridians turn into menses when it descends, and transform into milk when it ascends. The delayed or insufficient secretion of milk after delivery is due to the insufficiency of qi and blood. Those who have no milk secretion definitely suffer from the weakness of the Chong and Ren Meridians."
b) Liver qi stagnation:
It is caused by mental depression after delivery impaired dispersing of the liver qi, disorder of qi and blood, blockage of the

meridians, and obstructed flow of milk, finally bringing on the insufficient lactation. The book *The Literati's Care of Parents* goes, "Sobbing, crying, grief, anger, depression lead to obstruction of the milk passage."

Differentiation
a) Deficiency of qi and blood:
Main manifestations: Insufficient secretion of milk after delivery or even absence of milk, or decreasing secretion during lactation period, no distending pain in the breast, pale complexion, dry skin, palpitation, lassitude, poor appetite, loose stools, pale tongue with little coating, weak and thready pulse.

Analysis: Because of the deficiency of qi and blood, the weakened transforming source of milk leads to scanty secretion without distension in breasts. Insufficient qi and blood makes pale face and dry skin. Palpitation ensues on malnutrition of the heart and blood. Dysfunction of the spleen and insufficiency of qi in the middle jiao give rise to lassitude, poor appetite and loose stools. Pale tongue and weak thready pulse are signs of deficiency of both qi and blood.
b) Liver qi stagnation:
Main manifestations: Absence of milk secretion after delivery, distending pain in breast, mental depression, chest distress and hypochondriac pain, epigastric distension, loss of appetite, pink tongue and string-taut pulse.

Analysis: Liver carries out the dispersing function of qi. Mental depression after delivery impairs liver qi, which obstructs the milk flow, leading to the distending pain in the breast, and hypochondriac pain. Disharmony of the stomach causes epigastric distension and loss of appetite. String-taut pulse is another sign of stagnated liver qi.

Treatment

Method: Mainly select the points from the Foot-Yangming Meridian. Acupuncture is given with reinforcing method and moxibustion in case of deficiency of qi and blood to tonify the qi and blood so as to promote lactic secretion. Acupuncture with either reducing or even movement or with appropriate moxibustion in case of liver qi stagnation is to remove the stagnation of liver qi, free obstruction from the meridians and promote secretion of milk.

Prescription: Rugen (S 28), Tanzhong (Ren 17), Shaoze (S I 1).

Supplementary Points:

Deficiency of qi and blood: Pishu (B 20), Zusanli (S 36), Sanyinjiao (Sp 6).

Liver qi stagnation: Qimen (Liv 14), Neiguan (P 6), Taichong (Liv 3).

Explanation: Since breast is where Foot-Yangming Meridian passes and Rugen (S 28) is located on the Stomach Meridian of Foot-Yangming at the breast, Rugen (S 28) is used here to restore the free flow of qi in the Yangming Meridian so as to promote the lactic secretion. Tanzhong (Ren 17), the Confluential Point of qi, serves to regulate qi and promotes the flow of milk. Shaoze (S I 1) is an effective and empirical lactogenic point. Pishu (B 20), Zusanli (S 36) and Sanyinjiao (Sp 6) are used to regulate and tonify spleen and stomach, promote the transformation of milk from blood. Qimen (Liv 14) and Taichong (Liv 3) are to remove stagnation of liver qi. Neiguan (P 6) is added to regulate qi flow in the chest and restore the free flow of milk.

Remarks

While receiving acupuncture for insufficient lactation, the mother should also be advised to have nutrient diet, to take plenty of soup, and to apply correct nursing method.

Appendix: Lactifuge

Those who do not want to nurse the infant after delivery can check milk secretion by acupuncture.

Point selection: Zulinqi (B 41), Guangming (B 37).

Ten-minute moxibustion is applied to each point after acupuncture. Treatment is given once every day, three to five treatments in the following day.

9. Prolapse of Uterus

Prolapse of uterus refers to descent of the uterus into the vagina, or descent of the front wall of the vagina with the uterus. Usually it is the result of the sinking of inadequate qi, kidney qi deficiency, instable Chong and Ren Meridians, and the loss of restriction by Dai Meridian.

Etiology and Pathogenesis

Its occurrence is often due to insufficiency of the qi in the middle jian caused by weak constitution, or early physical labour after delivery before qi and blood are fully restored, or exhaustion in delivery, or overstrain to counteract constipation, all of which bring about sinking of qi, which fails to keep the uterus in position. Another cause is frequent pregnancy and delivery, and indulgence in sexual life overconsuming the kidney qi and incur the loss of restriction by the Dai Meridian and weakened functioning of the Chong and Ren Meridians, hence prolapse of uterus.

Differentiation

a) Qi deficiency:

Main manifestations: Drop of the uterus in the vagina or out of the vulva several inches, sinking sensation in the lower abdomen, lassitude, palpitation, shortness of breath, frequent urine, leukorrhagia, pale tongue with thin coating, weak pulse.

Analysis: Since the qi is too weak to conduct its sustaining function of uterus, prolapse of uterus appears. It is relieved by lying down and aggravated by prolonged standing, with a sinking sensation in the lower abdomen and frequent urine. The weakened spleen and stomach lead to lassitude. Malnutrition of heart results in palpitation and shortness of breath. The downward going of pathogenic damp turns to excessive leukorrhea. Pale tongue and weak pulse are signs of qi deficiency.

b) Kidney deficiency:

Main manifestations: Prolapse of uterus, sore and weak low back and legs, bearing sensation in the lower abdomen, dryness in the vagina, frequent urine, dizziness, tinnitus, pink tongue, deep weak pulse.

Analysis: The kidney is located at the low back. With the kidney in deficiency, the Chong and Ren Meridians become weakened, and the Dai Meridian loses its restricting function, thus there appear the prolapse of uterus, frequent urine, sore and weak low back and legs. Dizziness, tinnitus and dry vagina derive from the insufficiency of essence and blood. Deep weak pulse and pink tongue are signs of kidney deficiency.

Treatment

a) Qi deficiency:

Method: Points are chiefly chosen from the Ren and Foot-Yangming Meridians. Acupuncture is applied with reinforcing method and moxibustion to replenish qi, and restore the prolapsed uterus in place.

Prescription: Baihui (Du 20), Qihai (Ren 6), Zhongwan (Ren 12), Zusanli (S 36), Guilai (S 29).

Explanation: Baihui (Du 20) is located at the vertex on the Du Meridian. Its selection indicates to "use upper points for the lower disorders." Qihai (Ren 6) is selected to replenish qi so as to strengthen its sustaining function. Zhongwan (Ren 12) and Zusanli (S 36) are used to build up the qi of the middle jiao. Guilai (S 29) is used as a local point to lift the uterus.

b) Kidney deficiency:

Method: Points are mainly selected from the Ren and Foot-Shaoyin Meridians. Acupuncture is given with the reinforcing method and moxibustion to replenish the kidney qi so as to keep the uterus in position.

Prescription: Guanyuan (Ren 4), Zigong (Extra), Ququan (Liv 8), Zhaohai (K 6).

Explanation: Guanyuan (Ren 4) is a point concerning with the primary qi, and functions to benefit kidney and lift the uterus. Zigong (Extra) is an extra point effective for prolapse of uterus. Ququan (Liv 8) and Zhaohai (K 6) paired together can tonify the kidney, nourish the tendons and sustain the uterus.

Remarks

The patient should be advised to avoid overstrain when receiving acupuncture treatment. Rest can amplify the therapeutic effect.

II. PEDIATRIC DISEASES

1. Infantile Convulsion

Infantile convulsion is commonly seen in pediatrics, manifested by series of muscle contractions accompanied by impairment of consciousness.

It can be brought about by various causes, including invasion of seasonal pathogenic factors, accumulation of internal phlegm-heat, protracted vomiting and diarrhoea, deficiency condition of the spleen with hyperfunction of the liver. It occurs in any season, mostly in those aged from one to five. Since the onset may be either sudden or gradual and the symptoms may show a deficiency condition or an excess condition, infantile convulsion can be classified into two types: acute and chronic.

Etiology and Pathogenesis

a) Acute infantile convulsion:

i) Invasion of seasonal pathogenic factors:

The skin and muslces of infants are frail, hence they are easily attacked by external pathogenic wind, which turns into fire in the interior. Infants always have excess activity of the liver, the heat therefore is liable to stir up liver wind, thus wind and fire bring about the impairment of consciousness and convulsion. The exogenous pathogenic heat can also penetrate deep into the pericardium, or the body fluid is consumed by heat and turned into phlegm which blocks the mind, resulting in loss of consciousness and convulsion.

ii) Accumulation of phlegm fire:

Irregular food intake leads to stagnation in the stomach and intestines, obstructing the flow of qi and producing phlegm heat which turns into wind, hence the disease.

iii) Sudden fright:

Infants have weak mind with insufficient vital qi. Sudden seeing of strange things and hearing of strange sounds may disturb their qi and blood and stir their mind, causing convulsion.

b) Chronic infantile convulsion:

Its onset is gradual. In most cases it is associated with a deficiency condition, such as persistent dysentery, severe vomiting and diarrhoea, or excessive administration of purgatives cold or cool in nature that injures the spleen and stomach, damaging the source of essential nutrients, and leading to deficiency of blood which fails to nourish the liver. As a result, the wind caused by the condition of deficiency is stirred up internally, giving rise to convulsion. In addition, the chronic infantile convulsion can also be the result of the acute cases that have not been treated properly.

Differentiation

a) Acute infantile convulsion:

Main manifestations: Unconsiousness, upward gazing, lockjaw, neck rigidity, opisthotonos, contracture of limbs, rapid and string-taut pulse.

If fever, headache, cough, congested throat, thirst, and irritability are present, the convulsion is due to the invasion of exogenous pathogenic heat.

If fever, anorexia, vomiting, abdominal distention and pain, sputum gurgling in the throat, constipation or defecation with stinking smell are present, it is due to phlegm heat.

If there is no fever, but cold limbs, disturbed sleep or lethargy, crying and fearing after waking, and intermittent contraction of muscles, the convulsion is probably caused by sudden fright.

Analysis: Invasion of pathogenic heat can be transmitted internally to the pericardium, so the fever is accompanied with irritability or impaired consciousness. Since there is constitutional excess of liver in infancy, the pathogenic heat can induce the liver wind. With the help of the fire the liver wind stirs upwards, resulting in upward gazing, lockjaw, and neck rigidity. Accumulation of phlegm heat and turbid dampness in the stomach and intestines obstructs the circulation of qi, thus causing anorexia, vomiting, abdominal distention and pain, and constipation. Fright harms the mind, hence there is crying with fear.

b) Chronic infantile convulsion:

Main manifestations: Emaciation, pale complexion, lasssitude, lethargy with eyes open, intermittent convulsion, cold limbs, loose stool containing undigested food, clear and profuse urination, deep and weak pulse.

Analysis: Chronic illness damages the spleen and stomach, causing disorders in digestion and transportation, thus there are emaciation, pallor and lassitude. Insufficiency of the source of essential nutrients gives rise to the deficiency of yin and blood, so that the liver fails to be nourished, and consequently the wind caused by the condition of deficiency is stirring. Therefore, the victim has lethargic sleep with open eyes and intermittent convulsion. The kidney is also involved in a long-standing case. Yang deficiency of the kidney and spleen is manifested by loose stools with undigested food, profuse and clear urination, cold limbs and deep forceless pulse.

Treatment

a) Acute infantile convulsion:

Method: Points of the Du Meridian and the Liver Meridian of Foot Jueyin, are selected as the principal points. The reducing method is applied to promote the restoration of consciousness, eliminate heat and suppress wind.

Prescription: Yintang (Extra), Shuigou (Du 26), Taichong (Liv 3).

Supplementary points:

Invasion of pathogenic heat: Dazhui (Du 14), Quchi (L I 11), Twelve Jing-(Well) Points (L 11, L I 1, H 9, S I 1, P 9, S J 1).

Convulsion due to phlegm heat: Qimai (S J 18), Zhongwan (Ren 12), Hegu (L I 4), Fenglong (S 40).

Convulsion due to fright: Sishencong (Extra), Laogong (P 8), Yongquan (K 1).

Explanation: Yintang (Extra) has a sedative action, while Shuigou (Du 26) can regulate the Du Meridian and promote resuscitation. Puncturing Taichong (Liv 3) with reducing method is to subdue the liver wind. An excess of pathogenic heat can be brought down by puncturing Dazhui (Du 14) and Quchi (L I 11). The application of Twelve Jing-(Well) Points can eliminate the heat from all the meridians. For those with excessive phlegm heat, Zhongwan (Ren 12), Fenglong (S 40) and Hegu (L I 4) are used to regulate the spleen and stomach for removing the phlegm heat. Combination with Qimai (S J 18) clears away the heat from the Sanjiao Meridian to relieve convulsion. Sishencong (Extra) has the action of tranquilization for those suffering from fright. The supplementary points, Laogong (P 8) and Yongquan (K 1), are used to calm down the mind and stop convulsion.

b) Chronic infantile convulsion:

Method: Points of Ren and Du Meridians are selected as the principal points. The reinforcing method and moxibustion are applied to adjust yin and yang for sedation and relief of convulsion.

Prescription: Baihui (Du 20), Shenting (Du 24), Guanyuan (Ren 4), Sanyinjiao (Sp 6), Zusanli (S 36).

Supplementary points:

Yang deficiency of the spleen and kidney: Pishu (B 20), Shenshu (B 23), Zhongwan (Ren 12).

Deficiency of blood: Taichong (Liv 3), Rangu (K 2).

Explanation: Since chronic infantile convulsion is due to the condition of deficiency, Baihui (Du 20) and Shenting (Du 24) are used for tranquilization, and Guanyuan (Ren 4), Sanyinjiao (Sp 6) and Zusanli (S 36) to reinforce body resistance and alleviate convulsion. Application of Pishu (B 20) and Zhongwan (Ren 12) builds up the spleen and stomach and strengthens the source of essential nutrients. Shenshu (B 23) is combined with the above points to reinforce the kidney and invigorate the yang in order to dispel the cold. Taichong (Liv 3) and Rangu (K 2) nourish yin and blood to subdue the wind and stop convulsions.

Remarks

a) Acute infantile convulsion is involved in the infections of the central nervous system and toxic encephalopathies, e.g. epidemic cerebrospinal meningitis and pneumonia with toxemia. Acupuncture has a certain antipyretic and antispasmotic effect. However, it is necessary to make the diagnosis timely and adopt a comprehensive treatment.

b) Chronic infantile convulsion is mostly caused by long duration of vomiting and diarrhoea, metabolic disorders, malnutrition and chronic infections of the central nervous system, or transmitted from acute convulsion. So the comprehensive treatment should also be adopted.

2. Infantile Diarrhoea

Infantile diarrhoea is a common disease in pediatrics, characterized by disharmony of the spleen and stomach with frequent bowel movements, and loose or watery feces. Since the children's spleen and stomach are weak, this disease is easily caused by either invasion of exogenous pathogenic factors or internal injury of milk and food. It may occur in any season, but more frequently in summer and autumn.

Etiology and Pathogenesis

The weak spleen and stomach of childern are apt to be injured by irregular diet, contaminated food, or improper attending. Dysfunction of the spleen and stomach in transportation and transformation leads to indigestion. The undigested food and water can not be separated but go together into the large intestine. This accounts for the diarrhoea. It says in Chapter 43 of *Plain Questions*, "Overintake of milk and food will harm the intestines and the stomach." Therefore, internal damage by food is an important factor of diarrhoea. Since the zang-fu organs of infants are delicate, the attack of exogenous pathogenic factors can also give rise to impairment of transportation and transformation function of the spleen and stomach, and hence diarrhoea.

Differentiation

Main manifestations: Abdominal distension is accompanied by borborygmi and frequent fits of pain. The fit of pain is followed by bowel movements, and the pain will be relieved after defecation.

There are several times of defecation a day with sour and putrid feces. The diarrhoea caused by overfeeding is marked by presence of undigested milk and food in the fecal discharge, frequent eructation, anorexia, sticky tongue coating, rolling and full pulse. In diarrhoea caused by damp heat, there are loose stools with yellow colour and offensive smell, abdominal pain, fever and thirst, burning sensation at the anus, scanty and dark urine, yellow and stick tongue coating, rolling and rapid pulse.

Analysis: Undigested milk or food accumulated in the intestines and the stomach causes abdominal distension with borborygmi and frequent attacks of pain with the desire of emptying the bowels. The pain is relieved after defecation as the food stagnation is somewhat removed. Stagnation of food leads to putrefaction, making the feces sour and putrid. The weakened spleen and stomach fail to digest food, hence there is undigested milk or food in the feces. The putrid turbidity may ascend, so there is frequent eructation. Dysfunction of the spleen and stomach in transportation and transformation gives rise to anorexia. The sticky tongue coating and rolling pulse are both the signs of food retention.

The pathogenic damp heat accumulated in the stomach and the intestines causes impairment of transportation. When the damp heat flows downward, there are loose stools with yellow colour and offensive smell, and abdominal pain. Accumulation of damp heat in the stomach and intestines brings on fever and thirst. Burning sensation at the anus and scanty dark urine are also due to the downward flow of damp heat. Yellow sticky tongue coating and rolling rapid pulse are signs of damp heat.

Treatment

Method: Points of Foot Yangming Meridian are mainly recommended with in-and-out puncturing to adjust the spleen and stomach, eliminate damp heat and stop diarrhoea.

Prescription: Tianshu (S 25), Shangjuxu (S 37), Sifeng (Extra).

Supplementary points:

Diarrhoea due to overfeeding: Jianli (Ren 11), Qihai (Ren 6).

Diarrhoea due to damp heat: Quchi (L I 11), Hegu (L I 4), Yinlingquan (Sp 9).

Analysis: Tianshu (S 25) is a point of the Stomach Meridian of Foot Yangming, and also the Front-(Mu) Point of the large intestine, while Shangjuxu (S 37) is the Lower He-(Sea) Point of the large intestine. The combination of these two points can regulate the intestines and check diarrhoea. Sifeng (Extra) can promote digestion to remove the stagnation, and strengthen transportation to stop diarrhoea. If the diarrhoea is due to overfeeding, Jianli (Ren 11) and Qihai (Ren 6) are combined in order to remove the stagnation of food, alleviate abdominal distension and fullness, and reinforce the spleen and stomach. If the diarrhoea is caused by damp heat, Quchi (L I 11) Hegu (L I 4) are used to clear away the heat, and Yinlingquan (Sp 9) to eliminate dampness and check diarrhoea.

Remarks

a) Attention should be paid to severe diarrhoea which may lead to the critical condition of the damage of both yin and yang, collapse of qi and exhaustion of yin.

b) The diet should be restricted and a light diet of small quantity is preferable.

3. Infantile Malnutrition

Infantile malnutrition is characterized by emaciation, sparse hair, distended belly with outstanding blue veins, loss of appetite, and listlessness.

The cardinal causes of this disease are irregular intake of food, improper nursing, parasitosis, and general debility due to a chronic illness which injures the spleen and stomach.

Etiology and Pathogenesis

Irregular intake of food may impair the

spleen and stomach. It is important to feed the children regularly with suitable food. Irregular food intake with indulgent ingestion of greasy, sweet, raw and cold food usually leads to retention of undigested food. Long-standing food retention damages the spleen and stomach, so that the refined nutrient from food and milk fails to be transported. Thus the qi and blood in zang-fu organs are lack of nourishment, resulting in malnutrition and emaciation with insufficiency of qi and fluid. Malnutrition may also be due to improper feeding or feeding with indigestible food which in the long run will bring on emaciation, deficiency of qi and fluid, and retardation of development. In addition, improper nursing after a chronic disease or parasitosis may also impair the functions of the spleen and stomach and consumes body fluid. Thus food can not be digested, and stagnancy of undigested food will lead to transformation into heat and ultimately to malnutrition.

Differentiation

Main manifestations: Gradual onset of slight fever or tidal fever in the afternoon, dryness of the mouth, abdominal distension, diarrhoea with offensive odour, rice-water-like urine, crying with irritability, and anorexia. Then, distended belly with protruding umbilicus due to internal stagnation, sallow complexion, emaciation, scaly and dry skin, sparse hair, dirty and sticky coating of the tongue, or complete loss of coating, and weak pulse. The above symptoms are related to deficiency of the spleen and stomach. If there is abnormal intake of food with irregular hunger or satiety, or craving for unnatural articles of food, the malnutrition is probably due to parasitosis.

Analysis: Long retention of undigested food or milk causes production of heat, so there is slight fever or tidal fever in the afternoon and crying with irritability. When the spleen fails in transportation, the damp heat is liable to be accumulated, hence there are loose bowel movements with offensive odour, rice-water-like urine, dryness of the mouth and abdominal distension. Impairment of the spleen and stomach results in anorexia and the long time stagnation causes potbelly and protruding umbilicus. The impaired spleen and stomach fail to digest food and transport the refined nutrients to nourish zang-fu organs, qi and blood, skin, muscles and hair. This is manifested by sallow complexion, emaciation, scaly dry skin and sparse hair. The grimy and sticky tongue coating reveals the internal retention of food, while the complete loss of coating demonstrates exhaustion of body fluid. Weak pulse indicates impairment of the spleen and stomach. Parasites in the abdomen disturb the stomach and intestines, resulting in abnormality of food ingestion and craving for unnatural food.

Treatment

Method: Points of Foot Taiying and Foot Yangming Meridians are selected to reinforce the spleen and remove the stagnation. Superficial pricking with filiform needles is applied and the needles are not retained.

Prescription: Xiawan (Ren 10), Weishu (B 21), Pishu (B 20), Zusanli (S 36), Sifeng (Extra), Taibai (Sp 3).

Supplementary points:

Baichongwo (Extra) for parasitosis.

Analysis: Infantile malnutrition is after all due to dysfunction of the spleen and stomach in transportation and transformation. If the spleen and stomach are active in function, the food stagnation can be removed and the source of essential nutrients can be regained. So Xiawan (Ren 10) is applied to harmonize the stomach and eliminate heat. Zusanli (S 36), the Lower He-(Sea) Point of the stomach, is used to build up earth and to replenish the qi in the middle jiao. Taibai (Sp 3), the Shu-(Stream) Point of the Spleen Meridian, is employed to reinforce the spleen and remove the stagnation. Sifeng (Extra) is an extra point beneficial for treating infantile malnutrition. Application of Pishu (B 20) and Shenshu (B 23) can invigorate the qi of spleen and stomach and restore their function of transportation and transformation. Baichongwo (Extra) is a special point to treat parasitosis.

4. Infantile Paralysis

Infantile paralysis is in the range of "wei syndrome." What is stated here is the sequellae of poliomyelitis. The causative factor of this disease is the invasion of epidemic pathogenic factors, which injure the meridians.

Etiology and Pathogenesis

This disease is mainly due to invasion of pathogenic wind, dampness and heat. These epidemic pathogenic factors invading the lung and stomach through the mouth and nose, accumulate and turn into heat which gets into and obstructs the meridians. Consequently qi and blood fail to circulate normally to nourish tendons, vessels and muscles, hence there is paralysis of the limbs. Long-lasting illness will lead to deficiency of essence and blood and affect the liver and kidney, so the tendons and muscles are withered. This is the reason why in the later stage of this disease there are flaccidity of tendons, atrophy of muscules and deformity of bones.

Differentiation

Main manifestations: Paralysis may occur in any part of the body, especially in the lower limb with weakness of the muscles and cold skin. Paralysis of the abdominal muscles is revealed by bulging of the abdomen during crying. In a chronic case there is muscular atrophy of the affected part with deformity of the trunk, and the paralysis is intractable.

Analysis: All the limbs and the skeleton of the human body rely on the nourishment of qi and blood that circulate in the meridians and collaterals. When the pathogenic factors attack the meridians and collaterals, ying (nutrient qi) and wei (defensive qi), qi and blood lose their normal flow, and tendons, vessels and muscles fail to be nourished. Therefore, the limb becomes paralytic and the skin cold. Long standing of the disease not only leads to muscular atrophy by impaired qi and blood supply, but also exhausts the essence and blood, and affects the liver and kidney. The liver dominates tendons while the kidney is in charge of bones, so the injury of the liver and kidney causes poor nourishment of the tendons and bones. As the result, the tendons become flaccid while the bones deformed, and the paralysis is intractable.

Treatment

Method: Points of Hand and Foot Yangming Meridians are selected as the principal points to regulate the circulation of qi in the meridians so as to nourish the tendons and bones. The methods of reducing, reinforcing and even movement can be adopted in different cases. Points of diseased side are punctured usually, but in a long course of treatment, the healthy side and the affected side of the body can be needled alternatively.

Prescription:

Paralysis of the upper limb:

Jianyu (L I 15), Quchi (L I 11), Hegu (L I 4), Waiguan (S J 5), Dazhui (Du 14), Tianzhu (B 10).

Paralysis of the lower limb:

Biguan (S 31), Zhusanli (S 36), Jiexi (S 41), Huantiao (G 30), Yanglingquan (G 34), Xuanzhong (G 39), Sanyinjiao (Sp 6), Kunlun (B 60), Huatuojiaji points at the lumbar region (0.5 cun lateral to the lumbar vertebrae from the first to the fifth).

Paralysis of abdominal muscles:

Liangmen (S 21), Tianshu (S 25), Daimai (G 26), Guanyuan (Ren 4).

Supplementary points:

Contracted knee: Yinshi (S 33).

Reverse flexion of knee: Chengfu (B 36), Weizhong (B 40), Chengshan (B 57).

Inversion of foot: Fengshi (G 31), Shenmai (B 62), Qiuxu (B 40).

Eversion of foot: Zhaohai (K 6), Taixi (K 3).

Difficult intorsion and extorsion of hand: Yangchi (S J 4), Yangxi (L I 5), Houxi (S I 3), Sidu (S J 9), Shaohai (H 3).

Drop of wrist: Sidu (S J 9), Waiguan (S J 5).

Analysis: This prescription follows the principle in internal classic that "only select the points of Yangming Meridians for the treatment of paralysis" Yanglingquan (G 34), the Influential Point of tendons, and Xuanzhong (G 39), the Influential Point of bones, are used to enhance the function of nourishing the tendons and bones. Other points such as Dazhui (Du 14), Tianzhu (B 10), Waiguan (S J 5), Huantiao (G 30), Liangmen (S 21), Tianshu (S 25), Daimai (G 26), Sanyinjiao (Sp 9), Kunlun (B 60), are all local points to remove the obstruction of meridians for a smooth flow of qi. Huatuojiaji points, the extra points with the action of adjusting the functions of the zang-fu organs and removing the obstruction of meridians, are also used as the local points.

Remarks

This disease should be treated as early as possible, in combination with the functional exercises for strengthening the therapeutic effect.

5. Mumps

Mumps is an acute infectious disease characterized by painful swelling in the parotid region, caused by epidemic wind heat. It happens in all the seasons of a year, but mostly in winter and spring. It is more frequently seen among preschool children, but seldom in those under two years.

Etiology and Pathogenesis

Mumps is mainly due to invasion of the epidemic pathogen which enters the body via the mouth and nose. Together with phlegm fire it obstructs the collaterals of Shaoyang Meridians, causing abnormal circulation of qi and blood and bringing on pain and swelling in the parotid region, probably associated with chills and fever.

Differentiation

Main manifestations: At the onset there are chills and fever, redness, pain and swelling in unilateral or bilateral parotid regions, and dysmasesia. When the pathogenic heat is intense, the redness, pain and swelling in the parotid region are more marked, and there are pain and swelling of the testis, high fever with irritability, dryness of the mouth and constipation, dark urine, yellow tongue coating, and superficial and rapid pulse.

Analysis: Since the disease is caused by exogenous attack of the epidemic pathogenic heat, there is the exterior syndrome of chills and fever at the beginning. Agglomeration of the pathogenic heat in the Shaoyang collaterals results in the redness, pain and swelling in the parotid region, and dysmasesia. If the pathogenic heat is intense, it will consume the fluid of the Yangming collaterals, resulting in dryness of the mouth, constipation, dark urine, etc. The Shaoyang Meridians are interiorly-exteriorly related with the Jueyin Meridians and the Foot Jueyin Meridian winds around the genital organs, so when the pathogenic factor is transmitted internally to the Jueyin Meridian, there are redness, swelling and pain of the testis. Yellow tongue coating and superficial rapid pulse are signs of invasion of pathogenic heat.

Treatment
Method: Points of Shaoyang and Yangming Meridians are mainly recommended. The superficial puncturing with reducing method is adopted to expel wind and heat and remove the agglomeration.

Prescription: Jiache (S 6), Yifeng (S J 17), Waiguan (S J 5), Quchi (L I 11), Hegu (L I 4).

Supplementary points:

Chills and fever: Lieque (L 7).

High fever: Dazhui (Du 14), Twelve Jing-(Well) Points (L 11, L I 1, P 9, S J 1, H 9, S I 1).

Swelling and pain of testis: Taichong (Liv 3), Ququan (Liv 8).

Analysis: Mumps is located in the area pertaining to Shaoyang Meridians. Yifeng (S J 17), the meeting point of Hand and Foot Shaoyang Meridians, is used to resolve the local stagnation of qi and blood. Since the Hand Yangming Meridian travels up to the face, Jiache (S 6), Quchi (L I 11) and Hegu (L I 4) are applied to eliminate the pathogenic heat. Waiguan (S J 5), the meeting point of Hand Shaoyang Meridian and Yangwei Meridian, is employed in combination with the points from Yangming Meridian, to expel the wind, dissipate the agglomeration, and clear away the pathogenic heat. Lieque (L 7) is combined to disperse wind and alleviate the exterior symptoms for those suffering from chills and fever. Dazhui (Du 14) and Twelve Jing-(Well) Points are used to bring down the high fever. Taichong (Liv 3) and Ququan (Liv 8) regain the normal circulation of qi in Foot Jueyin Meridian for those with the pain and swelling of testis.

Remarks
a) Mumps is also called epidemic parotitis. Acupuncture and moxibustion provides satisfactory effect.

b) Moxibustion with Medulla Junci.

Point: Jiaosun (S J 20)

Method: Two pieces of rush pith soaked with vegetable oil are ignited and aimed at the point Jiaosun (S J 20). Remove them quickly as soon as there is a sound of burning of the skin. Usually the swelling will subside after one treatment. The treatment can be repeated the next day if the swelling is not completely gone.

III. EXTERNAL DISEASES

1. Urticaria

Urticaria is commonly seen in clinic. It is an eruption of the skin characterized by transitory, flat-topped wheals which look like measles or are as large as broad beans. It is apt to appear after exposure to wind, so traditional Chinese medicine terms it "wind wheal." Because it comes and goes, it is also named "hidden rash." In some cases it may repeatedly occur and have not been cured for months or years.

Its etiology and symptoms are described clearly in ancient literature, e.g. in the book of *Synopsized Prescriptions of Golden Chamber* it says, "If the pathogenic qi attacks the meridians, hidden rash with itching would appear."

Etiology and Pathogenesis

a) It is due to stagnation of dampness in the skin and muscles which are again attacked by wind heat or wind cold. The confrontation against dampness is going on between the skin and muscles, so there appears wind wheal.

b) It may be caused by accumulated heat in the stomach and intestines with further attack of the pathogenic wind which could neither be dispersed from the interior nor removed from the exterior. So pathogenic wind heat stays between the skin and muscles, and results in wind wheal.

c) It may also be due to intestinal parasitosis such as ascariasis, ancylostomiasis, fasciolopsis, etc, or due to intake of fish, shrimp or crab leading to dysharmony of the spleen and stomach with accumulation of damp heat in the skin and muscles.

Differentiation

Abrupt onset with itching wheals of various size or with pimples rising one after another. It might be aggravated or lessened by the changing of weather. Acute conditions subside quickly. It is divided into the following types according to clinical symptoms:

a) Wind heat:

Main manifestations: Red rashes with severe itching, superficial and rapid pulse.

Analysis: Red colour indicates heat; itching is caused by wind. Superficial and rapid pulse is a sign of wind heat.

b) Wind damp:

Main manifestations: White or light red rashes accompanied by heaviness of the body, superficial and slow pulse, white and sticky tongue coating.

Analysis: White or light red rashes and heaviness of the body indicate stagnation of wind damp in the skin and muscles. White sticky tongue coating and superficial slow pulse are signs of wind damp.

c) Accumulation of heat in the stomach and intestines:

Main manifestations: Red rashes complicated by abdominal or epigastric pain, constipation or diarrhoea, thin yellow tongue coating and rapid pulse.

Analysis: Red colour shows heat. Epigastric and abdominal pain with constipation suggests accumulated heat in the stomach and intestines, which causes the obstruction of qi in the fu organs. Rapid pulse and yellow tongue coating indicate existence of interior heat.

Treatment

Method: The reducing method is applied to disperse wind damp and eliminate heat in the blood. Points of the Spleen and Large Intestine Meridians are selected as the principal points. Tapping on the diseased area with a "plum-blossom" needle is advisable.

Prescription: Quchi (L I 11), Hegu (L I 4), Weizhong (B 40), Xuehai (Sp 10), Sanyinjiao (Sp 6).

Supplementary points:
Wind heat: Dazhui (Du 14).
Wind damp: Yinlingquan (Sp 9).
Accumulated heat in the stomach and intestine: Tianshu (S 25), Zusanli (S 36).

Explanation: Wind rash is mainly caused by stagnation of the pathogenic wind, heat or damp in the skin and muscles or due to accumulated damp heat in the stomach and intestine, so points Quchi (L I 11) and Hegu (L I 4) of Hand-Yangming Meridian are used to disperse the pathogenic factors from the skin and muscles. Xuehai (Sp 10) and Weizhong (B 40) are combined with the former points to eliminate heat in the blood, Sanyinjiao (Sp 6) is to remove dampness, Dazhui (Du 14), the point where all the yang meridian meet, is used to reduce heat, and Yinlingquan (Sp 9) removes damp. The reducing method applied to Tianshu (S 25) and Zusanli (S 36) is to dredge the accumulated heat from the stomach and intestines.

2. Erysipelas (*Appendix:* Herpes Zoster)

Erysipelas is an acute contagious infectious skin disease characterized by sudden onset of chills, fever, local redness and swelling which may take place on any site of the body and rapidly extend.

Etiology and Pathogenesis
Erysipelas is mostly due to accumulated damp heat in the spleen and stomach flowing downward to the leg; or due to obstruction of qi and blood in meridians caused by pathogenic wind and toxic heat. Therefore the pathogenic heat infects the blood, and then the skin and muscles. Or it is due to invasion of toxin into the wound in the skin. The erysipelas arising in face and head is mostly evoked by wind heat, that in the hypochondriac, lumbar and hip regions is usually caused by liver fire, that on the leg by damp heat, and in new-born babies by internal heat.

Differentiation
Main manifestations: Rapid onset of a well demarcated patch of redness, hotness and burning pain, rapidly extending in size; change in colour of the patch from bright red to dull red in several days and then healing with desquamation. If accompanied by chills, fever, acute headache, red tongue proper with thin yellow coating, and superficial rapid pulse, it is a wind heat syndrome. If accompanied by fever, irritability, thirst, stuffy sensation in the chest, poor appetite, constipation, dark urine, yellow sticky tongue coating, soft and rapid pulse, it is a damp heat syndrome. High fever, vomiting, delirium and convulsion indicate invasion of the pathogenic factors into the interior of the body.

Analysis: Erysipelas is caused by invasion of exogenous wind heat or damp heat from the stomach and intestines into the blood, skin and muscles. Therefore the affected skin is red and painful. If it is caused by exogenous wind heat stagnating in the skin and muscles, there are chills and fever. If it is caused by damp heat in the stomach and intestines, there are high fever, thirst, stuffy sensation in the chest, poor appetite, constipation and dark urine. When the pathogenic factor penetrates into the pericardium, delirium and convulsion occur.

Treatment
Method: Points of the Yangming Meridian are selected as the principal points. The reducing method is applied to eliminate

heat and relieve toxin, or prick the points to bleed.

Prescription: Quchi(L I 11), Hegu (L I 4), Quze (P 3), Weizhong (B 40), Xuehai (Sp 10), Ashi points.

Supplementary points:

Wind heat: Fengchi (G 20).

Damp heat: Zusanli (S 36), Yinlingquan (Sp 9).

Fever: Dazhui (Du 14).

Pathogenic toxin attacking the interior: Twelve Jing-(Well) points (L 11, L I 1, P 9, S J 1, H 9, S I 1), Laogong (P 8).

Constipation: Zhigou (S J 6).

Explanation: Quchi (L I 11) and Hegu (L I 4) disperse wind heat from the Yangming Meridians. Reducing Xuehai (Sp 10) and bloodletting of Weizhong (B 40), Quze (L I 11) and Ashi points are to clear off heat from the blood, i.e. "eliminating the accumulted heat by reducing method." The reducing method used to Zusanli (S 36) and Yinlingquan (Sp 9) is to dispel damp heat. Pricking the twelve Jing-(Well) points to cause bleeding and reducing Laogong (P 8) are to expel heat from the skin and heart. Reducing Dazhui (Du 14) and Fengchi (G 20) remove the pathogenic heat and relieve exterior symptoms. Zhigou (S J 6) is used for constipation by removing heat.

Remarks

Strict sterilization is necessary to avoid infection. If ulcer occurs due to mixed infection, or if there is septicaemia or pyemia, comprehensive treatment should be applied.

Appendix: Herpes Zoster

Herpes zoster occurs mainly in the lumbar and hypochondriac regions with small red vesicles like beads forming a girdle around the waist. It is mostly caused by endogenous damp heat, hyperactivity of fire in the liver and gallbladder or affection of exogenous toxin. At the onset there is stabbing pain of the affected skin, which soon becomes erythematous. Patches of blisters in the size of mump-beans or soybeans are evolved, forming a bandlike distribution with clearcut interspaces between the patches. The blisters are thick-walled and their contents are transparent at first, but turn turbid in five to six days. Resolution of the cutaneous lesions after decrustation without scar formation occurs in about ten days. In some cases pain lasts longer.

Treatment

Firstly, the head and the tail of the location of herpes zoster should be distinguished. The area where the skin lesions first appeared is considered as the tail, while the extending part of herpes as the head of its locality. Prick the skin around herpes zoster with a three-edged needle to cause a little bleeding: five pricks at 0.5 cun from the head of the herpes zoster area and then five pricks at 0.5 cun from the tail, and also several pricks along both sides. Then select Quchi (L I 11), Xuehai (Sp 10), Weizhong (B 40), Yanglingquan (G 34), Taichong (Liv 3).

Explanation: Pricking the skin around herpes zoster with a three-edged needle to cause bleeding is to reduce the pathogenic toxin. Quchi (L I 11) dispels wind and clears off heat. Xuehai (Sp 10) and Weizhong (B 40) eliminate heat in the blood. Yanglingquan (G 34) and Taichong (Liv 3) reduce damp heat from the liver and gallbladder.

3. Boil and "Red-Thread Boil"

Boil frequently occurs on the face, head and extremities. It has different names according to its location and form, e.g. "philtrum boil" if it is located at the median line of the upper lip, "snake-head boil" if it occurs at the finger tip which looks like the head of a snake, "red-thread boil" if there is a red line extending outward from the boil.

Etiology and Pathogenesis

Boil is usually caused by fatty and spicy food or contamination of the skin. The former may lead to accumulation of heat in zang-fu organs and then production of endogenous toxicity. The latter may result in invasion of the exogenous toxic factor and stagnation of qi and blood. It would be dangerous if the pathogenic toxic factor is transmitted into the meridians and the zang-fu organs.

Differentiation

Main manifestations: Boil on the head, face or extremity first appears like a grain of millet in yellow or purple colour. A blister or pustula with a hard base is formed, usually accompanied by tingling. Later there is increased redness, swelling and pain with burning sensation, often accompanied by chills and fever. Sometimes a red thread-like line extends proximally if the boil toxicity attacks the interior, there will be high fever, restlessness, dizziness, vomiting, impaired consciousness, reddened tongue with yellow coating, and rapid pulse, indicating that the toxicity is deeply rooted.

Analysis: When the toxic heat stays in the skin and muscles and drops into the meridians, resulting in stagnation of qi and blood, a swollen induration is formed. Since the stagnation is not severe, there is only mild tingling. Further accumulation of heat and toxicity causes aggravation of redness, swelling and burning pain. Since the pathogenic factors are in the exterior

portion of the body, there are chills and fever. Toxicity and heat travel along the vessels and bring about a red thread-like line extending proximally. High fever, restlessness and impairment of consciousness are due to invasion of the pathogenic heat and toxicity into the pericardium. Reddened tongue with yellow coating and rapid pulse are signs of toxic heat.

Treatment

Method: Points of the Du and Hand-Yangming Meridians are selected as the principal points. The reducing method or pricking with a three-edged needle to cause bleeding is used. For red-thread boil, prick with a three-edged needle to cause bleeding at two-inch intervals along the red line proximally towards the focus.

Prescription: Lingtai (Du 10), Shenzhu (Du 12), Ximen (P 4), Hegu (L I 4), Weizhong (B 40).

Supplementary points:

Points may be selected along the meridians related to the location of the boil, e.g. boil on the face: Shangyang (L I 1), Quchi (L I 11); on the tip of fingers: Quchi (L I 11), Yingxiang (L I 20); on temporal region: Yanglingquan (G 34), Zuqiaoyin (G 44); and on the fourth or fifth toe: Yanglingquan (G 34), Tinghui (G 2).

Explanation: Lingtai (Du 10) is an empirical point for the treatment of boil. Shenzhu (Du 12) readjusts the qi of all the yang meridians in order to disperse heat. Ximen (P 4), the Xi-(Cleft) Point of the Pericardium Meridian is effective for eliminating heat in the blood and stopping pain, and Hegu (L I 4) for removing the exogenous pathogenic factors from the exterior of the body. Weizhong (B 40) is effective for clearing away toxin from the blood. These points used together act on relieving toxicity and dispersing heat. Pricking the points to cause bleeding expels toxin and heat from the blood. Points combined with the main ones are used to remove the obstruction of qi and blood of the local meridians. The selection of points along the meridians related to diseased area is based upon the following theory: "The therapeutic effect will reach where the meridian is opened up."

Remarks

Another effective method for treating boil is to prick and tilt with a three-edged needle into small papules found alongside the thoracic vertebrae. Treatment is given once a day.

4. Breast Abscess

Breast abscess is an acute purulent disorder of the breast mostly found in lactation period after delivery. It is rare in the duration of pregnancy.

Etiology and Pathogenesis

It is caused by retention of milk in the breast due to mental depression affecting the qi of the liver or due to overtaking of fatty food that brings about stagnation of heat in the Stomach Maridian or due to obstruction of the milk duct after invasion of exogenous toxic fire into the breast through the rupture of the nipple.

Differentiation

Main manifestations: Redness, swelling and pain of the breast, mostly occurring after delivery. At the early stage when the abscess has not yet been formed, there is a lump in the breast accompanied by swelling, distension, pain, difficult lactation, chills, fever, headache, nausea, and dire thirst. Growing of the lump with local bright redness and intermittent throbbing pain indicates suppuration.

Analysis: Since the stagnated liver qi and obstructed lactation lead to producton of heat, there occurs redness, swelling, and pain of the breast with difficult lactation. The confrontation between the exogenous pathogenic factors and the body resistance causes chills, fever and headache. The pathogenic heat in the stomach disturbs the descending of the stomach qi, manifested by nausea and dire thirst. Unrelieved stagnation of milk may produce heat. "Extreme heat causes putrid muscle, and pus follows." So there is growing of the lump in the breast with bright redness, burning and intermittent throbbing pain.

Treatment

Method: The reducing method is applied to regulate the qi of the Liver and Stomach Meridians, remove stagnation and disperse heat. Points of Foot-Jueyin, Foot-Shaoyang and Foot-Yangming Meridians are selected as the principal points.

Prescription: Jianjing (G 21), Tanzhong (Ren 17), Rugen (S 18), Shaoze (S I 1), Zusanli (S 36), Taichong (Liv 3).

Supplementary points:

Chills and fever: Hegu (L I 4), Waiguan (S J 5).

Distension and pain in the breast; Zulinqi (G 41).

Explanation: The nipple is on the Liver Meridian, and the breast is located in the area where the Stomach Meridian is distributed. The breast abscess is caused by pathogenic heat in the stomach and the stagnation of liver qi. That is why Taichong (Liv 3) is used to remove the stagnation, Zusanli (S 36) and Rugen (S 18) are to lower the stomach fire in order to eliminate the accumulation of pathogenic factors in the Yangming Meridian. Tanzhong (Ren 17) is to regulate the activity of qi and remove obstruction of lactation. Foot-Shaoyang Meridian runs along the chest and hypochondriac regions, so Jianjing (G 21) is used to adjust qi circulation and remove obstruction of qi in the chest and hypochondriac regions, being an effective point in treating the breast abscess. Shaoze (S I 1) is an empirical point for the treatment of the breast abscess. Hegu (L I 4) clears the heat away from the Yangming Meridian. Waiguan (S J 5) connecting the Yangwei Meridian is used to treat chills and fever. Zulinqi (G 41) spreads qi and blood and removes obstruction of lactation so as to relieve distension and pain in the breast.

Remarks
This condition corresponds to acute mastitis in modern medicine.

5.   Intestinal Abscess

Intestinal abscess is an acute abdominal disorder occurring in the intestines. According to the ancient literature, it can be classified into large-intestinal abscess and small-intestinal abscess. The abscess with pain around Tianshu (S 25) is known as "large-intestinal abscess," while that with pain around Guanyuan (Ren 4) is named "small-intestinal abscess." Because extension of the right leg is limited, it is also called "leg-contracted intestinal abscess."

Etiology and Pathogenesis
Intestinal abscess is caused by irregular intake of food, retention of undigested food, undue cold and warmth, or running after a big meal. All these factors may give rise to dysfunction of the intestines in transmission with accumulation of damp heat and stagnation of qi and blood, which in combination will lead to suppuration and abscess formation.

Differentiation
Main manifestations: At the onset there is sudden paroxysmal pain in the upper abdomen or around the umbilicus. Soon the pain becomes continuous and localized in the right lower abdomen near Tianshu (S 25), accompanied by tenderness, mild contracture of the abdominal wall, difficulty in extension of the right leg, fever, chills, nausea, vomiting, constipation, dark urine, thin, sticky and yellow tongue coating, rapid and forceful pulse. If the pain is severe and there is contracture of the abdominal wall with marked tenderness or palpable mass, accompanied by high fever and spontaneous sweating, forceful and rapid pulse, the condition is serious.

Analysis: Intestinal abscess is due to accumulation of damp heat and stagnation of qi and blood that obstructs the pathway of the stomach and intestines. So it is manifested by localized abdominal pain and tenderness. Intestinal abscess mostly occurs in the appendix which is located in the right lower abdomen, and hence severe abdominal pain is present in this quadrant. Stagnation of qi and blood, imbalance between the nutrient qi and defensive qi, and confrontation between the pathogenic factors and the body resistance result in fever and chills. When the stomach qi fails to descend, there are nausea and vomiting. Yellow-sticky tongue coating and rapid, forceful pulse indicate an excess syndrome caused by accumulation of damp heat in the stomach and intestines. Sharp pain with contracture of the abdominal wall, tenderness, local mass, high fever, spontaneous sweating, and rapid forceful pulse indicate suppuration with collection of pus and extreme heat in the Yangming Meridians.

Treatment

Method: To disperse damp heat, regulate qi circulation and stop pain by reducing method. Points of the Yangming Meridians are selected as the principal points. Needles are retained for a long time from thirty to one hundred twenty minutes. Manipulation is given every ten minutes, and treat every six to eight hours. When the symptoms and signs are alleviated, treatment should be given once daily with needles retained for thirty minutes.

Prescription: Tianshu (S 25), Quchi (L I 11), Lanwei (Extra), Shangjuxu (S 37).

Supplementary points:

Fever: Dazhui (Du 14), Hegu (L I 4).

Vomiting: Neiguan (P 6), Zhongwan (Ren 12).

Explanation: Lanwei (Extra) is an empirical point in treating the intestinal abscess. Shangjuxu (S 37), the lower He-(Sea) Point of the large intestine, together with Tianshu (S 25), the Front-(Mu) Point of the large intestine, are used to remove accumulation of damp heat from the intestines and to promote qi circulation and stop pain. Quchi (L I 11), the He-(Sea) Point of the Large Intestine Meridian, is used to eliminate heat from the intestines. Dazhui (Du 14) and Hegu (L I 4) are used to strengthen the antipyretic action. Neiguan (P 6) and Zhongwan (Ren 12) are used to harmonize the stomach and stop vomiting.

Remarks

"Intestinal abscess" is chiefly referred to acute simple appendicitis in modern medicine, for which acupuncture treatment is considered effective. If there is appendicial abscess or tendency to perforate, other therapeutic measures should be resorted to. For chronic appendicitis, the above-mentioned points may also be used. Acupuncture is given once a day or every other day. Moxibustion may be applied locally at the same time.

6.   Goiter

Goiter denotes an enlargement of the thyroid gland, causing a swelling in the front part of the neck, which is not accompanied by pain, ulceration or skin discolouration. According to the records of ancient literature, it can be classified as "qi goiter," "flesh goiter" and "stone goiter." In this section only "qi goiter" and flesh goiter" are discussed.

Etiology and Pathogenesis

Goiter may be caused by exasperation, anxiety or mental depression which leads to stagnation of qi and accumulation of fluid forming phlegm. It also occurs in certain localities where the soil and water are not good. In the book *General Treatise on the Etiology and Pathogenesis*, it says: "Mountainous areas with black soil where the spring takes its source are not good for permanent dwelling, because drinking the spring water causes goiter." Generally speaking, qi goiter is mostly caused by drinking mountainous water and qi stagnation, and flesh goiter by stagnation of qi and accumulation of phlegm damp.

Differentiation

Main manifestations: Qi goiter is marked by diffusive swelling in the neck, soft, gradually increasing in size with unclear margins, normal colour, absence of pain; in some cases big and drooping, accompanied with dyspnea and hoarseness of voice. The size of the goiter usually changes with emotions.

Flesh goiter often occurs in individuals below forty , more frequently in women than in men, a few oval movable lumps below the Adam's Apple with smooth surface and without pain, accompanied by exophthalmos, hot temper, irritability, tremor of the hands, sweating, stuffiness in the chest, palpitation, string-taut, slippery and rapid pulse, and irregular menstruation.

Treatment

Method: Activiate blood circulation and remove blood stasis, and disperse the agglomeration through promoting the qi circulation by reducing method. Points of Hand Shaoyang and Yangming Meridians are selected as the principal points.

Prescription: Naohui (S J 13), Tianding (L I 17), Tianrong (S I 17), Tiantu (Ren 22), Hegu (L I 4), Zusanli (S 36).

Supplementary points:

Liver-qi stagnation: Tanzhong (Ren 17), Taichong (Liv 3) with even movement.

Palpitation: Neiguan (P 6), Shenmen (H 7) with the reinforcing method.

Exophthalmos: Sizhukong (S J 23), Zanzhu (B 2), Jingming (B 1), Fengchi (G 20) with even movement.

Hot temper, anxiety and sweating: Sanyinjiao (Sp 6) and Fuliu (K 7) with even movement.

Explanation: Naohui (S J 13) is a point of the Sanjiao Meridian of Hand-Shaoyang.

Sanjiao dominates the qi of the whole body. So Naohui (S J 13) is used to remove obstruction from the meridians in order to relieve qi stagnation and phlegm accumulation for the goiter. Tianding (L I 17), Tianrong (S I 17) and Tiantu (Ren 22) are located on the neck. Puncturing them is to regulate the local circulation of qi and blood, to remove blood stasis and disperse agglomeration. Hegu (L I 4) and Zusanli (S 36) belong respectively to the Hand and Foot Yangming Meridians, which pass through the neck region. They have the action of promoting qi circulation in the Yangming Meridians and eliminating stagnation of qi and blood. Tanzhong (Ren 17) is an Influential Point of qi, and Taichong (Liv 3) is the Yuan-(Primary) Point of the Liver Meridian. Both are used to regulate the circulation of the liver qi. Shenmen (H 7) is the Yuan-(Primary) Point of the Heart Meridian, and Neiguan (P 6), the Luo-(Connecting) Point of the Pericardium Meridian. They are effective for palpitation. Sizhukong (S J 23), Zanzhu (B 2) and Jingming (B 1) are local points. Fengchi (G 20) connects with the eye region. These four points are used together to readjust the circulation of qi and blood in the eye region so as to control exophthalmos. Sanyinjiao (Sp 6) and Fuliu (K 7) are used to reinforce yin and check yang in order to relieve irritability, boulimia and excessive perspiration.

Remarks

1. The morbid condition described here refers to simple goiter and hyperthyroidism in modern medicine.

2. The method of puncturing with several needles surrounding the goiter and with one needle in the center has a fairly good effect of reducing the goiter.

7. Sprain and Contusion
(*Appendix:* Torticollis)

Sprain and contusion here refer to the injury of soft tissues, such as skin, muscles and tendons of the trunk or limbs without fracture, dislocation or wound.

Main manifestations are pain and swelling of the injured areas, and motor impairment of the joints.

Etiology and Pathogenesis

Local stagnation of qi and blood in the meridians of diseased areas is due to injury of tendinous tissues and joints by violent movement, awkward posture of the body, bruise, falling, traction or overtwisting.

Differentiation

Main manifestations: Local swelling and pain, redness or ecchymosis. A new injury is slightly swollen with tenderness. Large area of swelling together with motor impairment of the joints is found in serious cases. Old injury is characterized by absence of marked swelling but repeated recurrence due to invasion of exogenous pathogenic wind, cold and damp. The injury mostly happens in the shoulder, elbow, wrist, back, hip, knee, and ankle.

Analysis: Sprain or contusion at any place of the body is due to tendinous injury with local qi stangation and blood stasis, manifested by swelling and pain with tenderness. In a protracted case, qi and blood are consumed, and their circulation in the meridians tends to be further obstructed by exposure to wind, cold and damp. That is why pain is exacerbated in bad weather.

Treatment

Ashi points are used as the principal points. Local and distal points of involved meridians may be combined to ease tendons and activiate blood circulation, relieving swelling and pain. Apply needling plus moxibustion to the local points and needling alone to the distal points.

Prescription: Ashi points.

Supplementary points:

Neck: Tianzhu (B 10), Houxi (S I 3).

Shoulder joint: Jianjing (G 21), Jianyu (L I 15).

Elbow joint: Quchi (L I 11), Hegu (L I 4).

Wrist joint: Yangchi (S J 4), Waiguan (S J 5).

Hip joint: Huantiao (G 30), Yanglingquan (G 34).

Knee joint: Dubi (S 35), Neiting (S 44).

Ankle joint: Jiexi (S 41), Qiuxu (G 40), Kunlun (B 60).

Explanation: Local and distal points from the affected meridians are selected to promote the circulation of qi and blood in the meridians. Moxibustion to the local points promotes the circulation of qi and blood by warmth so as to relieve swelling and pain, and to speed up the recovery of the injuried tissues.

Remarks

Needling can be applied to the healthy side at the area corresponding to the affected area. When manipulating the needle, ask the patient to move the sprained joint. Alleviation or subsidence of pain may be expected.

Appendix: Torticollis

Torticollis here refers to wry neck caused by an awkward sleeping posture or attack of wind cold on the nape that leads to disturbance of local circulation of qi in the meridians. Its main manifestations are stiffness and pain of the neck and nape, and wry neck towards one side with motor impairment.

Method: Points of the Du Meridian and Taiyang Meridians are selected as the principal points. The reducing method and moxibustion are applied to Dazhui (Du 14), Tianzhu (B 10), Jianwaishu (S I 14), Xuanzhong (G 39), Houxi (S I 3) to expel wind and disperse cold, and to relax tendons and activiate blood and qi circulation in the meridians. Kunlun (B 60) and Lieque (L 7) are added for inability of flexion and extension. Zhizheng (SI 7) is added for difficulty in rotating the neck so as to promote the qi circulation of Taiyang Meridians. Cupping may be applied after needling, or Laozhen (Extra) is used alone for stiff neck.

IV. DISEASES OF EYES, EARS, NOSE AND THROAT

1. Deafness and Tinnitus

Both deafness and tinnitus are auditory disturbances. Tinnitus is characterized by ringing sound in the ears felt by the patient and deafness is failing or loss of hearing. Because of the similarities between these two conditions in etiology and treatment, they are discussed together.

Etiology and Pathogenesis
Deafness and tinnitus can be divided into two types: deficiency and excess. The excess type is caused by fury or fright with upward rush of wind fire of the liver and gallbladder that obstructs the qi circulation in the Shaoyang Meridians or caused by invasion of pathogenic wind blocking the orifice. The deficiency type is due to deficiency of the

kidney qi and failure of essential qi to ascend to the ear.

Differentiation
a) Excess type:
Main manifestations: Sudden deafness, distension sensation and constant ringing in the ear that can not be eliminated by pressing. In the case of upward perversion of pathogenic wind fire of the liver and gallbladder, there are flushed face, dry mouth, irritability and hot temper, forceful and string-taut pulse. In the case of invasion by exogenous pathogenic wind, there appear headache and superficial pulse.

Analysis: The pathogenic fire of the liver and gallbladder that flames up along the related meridians results in deafness, tinnitus, headache, flushed face, bitter taste in the mouth and dryness of the throat. Hyperfunction of the liver causes hot temper, and irritability is brought about by the pathogenic heat disturbing the mind. Forceful and string-taut pulse indicates the excess condition of the liver and gallbladder. When the pathogenic wind attacks the exterior of the body and obstructs the orifices, deafness, tinnitus and headache occur. Superficial pulse is a sign of invasion of the exogenous pathogenic wind.

b) Deficiency type:
Main manifestations: Protracted deafness, intermittent tinnitus aggravated by strain and eliminated by pressing, dizziness, soreness and aching of the lower back, seminal emission, excessive leukorrhea, thready and weak pulse.

Analysis: Hypofunction of the kidney makes essential qi fail to ascend and fill up the orifices, so there are deafness, tinnitus and dizziness. The loin is the house of the kidney, so hypofunction of the kidney causes soreness and aching of the lower back. Deficiency of the kidney qi with impaired restraining function or deficiency of yin with flaming up of the asthenic fire that stimulates the seminal organs causes emission. Since the kidney loses its function of restricting the Dai Meridian, there is excessive leukorrhea. Thready and weak pulse are signs of deficiency condition.

Treatment
Method: Points of Shaoyang Meridians of Hand and Foot are used as the principal points. The reducing method is applied for excess condition, while the reinforcing method for deficiency condition. Moxibustion is also advisable.

Prescription: Yifeng (S J 17), Tinghui (G 2), Xiaxi (G 43), Zhongzhu (S J 3).

Fire preponderance in the liver and gallbladder: Xingjian (Liv 2), Zulinqi (G 41).

Invasion of exogenous pathogenic wind: Waiguan (S J 5), Hegu (L I 4).

Hypofunction of the kidney: Shenshu (B 23), Mingmen (Du 4), Taixi (K 3).

Explanation: The Shaoyang Meridians of Hand and Foot travel to the ear region, so points of Shaoyang Meridians are used, e.g. Zhongzhu (S J 3), Yifeng (S J 17) of Hand-Shaoyang, Tinghui (G 2) and Xiaxi (G 43) of Foot-Shaoyang, to regulate the qi circulation in the meridians. In the prescription, two local and two distal points are combined. Xingjian (Liv 2) and Zulinqi (G 41) are used to clear away the pathogenic fire from the liver and gallbladder, and to connect the upper and lower portions of the body. Waiguan (S J 5) and Hegu (L I 4) expel pathogenic wind. Shenshu (B 23), Mingmen (Du 4) and Taixi (Liv 3) reinforce the essential qi of the kidney.

Remarks
Tinnitus and deafness may be present in various diseases, most of which seen in acupuncture clinic are neural.

2. Congestion, Swelling and Pain of the Eye

Congestion, swelling and pain of the eye is an acute condition in various external eye disorders.

Etiology and Pathogenesis
This condition is mostly due to exogenous pathogenic wind heat causing obstruction of qi circulation in the meridians, or due to preponderance of fire in the liver and gallbladder which flares up along the related meridians, causing qi stagnation and blood stasis in the meridians.

Differentiation
Main manifestations: Congestion, swelling and pain of the eye, photophobia, lacrimation and sticky discharge. In the case of wind heat, there occur fever, superficial and rapid pulse. In the case of preponderance of fire in the liver and gallbladder, there are bitter taste in the mouth, irritability with feverish sensation, constipation and string-taut pulse.

Analysis: When the pathogenic wind heat attacks the eye, congestion, swelling and pain of the eye, photophobia, lacrimation and sticky discharge take place. Headache, fever and superficial-rapid pulse are also signs of exogenous attack of the pathogenic wind heat. The liver has its specific body opening in the eyes, and the Gallbladder Meridian starts at the outer canthus. Upward disturbance of fire in the liver and gallbladder may bring about congestion, swelling and pain of the eye, bitter taste in the mouth, and irritability. String-taut pulse is a sign of the liver trouble.

Treatment
Method: Distal and local points are used in combination to disperse wind heat. Needling is given with the reducing method.

Prescription: Jingming (B 1), Fengchi (G 20), Taiyang (Extra), Hegu (L I 4), Xingjian (Liv 2).

Supplementary points:

Wind heat: Waiguan (S J 5).

Fire preponderance in the liver: Taichong (Liv 3).

Explanation: The liver has its specific body opening in the eyes; Shaoyang, Yangming and Taiyang Meridians all run up to the eye region. Therefore Fengchi (G 20) and Hegu (L I 4) are used to regulate the qi circulation of the Yangming and Shaoyang Meridians in order to dispel wind and heat. Jingming (B 1) is where the Taiyang and Yangming Meridians meet, and is used to disperse the local accumulated heat. Xingjian (Liv 2), the Ying-(Spring) Point of the Liver Meridian, can conduct the qi of the Jueying Meridian downward so as to remove the heat from the liver. Taiyang (Extra), an adjacent point to the eye region, is pricked to bleed to reduce heat and relieve swelling. In case of wind heat, Waiguan (S J 5) is used to clear it away from the head and eyes. Taichong (Liv 3), the Yuan-(Primary) Point of the Liver Meridian, is selected to clear off the fire from the liver and gallbladder.

Remarks
This condition is involved in acute conjunctivitis, pseudomenbranous conjunctivitis, epidemic kerato-conjunctivitis, etc. in modern medicine.

3. Thick and Sticky Nasal Discharge

It is accompanied by nasal obstruction and loss of the sense of smell.

Etiology and Pathogenesis
Occurrence of thick sticky nasal discharge is related to the attack of pathogenic factors on the lung which has its specific body opening in the nose. Exogenous wind cold may transform into heat. Sometimes, the lung is directly attacked by wind heat. Both may lead to dysfunction of the lung and invasion of the pathogenic factors upon the nose through the upper respiratory tract.

Differentiation
Main manifestations: Nasal obstruction, loss of the sense of smell, yellow fetid nasal discharge, thick and sticky, accompanied by cough, dull pain in the forehead, rapid pulse, reddened tongue with thin, white and sticky coating.

Analysis: Pathogenic heat accumulated in the lung impedes the descending of the lung qi, then pathogenic heat rushes up to the nose, causing nasal obstruction. Pathogenic heat consumes the body fluid and changes it into phlegm and mucus, so there is turbid and fetid nasal discharge. Cough results from adverse flow of the lung qi. When extreme heat in the lung and stomach further disturbs the upper orifices, pain with distension occurs in the forehead. Reddened tongue and rapid pulse are signs of pathogenic heat in the lung.

Treatment
Method: Points of the Hand-Taiyin and Hand-Yangming Meridians are selected as the principal points to smooth the flow of the lung qi and expel pathogenic wind heat by applying the reducing method.

Prescription: Lieque (L 7), Yingxiang (L I 20), Bitong (Extia), Hegu (L I 4), Yintang (Extra).

Explanation: Lieque (L 7) smoothes the flow of the lung qi and eliminates the pathogenic wind. The Hand-Yangming Meridian is exteriorly-interiorly related to the Hand-Taiyin Meridian, and travels by the sides of nose. So Hegu (L I 4) and Yingxiang (L I 20) are selected to regulate the qi circulation in the Hand-Yangming Meridian and to clear away the heat from the lung. Yintang (Extra) is close to the nose, and Bitong (Extra) is located at the sides of the nose. Both have the action of removing the obstruction and eliminating heat from the nose.

Remarks

This condition corresponds to chronic rhinitis and chronic nasosinusitis in modern medicine.

4. Epistaxis

Etiology and Pathogenesis

The lung qi flows up to the nose. The Foot-Yangming Meridian starts at the side of the nose. If there is accumulated wind heat in the lung or pathogenic fire in the stomach, they would rush upward to the nose. If there is yin deficiency leading to upflaring of the asthenic fire, the blood would flow up together with the fire. All of these cause blood to rush out of the vessels, resulting in epistaxis.

Differentiation

a)   Extreme heat in lung and stomach:

Main manifestations: Epistaxis accompanied by fever, cough, reddened tongue, superficial and rapid pulse; or dire thirst with preference for cold drink, constipation, foul breath, reddened tongue with yellow coating, forceful and rapid pulse.

Analysis: Extreme heat in the lung goes up to the nose, forcing blood to rush out of the vessels. The heat also causes dysfunction of the lung in spreading and descending of qi. The reverse flow of qi results in cough. Reddened tongue and rapid pulse are signs of heat in the lung. Sometimes epistaxis occurs when the stomach fire flares up along the meridians to the nose, and injures the blood vessels. Thirst and preference for cold drinking are caused by the stomach heat consuming the fluid. Exhaustion of fluid causes constipation. The stomach heat makes foul breath. Irritability and restlessness are due to extreme heat in the Yangming Meridians disturbing the heart mind. Reddened tongue with yellow coating and forceful rapid pulse are signs of the stomach heat.

b)   Deficiency of yin with preponderance of fire:

Main manifestations: Epistaxis accompanied by malar flush, dryness of the mouth, feverish sensation of the palms and soles, afternoon fever, night sweating, thready and rapid pulse.

Analysis: When deficiency of the kidney yin causes the asthenic fire to flare up to the nose, blood vessels are injured, resulting in epistaxis. Malar flush, dryness of the mouth, feverish sensation of the palms and soles, and afternoon fever are manifestations of the asthenic fire associated with yin deficiency. Night sweating is also due to the asthenic fire that forces the moisture to be given off. Thready and rapid pulse is a sign of yin deficiency.

Treatment

Method: Points of the Hand-Yangming

and Du Meridians are selected as the principal points. The reducing method is applied to clear off the heat and stop bleeding for extreme heat in the lung and stomach. The even movement is used to nourish yin and descend the fire for deficiency of yin with preponderance of fire.

Prescription: Yingxiang (L I 20), Hegu (L I 4), Shangxing (Du 23).

Supplementary points:
Heat in the lung: Shaoshang (L 11).
Heat in the stomach: Neiting (S 44).
Deficiency of yin with preponderance of fire: Zhaohai (K 6).

Explanation: The Hand-Yangming Meridian and Hand-Taiyin Meridian are exteriorly and interiorly related. The Hand-Yangming Meridian connects with the Foot-Yangming Meridian. So Yingxiang (L I 20) and Hegu (L I 4) are seclected to clear off heat and stop bleeding. The Du Meridian is the sea of all the yang meridians. Extreme yang forces blood to rush out. So Shangxing (L I 20) is used to reduce heat of the Du Meridian. The lung has its specific body opening in the nose. Shaoshang (L 11), the Jing-(Well) Point of the Lung Meridian, is used to reduce heat of the lung. Neiting (S 44), the Ying-(Spring) Point of the Stomach Meridian, is good for eliminating the stomach fire. Zhaohai (K 6), one of the Confluential Points of the Eight Extra Meridians, has the action of nourishing yin and reducing fire.

Remarks
Epistaxis may be caused by trauma, nasal disorders and acute febrile diseases. In addition to acupuncture treatment, other therapeutic measures should be adopted according to its primary cause.

5. Toothache

Toothache is a common ailment. It may be due to wind fire, stomach fire, asthenic fire, and dental caries.

Etiology and Pathogenesis
The Hand and Foot Yangming Meridians go into the upper and lower gums respectively. Toothache may be due to flaring up along the meridians of the pathogenic fire transformed from pathogenic heat in the large intestine and stomach, or from exogenous pathogenic wind that attacks and accumulates in the Yangming Meridians. The kidney controls bones and the teeth are the odds and ends of the bones. Deficiency of the kidney yin with flaring up of the asthenic fire may also give rise to toothache. Sometimes toothache is due to dental caries caused by overintake of sour and sweet food.

Differentiation
a) Toothache due to stomach fire:
Main manifestations: Severe toothache accompanied by foul breath, thirst, constipation, yellow tongue coating, forceful and rapid pulse.
Analysis: Accumulated heat in the stomach and intestines results in constipation. Upsurging of the stomach heat causes yellow tongue coating and foul breath. Thirst is due to the exhaustion of body fluid by heat. Severe toothache is due to the stomach heat flaring up along the meridians. Forceful and rapid pulse also indicates the stomach fire.
b) Toothache caused by wind fire:
Main manifestations: Acute toothache with gingival swelling accompanied by chills and fever, superficial and rapid pulse.
Analysis: The exogenous pathogenic wind

invades the Yangming Meridians and turns into fire. Then occurs the toothache with gingival swelling. When the exogenous pathogenic factors struggle against the body resistance in the muscles and skins, there are chills and fever as exterior symptoms. Superficial and rapid pulse is a sign of wind-fire.

c) Toothache caused by deficiency of the kidney yin:

Main manifestations: Dull pain off and on, loose teeth, absence of foul breath, reddened tongue, thready and rapid pulse.

Analysis: The kidney controls bones and the teeth are the odds and ends of the bones. The kidney in deficiency state fails to keep the teeth strong, so they are loose. Flaring up of the asthenic fire leads to dull pain. Since nothing is accumulated in the stomach, there is no foul breath. Thready, rapid pulse and reddened tongue are due to heat caused by yin deficiency.

Treatment

a) Toothache due to stomach fire:

Method: The reducing method is applied to eliminate heat and stop pain. Points of Hand-Yangming Meridian are selected.

Prescription: Hegu (L I 4), Jiache (S 6), Neiting (S 44), Xiaguan (S 7).

Explanation: Hegu (L I 4) of the contralateral side is used to disperse pathogenic heat from the Hand-Yangming Meridian. Neiting (S 44), the Ying-(Spring) Point of the Stomach Meridian, is used to reduce the fire in the stomach. Xiaguan (S 7) and Jiache (S 6) are local points to stop pain and regulate the qi circulation in the Foot-Yangming Meridian.

b) Toothache caused by wind fire:

Method: The reducing method is applied to dispel wind and clear off heat. Points of the Sanjiao Meridian of Hand-Shaoyang are selected.

Prescription: Yemen (S J 2), Fengchi (G 20), Hegu (L I 4), Jiache (S 6), Xiaguan (S 7), Waiguan (S J 5).

Explanation: Waiguan (S J 5) is the Ying-(Spring) Point of the Sanjiao Meridian of Hand-Shaoyang. Fengchi (G 20) is used to dispel wind and clear off fire. Hegu (L I 4), Jiache (S 6) and Xiaguan (S 7) are selected to regulate the qi circulation in the Yangming Meridians of Hand and Foot and to eliminate heat for relieving pain.

c) Toothache caused by deficiency of the kidney yin:

Method: The even movement is applied to nourish yin and lower the fire. Points of the Foot-Yangming and Foot-Shaoyin Meridians are selected.

Prescription: Jiache (S 6), Xiaguan (S 7), Taixi (K 3).

Explanation: The teeth relate to the kidney and are situated at the place where the Stomach Meridian and Large Intestine Meridian go through. Thus Taixi (K 3) is used to nourish yin of the kidney and lower the asthenic fire. Jiache (S 6) and Xiaguan (S 7) relieve pain by regulating the qi in the meridians.

Remarks

Toothache described here is involved in acute and chronic pulpitis, dental caries, peridental abscess and pericoronitis.

6. Sore Throat

Sore throat is commonly seen. It can be divided into two types: excess and deficiency.

Etiology and Pathogenesis

The throat communicates with the

stomach and the lung through the esophagus and the trachea respectively. Sore throat of excess type (excess of heat) is due to exogenous pathogenic wind heat that scorches the lung system or due to the accumulated heat in the Lung and Stomach Meridians that disturbs upward. Sore throat of deficiency type (deficiency of yin) is due to the exhaustion of the kidney yin that fails to flow upward to moisten the throat, while the asthenic fire flares up instead.

Differentiation

a) Syndrome of excess of heat:

Main manifestations: Abrupt onset with chills, fever, headache, congested and sore throat, thirst, dysphagia, constipation, reddened tongue with thin yellow coating, superficial and rapid pulse.

Analysis: Exogenous pathogenic wind heat invades the exterior portion of the body, leading to chills, fever and headache. After having been transmitted to the lung system the pathogenic wind heat causes sore throat and dysphagia. The lung is exteriorly-interiorly related with the large intestine. Since the pathogenic heat consumes the body fluid, there are symptoms of thirst and constipation. Reddened tongue with thin yellow coating, superficial and rapid pulse are signs of the pathogenic wind heat invading the lung.

b) Syndrome of deficiency of yin:

Main manifestations: Gradual onset without fever or with low fever, slightly congested throat with intermittent pain or pain during swallowing, dryness of the throat, more marked at night, feverish sensation in the palms and soles, reddened and furless tongue, thready and rapid pulse.

Analysis: The Kidney Meridian of Foot-Shaoyin travels to the throat. Because the kidney yin is insufficient to run up to

moisten the throat, the throat is slightly congested with mild pain on and off and with dryness more marked at night. Feverish sensation in the palms and soles, reddened and furless tongue, thready and rapid pulse are signs of deficiency of yin that causes yang preponderance.

Treatment

a) Syndrome of excess of heat:

Method: To disperse wind and eliminate heat by puncturing the points of Hand-Taiyin and Foot-Yangming Meridians with the reducing method.

Prescription: Shaoshang (L 11), Hegu (L I 4), Neiting (S 44), Tianrong (S I 17).

Explanation: Pricking Shaoshang (L 11) to let a few drops of blood out is used to clear off the heat from the lung and relieve pain. Hegu (L I 4) disperses exterior pathogenic factors from the Lung Meridian and the accumulated heat from the Yangming Meridians. Neiting (S 44), the Ying-(Spring) Point of the Stomach Meridian, reduces heat in the stomach. Tianrong (S I 17) is a local point used to ease the pain of a sore throat.

b) Syndrome of deficiency of yin:

Method: To nourish yin and descend fire by puncturing with the reinforcing method at points of Shaoyin Meridians of Hand and Foot as the principal points.

Prescription: (a) Taixi (K 3), Yuji (L 10), Lianquan (Ren 23) (b) Zhaohai (K 6), Lieque (L 7), Futu (L I 18).

The above two prescriptions may be used alternatively.

Explanation: Taixi (K 3) is the Yuan-(Primary) Point of the Kidney Meridian which runs up to the throat. Yuji (L 10) is the Ying-(Spring) Point of the Lung Meridian. Combination of the two points nourishes yin and reduces the fire. Zhaohai (K 6) and Lieque (L 7), a pair of the Eight Confluent

Points, relieve sore throat by leading the asthenic fire downward. Futu (L I 18) and Lianquan (Ren 23) are local points for relieving pain.

Remarks

Sore throat as described here is involved in acute tonsilitis, acute and chronic pharyngitis.

7. Optic Atrophy

Optic atrophy is a chronic eye disorder marked by gradual degeneration of the vision acuity. At the early stage there is only blurring of vision, but at the late stage the eyesight may be totally lost.

Etiology and Pathogenesis

a) Deficiency of the kidney and liver yin leads to consumption of the essence and blood that nourish the eyes.

b) Dysfunction in transportation and transformation of the spleen due to irregular diet and overstrain results in inadequate supply of the essential nutrients for the eyes.

c) Dysfunction of the liver with stagnation of qi and blood in emotional troubles causes failure of the essential qi to flow upwards to nourish the eyes.

Differentiation

a) Deficiency of the liver and kidney yin:

Main manifestations: Dryness of the eyes, blurred vision, dizziness, tinnitus, nocturnal emission, aching of the lower back, thready and weak pulse, reddened tongue with scanty coating.

Analysis: Dryness of the eyes and blurred vision are due to failure of the essential vision are due to failure of the essential nutrients to nourish the eyes in deficiency of the liver and kidney yin. The lumbus is the seat of the kidney. When the kidney is in a deficiency state, there is aching of the lower back. Deficiency of the kidney yin may lead to nocturnal emission when there is hyperactivity of the asthenic fire, and to dizziness and tinnitus when there is yang preponderance. Thready and weak pulse, reddened tongue with scanty coating are signs of yin deficiency.

b) Deficiency of qi and blood:

Main manifestations: Blurred vision, weakness of breath, disinclination to talk, lassitude, poor appetite, loose stools, thready and weak pulse, pale tongue with thin white coating.

Analysis: The essential qi of all the zang-fu organs flows up to the eyes. When qi and blood in a deficiency state can not nourish the eyes, the vision becomes blurred. Qi deficiency of the spleen and stomach causes weakness of breath, disinclination to talk, lassitude, poor appetite and loose stools. Thready and weak pulse, pale tongue with thin and white coating are signs of deficiency of qi and blood.

c) Stagnation of the liver qi:

Main manifestations: Blurred vision, emotional depression, dizziness, vertigo, hypochondriac pain, bitter taste in the mouth, dry throat and string-taut pulse.

Analysis: The liver has its specific body opening in the eyes. Stagnation of the liver qi causes general obstruction of qi and blood which fail to ascend to nourish the eyes. So the vision is blurred. The Liver Meridian passes by the hypochondriac region, so there is hypochondriac pain when the liver qi is stagnated. Retarded qi may turn into fire, which flares up to cause dizziness, vertigo, bitter taste in the mouth and dry throat. String-taut pulse is the sign of a liver disease.

Treatment

Method: To reinforce the liver and kidney and nourish qi and blood by puncturing the points of the Foot-Shaoyang and Taiyang Meridians with reinforcing method for deficiency of the liver and kidney yin and deficiency of qi and blood. Even movement is applied to the same points to remove the stagnation of the liver qi.

Prescription: Fengchi (G 20), Jingming (B 1), Qiuhou (Extra), Guangming (G 39).

Deficiency of the liver and kidney yin: Taichong (Liv 3), Taixi (K 3), Ganshu (B 18), Shenshu (B 23).

Deficiency of qi and blood: Zusanli (S 38), Sanyinjiao (Sp 6).

Stagnation of the liver qi: Qimen (Liv 14), Taichong (Liv 3), Yanglingquan (G 34).

Explanation: The Foot-Shaoyang and Taiyang Meridians connect with the eye region, so Fengchi (G 20), Guangming (G 37), Jingming (B 1) are selected to regulate the qi circulation in the meridians and to improve the eyesight. Qiuhou (Extra) is an extra point effective for eye diseases. Ganshu (B 18), Shenshu (B 23), Taixi (K 3) and Taichong (Liv 3) are used to reinforce the yin of the liver and kidney. Zusanli (S 36) and Sanyinjiao (Sp 6) reinforce qi and blood. Qimen (Liv 14), Taichong (Liv 3) and Yanglingquan (G 34) remove stagnation of the liver qi.

EAR ACUPUNCTURE THERAPY

Ear acupuncture therapy treats and prevents diseases by stimulating certain points on the auricle with needles.

Ear acupuncture therapy has long been used in China, and is recorded in Chapter 24 of *Miraculous Pivot* that "Jue headache with the symptoms of acute pain in the head, and hot sensations in the vessels in front of and behind the ear should be treated by bloodletting in order to reduce the heat, then to be followed by needling at the points of Foot Shaoyang Meridian." In the twentieth chapter of *Miraculous Pivot* it says, "When the pathogenic factor attacks the liver, it will cause pain in the ribs on both sides . . . for the pain caused by internal blood stagnation . . . needle at the blue vessels around the ear to relieve the dragging pain." In other classical medical literature there are descriptions on stimulating certain auricular areas with needle, moxibustion, massage, and herbal suppository to treat and prevent diseases. Those methods are still used as folk remedies.

I. ANATOMICAL TERMINOLOGY OF THE AURICULAR SURFACE

Ear is an organ of hearing symmetrically on both sides of the head. The auricle is composed of a plate of elastic cartilage, a thin layer of fat and connective tissue supplied by numerous nerves. The main nerves are the great auricular and the lesser occipital derived from the second, third and fourth cervical spinal nerves, the auricule-temporal branch of the trigeminal nerve, vagus, the mixed branch of the facial nerve and the glossopharyngeal nerves, and sympathetic nerves.

To facilitate location of ear points, the anatomical structures of the auricular surface relating to ear acupuncture are briefly described as follows:

1. Helix: The prominent rim of the auricle.
2. Helix tubercle: A small tubercle at the posterior-inferior aspect of the helix.
3. Helix cauda: The inferior part of the helix, at the junction of the helix and the lobule.
4. Helix crus: A transverse ridge of helix continuing backward into the ear cavity.
5. Antihelix: An elevated ridge anterior and parallel to the helix. Its upper part branches out into the superior and inferior antihelix crus. It includes the principal part of antihelix.
6. The principal part of antihelix: The

roughly vertical portion of the antihelix.

7. Superior antihelix crus: The superior branch of the bifurcation of the antihelix.

8. Inferior antihelix crus: The anterior branch of the bifurcation of the antihelix.

9. Triangular fossa: The triangular depression between the two crura of the antihelix.

10. Scapha: The narrow curved depression between the helix and the antihelix.

11. Tragus: A small, curved flap in front of the auricle.

12. Supratragic notch: The depression between the helix crus and the upper border of the tragus.

13. Antitragus: A small tubercle opposite to the tragus and inferior to the ear lobe.

14. Intertragic notch: The depression between the tragus and antitragus.

15. Helix notch: The depression between the antitragus and antihelix.

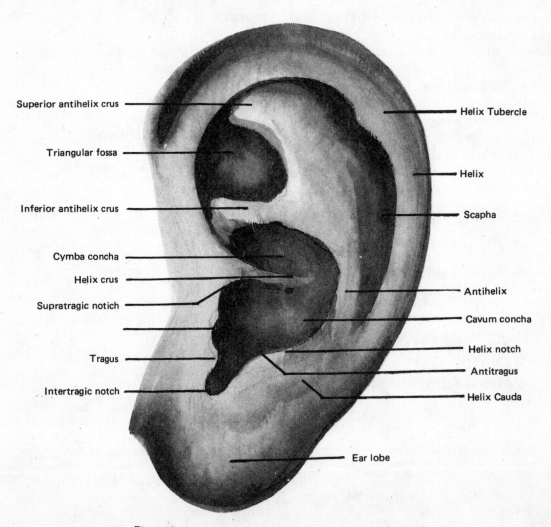

Fig. 163 Anatomical Structure of the Auricular Surface

16. Ear lobe: The lowerest part of the auricle where there is no cartilage.
17. Concha: The hollow formed by the antitragus, between the anterior part of the helix and inferior antihelix crus.
18. Cymba concha: The concha superio to the helix crus.
19. Cavum concha: The concha inferior to the helix crus.
20. Orifice of the external auditory meatus: The opening in the cavum concha shielded by the tragus.
21. The superior auricular root: The area where the superior border of auricle attaches to the scalp.
22. The inferior auricular root: The area where ear lobe attaches to the face.

(See Fig. 163)

II. AURICULAR POINTS

Auricular points are specific stimulating points on the auricle. When disorders occur in the internal organs or other parts of the body, various reactions may appear at the corresponding areas of the auricle, such as tenderness, decreased cutaneous electric resistance, morphological changes, and discoloration. Therefore, these sites are also referred to as tender spots, conductant points or reflex spots. Thus, making a diagnosis, those phenomena can be taken into consideration. Stimulating the sensitive sites serves to prevent and treat diseases.

1. Distribution of Auricular Points

Ear points are distributed on the auricle in a certain pattern. The following is a summary of the distribution of auricular points:

Points located on the lobule are related to the head and facial region, those on the scapha to the upper limbs, those on the antihelix and its two crura to the trunk and lower limbs, and those in the cavum and cymba conchae to the internal organs. (See Fig. 164)

1) Helix Crus and Helix: Points include Middle Ear on Helix Crus, Lower Rectum. Urethra, External Genitalia, Ear Apex and Helix 1-6 on helix.

2) Scapha: Points include Finger, Wrist, Elbow and the corresponding parts of the upper limbs.

3) Antihelix: It includes the corresponding site of the trunk and the lower limbs.

4) Tragus: Point Nose is on the outer aspect of Tragus. At its border are points Superior Tragic Apex and Inferior Tragic Apex. Points Throat and Internal Nose are on the inner aspect of Tragus.

5) Antitragus: Points Forehead, Occiput and Temple are on the outer aspect of Antitragus. At the tip of the border of Antihelix is the Point Middle Border. Point Brain is on the inner aspect of Antihelix.

6) Intertragic Notch: Point Intertragic Notch is inferior to the orifice of external auditory meatus and on the intertragic notch. The areas anterior-inferior and posterior-inferior to the intertragic notch orderly are points Anterior Intertragic Notch, Posterior Intertragic Notch and Inferior Intertragic Notch.

7) Triangular Fossa: Points include Ear-Shenmen, Triangular Depression and Superior Triangle.

8) Cymba Conchae and Cavum Conchae: They are the corresponding areas for various internal organs. Point Digestive Tract is around helix crus. Posterior to the external auditory meatus is the Mouth point, then respectively are points Esophagus, Cardiac Orifice, Stomach,

Duodenum, Small Intestine, Appendix, Large Intestine, etc. Point Stomach is at the area where helix crus terminates. Point Liver is at the posterior aspect to Points Stomach and Duodenum. Above Point Small Intestine is Kidney. Point Bladder is above

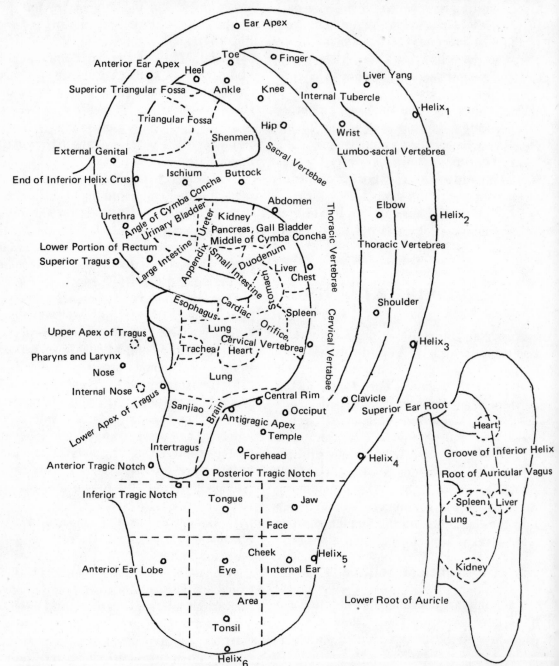

Fig. 164 Schematic Diagram of Distribution of Anricular Points

large intestine. Between Liver and Kidney is Point Pancreas. Point Spleen is inferior to Point Liver and close to the border of antihelix. In the centre of cavum is Point Heart. Between Point Heart and Point Mouth is Point Trachea. Among Points Intertragus, Brain and Lung there is Point Sanjiao.

9) Ear Lobe: In the middle of ear lobe is Point Eye. Above this Point is Point Tongue, in front of it are the four points of ear lobe. Posterior to Point Eye is Point Internal Ear, inferior to it is Point Tonsil, and at the posterior-superior aspect of Point Eye is Point Cheek.

10) The back of auricle: There are Points Groove of Inferior Antihelix Crus, Root of Auricular Vagus Nerve, Superior Root of Auricle and Inferior Root of Auricle, etc.

2. Location, Action and Indications of Ear Acupoints

Numerous writings about the name, location, action and indications of ear acupoints have been recorded in Chinese medical literature for centuries. In recent years new ear acupoints have been reported, but these reports vary. The table in the appendix for location, action and indications of ear acupoints is made according to the International Standardization of Ear Acupoints established by All-China Society of Acupuncture and Moxibustion.

Appendix: Location, Action and Indications of Ear Acupoints

Anotomical Portion	Name of Point	Former Name	Location	Action and Indications
	Middle Ear	Diaphragm	Helix crus.	Descending upward reversive qi of stomach, expelling wind and regulating the function of dia- phragm. Indications: hiccup, jaundice, symptoms and diseases of digestive system and skin.
	Lower Portion of Rectum		On the end of helix approximate to superior tragic notch.	Constipation, anus prolapse, external and internal hemarrhoids, tenesmus.
	Urethra		On helix at level with the lower border of inferior antihelix crus.	Enuresis, frequent, urgent and painful urination, retention of urine.
Helix Crus and Helix	Extenal Genitalia		On helix at level with the upper border of inferior antihelix crus.	Inflammation of external genital organs, eczema of the perineum, impotence.

	Front Ear Apex	Hemarr-hoidal Nucleus	Area between Ear Apex and Superior Root of Auricle.	External and internal hemarrhoids (It is used as assistant diagnosis for hemarrhoids).
	Ear Apex		At the tip of auricle and superior to helix when folded towards tragus.	Removing heat and wind, anti-spasmotism and analgesia, pacifying liver and clearing vision. Indications: fever, hypertension, inflammation of eyes, painful diseases.
	Liver Yang		At auricular tubercle.	Liver qi stagnation, liver yang preponderance.
	Helix 1-6		Region from lower border of auricular tubercle to midpoint of lower border of lobule is divided into five equal parts. The points marking the divisions are respectively Helix 1, Helix 2, Helix 3, Helix 4, Helix 5, Helix 6.	Clarifying heat and relieving pain, pacifying liver and removing wind. Indications: fever, tonsillitis, hypertension.
	Finger		At the top of scapha	Pain and dysfunction at corresponding area of the body.
	Interior Tubercle	Urticaria or Allergic Point	Midpoint between Finger and Wrist.	Expelling wind and stopping itching.
	Wrist		Midway between Elbow and Finger.	Pain and dysfunction at corresponding area of the body.
Scapha	Elbow		Midway between Finger and Clavicle.	Pain and dysfunction at corresponding area of the body.
	Shoulder		Midway between Elbow and Clavicle.	Pain and dysfunction at corresponding area of the body.
	Clavicle		On scapha at level with	Pain at corresponding

			helix-tragic notch.	area, peripheral arthritis of the shoulder, Takayashu's disease (pulseless disease).
Superior Antihelix Crus	Toe		Superior and lateral angle of superior antihelix crus.	Pain and dysfunction of corresponding area of the body.
	Heel		Superior and medial angle of superior of antihelix crus.	Heel pain.
	Ankle		Midway between heel and knee.	Ankle sprain, pain and dysfunction at corresponding area of the body.
	Knee		Middle portion at superior antihelix crus.	Pain and dysfunction at corresponding area of the body (such as sprain and arthritis of the knee joint).
Inferior Antihelix Crus	Hip		At inferior 1/3 of the superior antihelix crus.	Pain at corresponding area.
	Buttocks		At lateral 1/3 of the inferior antihelix crus.	Pain at corresponding area.
	Ischium	Sciatic Nerve	At medial 2/3 of the inferior antihelix crus	Sciatica
	End of Inferior Antihelix Crus	Sympathetic Nerve	The terminal of inferior antihelix crus.	Antispasmotism and analgesia, nourishing yin and supporting yang. Indications: pain of internal organs, palpitation, spontaneous sweating, night sweating; functional disorders of autonomous nerve system.
Antihelix	Cervical Vertebrae Thoracic Vertebrae Sacral Vertebrae		A curved line from helixtragic notch to the branching area of superior and inferior antihelix crus can be divided into 3 equal segments. The lower 1/3 of it is Cervical Vertebrae, the middle	Strengthening spine and nourishing marrow. Indications: pain at corresponding part of the spine.

			1/3 is Thoracic Vertebrae, and the upper 1/3 is Lumbosacral Vertebrae.	
	Neck		On the border of cavum conchae of Cervical Vertebrae.	Strained neck, wry neck, pain or dysfunction of the neck.
	Chest		On the border of cavum conchae of Thoracic Vertebrae.	Pain and stuffiness of the chest, or pain at the corresponding part of the body.
	Abdomen		On the border of cavum conchae of Lumbosacral Vertebrae.	Abdominal or gynecological diseases, lumbago.
	Ear-Shenmen		At bifurcating point between superior and inferior antihelix crus, and at the lateral 1/3 of triangular fossa.	Sadation, easing mind, relieving pain, clearing heat.
Triangular Fossa	Triangular Depression	Tiankui Uterus Seminal Palace.	In the triangular fossa and in the depression close to the midpoint of helix.	Supporting yang and nourishing essence, regulating menstruation and harmonizing blood. Indications: gynecological diseases and symptoms, impotence, prostatis, etc.
	Superior Triangle	Lowering Blood Pressure	At the superior-lateral angle of Triangular Fossa.	Pacifying liver and removing wind. Indication: hypertension.
	Superior Tragus	Ear	On the supratragic notch close to helix.	Nourishing kidney-water, subduing liver yang. Indications: ear disease, dizziness and vertigo.
	Nose	External Nose	In the centre of lateral aspect of tragus.	Removing obstructions from the meridians in the nose region. Indications: brandy-nose or nose furuncles,

				nasal obstruction, and other nose problems.
Tragus	Supratragic Apex	Tragic Apex	At the tip of upper protuberance on border of tragus.	Reducing heat and relieving pain.
	Infratragic Apex	Adrenal	At the tip of lower tubercle on border of tragus.	Reducing heat and relieving pain, antispasmotism and expelling wind.
	Pharynx-Larynx		Upper half of medial aspect of tragus.	Clarifying obstructions of the pharynx and largnx. Indications: acute and chronic pharyngitis and chronic laryngitis and tonsillitis.
	Internal Nose		Lower half of medial aspect of tragus.	Removing obstructions of the nose. Indications: allergic rhinitis and other nose diseases.
	Antitragic Apex	Soothing Asthma or Parotid	At the tip of antitragic.	Strengthening the lung and stopping asthma, clearing up heat and antitoxic, and expelling wind. Indications: asthma, bronchitis, parotitis and itching skin.
	Middle Border	Brain	Midpoint between antitragic apex and helix-tragic notch.	Replenishing brain and easing mind. Indications: oligophrenia (incomplete development of intelligence), enuresis, etc.
	Occiput		At posterior superior corner of lateral aspect of antitragus.	Sedation and analgesia, easing mind and removing wind. Indications: dizziness, headache, insomnia, etc.
Antitragus	Temple	Taiyang	On antitragus between Forehead and	Sedation and analgesia.

			Occiput.	Indication: Shaoyang headache.
	Forehead		At anterior inferior corner of lateral aspect of antitragus.	Sedation and analgesia. Indication: Yangming headache.
	Brain	Subcortex		Reinforcing marrow and replenishing brain, relieving pain and easing mind. Indications: oligophrenia, insomnia, dream disturbed sleep, tinnitus due to kidney deficiency.
	Mouth		Close to posterior and superior border of orifice of external auditory meatus.	Clearing up heart fire, removing pathogenic wind. Indications: facial paralysis, stomatitis, etc.
Periphery helix crus	Esophagus		At medial 2/3 of inferior aspect of helix crus.	Regulating function of diaphragm and harmonizing stomach. Indications: dysphagia, esophagitis, etc.
	Cardiac Orifice		At area where helix crus terminates.	Harmonizing stomach and replenishing spleen, reinforcing middle jiao and easing mind. Indications: insomnia, gastritis, gastroduodenal ulcer and other diseases and symptoms of gastric region.
	Duodenum		At lateral 1/3 of superior aspect of helix crus.	Warming middle jiao and harmonizing stomach. Indications: duodenal ulcer, pylorospasm, etc.
	Small Intestine		At middle 1/3 of superior aspect of helix crus.	Reinforcing spleen and harmonizing middle jiao, nourishing heart and

			producing blood. Indications: indigestion, palpitation, etc.
	Appendix	Between Small Intestine and Large Intestine	Clearing up damp heat from lower jiao. . Indications: appendicitis, diarrhoea, etc.
	Large Intestine	At medial 1/3 of superior aspect of helix crus.	Clearing up lower jiao, replenishing lung-qi. Indications: diarrhoea, constipation.
	Liver	At posterior aspect of Stomach and Duodenum.	Clearing up liver and brightening vision, promoting smooth circulation of qi and blood to relax muscles and tendons. Indications: liver-qi stagnation, eye diseases and disorders of lateral-lower abdomen.
Cymba Conchae	Pancrease	Between Liver and Kidney.	Replenishing gallbladder and building up stomach, removing liver-qi stagnation and liver-wind. Indications: diseases and symptoms of bile duct, pancreasitis, migraine, etc.
	Kidney	On the lower border of inferior antihelix crus, directly above Small Intestine.	Reinforcing kidney and promoting hearing, strengthening bone and filling up marrow. Indications: nephritis, lumbago, tinnitus, diplacusis, spermatorrhea, impotence, etc.
	Ureter	Between Kidney and Bladder.	Stone and colic pain of ureter.
	Bladder	On the lower border of inferior antihelix crus, directly above Large Intestine.	Replenishing lower jiao and reinforcing lower sap. Indications: lower back pain, sciatica, cystitis, enuresis, retention of urine.
	Angle of Cymba Conchae	At medial superior angle of Cymba	Clarifying lower jiao, removing obstruction

			Conchae.	from the urethra Indication: prostatitis.
	Middle Cymba Conchae	Periphery Umbilicus	In the center of Cymba Conchae.	Regulating middle jiao and harmonizing spleen. Indications: low fever, abdominal distension, ascariasis of bile duct, impaired hearing, parotitis, etc.
Cavum Conchae	Heart		In the central depression of cavum conchae.	Tranquilizing heart and easing mind, regulating ying-blood, relieving pain and itching. Indications: insomnia, palpitation, hysteria, night sweating, angina pectoris, etc.
	Lung		Around Heart.	Promoting smooth circulation of qi and blood, diuresis, reinforcing deficiency and clearing up heat, nourishing skin and hair. Indications: cough and asthma, skin diseases, hoaseness of voice; commonly used point of acupuncture anesthesia.
	Trachea		In the area of Lung, between Mouth and Heart.	Stopping cough and dispelling phlegm. Indications: cough and asthma.
	Spleen		Inferior to Liver, at lateral and superior aspect of cavum conchae.	Digesting food, producing ying-blood, nourishing muscles, building up spleen qi. Indications: abdominal diarrhoea, distension, chronic indigestion, stamotitis, functional uterus bleeding, etc.
	Sanjiao		Superior to Intertragus.	Removing obstruction from the water pass-

				ages, clearing up heat and stopping itching.
	Intertragus	Endocrine	At the base of cavum conchae in the inter-tragic notch.	Removing liver-qi stagnation, regulating menstruation and ac-tiviating blood circu-lation, expelling pathogenic wind, rein-forcing lower jiao. Indications: skin dis-eases, impotence, ir-regular menstruation, climacteric syndrome, dysfunction of endo-crine, etc.
	Frontal Tragic Notch	Eye 1	On lateral and anterior side of intertragic notch.	Clearing up liver and brightening vision. In-dications: glaucoma, pseudomyopia and other eye diseases.
	Lower Tragic Notch	Elevating Blood Pres-sure Point	On the inferior aspect of intertragic notch.	Reinforcing qi and elevating yang. Indication: hypoten-sion.
Ear Lobule	Back Tragic Notch	Eye 2	On lateral and inferior aspect of intertragic notch.	Clearing up liver fire and brightening vision. Indications: ame-tropia, external eye inflamation, etc.
	Cheek		On the ear lobe, at posterior and superior aspect of Eye.	Removing obstruc-tions from the meridians on facial region. Indications: facial par-alysis and other facial problems.
	Tongue		In the centre of 2nd section of lobule.	Clearing up heart fire. Indication: glossitis.
	Jaw		In the centre of 3rd section of lobule.	Toothache, submandi-bular arthritis, etc.
	Section 4 of Ear Lobe	Neurasthenic Point	In the 4th section of ear lobe.	Communicating water with fire, tranquilizing heart and easing mind.

			Indications: tooth-ache, neurasthesnia.
Eye		In the 5th section of ear lobe.	Brightening vision. Indications: acute conjunctivitis, electric ophthalmia, myopia and other eye diseases.
Internal Ear		In the 6th section of the ear lobe.	Relieving vertigo and improving hearing. Indications: tinnitus, impaired hearing, auditory vertigo, etc.
Tonsil		In the 8th section of the ear lobe.	Relieving throat problems. Indication: acute tonsillitis.
Upper Root of Auricle	Middle Stasis or Spinal Cord	At the upper border of the auricular root.	Relieving pain and asthma. Indications: headache, abdominal pain, asthma.
Lower Root of Auricle	Spinal Cord	On the lower border of the juncture between the ear lobe and the cheek.	Relieving pain and asthma. Indications: headache, abdominal pain, asthma.
Root of Auricular Vagus Norve		At the junction of retroauricle and mastoid, level with helix crus.	Openning orifice and relieving pain, easing zang-fu organs. Indications: headache, nasal obstruction, ascariasis of bile duct, etc.
Back Auricle	Groove of Inferior Helix Crus	Groove for Lowering Blood Pressure	Through the backside of superior antihelix crus and inferior antihelix crus, in the depression as a "Y" form.	Pacifying liver and descending reversing qi of the liver, relieving skin disease. Indications: hypertension, skin diseases.
	Heart		At the upper back of the ear.	Clearing and reducing heart fire, tranquilizing heart and easing mind, relieving pain. Indications: furuncles,

			insomnia, dream-disturbed sleep, hypertension, headache. etc.
Spleen		In the middle at the back of the ear.	Building up spleen and harmonizing stomach, producing ying-blood and nourishing muscles. Indications: abdominal distension, diarrhoea, indigestion, etc.
Liver		On the back of ear, at lateral aspect of Spleen.	Removing liver-qi stagnation and harmonizing stomach, nourishing tendons and activiating blood circulation. Indications: distension and fullness of chest and hyperchondriac region, acute appendicitis, soreness and aching of the lower back, etc.
Lung		On the back of the ear, at medial aspect of Spleen.	Reinforcing lung and soothing asthma, clearing up heat, relieving problems of skin and hair. Indications: asthma, diseases and symptoms of digestive system, fever, etc.
Kidney		At the lower part of the retroauricle.	Nourishing kidney water, improving hearing, strengthening bone, filling up marrow. Indications: headache, insomnia, dizziness, vertigo, irregular menstruation.

3. Examination Methods of Ear Acupuncture

When an internal organ or a part of the body is diseased, reactions can be detected at the corresponding areas on the auricle. For example, a reaction can be detected at Point Stomach when the stomach is ill. Clinical practice has proven that stimulating these reaction points yields good therapeutic results. Therefore, detecting reaction points should be combined with consulting an auricular acupoint chart in the application of ear acupuncture. The following are commonly used methods of detection:

1) Detecting the tender spot Press with a probe or the handle of a filiform needle the disease-related corresponding area, to ascertain the most sensitive point.

2) Observing by naked eye Look for any abnormality or discoloration of the auricle such as scaling, blisters, papulae, hard nodules, pigmentation, or morphological changes such as in blood vessels of the auricle.

3) Detecting electrical changes Observing changes in electrical resistance, capacity, and potential at auricular points. The most commonly used method is to determine the conductant point of skin resistance by instrument. Those auricular points with low electrical resistance can be displayed on a screen, or by an indicator, or by sound, through the apparatus. This is used for clinical diagnosis.

III. CLINICAL APPLICATION OF EAR ACUPUNCTURE

Ear acupuncture is used for prevention and treatment of disease, and also for acupuncture anesthesia. This chapter mainly deals with its application to clinical treatment and disease prevention.

1. Principles for Selection of Points

Point selection can be on the following bases:

1) Selection of points according to disease location Auricular points corresponding to the diseased areas are selected for treatment, e.g. Point Stomach for gastralgia, Point Shoulder for shoulder pain.

2) Selection of points according to the theories of traditional Chinese medicine According to the theories of zang-fu or meridians and collaterals, corresponding auricular points are selected for treatment, e.g. Point Lung can be selected for skin diseases because the lung dominates the skin and hair; Point Small Intestine for arrythmia as the heart is exteriorly-interiorly related to the small intestine; Point Gallbladder for temporal headache as the temporal region is supplied by the Gallbladder Meridian of Foot-Shaoyang; Point Liver for pain, redness and swelling of the eyes, since the liver opens to the eyes.

3) Selection of points according to clinical experience e.g. Point Ear Apex can be selected for pain, redness and swelling of the eyes; Points Helix 2,4, and 6 for pain and swelling of the throat.

2. Manipulation Methods of Ear Acupuncture

Different methods have been developed on the basis of filiform needling, such as embedding needles and needling with electrical stimulation. However, filiform needling remains the most widely used.

The technique is performed as follows:

1) Probing the sensitive spot and aseptic procedure After diagnosis and point prescription detect the sensitive spots by probing or by an electric acupoint detector. When tenderness or low electrical resistance areas are found, then mark the spot for needling. Auricular points should be swabbed with 75% alcohol or 20% iodine as routine asepsis.

2) Method of needle insertion Stabilize the auricle with the left hand. Hold the filiform needle of 0.5 or 1 cun with the right hand and insert swiftly and perpendicularly into the point avoiding penetration through the ear. Generally, a sensation of pain, and occasionally heat, distension, soreness, or heaviness are felt. Patients experiencing these sensations usually obtain satisfactory therapeutic results. If acupuncture sensation does not appear, then the direction of needling should be adjusted to obtain sensation.

3) Retention and removal of needles Needles are usually retained for 25 to 30 minutes, but in cases with severe pain or chronic seizures, needles may be retained for a longer period, or needle embedding may be applied. After the needle is removed, press the puncture hole with a dry cotton ball to avoid bleeding, swab with iodine at once to avoid infection.

3. Prescriptions for Common Diseases

1) Headache Selection of points: Forehead, Occiput and Brain, Middle Border, Ear Apex. Apply strong stimulation with filiform needles. Needles are retained for 30 to 60 minutes. Ten treatments constitute a course.

2) Migraine Selection of points: Forehead, Temple, Occiput, Ear-Shenmen.

Secondary points: Neck, Heart, Liver, Ear Apex and Helix 6. Apply electric acupuncture once every other day. Select 3 to 5 points for each treatment. During an attack, bloodletting on Helix 6 and Ear Apex can be added.

3) Stiff neck Find tenderness or most sensitive spot at Forehead and Cervical Vertebrae. Apply strong stimulation. Needles are retained for 60 minutes, during which the patient should exercise the neck by moving it about. Apply needling plus moxibustion on the tender spot of the neck region. Alleviation or subsidence of pain may be expected. Treat once daily.

4) Acute sprain Selection of points: Ear-Shenmen, Brain, and Tender spots corresponding to sprained areas. Apply strong stimulation with filiform needle. Needles are retained for 30 to 60 minutes, treat once daily. After needle insertion, patient may have congestion or heat sensation of the auricle; the patient should then exercise the affected area. At the same time, warm moxibustion or massage can be added to enhance the therapeutic effect.

5) Sciatica Selection of points: Ischium. Puncture the affected side first. If there is not much improvement, needle the same auricular point of the healthy side. Apply strong stimulation. Needles are retained for 1 to 2 hours, treat once daily or every other day.

6) Phantom limb pain Selection of points: Ear-Shenmen, Forehead, Brain, other auricular points of corresponding areas. Several needles may be inserted at one point. Give strong stimulation with a filiform needle. If necessary, treatment can be increased twice or three times per day, with 3 to 5 days constituting a course.

7) Postoperative incision pain Selection of points: Ear-Shenmen, Brain, Ear Apex, Lung and other ear points corresponding to operative incision. Apply strong stimulation with a filiform needle or electric acupuncture. Needles are retained 1 to 2 hours, treat once daily.

8) Postoperative abdominal distension Selection of points: Large Intestine and Small Intestine, Stomach, End of Inferior Helix Crus, and Spleen. Apply strong stimulation with intermittent rotation of needles or with electric acupuncture. Needles are retained for one to two hours.

9) Perifocal inflammation of the shoulder Selection of points: Shoulder, Clavicle, Infra Tragic Apex.

Secondary points: Liver, Spleen and Brain, Tender spots in the cavum conchae. Treat once daily with a filiform needle or electric acupuncture. Choose 3 or 4 points for each treatment. Treatment course varies according to the individual disease condition.

10) Acute cholecystitis and gallstones Selection of points: Penetrating the right Ear-Shenmen towards Abdomen, End of Inferior Helix Crus and Gallbladder; penetrating Gallbladder 0.2 cm below towards Duodenum, and the left Gallbladder penetrating towards Duodenum. Give electric stimulation for 20 to 40 minutes once a day. Three to 5 treatments are considered as a course.

11) Ascariasis in the biliary duct Selection of points: Liver, Gallbladder, Duodenum and Root of Auricular Vagus Nerve. Puncture right side first. Stimulate left side if there is not much improvement in pain. During retention, rotate the needles once every five to ten minutes. After abdominal pain stops, western medication or Chinese medicinal herbs should be administered.

12) Colic pain due to ureteral calculus Selection of points: Kidney, Abdomen, End of Inferior Antihelix Crus and Brain. Puncture the affected side first, then the healthy side. If there is not much relief, apply strong stimulation with retention of needles for 20 to 40 minutes or with electric acupuncture.

13) Pain caused by cancer or tumor Selection of points: Brain, Heart, Ear Apex and other auricular points corresponding to the pathological areas.

Secondary points: End of Inferior Antihelix Crus, Liver and Ear-Shenmen. Choose 4 to 6 points for each treatment; use both sides alternatively. Treat once daily. Or apply acupoint injection with 0.1-0.3 ml Dolantin subcutaneously and obliquely from Ear-Shenmen to the anterior and inferior aspect of this point. After injection, remove the needle slowly in order to avoid the out flow of drug from the needle hole.

14) Transfusion reaction Selection of points: Ear-Shenmen, Infratragic Apex and Brain. Apply strong stimulation with a filiform needle. Continue the retention of needles for 30 minutes after the stopping of chills.

15) Acute bacterial dysentery Selection of points: Large Intestine, Small Intestine and Lower Portion of Rectum. Apply strong stimulation with a filiform needle. Treat once or twice a day for 3 to 7 days.

16) Tertian malaria Selection of points: Infratragic Apex, Brain and Intertragus. Treat once daily or every other day or two hours before estimated time of attack. Retain needles until the attack is over. Rotate the needles twice or three times during retention.

17) Epidemic parotitis (mumps) Selection of points: Antitragic Apex,

Cheek, Subcortex and Brain. Apply strong stimulation with a filiform needle. Treat once or twice daily. Three days constitute a treatment course. Scorching moxibustion with oily herbal lampwick also can be applied on Ear Apex or between Small Intestine and Kidney. Moxibustion can be applied on the affected side for swelling of one side, or bilaterally for mumps of both sides. Moxibustion is given once a day until swelling subsides.

18) Bronchial asthma Selection of points: Lung, Trachea, Infratragic Apex, Antitragic Apex and Ear-Shenmen.

Secondary points: Root of Auricular Vagus Nerve, Kidney, Sanjiao and Large Intestine. Apply strong stimulation with a filiform needle. One treatment is given daily during an attack. Choose 4 or 5 points bilaterally or unilaterally for each treatment with retention of needles for 30 minutes. After the stabilization of condition, treatment is reduced to once every other day. During remission needle embedding can be applied to consolidate effectiveness.

19) Acute bronchitis Selection of points: Lung, Trachea and Ear-Shenmen.

Secondary points: Occiput, Infratragic Apex and Root of Auricular Vagus Nerve. Treat once daily or every other day with a filiform needle. Choose 3 or 4 points bilaterally for each treatment.

20) Paroxysmal tachycardia Selection of points: Heart, End of Inferior Antihelix Crus, Ear-Shenmen and Brain. Apply mild stimulation. Retain needles for 30 to 60 minutes. Rotate needles twice or three times during needle retention. Treat once daily.

21) Hypertension Selection of points: Infratragic Apex, Groove of Inferior Antihelix Crus, Helix and Ear-Shenmen.

Secondary points: Intertragus, Forehead, Temple, Liver and Kidney. Filiform

needle, electric acupuncture or needle embedding can be used according to different conditions. Treat once daily or every several days. Choose 4 or 5 points for each treatment. Ten treatments are considered as a course. A one-week rest interval is instituted between courses.

22) Hiccough Selection of points: Sensitive spots near Middle Ear or Root of Auricular Vagus Nerve. Puncture with strong stimulation. For refractory cases needle embedding is applied following filiform needling.

23) Vomiting Selection of points: Stomach, Liver, Spleen and Ear-Shenmen. Treat once daily, for severe cases twice or three times per day. One course is composed of 3 to 5 treatments. Use mild stimulation during early stage of treatment.

24) Chronic gastritis Selection of points: Stomach, End of Inferior Antihelix Crus and Lung.

Secondary points: Liver, Spleen, Mouth and Intertragus. Embedding method with herbal seeds or any kind of granules is applied after filiform needling or electric acupuncture. Needle once daily with 3 to 5 points each time.

25) Gastric or duodenal ulcer Selection of points: Stomach or Duodenum, End of Inferior Antihelix Crus, Brain and Mouth.

Secondary points: Sanjiao, Ear-Shenmen, Liver, Spleen and Middle Ear. Filiform needling is applied at 3 to 5 points each time. In the acute stage treat once daily, and during remission once every other day.

26) Acute diarrhoea Selection of points: Large Intestine (puncture three needles) and Stomach. Stimulation is given according to the patient's constitution. For severe cases treat once every 2 to 4 hours, and reduce to once every other day or twice a week after relief of symptoms. Retain needles for 30 minutes.

27) Enuresis Selection of points: Kidney, Bladder, Liver and Brain. A filiform needle or electric acupuncture is applied at 3 or 4 points for each treatment. Treat once daily or once every other day, and reduce to once a week after therapeutic effect is stable.

28) Neurasthenia Selection of points: Ear-Shenmen, Heart, Brain and Middle Border.

Secondary points: Kidney, Liver and Intertragus. Apply mild stimulation with a filiform needle or electric acupuncture once daily. Choose 4 or 5 points and use alternatively at each treatment.

29) Hysteria Selection of points: Heart, Brain, Occiput and Middle Border.

Secondary points: Liver, Intertragus. Ear-Shenmen and other corresponding points. During an attack apply strong stimulation with a filiform needle or electric acupuncture. Choose 3 or 4 points on both ears according to different symptoms. Retain the needles for 20 minutes. Treat once every other day. Ten treatments constitute a course. Mild stimulation should be given during the recovery stage.

30) Facial neuritis Selection of points: Eye, Cheek, Liver and Mouth.

Secondary points: Spleen, Forehead, Ear-Shenmen and Infratragic Apex. During acute stage apply mild stimulation with a filiform needle to 3 to 5 points on the affected side for each treatment. After being treated for several days, change to electric acupuncture with low frequency or dense-dispersion wave-form. Treat once daily or once every other day.

31) Sequelae of cerebrovascular accident Selection of points: Brain, Middle Border, Liver, Sanjiao, and other auricular points corresponding to the paralytic sides of the body. Secondary points are added according to different symptoms. For aphasia add Heart and Spleen, and for dysphagia add Mouth, Root of Auricular Vagus Nerve, and Throat. Treat once every other day after stabilization of diseased condition and recovery from unconsciousness. One course of treatment is composed of 15 to 20 sessions.

32) Dysmenorrhea Selection of points: Depression in Triangular Fossa, Intertragus and Root of Auricular Vagus Nerve. Choose one or two pairs of points and treat once daily by strong stimulation with a filiform needle or electric acupuncture. Retain the needles until acute pain is relieved.

33) Functional bleeding of uterus Principal points: Depression in Triangular Fossa, Intertragus and Ear-Shenmen.

Secondary points: Spleen, Brain, Liver and Middle Ear. Treat once daily with a filiform needle at 3 to 5 points. Retain the needles for 30 to 60 minutes. Ten treatments constitute one course.

34) Insufficient lactation Selection of points: Puncture the most painful spot at Chest with mild stimulation. Retain the needles for 15 minutes. Treat once or twice daily for 1 to 3 days.

35) Itching of the skin Selection of points: Ear-Shenmen, Lung, Brain, Infratragic Apex and Interior Tubercle.

Secondary points: Liver, Spleen, Heart, Intertragus, Pancreas and Gallbladder. Treat once every other day by filiform needling or electric acupuncture. Choose 3 to 5 pairs of points at each treatment, five to ten treatments constitute a course. If it is necessary to continue the treatment, one week of rest should be instituted after one course of treatment. Embedding method with herbal seeds or other granules is also applicable once every week.

36) Urticaria Selection of points:

Interior Tubercle, Infratragic Apex, Anti-tragic Apex and Liver. Apply strong stimulation with a filiform needle. Treat once daily or every other day. Ten treatments are considered one course. Severe itching may be treated twice or thrice per day. For chronic urticaria, patients should persist in a prolonged course of therapy.

37) Neurodermatitis Selection of points: Lung, Infratragic Apex, Intertragus and other corresponding points. Treat once daily or every other day. Retain the needles for one to two hours. Needle embedding is also applicable. For severe itching treatment may be applied twice daily. One additional course of treatment should be administered after symptoms are controlled in order to consolidate the therapeutic effect.

38) Herpes zoster Selection of points: Lung, Brain, Intertragus and other corresponding points. Apply strong stimulation with a filiform needle. Retain the needles for two hours. Treat once or twice daily, and reduce to once every other day after relief of symptoms. Ten treatments constitute a course.

39) Verruca plana Selection of points: Ear-Shenmen, Lung, Brain, Large Intestine, Occiput and Intertragus. Use needle embedding at two or three points for each treatment. Retain the needles one to three days. Ten treatments constitute one course.

40) Stye Selection of points: Ear Apex. Apply strong stimulation with a filiform needle. Retain the needle for 15 to 20 minutes. Treat once or twice daily. Or select Anterior Tragic Notch, Posterior Tragic Notch and Liver of the affected side. Electric acupuncture is applied once daily with retention of needles for 15 to 20 minutes. Treatment should be administered promptly after the onset of stye, to ensure swifter

subsidence.

41) Acute conjunctivitis Selection of points: Bloodletting on Ear Apex or on minor veins of retroauricle. Treat once or twice daily. Or puncture Eye, Ear-Shenmen and Ear Apex with a filiform needle and strong stimulation. Retain the needles for 30 minutes.

42) Electric ophthalmalgia and snow blindness Selection of points: Puncture Eye with a filiform needle and strong stimulation. Retain the needle for 15 to 30 minutes. Or use electric acupuncture on Eye, Liver and Kidney for 15 to 20 minutes.

43) Congestive glaucoma Selection of points: Bloodletting on Groove of Lowering Blood Pressure or Ear Apex. Treat once daily or every other day. Or select Eye, Liver, Anterior Tragic Notch or Posterior Tragic Notch. Use filiform needles or embedding granules at these points.

44) Tinnitus and impaired hearing Selection of points: Ear, Liver and Kidney, unilateral or bilateral. Apply strong stimulation with a filiform needle or electric acupuncture once daily or every other day. Retain the needles for 30 to 60 minutes. One course consists of 15 to 20 treatments.

45) Acute tonsillitis Selection of points: Bleeding the veins of retroauricle Ear Apex, or Helix 3,4, and 6 once every day. Or needling Throat and Helix 4 and 6 with strong stimulation once or twice per day. Retain the needles for one hour. Needle embedding can be added after filiform needling.

46) Hoarseness Selection of points: Lung, Throat, Neck, Trachea, Heart, Large Intestine and Kidney. Apply mild stimulation at 2 or 3 pairs of points. Five treatments compose one course.

47) Toothache Selection of points: Apply strong stimulation at Ear Apex with a filiform needle. Retain the needle for 20 minutes. Or apply strong stimulation at Cheek with a filiform needle. Retain the needle for 30 minutes.

IV. PRECAUTIONS

1. If sudden dizziness, nausea, stuffiness of the chest or other fainting symptoms occur during treatment, the patient should be managed in the same manner as during ordinary body acupuncture. During initial visits, patients should be in a reclining position in order to avoid fainting.

2. Strict antisepsis is necessary to avoid infection of the auricle. In case of inflammation or redness of the needle hole or distension and pain of the auricle, timely and appropriate measures should be taken such as applying 2% iodine or oral administration of anti-inflammation drugs. Needling is contraindicated if frost-bite or inflammation is present on the auricle in order to avoid diffusion or inflammation.

3. Ear acupuncture is not advisable for women during pregnancy if there is a history of miscarriage. Aged and weak patients with hypertension and arteriosclerosis should have proper rest before and after needling.

4. While there are extensive indications for ear acupuncture, it still has its limitations. The therapeutic effects for some diseases are not satisfactory, or only symptomatic relief is achieved, therefore, in treating some disorders, it is necessary to combine some other therapies.

ACUPUNCTURE ANALGESIA

Acupuncture analgesia (abbreviated to A.A.) is an analgesic method built on the basis of relieving pain and regulating the physiological function of the human body by needling. The procedure produces an absence of pain by stimulating certain points when the patient undergoes an operation in full consciousness. It is considered an important achievement in the successful integration of traditional Chinese and Western medicine.

I. THE CHARACTERISTICS OF ACUPUNCTURE ANALGESIA

1. Safe in Wide Indications

Extensive clinical practice has proven that acupuncture analgesia is completely safe. Millions of surgical operations with acupuncture analgesia have been carried out in China and none of them led to death attributed to needling. Acupuncture analgesia does not produce any side-effects and accidents which might happen when drug anaesthesia is employed. What is more, it does not result in respiratory tract infection, gastrointestinal dysfunction, abdominal distension and retention of urine. It, therefore, is more suitable to the aged patients with weak constitution, and the patients with cardiac, pulmonary, hepatic or renal condition and those who are too sick to sustain drug anaesthesia.

2. Reduced Physiological Disturbance and Rapid Recovery

As acupuncture functions to regulate the physiological condition of the human body, doctors are able to take immediate measures with acupuncture according to the subjective signs of the patient to avoid the physiological disturbance caused by severe pain. Blood pressure, pulse and respiration rates during the operation remain relatively stable in most cases. After the operation, patients' physiological state remain normal, as manifested in early regaining of appetite and ambulatory activities, and satisfactory healing of wound. All these are conducive to an early recovery.

3. Subjective Cooperation of the Patient and Improvement of Operative Results

The patient under acupuncture analgesia is mentally alert and able to communicate with the surgeons. This enables the surgeon to judge operative results as the operation proceeds. During thyroidectomy, for instance, the patient's phonation may be tested; in total laryngectomy, the swallowing movement can be checked; in eye surgery for strabismus, eyeball movement can be examined; in amputation of trigeminal sensory root and craniocerebral operation, the limits of facial anesthetic region can be observed. The close coordination between the patient and surgeon ensures the desirable operative results.

4. Simple Apparatus and Easy to Popularize

Acupuncture analgesia does not require any sophisticated medical equipment and is not restrained by preferential environment. The only requisites for success are to observe the patient's pain endurance carefully, select well-indicated cases, locate the points accurately and puncture skillfully. The practice across the nation has proven that acupuncture analgesia is more practical in backward regions where emergency surgery is possibly delayed due to lack of necessary medical equipment.

Acupuncture analgesia was created in the 1950's in China. With researching for more than twenty years, some noteworthy experiences have been accumulated. Like any other science and technology, acupuncture analgesia has a long way to go from imperfection to perfection. Though the mechanism of acupuncture analgesia has been preliminarily outlined, further studies are still needed to reach a thorough explanation. Acupuncture analgesia is able to raise pain threshhold and endurance, but there still exist some drawbacks, such as incomplete analgesia and muscular tension which is likely to cause discomforts due to

retraction of internal organs in an introabdominal operation. In this case, administrating a small dose of anesthetic drug or puncturing some acupoints will relieve the pain and discomforts of the patients.

II. PREOPERATIVE PREPARATIONS FOR ACUPUNCTURE ANALGESIA

1. Explanatory Work to the Patient

As the patient under acupuncture analgesia is mentally alert during the surgical operation, it is essential to consider his attitude toward acupuncture analgesia and his spiritual behaviour because these may affect his physiological function, pain endurance and ability to accept the operation. It is necessary to let the patient know in detail the characteristics, methods, process, effects of acupuncture analgesia, the operative procedures, and the reaction and sensation caused by needling. It is also important to make the patient mentally relaxed so that he can cooperate with the surgeons to ensure the successful operative results.

2. Preliminary Test of Needling and Pain Endurance

Before acupuncture analgesia, one or more points may be selected on the body of the patient for preliminary test of needling. With this, the patient can experience the needling sensation, free his nervousness from acupuncture analgesia and adapt himself to the needling stimulation. On the other hand, when he knows the tolerance of the patient, the surgeon can decide the method and intensity of stimulation in the operation. Also, physical or chemical stimulation can be applied to measure the patient's pain endurance. Anyway, the purpose of pain endurance test is for precise determination of the stimulation intensity in acupuncture analgesia.

3.   Practice of Deep Breathing

Instruct the patient under thoracic-abdominal operation to practise slow, deep abdominal breathing before operation. It can relieve stuffiness of the chest, heavy sensation and dyspnea after the chest is opened up. In abdominal surgery, deep breathing helps to ease the patient of the muscular spasm, nausea and vomiting caused by retraction of internal organs.

4. Preoperative Plan of Acupuncture Analgesia

The close cooperation between the acupuncturists, surgeons and nursing staff is indispensable for successful operation with acupuncture analgesia. The patient's psychological state, case history and focus of infection should be brought to thorough analysis and discussion. Prediction of the problems possibly occuring under operation and corresponding emergency measures will guarantee a safe operation on a fully conscious patient.

III.   PRINCIPLES OF SELECTING POINTS FOR ACUPUNCTURE ANALGESIA

Since it is through stimulating certain particular acupoints of the body that the acupuncture analgesia works, it is important for the operators to be well versed in the appropriate needling stimulation as well as the accurate point location.

The commonly used methods in selecting points are summarized as follows:

1.   Selecting Points According to the Theory of Meridians

Traditional Chinese medicine holds that the twelve regular meridians connect interiorly with the zang-fu organs and exteriorly with the four limbs. Each of the meridians has its own pathway and connects with the other in view of the exterior-interior relationship. The method of selecting points along the meridians is therefore based on the concept embodied in the theory of the meridians "where a meridian traverses, there is a place amenable to treatment."

2.   Selecting Points According to Syndrome Differentiations.

Traditional Chinese medicine emphasizes the concept of the organic integrity of the human body. When any portion of the body is diseased, various symptoms and signs may be manifested through the meridians connecting with that portion. In acupuncture therapy, it is important to apply the theory of zang-fu organs and theory of meridians to syndrome differentiations, so is it in acupuncture analgesia. Before selecting the points, symptoms and signs of a disease must be differentiated and then their relation with the zang-fu organs and meridians be found out. Attention should also be paid to the patient's responses that may be elicited in the operative procedure. For example, in the chest operation, the patient is likely to experience palpitation, shortness of breath and anxiety in the preoperative period or during the operation. According to the theory of traditional Chinese medicine, these symptoms are caused by the disturbance of heart qi. Thus, Ximen (P 4) and Neiguan (P 6) are usually selected to tranquilize the heart, sedate the mind and regulate the heart qi.

3. Selecting Points According to Segmental Innervation

Clinical practice and scientific experiments with acupuncture analgesia show that the nervous system is involved in pain suppression and physiological regulation of acupuncture analgesia. In other words, the functional integrity of nervous system is a prerequisite to produce needling sensation and analgesic effect. Based on the relation of the segmental innervation between the puncturing site and the operative site, there are three ways to select points, i.e. 1) selecting points in the adjacent segmentation, or in an area that is supplied by the same spinal nerve or an adjacent nerve that supplies the operative site; 2) selecting points in a remote segmentation, that is in an area not supplied by the same or adjacent spinal nerve of the operative site; 3) stimulating the nerve trunk within the same segmentation, that is to stimulate directly the peripheral nerve which supplies the operative site. For

instance, Hegu (L I 4) and Neiguan (P 6) are points of the adjacent segmentation in thyroidectomy, while Neiting (S 44) and Zusanli (S 36) are points in the remote segmentation. Futu (L I 18) is regarded as a point for direct stimulation of the cutaneous cervical nerve plexus, known as stimulating the nerve trunk within the same segmentation. The implication of selecting points in the adjacent and remote segmentation in acupuncture analgesia is different from that of selecting the neighbouring and distal points in acupuncture therapy. The latter only denotes the relative distance between the location of the points chosen and the affected area to be treated. Selecting points far from the affected site is known as the method of selecting distant points, while selecting points near the affected site is known as the method of selecting adjacent points. Neither method is related to segmental nerves of the puncturing site and operative site. For example, for analgesia in thyroidectomy, Hegu (L I 4) and Neiting (P 6) are chosen as adjacent points according to segmental innervation; but from the point of view of the relative distance between these points and the operative site on the neck, they are considered as distant points.

4. Selecting Auricular Points

This is to select the corresponding auricular areas according to the operative site and its involved internal organs. For example, auricular Stomach Point is chosen for subtotal gastrectomy. Auricular points are also selected according to the theory of zang-fu organs. For instance, "the lung dominates skin and hair; and Lung Point is often chosen in various operations; while the kidney dominates the bone," and Kidney Point is often selected in orthopedic surgery.

Moreover, reaction spots on the auricle may be selected as well. When an internal organ or area of the body is affected, some reaction spots with tenderness, reduction of electro-resistance, deformation of auricular structure and discoloration may occur on the corresponding auricular areas. These reaction spots may be chosen for acupuncture analgesia.

According to therapeutic experience, Ear-Shenmen and Inferior Crus, i.e. Sympathetic Nerve Point are effective for sedation and pain suppression. They are therefore widely used in auricular acupuncture analgesia.

IV. MANIPULATION TECHNIQUES

Based on the arrival of qi, hand-manipulation and electro-pulsating stimulation are commonly used in acupuncture analgesia.

1. Hand Manipulation

This is the basic stimulative method. Even if electro-stimulation is applied, it is also started with hand manipulation. The electro-apparatus is not employed until the patient feels the needling sensation. Hand manipulation is to lift-thrust and twist-rotate

2. Electric Stimulation

After the desired needling response is obtained by the hand manipulation, the outlet of the electric acupuncture apparatus is attached to the handle of the filiform needle, and the current will get through to the body. Clinically, the electric pulsating is divided into continuous, sparse-dense and intermittent three kinds, mostly in the form of biphasic spike or rectangular wave 0.5 to 2 msc. in width. But biphasic sinusoid or irregular sound wave may also be used. The frequencies of electric pulse are of two kinds: two to eight times per second and forty to two hundred times per second. The stimulation force should be adjusted according to the patient's tolerance. Generally, acupuncture analgesia requires powerful stimulation which may be increased gradually up to the highest limit, the one which the patient can stand. Each time of continuous electro-stimulus can not be too long, in case it produces too much stimulation to destroy patient's needling sensation. If a longer electro-stimulus is needed, the intermittent electric pulsating can be selected. The stimulation should be started from zero and added to the desired level gradually and when it is turned down, it should be reduced slowly. It is not advisable to produce abrupt stimulus, which may make the patient unbearable.

3. Induction and Retaining of the Needle

Needling or electric stimulation manipulated on the selected points for a desirable length of time prior to the operation is known as induction. The intensity of needling stimulation should be proper and induction period is about twenty minutes, or longer if the result of pain endurance test is unfavourable. By means of induction, the patient may adapt himself to the stimulus of acupuncture analgesia. At the same time, it can also regulate the function of various internal organs of the body, preparing the patient for surgical operation. At certain operative stages when the operative stimulus is mild, hand manipulation may be stopped or the current for electric stimulation cut off. This is so called retaining of the needle. Before the operation proceeds to a stage of vigorous stimulation, it is necessary to restart the hand manipulation or electric stimulation so as to maintain and strengthen the analgesic effect.

V. ADJUVANTS

In order to enhance the effect of acupuncture analgesia and guarantee the operation to go on smoothly, some adjuvants in small doses should be given to almost every case of acupuncture analgesia. Though some operation with acupuncture analgesia can be done without the help of any adjuvants, the analgesia effect will be more favourable if small doses of adjuvants are administered before or during the operation.

1. Adjuvants for preoperative administrations: Usually Dolantin is given intramuscularly or dropped intravenously fifteen to thirty minutes prior to an operation, generally 50 mg dose each time for adults, and 0.5 mg each kg body weight for children. When necessary, Promethazine (Phenergan) is added at the same time, 25 mg for adults, and 0.5 mg each kg body weight for children; or Chlorpromazine (Wintermin) 12.5 mg for adults, and 0.5 mg each kg body weight for children.

Atropine and Hyoscine (Scopolamine) are used in order to keep the respiratory tract unblocked. Atropine is given 0.5 mg for adults, and 0.01 mg each kg body weight for children subcutaneously or intramuscularly; Hyoscine is given 0.3 mg for adults subcutaneously or intramuscularly with the exception of the aged and infants.

2. Adjuvants during operations: Some proper adjuvants are given according to different stages of operations and different reactions the patients show. Adjuvants for local analgesia are mainly administered, for instance, Neocaine (Procaine Hydrochloride), Lidocaine (Xylocaine), Dicaine (Pantocaine), etc., for local infiltration and blockage. The amount of the adjuvants being used should be as small as possible so as to lessen patients' discomforts. Heavy doses of some sedatives will not only do harm to the health of the patient, but also cause unconsciousness or hypnotism. The patient will be unable to communicate and cooperate with the surgeons, and thus the result of the acupuncture analgesia and the operation will be affected.

VI. REMARKS

1. Because the patient is fully conscious during the operation under acupuncture analgesia, surgeons should preoperatively make the whole procedure of the operation known to the patient so as to gain the patient's cooperation. Surgeons should have an amiable attitude, well-prepared measures, observing blood pressure, pluse and respiration rate attentively during the operation, and reducing the patient's discomforts as far as possible.

2. The patient's chief complaint should be attended during the operation. When discomfort occurs, appropriate measures should be taken in time to relieve it, and the patient should be comforted to maintain his confidence. The amount of the adjuvants

should be proper, either overdose or under-dose is harmful to the patient's health or to the preceeding of the operation.

3. In order to promote the effect and lessen the subcortex bleeding, an appropriate dosage of physiological saline with the addition of a little adrenal may be used subcutaneously in the incision region before the skin incision in some operations.

4. Patients may regain appetite and ambulatory activity soon after an operation under the guidance of the medical workers besides general nursing care, and those are conducive to an early recovery.

SOME EXAMPLES OF SELECTING POINTS FOR ACUPUNCTURE ANALGESIA

Operation	Selecting Points
Cranial operation	A. Xiangu (S 43), Zulinqi (G 41), Taichong (Liv 3), Quanliao (S I 18). (All on the diseased side.) B. Hegu (L I 4), Neiguan (P 6), Quanliao (S I 18).
Retina Detachment	A. Hegu (L I 4), Zhigou (S J 6). (Both on the diseased side.) B. Auricular points: Forehead towards Eye 1 (Anterior Intertragic Notch), Eye 2 (posterior Intertragic Notch), Yangbai (G 14) towards Yuyao (Extra). (All on the diseased side.)
Operations of trichiasis for entropion Correction of strabismus	A. Hegu (L I 4) (Bilaterally) B. Taichong (Liv 3). Guangming (G 37). A. Hegu (L I 4), Zhigou (S J 6), Yangbai (G 14) towards Yuyao (Extra), Sibai (S 2) towards Chengqi(S 1). (All on the diseased side with electric stimulation.) B. Hegu(L I 4), Zhigou (S J 6), Houxi(S I 3), Jingmen (G 25).
Cataract couching	A. Hegu(L I 4), Waiguan (S J 5) towards Neiguan (P 6). (Both on the diseased side.) B. Hegu(L I 4), Zhigou(S J 6). (Both on the diseased side.)
Enucleation of eyeball	A. Hegu(L I 4), Waiguan(S J 5), Houxi (S I 3). (All on the diseased side. If the eyeball is sensitive, administer 1% dicaine for surface anaesthesia during the operation.) B. Auricular points: Lung, Liver, Kidney, Eye 1, Eye 2, Ear-Shenmen, Sympathetic Nerve (Inferior Antihelix Crus).
Iridectomy	A. Hegu(L I 4), Waiguan (S J 5), Neiting (S 44). (All

bilaterally. At the first two points, give hand manipulation. For the last one, retain the needle after needling sensation is produced.)

Shortening of sclera	A. Hegu(L I 4), Zhigou (S J 6), Yangbai(G 14) towards Yuyao(Extra), Sibai(S 2) towards Chengqi(S 1). (All on the diseased side with electric stimulation.) B. Hegu (L I 4), Zhigou (S J 6). (Both on the diseased side with electric stimulation.)
Replantation of pterygium	A. Auricular points: Eye, Liver. (Both on the diseased side.)
Exenteration of orbit	A. Hegu(L I 4) (Bilaterally), Zhigou (S J 6). Auricular points: Forehead towards Eye 1, Ear-Shenmen towards Sympathetic Nerve. (Both bilaterally.)
Resection of tumour in parotid glands	A. Fenglong(S 40), Yangfu(G 38), Fuyang (B 59), Xiangu(S 43), Taichong (Liv 3), Xiaxi (G 43). (All bilaterally. Needles are retained after needling sensation is produced.) B. Neiting(S 44), Neiguan(P 6) towards Waiguan(S J 5).
Operation in the submaxillary region	A. Fenglong(S 40), Yangfu(G 38), Fuyang(B 59), Taichong(Liv 3), Gongsun(Sp 4), Neiguan(P 6). (All on the diseased side.) B. Auricular points: Maxillary, Kidney, Ear-Shenmen towards Sympathetic Nerve, Lung.
Plastic operation of the tempromendibular joint	A. Fenglong(S 40), Yangfu(G 38), Fuyang(B 59), Taichong(Liv 3), Gongsun(Sp 4), Hegu (L I 4). (The first four points on both sides and the last two on the diseased side.)
Resection of the mixed tumour of the palate	A. Hegu(L I 4), Neiguan(P 6), Gongsun(Sp 4).
Radical mastoidectomy	A. Waiguan(S J 5), Yanglingquan(G 34). (Both bilaterally with electric stimulation.) B. Hegu(L I 4), Zhigou(S J 6). (Both on the diseased side.) Auricular points: Ear-Shenmen, Lung, Kidney, Ear(Tragion). (All on the diseased side. In the induction period use the auricular points only.)
Operation to expose the tympanic	A. Hegu(L I 4), Houxi(S I 3), Waiguan(S J 5). (All on

cavity	both sides.)
Tympanotomy	A. Hegu(L I 4). (Bilaterally or on the diseased side.) B. Waiguan(S J 5) towards Neiguan(P 6), Yang-lingquan(G 34), Hegu(L I 4).
Total laryngectomy	A. Auricular points: Ear-Shenmen towards Sympathetic Nerve, Forehead towards Ear-Asthma(at the apex of antitragus), Adrenal (at lower tubercle on border of Tragus), Hegu(L I 4), Zhigou(S J 6). (All on the left side.) B. Hegu(L I 4), Neiguan(P 6), Renying(S 9).
Tonsillectomy	A. Auricular points: Throat, Tonsil. (Both bilaterally.) B. Hegu(L I 4). (Bilaterally).
Tooth extraction	A. For upper teeth: Jiache(S 6), Quanliao(S I 18). For lower teeth: Daying(S 5).
Lateral nasal incision	A. Hegu(L I 4), Zhigou(S J 6), Juliao (S 3) towards Sibai(S 2). (All on the diseased side.)
Radical maxillary sinusotomy	A. Hegu(L I 4), Zhigou(S J 6). (During the induction period, Juliao(S 3) towards Dicang is added.) B. Hegu(L I 4), Neiguan(P 6), Neiting(S 44), Yingxiang(L I 20).
Radical frontal sinusotomy	A. Yangbai(G 14) towards Zanzhu(B 2), Juliao (S 3) towards Sibai(S 2), Hegu(L I 4), Zhigou(S J 6). (All on the diseased side.)
Nasal polypectomy	A. Hegu(L I 4) or Yingxiang(L I 20). (Bilaterally or on the diseased side.) B. Auricular points: Lung, Nose, Ear-Shenmen towards Sympathetic Nerve.
Resection of thyroid adenoma	A. Hegu(L I 4), Neiguan(P 6). B. Futu(L I 18). Auricular points: Ear-Shenmen, Lung, Neck, Endocrine(Intertragus).
Separation of mitral valve	A. Neiguan(P 6), Hegu(L I 4), Zhigou(S J 6). (All on the diseased side.)
Resection of pericardium	A. Hegu(L I 4), Neiguan(P 6). (Both bilaterally.)

Pneumonectomy	A. Binao(L I 14). (On the diseased side.) B. Hegu(L I 4), Neiguan(P 6) or Waiguan(S J 5) towards Neiguan (P 6), Sanyangluo(S J 8) towards Ximen(P 4).
Gastric operation	A. Zusanli(S 36), Shangjuxu(S 37). (Bilaterally or on the diseased side.) B. Auricular points: Ear-Shenmen, Lung, Sympathetic Nerve, Gastric. (All on the left side.)
Splenectomy	A. Hegu(L I 4), Zusanli(S 36), Sanyinjiao (Sp 6), Taichong(Liv 3). (All on the diseased side.) B. Auricular points: Lung, Spleen, Sympathetic Nerve, Ear-Shenmen, Sanjiao.
Appendectomy	A. Shangjuxu(Sp 37), Lanwei(Extra). (All bilaterally.) B. Hegu(L I 4), Neiguan(P 6), Gongsun(Sp 4). (All bilaterally.)
Herniorrhaphy	A. Zusanli(S 36), Weidao(G 28). (Both bilaterally.) B. Yinlingquan(Sp 9), Sanyinjiao(Sp 6). (Both on the diseased side.)
Cesarean section	A. Zusanli(S 36), Sanyinjiao(Sp 6), Daimai (G 26), Neimadian(Extra), located at the midpoint of the line joining Yinlingquan (Sp 9) and internal malleolus. (All bilaterally.) B. Auricular points: Ear-Shenmen, Lung, Uterus (Triangular fossa), Abdomen.
Panhysterectomy with resection of appendixes of the uterus	A. Yaoshu(Du 2), Mingmen(Du 4), Daimai (G 26), Zusanli(S 36), Sanyinjiao(Sp 6), Zhongliao(B 23) or Ciliao(B 22). (All bilaterally.) B. Auricular points: Uterus, Lung, Ear-Shenmen, Abdomen, Endocrine(in cavum conchae), External Genitals.
Tubal ligation	A. Zusanli(S 36), Foot-Zhongdu(Liv 6). (Both bilaterally.) B. Zusanli(S 36), Sanyinjiao(Sp 6), Daimai(G 26), Qiecou(peri-incision acupuncture).
Hemorrhoidectomy	A. Sanyinjiao(Sp 6), Ciliao(B 22), Chengshan(B 51). B. Auricular points: Lung, Lower Portion of Rectum. (Both on the diseased side with electric stimulation.)

Nephrectomy	A. Hegu(L I 4), Neiguan(P 6), Zusanli(S 36), Sanyinjiao(Sp 6), Taichong(Liv 3). (All on the diseased side.) B. Auricular points: Ear-Shenmen, Lung, Waist, Ureter. (All on the diseased side.)
Clore-reduction of shoulder joint	A. Auricular points: Shoulder towards Shoulder Joint, Ear-Shenmen, Sympathetic Nerve, Kidney. (All on the diseased side.) B. Hegu(L I 4). (Bilaterally.) Auricular points: Shoulder, Arm. (Both bilaterally.)
Open-reduction of fracture of the humerus	A. Jianzhen(S I 9), Jianyu(L I 15), Houxi (S I 3), Hegu(L I 4), Neiguan(P 6). B. Auricular points: Ear-Shenmen, Lung, Arm, Elbow.
Amputation of forearm	A. Chize(L 5), Qingling(H 2). (Both bilaterally.)
Internal fixation of fractures of the femoral neck with three-flanged nail	A. Zusanli(S 36), Fenglong(S 40), Fuyang (B 59), Waiqiu(G 36), Juegu(Xuanzhong G 39), Sanyinjiao (Sp 6), Qiuxu(G 40), Xiangu(S 43). (All on the diseased side with electric stimulation.) B. Auricular points: Ear-Shenmen, Sympathetic Nerve, Coxa, Ischium Lung, Kidney.
Resection of valvula semilunaris and fusion of articulatio genus	A. Futu(S 32), Yinlingquan(Sp 9), Yanglingquan(G 34), Xuehai(Sp 10), Liangqiu(S 34), Sanyinjiao(Sp 6), Huantiao (G 30), Fengshi(G 31). B. Auricular points: Sympathetic Nerve, Kidney, Knee, Lung.
Amputation of lower portion of leg	A. Huantiao(G 30), Zhibian(B 54), Fengshi(G 31), Yanglingquan(G 34), Yinglingquan(Sp 9), Sanyinjiao(Sp 6). B. Auricular points: Ear-Shenmen, Lung, Kidney, Ischium towards Sympathetic Nerve. (All on the diseased side with electric stimulation.)

BIBLIOGRAPHY

Historical Publications

Huangdi's Internal Classic (黄帝内经)
Miraculous Pivot (灵枢)
Plain Questions (素问)
Classic on 81 Medical Problems (八十一难经)
Classic on Pulse (脉经)
Complete Collection of Acupuncture and Moxibustion
Synopsis of Prescriptions from the Golden Chamber (金匮要略)
Treatise on Febrile Disease (伤寒论)
Treatment of Different Kinds of Diseases (诸病源候论)
Exposition of the Fourteen Meridians (十四经发挥)
Emergency Moxibustion Therapy (备急灸法)
Highlights of Acupuncture (针灸聚英)
Compendium of Acupuncture and Moxibustion (针灸大成)
Guide to the Classic of Acupuncture (针灸指南)
Illustrated Appendices to the Classic of Categories (类经图翼)
Illustrated Manual of Acupoints on Bronze Figure (铜人输穴针灸图经)
Elementary Medicine (医学入门)
Medical Highlights (外台必要)
Popular Prescriptions (普济方)
Questions and Answers Concerning Acupuncture and Moxibustion (针灸问答)
A Medical Book by Master Danxi (丹溪心法)

Imperial Encyclopaedia of Medicine (圣经总录)
Medical Records as a Guide to Diagnosis (临证指裁)
Recipes for Saving Lives (济生方)
Systematic Classic of Acupuncture (针灸甲乙经)
A Treatise on the Three Categories of Pathogenic Factors of Disease (三因方)
Ye Tianshi Gynecology (叶天士妇科)
Secrets for Delivery Methods (胎产心法)

Recent Publications

Acupuncture and Moxibustion (针灸学), first edition, edited by Shanghai College of Traditional Chinese Medicine, published by People's Medical Publishing House, 1974, Beijing.

A Textbook on Acupuncture and Moxibustion (针灸学讲义), first edition, edited by Acupuncture Teaching Group, Shanghai College of Traditional Chinese Medicine, published by Shanghai Science and Technology Publishing House, 1960, Shanghai.

Acupuncture and Moxibustion (针灸学), first edition, edited by Nanjing College of Traditional Chinese Medicine, published by Shanghai Science and Technology Publishing House, 1979, Shanghai.

Annotations on Systematic Classic of Acupuncture (针灸甲乙经校释), Vol.

1, first edition, edited by Shandong College of Traditional Chinese Medicine, published by People's Medical Publishing House, 1979, Beijing.

Anatomical Charts for Acupuncture and Moxibustion （针灸解剖学图谱）, first edition, charted by Editorial and Charting Group of Anatomical Charts for Acupuncture and Moxibustion, Zhejiang Medical University, Zhejiang College of Traditional Chinese Medicine, published by Zhejiang People's Publishing House, 1979, Hangzhou.

Paper Abstracts of the National Symposium on Acupuncture and Moxibustion and Acupuncture Anesthesia （全国针灸针麻学术讨论会论文摘要）, edited by Academic Section, National Symposium on Acupuncture and Moxibustion and Acupuncture Anesthesia, 1979, Beijing.

Anatomical Charts of Acupoints of the 14 Meridians （十四经穴位解剖挂图）, edited and charted by Shanghai College of Traditional Chinese Medicine, Shanghai Research Institute of Trad-

itional Chinese Medicine, published by Shanghai People's Publishing House, 1975, Shanghai.

Acupuncture and Moxibustion, Vol. 1 Meridian Theory （针灸学第一册经络学说）, first edition, edited by Shanghai College of Traditional Chinese Medicine, published by People's Medical Publishing House, 1962, Beijing.

Acupuncture and Moxibustion, Vol. 2 Acupoints （针灸学第二册输穴学）, edited by Shanghai College of Traditional Chinese Medicine, published by People's Medical Publishing House, 1962, Beijing.

Meridians and Collaterals—A Course of 10 Lectures （经络十讲）, first edition, edited by Editorial Group of "Meridians and Collaterals"—A Course of 10 Lectures, published by Shanghai People's Publishing House, 1976, Shanghai.

Essentials of Chinese Acupuncture （中国针灸学概要）, published by People's Medical Publishing House, 1979, Beijing.

CROSS INDEX OF ACUPOINTS (*PINYIN*)

A

Anmian (Extra 13)

B

Bafeng (Extra 40)
Baichongwu (Extra 35)
Baihuanshu (B 30)
Baihui (Du 20)
Bailao (Extra 16)
Benshen (G 13)
Biguan (S 31)
Binao (LI 14)
Bingfeng (LI 12)
Bitong (Extra 10)
Bizhong (Extra 32)
Bulang (K 22)
Burong (S 19)

C

Changqiang (Du 1)
Chengfu (B 36)
Chengguang (B 6)
Chengjiang (Ren 24)
Chengjin (B 56)
Chengling (G 18)
Chengman (S 20)
Chengqi (S 1)
Chengshan (B 57)
Chize (L 5)
Chongmen (Sp 12)
Chongyang (S 42)
Ciliao (B 32)

D

Dabao (Sp 21)
Dachangshu (B 25)
Dadu (Sp 2)
Dadun (Liv 1)
Dahe (K 12)
Daheng (Sp 15)
Daimai (G 26)
Daju (S 27)
Daling (P 70)
Dannangxue (Extra 39)
Danshu (B 19)
Dazhu (B 11)
Daying (S 5)
Dazhong (K 4)
Dazhui (Du 14)
Dicang (S 4)
Diji (Sp 8)
Dingchuan (Extra 14)
Diwuhui (G 42)
Duiduan (Du 27)
Dubi (S 35)
Dushu (B 16)

E

Erbai (Extra 31)
Erheliao (SJ 22)
Erjian (Extra 4)
Ermen (SJ 21)

F

Feishu (B 13)

Feiyang (B 58)
Fengchi (G 20)
Fengfu (Du 16)
Fenglong (S 40)
Fengmen (B 12)
Fengshi (G 31)
Fuai (Sp 16)
Fubai (G 10)
Fufen (B 41)
Fujie (Sp 14)
Fuliu (K 7)
Fushe (Sp 13)
Futonggu (K 20)
Futu (S 32)
Futu (LI 18)
Fuyang (B 59)
Fuxi (B 38)

G

Ganshu (B 18)
Gaohuang (B 43)
Geguan (B 46)
Geshu (B 17)
Gongsun (Sp 4)
Guanchong (SJ 1)
Guangming (G 37)
Guanmen (S 22)
Guanyuan (Ren 4)
Guanyuanshu (B 26)
Guilai (S 29)

H

Hanyan (G 4)
Heding (Extra 38)
Hegu (LI 4)
Henggu (K 11)
Heyang (B 55)
Houding (Du 19)
Houxi (SI 3)

Huagai (Ren 20)
Huangmen (B 51)
Huangshu (K 16)
Huantiao (G 30)
Huanmen (B 47)
Huanzhong (Extra 34)
Huaroumen (S 24)
Huatuojiaji (Extra 15)
Huiyang (B 35)
Huiyin (Ren 1)
Huizong (SJ 7)
Hunmen (B 47)

J

Jiache (S 6)
Jiachengjiang (Extra 8)
Jianjing (G 21)
Jianli (Ren 11)
Jianliao (SJ 14)
Jianqian (Extra 23)
Jianshi (P 5)
Jianwaishu (SI 14)
Jianyu (LI 15)
Jianzhen (SI 9)
Jianzhongshu (SI 15)
Jiaosun (SJ 20)
Jiaoxin (K 8)
Jiexi (S 41)
Jimai (Liv 12)
Jimen (Sp 11)
Jinggu (B 64)
Jingmen (G 25)
Jingming (B 1)
Jingqu (L 8)
Jinjin (Extra 9)
Jinmen (B 63)
Jinsuo (Du 8)
Jiquan (H 1)
Jiuwei (Ren 15)

Jizhong (Du 6)
Juegu (G 39)
Jueyinshu (B 14)
Jugu (LI 16)
Juliao (S 3)
Juliao (G 29)
Juque (Ren 14)

K

Kongzui (L 6)
Kouheliao (LI 19)
Kufang (S 14)
Kunlun (B 60)

L

Lanweixue (Extra 37)
Laogong (P 8)
Liangmen (S 21)
Liangqiu (S 34)
Lianquan (Ren 23)
Lidui (S 45)
Lieque (L 7)
Ligou (Liv 5)
Lingdao (H 4)
Lingtai (Du 10)
Lingxu (K 24)
Lougu (Sp 7)
Luoque (B 8)
Luozhen (Extra 28)
Luxi (SJ 19)

M

Meichong (B 3)
Mingmen (Du 4)
Muchuang (G 16)

N

Naohu (Du 17)

Naohui (SJ 13)
Naokong (G 19)
Naoshu (SJ 10)
Neiguan (P 6)
Neiting (S 44)

P

Pangguangshu (B 28)
Pianli (LI 6)
Pigen (Extra 20)
Pishu (B 20)
Pohu (B 42)
Pushen (B 61)

Q

Qianding (Du 21)
Qiangjian (Du 18)
Qiangu (SI 2)
Qianzheng (Extra 11)
Qichong (S 30)
Qihai (Ren 6)
Qihaishu (B 24)
Qihu (S 13)
Qimai (SJ 18)
Qimen (Liv 14)
Qinglengyuan (SJ 11)
Qingling (H 2)
Qishe (S 11)
Qiuhou (Extra 7)
Qiuxu (G 40)
Qixue (K 13)
Quanliao (SI 18)
Qubin (G 7)
Quchai (B 4)
Quchi (LI 11)
Quepen (S 12)
Qugu (Ren 2)
Ququan (Liv 8)
Quyuan (SI 13)

Quze (P 3)

R

Rangu (K 2)
Renying (S 9)
Renzhong (Du 26)
Riyue (G 24)
Rugen (S 18)
Ruzhong (S 17)

S

Sanjian (LI 3)
Sanjiaoshu (B 22)
Sanyangluo (SJ 8)
Sanyinjiao (Sp 6)
Shangguan (G 3)
Shangjuxu (S 37)
Shanglian (LI 9)
Shanglianquan (Extra 3)
Shangliao (B 31)
Shangqiu (Sp 5)
Shangqu (K 17)
Shangwan (Ren 13)
Shangxi (Du 23)
Shangyang (LI 1)
Shaochong (H 9)
Shaofu (H 8)
Shaohai (H 3)
Shaoshang (L 11)
Shaoze (SI 1)
Shencang (K 25)
Shendao (Du 11)
Shenfeng (K 23)
Shenque (Ren 8)
Shenmai (B 62)
Shenmen (H 7)
Shenshu (B 23)
Shentang (B 44)
Shenting (Du 24)

Shidou (Sp 17)
Shiguan (K 18)
Shimen (Ren 5)
Shiqizhui (Extra 18)
Shixuan (Extra 24)
Shousanli (LI 10)
Shouwuli (LI 13)
Shuaigu (B 8)
Shufu (K 27)
Shugu (B 65)
Shuidao (S 38)
Shuifen (Ren 9)
Shuigou (Du 26)
Shuiquan (K 5)
Shuitu (S 10)
Sibai (S 2)
Sidu (SJ 9)
Sifeng (Extra 25)
Siman (K 14)
Sishencong (Extra 6)
Sizhukong (SJ 23)
Suliao (Du 25)

T

Taibai (Sp 3)
Taichong (Liv 3)
Taixi (K 3)
Taiyang (K 1)
Taiyuan (L 9)
Tanzhong (Ren 17)
Taodao (Du 13)
Tianchi (P 1)
Tianchong (G 9)
Tianchuang (SI 16)
Tianding (LI 17)
Tianfu (L 3)
Tianjing (SJ 10)
Tianliao (SJ 15)
Tianquan (P 2)

Tianrong (SI 17)
Tianshu (S 25)
Tiantu (Ren 22)
Tianxi (Sp 18)
Tianyou (SJ 16)
Tianzhu (B 10)
Tianzong (SI 11)
Tiaokou (S 38)
Tinggong (SI 19)
Tinghui (G 2)
Tongli (H 5)
Tongtian (B 7)
Tongziliao (G 1)
Toulinqi (G 15)
Touqiaoyin (G 11)
Touwei (S 8)

W

Waiguan (SJ 5)
Wailing (S 26)
Waiqiu (G 36)
Wangu (G 12)
Wangu (SI 4)
Weicang (B 50)
Weidao (G 28)
Weiguanxiashu (Extra 17)
Weishu (B 21)
Weiyang (B 39)
Weizhong (B 40)
Wenliu (LI 7)
Wuchu (B 5)
Wushu (G 27)
Wuyi (S 15)

X

Xiguan (Liv 7)
Xiyan (Extra 36)
Xiyangguan (G 33)
Xiaguan (S 7)

Xiajuxu (S 39)
Xialian (LI 8)
Xialiao (B 34)
Xiawan (Ren 10)
Xiaxi (G 43)
Ximen (P 4)
Xiangu (S 43)
Xiaochangshu (B 27)
Xiaohai (SI 8)
Xiaoluo (SJ 12)
Xingjian (Liv 2)
Xinhui (Du 22)
Xinshu (B 15)
Xiongxiang (Sp 19)
Xuanji (Ren 21)
Xuanli (G 6)
Xuanlu (G 5)
Xuanshu (Du 5)
Xuanzhong (G 39)
Xuehai (Sp 10)

Y

Yamen (Du 15)
Yangbai (G 14)
Yangchi (SJ 4)
Yangfu (G 38)
Yanggang (B 48)
Yanggu (SI 5)
Yangjiao (G 35)
Yanglao (SI 6)
Yanglingquan (G 34)
Yangxi (LI 5)
Yaoqi (Extra 19)
Yaoshu (Du 2)
Yaotongxue (Extra 29)
Yaoyan (Extra 21)
Yaoyangguan (Du 3)
Yemen (SJ 2)
Yifeng (SJ 17)

INDEX

图书在版编目(CIP)数据

中国针灸学:英文/程莘荥等编著;谢竹藩等译.
—北京:外文出版社,1987(1996年重印)
ISBN 7－119－00378－X

Ⅰ.中… Ⅱ.①程… ②谢… Ⅲ.针灸学－英文 Ⅳ.R245

中国版本图书馆 CIP 数据核字 (96) 第 06505 号

中国针灸学

程莘农等　著

谢竹藩等　译

*

ⓒ外文出版社

外文出版社出版

(中国北京百万庄大街 24 号)

邮政编码 100037

中国科学院印刷厂印刷

中国国际图书贸易总公司发行

(中国北京车公庄西路 35 号)

北京邮政信箱第 399 号　邮政编码 100044

1987 年(16 开)第 1 版

1998 年第 1 版第 6 次印刷

(英)

ISBN 7－119－00378－X /R·6(外)

11000

14－E－2121S